PRINCIPLES & ISSUES IN NUTRITION

PRINCIPLES & ISSUES IN
NUTRITION

Y. H. Hui, Ph.D.

HUMBOLDT STATE UNIVERSITY
ARCATA, CALIFORNIA

Wadsworth Health Sciences Division
Monterey, California
A Division of Wadsworth, Inc.

Wadsworth Health Sciences Division
A Division of Wadsworth, Inc.

Printed in the United States of America

10 9 8 7 6 5 4 3 2 1

Library of Congress Cataloging in Publication Data
Hui, Y. H., (Yiu H.)
    Principles and issues in nutrition.

    Includes bibliographies and index.
    1. Nutrition. 2. Malnutrition. I. Title. [DNLM:
1. Nutrition—popular works.   QU 145 H899p]
QP141.H7724   1985   612'.3   84-27051

ISBN 0-534-04374-7

Sponsoring Editor: James Keating
Production Services Coordinators: Marlene Thom and David Hoyt
Production: Del Mar Associates
Manuscript Editor: Lillian Rodberg
Interior and Cover Design: E. Paul Slick
Illustrations: E. Paul Slick
Typesetting: Thompson Type, San Diego, California
Printer and Binder: R. R. Donnelley and Sons, Crawfordsville, Indiana

Cover Painting: John Johnston, *Still Life,* 1810.
Courtesy of The St. Louis Art Museum,
anonymous gift.

With the special assistance of

James A. Hamby, M.A.

Preface

One of the wisest people I have known once told me: "If you never do anything else for yourself, do everything you can to be healthy." This text, designed for introductory courses, offers you not only the opportunity to learn about nutrition but also the opportunity to take a major step in providing for your health. Nutrition is the heart of health, and education lies at the heart of nutrition.

Certainly you already know that you live in one of the most health-conscious ages we have known. New information regarding nutrition has been virtually exploding for the last several years, and this text presents you with the opportunity to engage that knowledge at a reasonable depth and with meaningful insight. This text is written specifically for students in all disciplines. Those with no previous training in college biology, chemistry, nutrition, or related sciences will not be at a disadvantage.

You will find that nutritional principles have brought a recent improvement in dental health, one of the most widespread health concerns in the world. You will encounter important subjects so new you may not previously have heard of them—topics such as orthomolecular psychiatry, starch blockers, and laetrile poisoning. As interesting as these insights will be, the basic purpose of this text remains the provision of a broad-based yet thorough understanding of the basics for bringing health and vigor to your life. You will discover in these chapters that no special diet, no combination of pills, no magic nutrition potion, can ever take the place of a balanced diet. Remember that fact always, for it is the most central of all nutritional principles. Learn to make foods work for you to bring you the state of health and well-being you richly deserve.

The text is organized into five parts. Part One, "The Study of Human Nutrition," has two objectives. First, it gives you a broad picture of major issues in food, nutrition, and diet that are of special concern to Americans. Second, it provides you with a basic understanding of materials common to most chapters—subjects such as human physiology; and fundamental nutritional concepts such as food guides, dietary goals, food exchanges—in general, a frame of reference that will facilitate your progress in studying the various topics addressed.

Part Two, "Nutrition Basics," provides three sets of information. The major discussion relates to nutrients, as indicated in Figure 1 (numbers in parentheses refer to chapters). In addition, Chapters 3 and 4 study energy and body composition. Because these two subjects contain integrated materials, they may be taught before or after a student has become familiar with the role of nutrients. This part addresses the principles of nutrition in terms of the dynamics of life, and, of

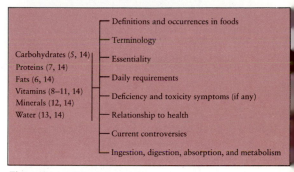

Carbohydrates (5, 14)
Proteins (7, 14)
Fats (6, 14)
Vitamins (8–11, 14)
Minerals (12, 14)
Water (13, 14)

- Definitions and occurrences in foods
- Terminology
- Essentiality
- Daily requirements
- Deficiency and toxicity symptoms (if any)
- Relationship to health
- Current controversies
- Ingestion, digestion, absorption, and metabolism

Figure 1

equal importance, it does so within the focus of meaningful nutritional issues. For example, vitamins are reviewed in relation to the supplement question. This is a hot topic, one around which a multi-million dollar industry has developed. Fats are examined in regard to one of the leading killers, heart disease. The role of proteins in a vegetarian diet is explored.

You will find that Part Three traces nutrition through the cycles of your life as illustrated in Figure 2. We will investigate the special nutritional needs of pregnant women, the variations between infant nutrition and child nutrition, adolescent nutrition as a bridge to adult nutrition, and the special nutritional needs of the elderly. Thus, Part Three analyzes the life cycle by discussing the nutritional needs and requirements, nutritional status, and nutrition-related health problems and controversial issues of each stage.

There are certain unique nutritional situations that are of sufficient significance to

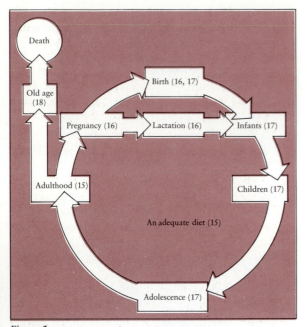

Figure 2

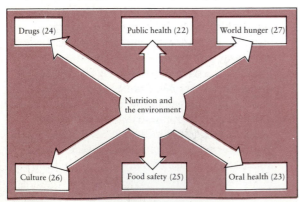

Figure 3

deserve special attention. Part Four focuses on three such unique human conditions. Nutrition for the undernourished, for the overweight, and for the athlete provide timely and important insights.

Part Five, "Nutrition and Public Health," relates nutrition to our environment, as indicated in Figure 3. Cultural, ethnic, and geographical backgrounds have always played an important part in our preferences for certain

foods. Now scientists believe that some of our eating practices benefit our health, whereas others have a negative impact. Similarly, nutritionists believe that many degenerative diseases in our old age result from bad eating habits adopted since childhood, habits that may be corrected through nutrition education. Our concern for food safety has traditionally emphasized biological food poisoning. However, the public has recently begun to express alarm about food and color additives and accidental chemical contamination of our food supply. In the same context, the public is increasingly aware of the multiple consequences of prescription, over-the-counter, and illicit drugs, especially their profound relationship to food and our nutritional status. Part Five attempts to explore the complicated relationships between our nutritional well-being and our environment.

The chapter on public health nutrition is one of the highlights of this book. It addresses the health of population groups and discusses the various approaches that can be used to assess the nutritional status of groups, along with insights into the limitations associated with those assessment tools. Examples of community nutrition programs are provided. Nutrition and cancer, one of the most controversial issues of public health nutrition in this country, is also explored.

The text concludes with a fascinating yet disturbing look at the world's health and hunger. You will have opportunities to see health and nutrition in relation to cultural differences and to grasp the issues inherent in one of the most fruitful research topics, nutrition and drugs.

This book has some unique features that should be emphasized here:

The appendix presents tables of major reference data, including food composition tables, growth curves, and Recommended Daily Dietary Allowances. These tables serve two important purposes: They assist a student in completing classroom assignments, and together with the text materials, they serve as a useful reference source for health professionals who may be directly or indirectly responsible for the nutritional and dietary care of a patient.

Wherever applicable, each chapter is introduced by an appropriate clinical case history. Each is an actual case history, with the identity of the patient changed for obvious reasons. The case history will serve to illustrate the principles and issues of the chapter.

Interesting and appropriate materials have been drawn from leading nutritional literature. Such materials will include:

Actual incidents that illustrate a particular point discussed. For example, you will read about a writer who investigated cellulite by having a cellulite treatment.

Public health and field programs as a teaching aid. For example, you will learn of a food relief program for an underdeveloped country.

Discoveries and scientific advancement. For example, the "DMF" index facilitates dental health comparison on an international basis.

Interesting and illustrative court cases are presented. For example, you will see how the government restrained a company from selling its products because it made false claims about its vitamin capsules.

There are various teaching and learning aids for this text. Carefully designed and developed computer testing programs will accompany the book. These computer programs will enable you and your instructor to evaluate your learning. An instructor's manual will accompany the text.

Apart from specific text references provided for each chapter, listings of additional references are included in the instructor's manual. The manual also provides additional food composition tables to supplement those in the appendix of this book. The instructor is given permission to reproduce both the references and the food composition tables in the instructor's manual in any format for use by the students. It is expected that such additional information will facilitate the teaching-learning process.

Whether your interest in nutrition derives from curiosity about your body's health or from a fervent belief that your body is the temple of your soul, nutritional education will benefit you. It will offer you the understandings that open the way to health. You are to be congratulated for doing this for yourself.

Theodore Roethke, an American poet, wrote in his poem "The Waking" that we take our waking slow and learn by going where we have to go. May your journey into nutrition and health be sure, solid, and sound. Let education dispel the mystery that too often surrounds nutritional health.

Acknowledgments

I wish to express my sincere appreciation to all my colleagues and friends for the generous help given during the preparation of this book, and to various investigators and authors for permission to use material from their research and work. Special commendation goes to those thousands of students who have taken my classes in basic nutrition and other specialties of the field—they have taught me so much. Their input has helped shape the objectives, content, style, and practically every aspect of this book.

Mr. James Hamby, a professional writer and an author himself, has taken the scientific information I provided and transformed it into an effective tool for teaching the basics of nutrition to nonmajors. His excellent work has produced a text useful to students of all disciplines.

Mrs. Mary Farr, Miss Dorothy Bissell, and Dr. Darlena Blucher are three friends who have stood by me year after year. Whenever possible, they have helped me in all aspects of my research and writing. I will always be grateful to them. In addition, the entire staff of reference librarians at Humboldt State University is always there to provide assistance whenever I need it. They have my sincere appreciation.

I would like to thank two persons for their special help: Ms. Leona Avidiya, a dental hygienist consultant for the State of California clarified a number of points for me in Chapter 23, and Professor Samuel Dreizen, M.D., D.D.S., of the University of Texas Dental Branch, has been most generous with his wonderful collection of slides on nutritional deficiency symptoms. Without their contribution, the educational value of this book would be reduced.

No matter how many times I might express my thanks to Mr. James Keating, the sponsoring editor for this book, I feel that it would never be enough. Mr. Keating has played an important part in my professional life. We will always be good friends.

This book has been produced under the management of Del Mar Associates Publishing Services of Del Mar, California. Their quality work and professionalism is self-evident. Special thanks to Miss Frankie Wright who took care of the plethora of details that go with the tedious process of producing a book. Of course, you want to know who did the illustrations. The artist, Paul Slick, deserves an A.

Finally, I am deeply grateful to my family for their long-enduring patience and indispensable support.

To all who have assisted in the preparation of this textbook, I express gratitude and recognize that if any factual errors appear in the text, they are solely my responsibility.

Y. H. Hui

Contents

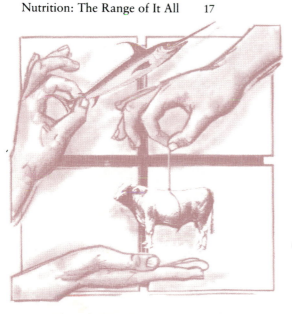

CHAPTER 23

Nutrition and Oral Health:
Not Just Teeth   521

CHAPTER 24

Nutrition and Drugs:
Drug-Caused Deficiencies   541

CHAPTER 25

Food Safety:
Are Food Chemicals Safe?   563

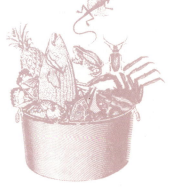

Case Studies

PRINCIPLES & ISSUES IN NUTRITION

ONE

The Study of Human Nutrition

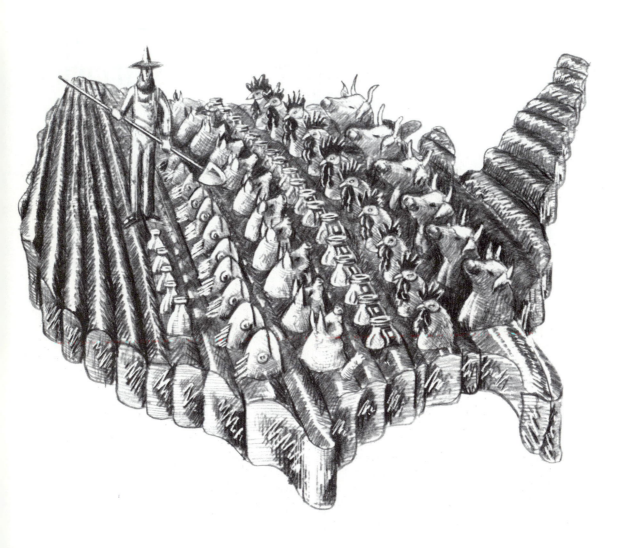

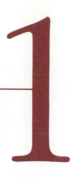

1

NUTRITION, DIET, AND HOW AMERICANS LIVE

NUTRITION:
A WORLD ISSUE,
A PERSONAL CONCERN

Susan is a diabetic who must follow a precise diet to keep her blood sugar levels in the normal range; she is allowed no foods that contain sugar. She uses "diet" soft drinks made with saccharin or aspartame to satisfy her desire for sweets. But she worries about reports that saccharin has caused cancer in lab animals—and that aspartame, a relatively new product, has not been fully proved safe. . . . Jim and his family operate two subsistence farms in the hills of Northern California. He worries that the aerial application of herbicides to adjacent forests may introduce health hazards to their food supply. . . . Jackie has changed to part-time work so she can care for her new baby. When she worked full time as a waitress, riding a bicycle to the restaurant every day, she was continually on the go. Now that she works only two days a week and uses "fast foods" to save time, she has gained 10 pounds in a few months. . . . Rusty has high blood pressure, and his doctor has told him to cut out coffee. He'd like to switch to a decaffeinated brand—but what about reports that the chemicals used in decaffeination are dangerous?

Why Study Nutrition?

Many health experts have for years found it hard to believe that so little attention has been given to nutrition and health. Those health scientists have had legitimate reasons for concern. For example, only in recent years has clinical nutrition been included as a subject in some medical schools.

Despite this lack of attention to nutrition, health professionals, as well as the general public, have been aware that water and food are second only to air in being central to life. As we become more aware of just how important water and food are to health, nutrition is coming into its own as a field of study central to our health and well-being.

As nutrition has drawn the attention of scientists and health experts, it has also drawn the attention of both government and industry. State and federal governments try to regulate for your good. Industry creates products, advertises them, and stimulates your interest as a consumer. Scientists investigate such important subjects as the possible links between food and cancer, the potential dangers or benefits of large doses of vitamins, and the cultural forces and physical reasons behind a pregnant woman's eating such nonfood substances as clay. Internationally, governments meet to consider world hunger, and we read about or hear projections of the world running out of food or water by a certain date. These are all valid subjects of nutrition. Let us consider some of the topics that currently hold the spotlight in discussions of nutrition and health.

The Food Supply: A Giant Buffet

Imagine that you have decided to have a large party. You want to be certain that all your guests have a good time, and you know that the food you serve will play a central role in your guests' enjoyment. So you will have available a variety of foods and beverages to satisfy the range of tastes and needs that will characterize your guests.

You know that some of your guests will want to eat only vegetables. Others would be disappointed if there were not some sliced meats and cheeses. Some of your guests will consume only beverages, but not all of those will want alcohol.

The evening of your party has arrived. As you scan the room observing your guests, what do you see? Some of them seem to be eating only chips and dip, or crackers covered with spreads. You see two or three dieters who are concentrating on vegetables; among them is one of your friends who is a strict vegetarian. Several of your friends seem to only drink.

You know, of course, that your friends' eating habits cannot be fully understood on the basis of their selections at your party, yet certain differences in eating habits do surface. You can see differences in quantities consumed, in varieties of food chosen, in frequency of consumption, and in the proportions of liquids to solids consumed. Can you draw valid conclusions about the nutritional health of your guests? What additional choices might you have offered as host? These are some of the considerations we each face in regard to nutrition. While your concern is your party, your state government may be concerned about the health and diet of schoolchildren, whereas the federal government is concerned about malnutrition in a whole region of our nation.

The range of nutritional concerns encompasses world hunger and malnutrition at one end of the spectrum and the relationship between health and decaffeinated coffee at the other end. Both concerns are important.

"Eat Right and Be Healthy": Are We What We Eat?

Current nutritional research tends to focus on the relationship between food choices and health (USDA, 1981). We know that the average American diet contributes to some of the diseases that characterize our population, especially the elderly. Yet scientists and other nutritional experts hold varying opinions as to the extent of the connection between diet and disease. Many experts claim that our consumption of calories, fats, cholesterol, sugar, and salt significantly exceeds our need. They contend that a greater consumption of whole grains, fruits, and vegetables will yield a reduction in heart disease, various forms of cancer, and strokes. For each expert who makes such claims, you can find another who says the evidence does not sufficiently support such conclusions.

You, as a consumer, have probably felt overwhelmed by the food choices before you. The typical American supermarket presents you with thousands of food products. If you could read both the advertising for those products and the criticisms of them, you would find a mix of good and bad claims. If you are a typical consumer, you have never tried many of the food products available. Factors such as your food budget, how much time you have to prepare food, the tastes you have developed over the years, and your weight gain or loss goals have shaped your food choices.

Although the array of choices may be confusing, that array is beneficial. Nutritional research has demonstrated that our nutrient and energy needs are best met if we eat a variety of foods. Our food supply is characterized by both abundance and variety, and that food supply is spread across a wide price range. We are blessed with foods fresh, frozen, canned, or dehydrated. Partially or fully prepared meals are readily available. Many of the foods available to us have been fortified with additional nutrients, taking us one step closer to an acceptable nutritional status.

To further guide us toward nutritional health, scientists have developed recommended dietary allowances (RDAs) for nutrients and calories for various age groups. As Unit Three will demonstrate, nutritionists have taken these recommendations and translated them into kinds and amounts of food. These translations are known as food guides, and they provide an easy way to make wise and beneficial food choices.

Learning to select foods that bring both enjoyment and health is to our advantage. The abundance and variety of our food supply opens various food paths—paths that will accommodate our differences in budget, tastes, religious beliefs, lifestyles, and preparation time, yet will still lead us to the same nutritional goal. The goal of good nutrition is attainable, and it will bring us joy in living while making us feel, look, and perform at our best.

Health Foods: Are They Better for Me?

"How can I attract girls with this complexion?"
"My brother solved his complexion problem by taking protein capsules."

The advantage of health foods over conventional food products is a matter of significant debate. Proponents of health foods, organic foods, and natural foods claim such foods are safer for our bodies and are more nutritious than conventionally grown and processed foods. Such claims have struck a responsive chord among American consumers, who have shown an increasing concern in the safety and nutritional value of the typical American diet (Herbert, 1980). If you have priced health foods, organic foods, and natural foods, you have discovered that they can cost from two to five times as much as conventional foods. Are they worth the extra cost?

We have been flooded with news that certain food types or additives contribute to heart disease or cause cancer in laboratory animals. Alarmists have fueled our fears. From the mix of information available to us, we tend to select a set of nutritional beliefs that are part truth and part fiction. We are tempted by claims for "anticancer" foods, "no-aging" diets, and "wonder foods" because we all want to avoid disease and feel and look our best.

We wonder whether natural vitamins are superior to synthetic ones, whether organic fertilizer yields better, more nutritious vegetables than manufactured fertilizer, whether raw milk is better than pasteurized milk. We may be drawn to such health foods partially because they speak of a simpler time, a pretechnology way of life when the chemical dangers were not present.

For all the lure that health foods, organic foods, and natural foods may have, we know that we cannot hold a stalk of celery in our hand and determine whether it was raised in organic fertilizer or manufactured fertilizer. Since plant roots absorb nutrients regardless of the source, no scientific basis exists for claiming organic foods are more nutritious than conventional foods. What scientists have determined, however, is that the nutrient content within a specific food—vitamin A in carrots, for example—can vary according to the genetic nature of the plant, the climate, nutrients available during growth, and age at harvesting.

One claim for organic foods relates to the absence of pesticides, but we realistically know that pesticides can affect foods even if a particular farmer did not use them. Pesticides remain in the soil from being used years ago. They can be carried in the air from adjoining farms, or they can fall with the rain. Chemical analysis shows that pesticides find their way into both organic and conventional food, but such residues are normally below levels considered dangerous.

Because chemicals work their way into our food supply, and because we really cannot tell the difference between organic and conventional foods in the produce bin of the grocery store, our best approach still remains the consumption of a variety of foods to ensure a balanced diet. Eating too much of any single food can often be a nutritional mistake, so it is always nutritionally wise to have a balanced diet obtained from a variety of foods. Thus, health foods are a subject of significant interest.

Food Safety: A Real Concern

The present universal fear has been the result of a forward surge in our knowledge and manipulation of certain dangerous factors in the physical world.
John Steinbeck, Nobel Prize Acceptance Speech, 1962

Our concerns about the safety of our food supply are increasing in almost direct proportion to our expanding knowledge. Consider the

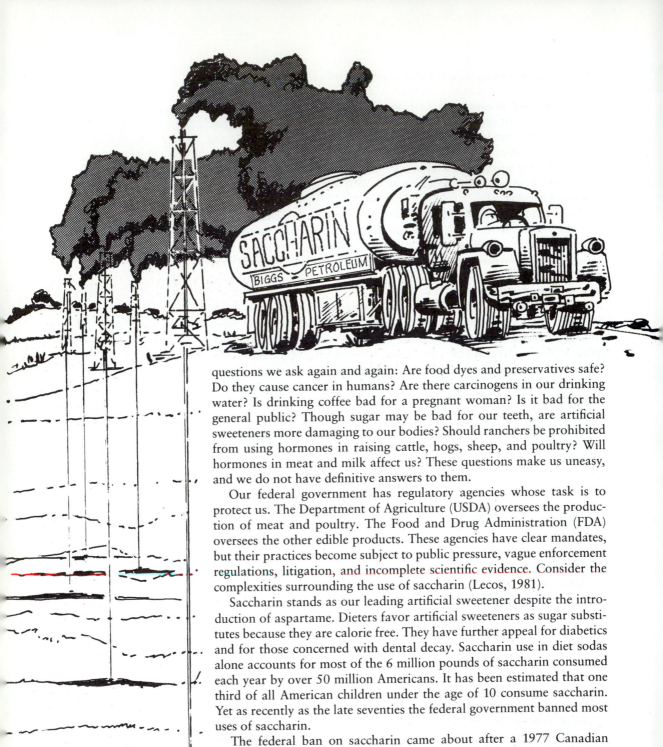

questions we ask again and again: Are food dyes and preservatives safe? Do they cause cancer in humans? Are there carcinogens in our drinking water? Is drinking coffee bad for a pregnant woman? Is it bad for the general public? Though sugar may be bad for our teeth, are artificial sweeteners more damaging to our bodies? Should ranchers be prohibited from using hormones in raising cattle, hogs, sheep, and poultry? Will hormones in meat and milk affect us? These questions make us uneasy, and we do not have definitive answers to them.

Our federal government has regulatory agencies whose task is to protect us. The Department of Agriculture (USDA) oversees the production of meat and poultry. The Food and Drug Administration (FDA) oversees the other edible products. These agencies have clear mandates, but their practices become subject to public pressure, vague enforcement regulations, litigation, and incomplete scientific evidence. Consider the complexities surrounding the use of saccharin (Lecos, 1981).

Saccharin stands as our leading artificial sweetener despite the introduction of aspartame. Dieters favor artificial sweeteners as sugar substitutes because they are calorie free. They have further appeal for diabetics and for those concerned with dental decay. Saccharin use in diet sodas alone accounts for most of the 6 million pounds of saccharin consumed each year by over 50 million Americans. It has been estimated that one third of all American children under the age of 10 consume saccharin. Yet as recently as the late seventies the federal government banned most uses of saccharin.

The federal ban on saccharin came about after a 1977 Canadian study showed that the product could cause bladder tumors in rats. The American ban was removed after the saccharin-using public demanded that saccharin be returned to the market place.

Saccharin represents a truly fascinating study in food safety. It is a product with no nutritional value. It is made from petroleum materials and is manufactured by one company, the Sherwin-Williams Paint Company. The product has been in use since 1899, predating most consumer-protecting food laws. Saccharin advocates are staunch supporters. In 1907, when President Theodore Roosevelt was warned of the potential dangers of saccharin, he retorted: "My doctor gives it to me every day. Anybody who says saccharin is injurious to health is an idiot."

Saccharin users continue to support the product. Canada has banned its use except as a sugar substitute sold with a warning label in drug stores. When the FDA tried a similar ban in 1977, the public outcry was sufficiently influential to force Congress to pass a moratorium on the ban until more research becomes available. Research results have not been conclusive.

The National Academy of Sciences has concluded that saccharin is a weak carcinogen in animals and a potential carcinogen in humans; it may be a potentiator of cancer-causing effects of other carcinogens. A study by the National Cancer Institute has determined that saccharin increases the risk of cancer for two subgroups—heavy saccharin users and heavy saccharin users who are also heavy smokers. Two other population studies failed to link cancer and saccharin use for any category of users.

As we try to understand food safety, what should we conclude about saccharin? Can we conclude that it causes cancer in animals but not in humans? Or can we conclude that it is such a weak carcinogen that its effect is imperceptible? Or have we simply not been using it enough for the danger to become clear? Obviously, we can be no more conclusive than experts can. What we can conclude, however, is that saccharin presents an excellent example of the problems inherent in food safety. Chapter 26 will further explore issues in food safety.

Food Is a Fuel: You Burn It

Let us go then, you and I,
. . . Like a patient etherised upon a table.
T. S. Eliot, "The Love Song of J. Alfred Prufrock"

Many of us go through life at an activity level low enough to give the impression we are under ether. Our sedentary lifestyles present significant health risk. While we tend to eat foods high in calories, we favor a lifestyle that utilizes few calories. That combination adds up to excessive weight gain, a condition that contributes to poor health (Katch and McArdle, 1983).

Our contemporary lifestyle has been fostered by technology. We travel by automobile, subway, train, or plane. Electrical appliances save labor. We expend less energy, thereby burning fewer of our calories. The average person's ordinary activities burn approximately 2,000 kilocalories, but we typically consume more than that. If our daily caloric intake is 3,200 kcal, while our activity level burns 2,000 kcal, we will gain over 3 pounds per month. We can restore the balance by exercising.

Half of Americans take advantage of the opportunity for caloric balance through exercise. The other half spends leisure time in spectator activities. According to the President's Council on Physical Fitness and Sports, exercising Americans favor running and jogging, bicycling, swimming, and racquet sports in providing weight control benefits. For example, if a person who is 20 pounds overweight begins to jog 30 minutes per day, 4 days per week, the excess weight will be gone in 9 months. Weight loss will be quicker if the exercise occurs just prior to a meal, since moderate exercise diminishes appetite. If vigorous exercise is used, caloric burning can persist after the exercise is concluded. For example, someone who runs for 30 minutes will continue to burn calories for up to 6 hours. Further, fitness brings with it a decrease in appetite.

Weight loss represents but one of the benefits of exercise. You can feel better, look better, need less sleep, and have more energy. As you gain in both strength and flexibility, you experience less depression and less anxiety. Unhealthy habits tend to be dropped.

Research has additionally shown that exercise serves a preventive function as well. Less incidence of cardiovascular disease occurs among those who exercise regularly. Blood pressure and serum cholesterol fall, while favorable high density lipoproteins (see Chapter 6) rise. Lung capacity increases, and blood sugar levels decrease. This latter benefit has enabled diabetics to rid themselves of diabetes.

Given the positive aspects of exercise, 15 to 30 minutes of exercise for 3 days of the week can be a very reasonable level of effort for our health. We need to constantly remind ourselves that we burn our calories and that our burning level should not drop to that of a patient "etherised upon a table."

World Hunger: A Challenge to Us All

The fields are left weedy/And the granaries empty.
The Tao-Te King, "The Great Way"

While many of us look for an exercise that will help us burn excess calories, many in the world go to sleep hungry (Presidential Commission on World Hunger, 1980). In third world countries, malnutrition is severe. When we think of world hunger, we first think of famine, perhaps a lack of food as a result of flood, crop failure, or war. Certainly famine has its role in world hunger. For example, during the years from 1876 to 1879, approximately 10 million people starved to death in China. Fortunately, national and international planning have helped to reduce the effects of famine, but world hunger also has other forms.

Chronic undernutrition lacks the drama of famine, but it is far more widespread. The World Bank has estimated that one fourth of the world's population can be classified as undernourished. That classification means that one of every four people lacks the protein and calories necessary for health and activity. Even more have nutritional deficiencies due to a lack of essential vitamins and minerals. Such problems as iron-deficiency anemia sap the energy of otherwise productive workers, cause high infant mortality, and open the door to infectious diseases. Undernourished populations are exposed to gastrointestinal and respiratory epidemics, nutrition-related events that can claim large segments of the population.

The damage done by chronic undernutrition lacks high visibility. The condition drains energy, destroys motivation, limits concentration and learning ability, and prevents developing nations from realizing potential. Over half of the malnourished are children under the age of 5, and far more women suffer the condition than men.

Countries such as the United States attempt to alleviate world hunger. In 1980 a Presidential Commission on World Hunger concluded that chronic undernutrition is the world's major hunger problem. Predictions indicate there may be a world food-supply crisis by the year 2000. The solution does not reside simply in productivity but rather in equal access to food. Further, the central cause of hunger is poverty, a problem rooted in political, economic, and social realities. The commission determined that the challenge to us lies in attacking the interrelated causes of world hunger. As the commission's report noted, "There is no ideal food, no perfect diet, no universally acceptable agricultural system waiting to be transplanted from one geographic, climatic, and cultural setting to another."

Despite obstacles, we know world hunger can be successfully combatted. As the largest producer, consumer, and trader of food, the United States can be a major factor in the war against world hunger. Such programs as food stamps, school lunches, and Aid to Families with Dependent Children (AFDC) have shown that hunger and malnutrition can be reduced. Certainly our nation cannot, and should not, single-handedly battle world hunger. A concerned effort among the world's nations could, however, accomplish the goal. The Presidential Commission's report concluded, "The outcome of the war on hunger, by the year 2000 and beyond, will be determined not by forces beyond human control, but by decisions and actions well within the capability of nations and people working individually and together." Chapter 28 will provide you with a more thorough understanding of world hunger, another of the leading topics of nutrition.

Do Yourself a Favor: Learn About Nutrition

Only where love and need are one,
And the work is play for mortal stakes . . .
Robert Frost, "Two Tramps in Mud Time"

By gaining knowledge about nutrition, you enable yourself to make informed choices. You are taking advantage of an opportunity to improve not only your present health but also your future well-being.

Recent studies have confirmed that even many health professionals do not have an adequate knowledge of food and nutrition (USDA). That realization gives cause for concern when we realize that nutrition is central to health. While efforts are under way to bring nutrition education to doctors, nurses, dentists, and other health professionals, those educational efforts can never replace the advantage of your own knowledge.

Current belief holds that an improper diet and a sedentary life are two of the major risk factors leading not only to disease but also to a shorter life span. Both appropriate, beneficial diet and sufficient exercise must therefore become our goals as individuals. In the case of nutrition, we are, as Robert Frost says, involved in mortal stakes.

Pregnancy and the Mystery of "Pica"

Pagophagia: ice cravings
Geophagia: dirt and clay cravings
Amylophagia: laundry starch cravings

We humans sometimes do strange things. The history of the human race records many cases of individuals and groups of individuals compulsively ingesting nonfood substances, a behavior known as "pica." You may have heard of such practices, especially among pregnant women. Such habits must concern us, for pica constitutes a nutritional abuse (Danford, 1982).

The list of nonfood substances that have been consumed includes most anything physically capable of being eaten: dirt and clay, charcoal and soot, ice, cigarette ashes, laundry starch, hair, corn starch, baking soda, coffee grounds, mothballs. The question we immediately ask is, why do people do that?

Research has given us some answers about pica. Studies of the incidence of pica among pregnant women in the United States have primarily focused on the southern states. The level of abuse may be startling to you. Among pregnant black women in rural Mississippi, over 40 percent ate starch, and over 25 percent ate clay. The practice is not, however, limited to the South. Studies in New York, Illinois, Pennsylvania, and California have confirmed the habit, with levels of incidence among pregnant women ranging from one fourth to one third of those surveyed. What are the medical implications of the practice?

Research has tended to focus on blood studies, seeking to determine how anemia, a common ailment of pregnant women, might be linked to pica. Unfortunately, most people who practice pica do not have blood tests before they begin. Rather, the tests are done after the practice has started, and usually because the practice has resulted in ill health.

As you might expect, eating nonfood substances can substitute for a nourishing diet, leading to malnutrition. Additionally, toxicity may result. For pregnant women, an additional concern is that the foreign matter can cross over to the fetus. Especially among clay eaters, a high incidence of toxemia has been confirmed among pregnant women. Among children born to clay eaters, cases of infants born with fecal impaction have been reported.

Studies have demonstrated a relationship between iron deficiency and pica. For example, pica practitioners have been cured of the practice

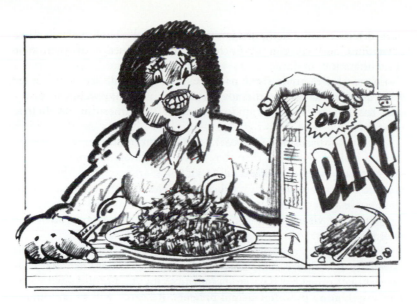

through the administration of iron, especially in cases involving the consumption of clay, dirt, and ice. Yet studies have also confirmed that the *practice* of pica can cause iron-deficiency anemia. So we see, iron deficiency may be a factor in causing pica, or it may be a result of pica.

Pica remains a nutritional abuse not fully understood. Some forms of pica may cause little damage, but others endanger both the practitioners and, in the case of a pregnant woman, the child she carries. Certainly one conclusion that we can draw is that pica stands as one of the more unusual dietary practices, one that the current interest in nutrition may help resolve.

When Is a Vitamin a Drug?

Nurse: *I can remember when mental patients were kept almost unconscious by drugs. Now we give them massive doses of vitamins.*

Although vitamins are essential nutrients needed in small amounts by our bodies, in some cases vitamin dosage far beyond recommended dietary allowances may occur. In such instances, the dosage, which may be from 4 to 1,000 times greater than the normal intake, becomes a pharmacological dosage. The vitamin is then being used as a drug, a treatment known as megavitamin therapy (Fried, 1984).

Megavitamin therapy, or orthomolecular psychiatry as it is called in the treatment of mental disease, is a medical practice that generally is not utilized except after diagnostic testing. As you will see in Chapter 9, a deficiency in niacin (a B vitamin) can result in pellagra, a disease characterized by neurological, gastrointestinal, and dermatologic (skin) symptoms. In view of some similarity between these symptoms and those of schizophrenics, niacin megavitamin therapy is used by some doctors to treat schizophrenics. Some patients benefit from such treatment.

In addition to niacin, megavitamin therapy also involves other B vitamins and vitamin C. Such vitamins are used individually or in combination in large doses to treat mental retardation, learning disorders, hyperactivity, and psychosis. As you will see in Chapter 8, the use of megavitamin therapy for the treatment of psychiatric problems has not received the endorsement of the American Psychiatric Association.

As you will discover in Chapters 9 and 10, our bodies react differently to water-soluble vitamins than they do to fat-soluble vitamins. Because excessive amounts of water-soluble vitamins are excreted, those who practice megavitamin therapy believe that patients are not endangered by massive doses. Since negative side effects have been reported for megadoses of vitamins C, B_6, and niacin, safety questions are being raised.

While the practice of megavitamin therapy or orthomolecular psychiatry is rather recent, there is mounting evidence that the practice may be somewhat dangerous nutritionally, despite the positive results experienced by some mental patients. Research will be continuing in regard to vitamins used as drugs, a topic of increasing nutritional interest.

Cancer: Diet May Cause It; Diet May Prevent It

. . . the injustice of it lit up the buildings . . .
From W. S. Merwin, "Departure's Girl-Friend"

Perhaps no single health issue more dominates our thinking than does the subject of cancer, the killer that strikes all ages, all walks of life. When we think of cancer, we certainly think of the injustice of it. The search for a cancer cure has taken researchers down many paths. The one that concerns us here is the relationship between nutrition or diet and cancer (White, 1982).

When you think about nutrition and cancer, you must keep in mind that cancer *prevention* attracts attention as well as does cancer cure. When analyzing the relationship between diet and cancer, two issues are generally explored: Is the incidence of cancer closely associated with any particular foods or dietary practices? Is the absence of cancer closely associated with any particular foods or dietary practices?

Researchers have found, for example, that the incidence of cancer is more associated with high fat intake than with any other dietary component. It may surprise you to realize that some correlation has also been found between high protein intake and an increased risk of cancer. Similar studies have been done in regard to carbohydrates, total caloric intake, and cholesterol, but the findings are too limited to be conclusive.

On the prevention side of the picture, attention has been directed toward fiber. Research has failed to confirm that fiber prevents cancer in humans. When vitamins have been the focus of attention, findings have been somewhat more definitive. For example, there appears to be a positive relationship between the lack of cancer and the dietary intake of foods rich in vitamin A—foods such as liver, yellow vegetables, and green vegetables. Though that relationship has been determined, it remains to be seen whether vitamin A itself is the beneficial factor, or if it is something else.

Findings in regard to vitamin C suggest that it can be beneficial in preventing the formation of certain carcinogens. No conclusions have been drawn regarding vitamins B and E.

When we turn our attention to minerals, we find that selenium appears to have a positive benefit. Iron deficiency appears to increase cancer susceptibility, though no firm conclusions can yet be drawn. Diet research has not firmly established that dietary lead, arsenic, or cadmium can increase the risk of cancer, but it is known that occupational exposure to each of these elements yields an increased risk of cancer.

Obviously, research about cancer and diet continues. Studies address not only particular foods but also chemicals within foods. Additives are being studied, as are environmental contaminants that invade our food supply. Because cancer draws the level of attention it does, we can regularly expect new insights regarding its relationship to diet. It could be that victory over that disease lies not in the discovery of some new medicine but in our diet.

The Brain: Food Affects Its Function

. . . and ye shall eat, and not be satisfied.
Leviticus 26:26

A most interesting topic of nutritional research concerns the relationship between diet and the functions of the brain (Fernstrom, 1979; Wurtman, 1983). Our nervous system, including the brain, functions via the transmission of electrical signals between neurons (nerve cells), and it is believed that these "messages" control our body functions and our behavior. It has been found that these transmissions involve chemical processes in utilizing compounds called neurotransmitters. More than a dozen compounds have been identified as neurotransmitters, and researchers have been exploring how diet affects them.

Findings demonstrate that the availability of certain dietary components will in turn affect the formation of neurotransmitters. For example, an increase or decrease of tryptophan (a chemical component of protein with a general name of amino acid) will stimulate or reduce the formation of serotonin, one of the neurotransmitters. Choline and lecithin—components in fats—can raise the level of blood choline in the brain, stimulating the formation of acetylcholine, a neurotransmitter. Tyrosine, an amino acid of protein, affects the synthesis of norepinephrine, another neurotransmitter.

The relationship between brain function and food represents a truly fascinating field of study. For example, research has found that the neurotransmitter serotonin causes us to be sleepy. The amino acid tryptophan stimulates the release of serotonin. Eating carbohydrate before bedtime helps clear other amino acids (protein) from the bloodstream, enabling tryptophan to stimulate the brain and thus make us more sleepy. Conversely, if you eat protein before going to bed, count on some sleeplessness.

Tryptophan has also proved effective in reducing the sensation of pain. Experiments used a high-carbohydrate, low-protein, low-fat diet, coupled with tryptophan in tablet form, to effectively reduce pain. Similarly, lecithin stimulates acetylcholine, which improves memory. Such findings hold the promise that we may one day be able to purchase foods with additives that help us sleep, experience less pain, or improve our memory.

Thus far the relationship between diet and brain function has primarily concentrated on the treatment of mental disease. We can, however, expect new insights to come from such research. For example, could an excessive amount of neurotransmitter cause overeating? Could a lack of a particular neurotransmitter cause overeating? Such questions have the potential for leading researchers to a new approach in the treatment of obesity.

Decaffeinated Coffee: A Solution or a New Problem?

"I sat long, sipping black coffee and smoking. And thinking . . . "
Mark Twain, "The Great Dark"

Dietary trends always hold an interest for researchers and other nutritional experts. For the last several years, our consumption of regular coffee has been decreasing, while the consumption of decaffeinated coffee has been increasing. This trend has caused researchers to focus their studies on the effects of caffeine and on the decaffeination process (Lecos, 1980).

Caffeine is a drug that stimulates our central nervous system. It is a natural substance in coffee, tea, chocolate, and cocoa, and it is an additive to soft drinks such as colas, to medicines such as cold remedies, and to foods such as baked goods. Since it is a drug that reaches all age groups, it has been the subject of some concern, to the point that consumer groups have questioned its safety, especially for pregnant women.

Decaffeination has brought concern because the most common decaffeination process uses chemicals to remove the caffeine. One chemical that was widely used, trichloroethylene, became suspect when it caused liver cancer in mice. Methylene chloride is the solvent now used to remove caffeine from coffee beans. Because it belongs to the same chemical family as trichloroethylene, it is still undergoing research. Industry also strives to leave as little solvent residue as possible.

Research into caffeine and decaffeination processes continues, and industry may ultimately go to a decaffeination process that uses only water, no solvents—a process already in use on a small scale. In the meantime, our dietary trends will continue to give shape to both research and consumer movements.

Nutrition: The Range of It All

You can see that the subject of nutrition is far-reaching. It involves the world and world hunger, the planning of nations. It involves the necessity of nutritional education, for many of our existing national problems can be resolved if the general public's knowledge, and that of health practitioners, is improved.

Nutritional health concerns balance, not only the balance of diet, the mix of nutrients, but also the balance between calories consumed and energy expended. The valid subjects of nutrition range from improving dental condition and complexion to the chemical and electrical processes of your brain, from the use of vitamins as drugs to the use of solvents in removing caffeine from coffee beans.

At first the breadth of the issues within nutrition may seem overwhelming, but it is not. When you understand the basic principles involved, you will gain insights that will have far-reaching implications for your life.

REFERENCES

Danford, D. E. "Pica and Nutrition." *Ann. Rev. Nutr.* 2 (1982): 303.

Fernstrom, J. D. "Food and Brain Function." *Professional Nutritionist*" 11 (Summer 1979): 5.

Fried, J. *Vitamin Politics.* New York: Prometheus, 1984.

Herbert, V. *Nutrition Cultism: Facts and Fictions.* Philadelphia: George F. Stickley, 1980.

Katch, F. I., and W. D. McArdle. *Nutrition, Weight Control, and Exercise.* 2nd ed. Philadelphia: Lea & Febiger, 1983.

Lecos, C. "More Cups Lifted Sans Caffeine." *FDA Consumer* 14 (May 1980): 23.

Lecos, C. "The Sweet and Sour History of Saccharin, Cyclamate, and Aspartame." *FDA Consumer* 15 (September 1981): 8.

Presidential Commission on World Hunger. *Overcoming World Hunger: The Challenge Ahead.* Washington, D.C.: Government Printing Office, 1980.

United States Department of Agriculture. "Food." Home and Garden Bulletin No. 228. Washington, D.C.: Government Printing Office, 1981.

White, K. "Diet and Cancer." *Medical World News* 23 (August 1982): 52.

Wurtman, J. J. "Obesity and the Brain: A Carbohydrate Connection." *Professional Nutritionist* 15 (Spring 1983): 1.

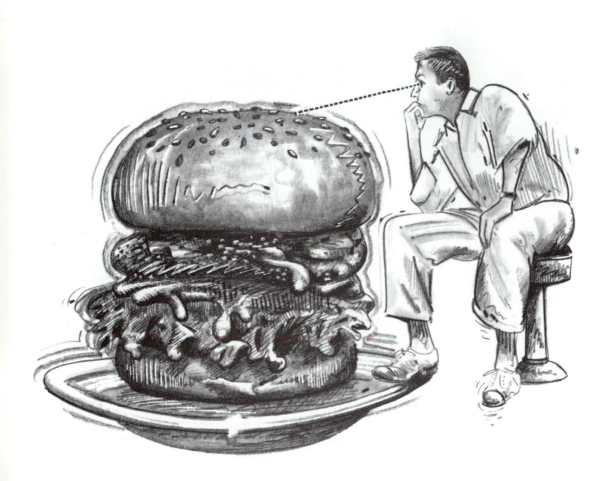

2

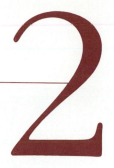

The Study of Human Nutrition:

TOOLS AND PREMISES

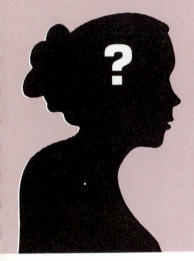

WHOM SHOULD SARAH BELIEVE?

Sarah's arthritis is hurting her again—it seems all she can do without hurting is to watch TV and read. Just yesterday she asked her doctor for advice—and now she's more confused than ever. "Get your weight down," he said. "And while you're at it, cut out the fats and sugars. You're putting too much strain on those joints." Fats? Well, butter is a fat. And margarine. But what are the "low-fat foods" the doctor talks about? Sugars? Does that mean the sugar in her morning coffee? And what about the coffee? Then there's the author—he calls himself "doctor"—on TV just this morning, saying that alfalfa tea and cutting out orange juice is the answer, that "acids erode the joints." And that ad in the paper for "miracle vitamin discovery—especially for senior citizens." The ad says "aches and pains disappear like magic!" Maybe if she combines that with the "overnight miracle weight loss plan" featuring "herb teas brewed by South American Indian tribes" . . .

Studying Nutrition: Is It for Me?

Probably the most common question that students ask their nutrition teacher is: What do we study in nutrition? There is one general answer to that question, one you can probably give right now. But that answer can be broken down into several components related to the tools and premises of the study of human nutrition. In general, we can say that you are studying basic nutritional concepts. But we would also want to say that nutrition involves our optimal requirements of certain essential nutrients; and that nutrition includes positive food choices, choices involving such issues as food guides, food exchange lists, and government guidelines for healthy eating. We will be addressing food composition so that we can understand how certain foods differ in nutrient content. And to evaluate the wealth of information about health and nutrition that surrounds us, we also want to talk about nutrition information and nutrition misinformation.

Nutrition is an exciting field, probably one of the most important you will ever study in terms of your health and well-being. Fortunately, it is a field you can approach at varying levels of complexity. You need not, for example, study nutrition with the same level of biological, chemical, and physiological background that a medical student would have, yet medical students, indeed even medical doctors, increasingly study nutrition. In these pages you will gain understanding of how your body functions. What you will ultimately acquire from your study of nutrition is a knowledge of positive nutritional choices that will improve your life.

Nutrition: What Is It?

According to *Webster's Third International Dictionary,* nutrition is "the sum of the processes by which an animal or plant takes in and utilizes food substances . . . typically involving ingestion, digestion, absorption, and assimilation." The Council on Foods and Nutrition of the American Medical Association defines nutrition as the "science of food, the nutrients and other substances therein, their action, itineration, and balance in relation to health and disease and the processes by which the organism ingests, absorbs, transports, utilizes, and excretes food substances." These definitions outline the area covered in this text.

In 1975, S. J. Ritchey briefly discussed the history of nutrition in that year's *Agricultural Yearbook,* published annually by the United States Department of Agriculture (USDA). The following is a brief summary of that discussion.

A relatively new science, nutrition evolved from the basic sciences of chemistry and physiology. Early investigators, primarily Europeans, initiated nutrition studies as they attempted to understand the physiological utilization of food in supporting the essential processes of life, including growth, reproduction, and lactation. The saga of human nutrition and the improvement of human health in the United States is reflected in the efforts of those scientists who have believed that human performance and well-being—both mental and physical—depend primarily on what one eats.

During the last hundred years, the science of nutrition has progressed from a meager understanding to the point that most of the essential nutrients appear to have been identified. Most nutrients have been isolated in purified form, and the biological functions of many are now reasonably well understood. Nutritionists have speculated that life could be sustained, although probably not enjoyably, by a supply of purified nutrients.

Nutritional deficiency diseases that were common in the past, such as scurvy, rickets, goiter, and pellagra, have been either eliminated or greatly reduced in incidence. Another measure of the progress made in the field of nutrition is that the life expectancy of the average American has increased from around 40 years at the turn of the century to over 70 in the 1980s—an increase that can be at least partially attributed to improvements in nutritional knowledge. Newborn babies have profited from advances in nutrition, and methods for preventing and managing such disorders as anemia have provided a better chance for children to experience normal growth and to develop their full physical and mental potential. Tremendous progress has been made in agriculture as well as in food science and technology to assure a safe, wholesome food supply for the American people. But the search for even more knowledge about nutrition continues.

Today, many people are paying considerable attention to what they eat, with the idea that food intake is closely related to health and a sense of well-being. In some cases, this concern is exaggerated by people who tend to link every dietary factor with some form of human disease, without good scientific evidence. Nevertheless, knowing how nutrition influences our well-being can help us decide what kind of life to lead.

Nutrition Concepts: Which Are Basic?

In 1964, the USDA formed the Interagency Committee on Nutrition Education. This committee developed four basic concepts to be used in implementing nutrition education programs. In 1969, the White House Conference on Food, Nutrition, and Health used these concepts to develop a framework that included seven nutrition concepts for use in planning nutrition curricula in public school systems. The language and content of these concepts are simple to understand and are applicable to all who want to be in good health. The concepts are as follows:

I. Nutrition is the process by which food and other substances eaten become you. The food we eat enables us to live, to grow, to keep healthy and well, and to get energy for work and play.

II. Food is made up of certain chemical substances that work together and interact with body chemicals to serve the needs of the body.
   (a) Each nutrient has specific uses in the body.
   (b) For the healthy individual, the nutrients needed by the body are usually available through food.
   (c) Many kinds and combinations of food can lead to a well-balanced diet.
   (d) No natural food by itself has all the nutrients needed for full growth and health.

III. The way a food is handled influences the amount of nutrients in the food, its safety, appearance, taste, and cost; handling means everything that happens to food while it is being grown, processed, stored, and prepared for eating.

IV. All persons, throughout life, have needs for about the same nutrients but in varying amounts.
   (a) The amounts needed are influenced by age, sex, size, activity, specific conditions of growth, and state of health, altered somewhat by environmental stress.
   (b) Suggestions for kinds and needed amounts of nutrients are made by scientists who continuously revise the suggestions in the light of the findings of new research.
   (c) A daily food guide is helpful in translating the technical information into terms of everyday foods suitable for individuals and families.

V. Food use relates to the cultural, social, economic, and psychological aspects of living, as well as to physiological aspects.
   (a) Food is culturally defined.
   (b) Food selection is an individual act, but it is usually influenced by social and cultural sanctions.

(c) Food can be chosen to fulfill physiological needs and at the same time satisfy social, cultural, and psychological wants.

(d) Attitudes toward food are a culmination of many experiences, past and present.

VI. The nutrients, singly and in combination of chemical substances simulating natural foods, are available in the market; these may vary widely in usefulness, safety, and economy.

VII. Food plays an important role in the physical and psychological health of a society or a nation just as it does for the individual and the family.

(a) The maintenance of good nutrition for the larger units of society involves many matters of public concern.

(b) Nutrition knowledge and social consciousness enable citizens to participate intelligently in the adoption of public policy affecting the nutrition of people around the world.

These concepts directly lead us to an examination of the premises underlying nutrition. One of these is nutrient need.

Nutrient Requirements: How Much Is Enough?

One basic premise in the study of nutrition is the need to know what nutrients are and how much of each we should consume each day. Unit One discusses those essential nutrients. Although our understanding of the human body's minimal and optimal needs for each essential nutrient is incomplete, the National Research Council of the National Academy of Sciences in the United States has established some standard guidelines. Its Food and Nutrition Board is composed of physicians, nutritionists, and scientists highly knowledgeable in the field. This group studies and evaluates scientific data and develops the Recommended Daily Dietary Allowances (RDAs) for a number of nutrients for people in different age and sex categories.

First published in 1943, the RDAs have already been revised eight times. All editions have carried a tabulation of the daily amounts of kilocalories and selected nutrients required for different age and sex groups, a text discussion of the basis for the tabulated allowances, and a consideration of nutrients not tabulated.

The number of nutrients tabulated has grown considerably over the years. In the 1943 edition, recommended daily allowances were given only for calories; protein; vitamins A, D, B_1, B_2, and C; niacin; calcium; and iron. By contrast, the 1980 edition gives recommended daily allowances for calories; protein; vitamins A, D, E, B_1, B_2, B_6, B_{12}, and C; niacin; folacin; calcium; phosphorus; magnesium; zinc; iodine; and iron, as well as ranges of estimated safe and adequate daily dietary intakes (recommended) of vitamin K, biotin, pantothenic acid, molybdenum, selenium, chromium, copper, manganese, fluoride, and the electrolytes sodium, potassium, and chloride. The complete 1980 RDAs are reproduced in Table 1 of the Appendix.

How adequate are the RDAs? According to the latest available scientific evidence, the RDAs represent those levels of essential nutrient intake that will adequately provide normal, healthy individuals with their known nutritional needs. Since each person has different requirements for various essential nutrients, the RDAs are intended to exceed the requirements of most normal, healthy persons and thus meet their varying needs. However, the RDAs are not considered adequate for people with clinical conditions such as hereditary diseases, illness, or trauma.

If the nutrient intakes of normal, healthy people are equal to or somewhat above the RDAs, their bodies should be nutritionally sound according to current scientific knowledge. If people are consuming the essential nutrients at levels below the RDAs, they are not necessarily deficient in those nutrients. However, their risk of becoming deficient in any particular essential nutrient is increased if such intake levels continue to drop below the RDAs for a prolonged period.

Nutritionists believe that the safest and most appropriate way to evaluate the nutritional status of a person is through a combination of methods: (1) an analysis of the person's nutrient intake based on a record of food eaten, using the RDAs as a guide; (2) physical examination; (3) clinical evaluation; and (4) blood, urine, and other laboratory and biochemical studies.

Food Guides: Deciding What to Eat

Translating the RDA guidelines into daily meal plans takes time and training. Accordingly, nutritionists and home economists in the USDA have translated the scientific recommendations into specifications of the kinds and amounts of food needed for good nutrition. These translations—known as *daily food guides*—provide an easy way to make good food choices.

Scientists are not aware of any one "perfect" food that can supply all the RDAs. To meet all our nutritional needs—including those yet to be determined and incorporated into future RDAs—we must eat a variety of foods. The daily food guides thus recommend a large number of nutritious foods, grouped into four broad categories. These **four food groups** are (1) milk and milk products, (2) meats or meat equivalents, (3) fruits and vegetables, and (4) breads and cereals. Each group contributes a substantial amount of the major nutrients needed for health.

Recently, the USDA introduced a fifth food group: fats, sweets, and alcohol. Because this new group has not yet been widely adopted, this book will adhere to the four food groups previously mentioned and will consider fats, sweets, and alcohol, along with a number of other items, as **supplementary foods** (see later discussion).

In addition to sorting nutrient-dense foods into four basic groups, the USDA has suggested an appropriate number of servings from each group to be consumed daily (Table 2-1). These recommendations are widely used by nutritionists, physicians, home economists, health agencies, government programs, and hospitals—as well as by individuals—as general guides to planning well-balanced and nutritious diets.

However, the food guides and the RDAs are neither iron-clad rules nor perfect instruments. Both criteria must be considered along with other variables in order to be applied optimally. Currently, the food guides in the United States take into account the availability of food supplies, food preferences, incomes, religious beliefs, ethnic origins, seasonal variations, and geographical distributions. In other words, the food guides tend to reflect the "standard American diet."

Chapter 15 will look at the foods we commonly choose from each food group and the nutrients these foods provide. The same chapter will also study supplementary foods not included in the more nutrient-dense four food groups. Chapter 7 discusses food guides for a vegetarian diet.

Table 2-1
Recommended Numbers of Servings from the Four Food Groups

FOOD GROUP	SERVING SIZE	NO. OF DAILY SERVINGS
Milk and milk products		
Fluid milk	1 c, 8 oz, ½ pt, ¼ qt	Children under 9: 2–3 Children 9–12: ≥3 Teenagers: ≥4 Adults: ≥2 Pregnant women: ≥3 Nursing mothers: ≥4
Calcium equivalent	1 c milk 2 c cottage cheese 1 c pudding 1¾ c ice cream 1½ oz cheddar cheese	
Meat and meat equivalents	2–3 oz cooked lean meat without bone 3–4 oz raw meat without bone 2 oz luncheon meat (e.g., bologna) ¾ c canned baked beans 1 c cooked dry beans, peas, lentils 2 eggs 2 oz cheddar cheese ½ c cottage cheese 4 T peanut butter	≥2
Fruits and vegetables	Varies by item: ½ c cooked spinach 1 potato 1 orange ½ grapefruit	≥4, including 1 of citrus fruit and another fruit or vegetable that is a good source of vitamin C and 2 of a fair source 1, at least every other day, of a dark green or deep yellow vegetable for vitamin C ≥2 or more of other vegetables and fruits, including potatoes
Bread and cereals	1 slice of bread, 1 oz ready-to-eat cereal ½ to ¾ c cooked cereal, cornmeal, grits, macaroni, noodles, rice, or spaghetti	≥4

Food Exchange Lists: Making It Easier

One of the major causes of defeat for some dieters is the sheer boredom of repetitious meals. A second major cause of defeat is the complexity of measurement or calorie counting involved in some diets. Food exchange systems are designed to alleviate both problems. Probably one of the most popular systems is the one developed jointly by the American Diabetes Association and the American Dietetic Association. "The exchange lists are based on material in the *Exchange Lists for Meal Planning* prepared by Committees of the American Diabetes Association, Inc. and the American Dietetic Association in cooperation with the National Institute of Arthritis, Metabolism and Digestive Diseases and the National Heart and Lung Institutes of Health, Public Health Service, U.S. Department of Health and Human Services." Although it has been developed for diabetic patients, it has much wider application. This system is explained in detail below.

Exchange lists can be understood as groups of measured foods having the same value. Foods are divided into the six groups shown in Tables 2-2 and 2-3. Within each group, you may exchange an entry for any other entry. Each entry is called an exchange, and each exchange has approximately equal content in calories, carbohydrate, protein, and fat. The contribution of vitamins and minerals in each exchange is also fairly constant.

Because food exchange diets can be so helpful in dieting, we will briefly discuss their application. Table 2-4 provides specific examples of food items within each of the exchange lists. Complete contents of these lists may be obtained from the American Diabetes Association or from a more detailed reference text. Keep in mind that within each list, each item is equal in value to the other in terms of essential nutrients and calories.

We now need to consider the six food groups together in relation to a specific diet so that you can see how the food exchange system works. Table 2-5 shows the total food exchanges in an 1,800 calorie diet for a

Table 2-2
Outline of the 1976 American Diabetes Association Exchange Lists

FOOD EXCHANGE LIST	FOOD GROUP	CONTRIBUTION PER EXCHANGE OF FOOD GROUP			
		kcal	PROTEIN (g)	CARBOHYDRATE (g)	FAT (g)
1	Milk	80	8	12	Trace
2	Vegetables	25	2	5	0
3	Fruits	40	0	10	0
4	Bread	70	2	15	0
5	Meat				
	Lean	55	7	0	3.0
	Medium	80	7	0	5.5
	Fat	100	7	0	8.0
6	Fat	45	0	0	5.0

Table 2-3
Types of Food Included in the Exchange Lists

FOOD EXCHANGE LIST	FOOD GROUP	FOOD TYPES
1	Milk	Nonfat fortified milk and products; low-fat fortified milk and products; whole milk and products*
2	Vegetables	Various raw and cooked vegetables excluding starchy vegetables
3	Fruits	Various fresh, dried, canned, frozen, and cooked fruits†
4	Bread	Bread, cereal, starchy vegetables
5	Meat	Red meat, poultry, fowl, seafood, meat alternates
6	Fats	Butter, margarine, dressings, nuts, others

*Used with adjustments.
†All processed products are unsweetened.

Table 2-4
Specific Examples of Food Items Within Each of the Food Exchange Lists*

FOOD EX-CHANGE LIST	FOOD GROUP	SPECIFIC FOOD EXAMPLE (= MEANS THE TWO ITEMS ARE INTERCHANGEABLE)
1	Milk	1 c skim milk = 1 c yogurt made from whole milk
2	Vegetable	½ c celery = ½ c turnip
3	Fruit	½ small mango = ¼ c grape juice
4	Bread	1 slice whole wheat bread = ½ c bran flakes = 6 saltine crackers = ¼ c baked beans = 1 small white potato
5	Meat (lean)	1 oz sirloin beef = 3 sardines
	Meat (medium-fat)	1 oz boiled ham = 1 egg
6	Fat	1 t margarine = 2 t mayonnaise

*These are only examples from the original exchange lists. In actual implementation, the original lists must be used (Hui, 1983).

Table 2-5
Total Food Exchanges in an 1800-kcal Diet for a Diabetic Patient

FOOD LIST	NO. OF EXCHANGES	PROTEIN (g)	CARBOHYDRATE (g)	FAT (g)	kcal*
Nonfat milk	2	16	24	0	160
Vegetables	2	4	10	0	50
Fruits	5	0	50	0	200
Bread	9	18	135	0	630
Meat, lean	8	56	0	24	440
Fat†	7	0	0	35	315
Total		94	219	59	1,795

*Calories are obtained by using the following equivalencies: 1 g protein = 4 kcal; 1 g of carbohydrate = 4 kcal; 1 g fat = 9 kcal.
†From Table 2-2, we see that 7 exchanges of fat provide 7 × 0 = 0 g of protein, 7 × 0 = 0 g of carbohydrate, and 7 × 5 = 35 g of fat.

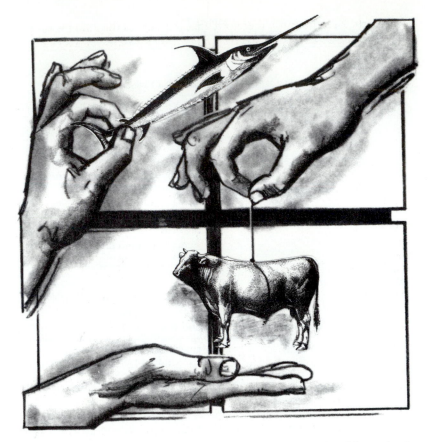

diabetic patient. The benefit of food exchange systems should now begin to become clear. Not only is it important for the diabetic to control calorie intake, but also to control the mix of protein, carbohydrate, and fat. Assume that you wish to maintain a certain level of caloric intake but that your body does not digest fats well. The food exchange system will enable you to control caloric intake *and* control fat intake, without having to learn the fat content of various foods.

Now assume that total caloric intake is the only concern and that any healthy balance of fats, carbohydrates, and protein is acceptable. Table 2-6 shows four different exchange combinations that yield the same number of calories. The first combination, method A, is the one from Table 2-5. Method B makes greater use of milk and fat exchanges and reduces others. Method C emphasizes meat exchanges. Method D balances the number of fat and meat exchanges.

To demonstrate how these 1,800-calorie food exchange plans relate to your actual meal planning, let us look at sample menus for Methods A and B. Table 2-7 presents possible meals for 2 days using the number of exchanges set out in Method A. Notice, for example, the milk exchange. Method A called for two milk exchanges (2 cups). If on the first day's menu you want milk with breakfast and lunch, and also with a bedtime snack, you could have it by splitting one exchange between breakfast and lunch. Keep in mind, therefore, that if 2 cups is the amount for the day, that can be accomplished by 4 half-cups, as in the first day's menu in Table 2-7.

Table 2-6
Four Ways of Assigning the Distribution of Food Exchanges in an 1800-kcal Diet

	NO. OF EXCHANGES			
	PROTEIN: 20% CALORIES FAT: 30% CALORIES CARBOHYDRATE: 50% CALORIES		PROTEIN: 26% CALORIES FAT: 34% CALORIES CARBOHYDRATE: 40% CALORIES	
FOOD LIST	METHOD A	METHOD B	METHOD C	METHOD D
Nonfat milk	2	4	2	4
Vegetables	2	2	2	2
Fruits	5	3	5	3
Bread	9	8	7	6
Meat, lean	8	6	11	9
Fat	7	10	7	9

Table 2-7
Sample Menus for Method A Exchange Distribution

BREAKFAST
Oatmeal, ½ c
Light cream, 4 T
Toast, whole wheat, 1 sl
Margarine, 1 t
Cantaloupe, small, ¼
Cottage cheese, ¼ c
Milk, skim, ½ c
Coffee or tea

LUNCH
Turkey sandwich:
  Bread, whole wheat, 2 sl
  Margarine, 1 t
  Turkey, 2 oz
String beans, ½ c
Margarine, 1 t
Yogurt, skim milk, ½ c
Grapefruit juice, ½ c
Salt, pepper
Coffee or tea

DINNER
Tomato juice, ½ c
Green salad:
  Lettuce
  Radish
  Italian dressing, 1 T
Salmon, broiled, 3 oz
Bagel, small, 1
Cream cheese, 1 t
Green peas, ½ c
Apple, small, 1
Salt, pepper, lemon
Coffee or tea

SNACK
Apple juice, ⅓ c
Bran flakes, ½ c
Raisins, 2 T
Milk, skim ½ c
Biscuit, plain, small, 1
Margarine, 1 t
Chicken, 1 oz
Milk, skim, ½ c

BREAKFAST
Yogurt, skim milk, ½ c
Pineapple, chunks, ½ c
Ham, 1 oz
Biscuits, 2
Butter, ½ t
Coffee or tea

LUNCH
Salad:
  Lettuce wedge, 1
  Radish, sliced, 1
  Tomato, sliced, ½ c
  Crab, canned, ¼ c
  Shrimp, 1 oz
  French dressing, 1 T
Matzo, 4″ × 6″, 1
Butter, 1 t
Peach, 1
Buttermilk, skim, ½ c
Salt, pepper
Coffee or tea

DINNER
Beef, tenderloin, 3 oz
French fries, 8
Vegetable medley:
  Zucchini, cooked, ½ c
  Corn, cooked, ⅓ c
Bread, rye, 1 sl
Margarine, 1 t
Honeydew, ⅛
Salt, pepper
Coffee or tea

SNACK
Banana, 1
Graham crackers, 2½ in. square, 4
Cream cheese, 2 T
Chicken, leg, cold, 1 oz
Milk, skim, 1 c

Table 2-8 presents two daily menus for Method B, the method that emphasizes fat exchanges. If you will look back over Tables 2-3 and 2-4, you will notice that certain foods are never mentioned. Some of those, such as candies, jams, cakes, cookies, pies, and soft drinks, are too high in calories to be safe for use in a diet plan. Others not mentioned, such as coffee, tea, and most seasonings, can be used in unlimited amounts.

Chapter 20 provides additional examples of dividing daily meals into exchanges to facilitate meal planning in weight reduction.

When using food exchange lists for meal planning, always keep in mind that the key to good nutrition lies in a balanced diet, one that does not rely on the same foods day after day. No single exchange group can meet nutrient need. All six must work together to provide you with adequate nutrition.

Government Guidelines: Aids to Healthy Eating

In recent years, intensive efforts have been made to develop a national nutrition policy to suggest nutritional patterns that would enable every American to achieve true preventive nutrition. The *Dietary Goals of the United States* was one such national policy proposed. However, its

Table 2-8
Sample Menus for Method B Exchange Distribution

BREAKFAST	LUNCH	DINNER	SNACK
Puffed rice, 1 c	Baked beans, 1 c	Pork, rump, roast, 2 oz	Tuna sandwich:
Banana, sliced, ½	Asparagus spears,	Sauerkraut, ½ c	Bread, whole wheat,
Light cream, 6 T	cooked, ½ c	Potatoes, mashed, ½ c	2 sl
English muffin, toasted, ½	Roll, plain, small, 1	Margarine, 1 t	Mayonnaise, 2 t
Margarine, 1 t	Butter, 1 t	Strawberries, sliced, ¾ c	Tuna, canned, ¼ c
Ham, 1 oz	Almonds, 10	Milk, skim, 1 c	Buttermilk, skim, 1 c
Milk, skim, 1 c	Pear, small, 1	Salt, pepper	
Coffee or tea	Milk, skim, 1 c	Coffee or tea	
	Salt, pepper		
	Coffee or tea		
BREAKFAST	LUNCH	DINNER	SNACK
Ham, 1 oz	Sandwich:	Veal, cutlet, 3 oz	Chicken, 1 oz
Pancakes, 2	Bread, whole wheat,	Brussels sprouts, ½ c	Bread, pumpernickel, 2 sl
Butter, 1 t	2 sl	Lima beans, ½ c	Margarine, 2 t
Applesauce, unsweetened,	Turkey, 2 oz	Butter, 1 t	Milk, skim, 1 c
½ c	Lettuce, leaf	Roll, small, 1	
Milk, skim, 1 c	Mustard	Butter, 1 t	
Coffee or tea	Mayonnaise, 1 t	Yogurt, skim milk, 1 c	
	Spinach, cooked, ½ c	Blueberries, ½ c	
	Mayonnaise, 1 t	Salt, pepper	
	Apricots, fresh, 2	Coffee or tea	
	Milk, skim, 1 c		
	Salt, pepper		
	Coffee or tea		

Selected Recommendations from the 1977 Dietary Goals for the United States

- To avoid being overweight, consume only as much energy (calories) as is expended; if overweight, decrease energy intake and increase energy expenditure.

- Increase the consumption of complex carbohydrates and naturally occurring sugars from about 28 percent of energy intake to about 48 percent.

- Reduce the consumption of refined and processed sugars by about 45 percent to account for about 10 percent of total energy.

- Reduce overall fat consumption from approximately 40 percent to about 30 percent of energy intake.

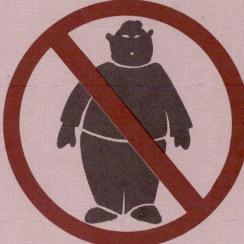

- Reduce saturated fat consumption to account for about 10 percent of total energy intake, and balance that with polyunsaturated and monounsaturated fats, each of which should account for about 10 percent of energy intake.

- Reduce cholesterol consumption to about 300 mg a day.

- Limit the intake of sodium by reducing the intake of salt to about 5 g a day.

release a few years ago started a controversy among health professionals and organizations, many of whom disagreed with the report's recommendations.

The U.S. Senate Select Committee on Nutrition and Human Needs released its second edition of *Dietary Goals for the United States* in 1977. The goals proposed were designed to ensure the best health for the American people. Selected recommendations from this report are listed in the box. To meet these goals, certain changes in food selection and preparation are recommended. Chapter 23 will provide a detailed discussion of the U.S. dietary goals and controversies about them.

Food Composition Tables: What and Where

One aspect of fitting foods into diet plans is learning what nutrients are in various foods and in what amounts. Food composition tables are convenient sources that provide much of the information that we need. Because of the magnitude of the task of developing these tables, most have been prepared by the federal government and international organizations, although a few are published by commercial companies.

Some of the major American food composition tables are listed in the accompanying box. Probably the most comprehensive of these is USDA Handbook No. 8: *Composition of Foods.* The first edition, published in 1963, gives data on 16 nutrients in 2,483 food items for both 100-g edible portions or for 1-lb measures as purchased.

Using USDA Handbook No. 8 as a source, the USDA developed Handbook No. 456 in 1975. It, too, provides data on 16 nutrients in 2,483 food items in household measures and market units. Home and Garden Bulletin No. 72 again used Handbook No. 8 to develop data for 16 nutrients in about 730 foods for average servings or common household units. This table is reproduced in full in the Appendix.

Handbook No. 8 is so heavily used as a standard reference by nutritionists, dietitians, nurses, physicians, and other scientists that the USDA is now massively revising it. The new edition is being released in stages. When complete, it will provide data on 61 nutrients found in about 4,000 foods. These data are presented for 100-g edible portions, common household measures, and 1 lb of the food as purchased. Sections of the revised edition released as of 1983 are listed in Table 2-9.

Another popular book of food composition tables is *Food Values of Portions Commonly Used.* Frequently updated, it is a compilation of information from various sources. These include manufacturers of processed foods, the USDA, and others. These tables give data on 26 nutrients, but the data are not complete for every product. Food products tabulated include regular and basic foods, mixed varieties, and many commercially processed items.

Table 2-9
Revised Sections of USDA Handbook No. 8 as of 1983

SECTION NO.	FOOD GROUP	YEAR ISSUED	NO. OF ITEMS
8-1	Dairy and egg products	1976	144
8-2	Spices and herbs	1977	43
8-3	Baby foods	1978	217
8-4	Fats and oils	1979	128
8-5	Poultry products	1979	304
8-6	Soups, sauces, and gravies	1980	214
8-7	Sausages and luncheon meats	1980	80
8-8	Breakfast cereals	1982	142
8-9	Fruits and fruit juices	1982	263
8-10	Pork products	1983	186

Although food composition tables are convenient, cheap, and widely used, they have some limitations. Nutrients found in a given kind of food vary according to the soil and climate in which the food is grown, the variety, and the season; how the food is harvested, packaged, and stored; and how it is prepared, served, and consumed. Different food composition tables may therefore give different data for the same food. Some of the foods we eat may not even be in the tables—they may be too new or too uncommonly used or too complex a mixture of processed foods. The task of updating a food composition table becomes increasingly difficult as new fresh or processed foods continually appear. The food producers may be the best source of information on the nutritional composition of these products.

Despite these drawbacks, food composition tables provide us with general guides and representative values. To minimize their limitations, the USDA is establishing a nutrient data bank to store information for revisions of the tables, for clinical application, and for professional meal planning. These data, supplied by producers of processed foods, include information required by increasingly stringent and comprehensive food labeling laws. In addition, foods not commonly found in the standard American diet may appear in food composition tables worked out for other areas of the world. Examples are provided in the references at the end of this book. Ethnic food compositions are also described in specialty books available at libraries and other conventional sources.

Facts and Fads: Information and Misinformation

MISINFORMATION IS EVERYWHERE

Fads, by definition, move quickly, and food fads prove no exception to this principle. Food and Drug Administration (FDA) estimates place the number of United States consumers who are attracted by food fads at nearly 18 million, and it is estimated that they annually spend $2 billion on nutritional supplements, diet books, special food products, and products such as weight-reducing devices (Herbert, 1980; Herbert, 1981; Herbert and Barrett, 1981).

Promoters of such products rely on emotional appeals, exaggerated claims, and such powers of persuasion as massive advertising campaigns to promote their products. Despite claims for such products that run counter to nutritional facts, the resultant fads are successful for various reasons.

Nutritionists must cope not only with food fads but also with basic misinformation regarding food. Virtually every population center has at least one health food store, and most large chain stores have at least a health food section. The existence of such businesses attests to both the health consciousness of Americans and their affluence, for health foods are some of the most expensive food items and supplements available.

The FDA tried to bring supplements under its regulatory authority. Those efforts were frustrated in 1977 by a health food lobby that successfully promoted legislation to deny the FDA that authority. The lobbying efforts were fueled by the realization that over three fourths of American households use dietary supplements of some kind. If our use of supplements were based upon our need, three fourths of us would be labeled as malnourished on the basis of our supplement use.

What the FDA found in regard to food quackery was that as fast as they closed down one operation, the promoters were at work on another product. Food fads tend to follow a predictable pattern. One characteristic is that they give almost magical properties to the product. Usually the products are claimed to cure a condition for which no cure exists— or one for which there are numerous sufferers. Cancer and arthritis prove popular conditions in that regard.

Some nutritionists have pointed out that food fads often conflict from one culture to another. For example, a food may be considered a cancer cure in one culture, a poison in another culture, and a source of sexual potency in a third culture. A current example of conflict within a single culture surrounds laetrile (see Chapter 11). Promoters herald it as a cancer cure, while nutritionists point out that it is a potentially lethal cyanide compound.

How Can I Tell It's a Fad?

Labeling on fad products often tends to be misleading. A common example would be a label that lists numerous ingredients and their benefit to a healthy existence but fails to advise that the product provides only a fraction of the recommended dietary allowances of the ingredients.

Fads can also use a negative approach. For example, the idea that enrichment of a food represents a chemical danger has caused some consumers to avoid such products as enriched white bread, despite the fact that enrichment of such products normally involves the addition of basic nutrients. What the fad promoters hope to do in such cases is to scare you away from a popular product so you will substitute theirs.

A current fad of far-reaching effect argues that all processed foods involve health risks. This fad stresses the use of organically grown or naturally grown products. Efforts to promote such naturally grown products go so far as to claim that food processing causes disease.

The organically grown trend promotes such food products as yogurt, honey, wheat germ, alfalfa sprouts, sunflower seeds, and herbal tea. Promoters argue that their products are free of the harmful effects of chemical fertilizers and pesticides. These products typically cost two to three times as much as their counterparts in grocery stores.

A sideline of health food promoters involves special food preparation equipment. Usually the claim is that the equipment processes food in such a way that little nutrient value is lost. The promoters use large gatherings such as fairs or department store sale days to take advantage of impulse buying.

Additives have given rise to a food fad of avoidance. Since some food additives have been found to have harmful side effects, suspicion surrounds all additives. This is, of course, an unfortunate attitude, for many additives prevent potentially harmful bacterial action. Others make food attractive and palatable. While additives must be constantly evaluated for both short-term and long-term effects, they are regulated ingredients and generally serve very positive purposes.

You may initially ask what the harm can be in people's spending their money for harmless products that fall far short of their claims. One concern is that some people—the elderly, for example—will be bilked out of money that they cannot afford to spend by promoters who exploit their natural fear of illness and dependency. Many promoters direct their appeals to the elderly knowing that segment of the population has such fears. A second concern is that individuals relying on worthless products for a cure are wasting valuable time and money that should be spent on known and effective treatments.

What Techniques Are Common to Most Quacks?

Food quacks appeal to the emotions of the consumers, but they do not stop there. Quacks will attempt to shroud their promotions in an air of medical or scientific knowledge. They use titles for themselves, and create their own professional organizations. These are all legal moves, but they are made to mislead consumers. Such efforts tend to be successful because most consumers are not able to distinguish between the legitimate professional groups and those that are strictly profit motivated.

A favorite technique of food quacks is to draw upon scientific fact and enlarge upon its significance. For example, quacks like to follow the findings of animal studies. If they found, for example, that a standard additive produced cataracts in laboratory mice after massive doses, quacks would rush to the market with a product that did not contain the additive. Their advertisements would argue that their competitors use cataract-causing additives whereas they do not.

Certain characteristics seem to be shared by most get-rich-quick food promoters. They generally claim to have information not available to the medical community, such as a secret formula, often from some primitive culture, and they claim their product can almost magically cure diseases or maladies that have proved medically difficult to resolve. We have previously mentioned cancer and arthritis as typical examples. Arteriosclerosis ("hardening of the arteries") also tends to be a popular disease for magical cures. Quacks will usually claim that the medical profession tries to silence them because they are cutting into the doctors' livelihood. Quacks also talk about soil depletion, food processing dangers, and contaminants. They argue that theirs is the only safe product. They also tend to try to enlarge their potential market by claiming that we are all undernourished, usually owing to such foods as refined sugars, pasteurized milk, or canned foods.

Sales techniques involve almost any approach possible. Food quacks use large crowds to take advantage of impulse buying. They sell door to door with evangelical enthusiasm, generally offering the consumer an opportunity to safeguard the family's health. Introductory offers in popular publications are a common approach. Public lectures and radio and television advertising are growing in popularity as merchandising techniques of food quacks. Books have become especially useful in launching food fads, especially those by authors who hold medical degrees. The authors often appear on talk shows and will frequently feature testimonials by popular figures like movie stars or athletes.

Many governmental agencies and community agencies devote significant effort to combatting food quackery. The FDA seeks to prevent mislabeling but must necessarily concentrate its efforts on dangerous products. The U.S. Postal Service can prosecute firms that use the mails to promote and sell worthless products by means of false advertising. The American Medical Association has initiated efforts to counter quackery and faddism. It issues statements on products and maintains its own Bureau of Investigation to respond to inquiries about products and fad promoters. The Federal Trade Commission (FTC) can prosecute for false advertising. Such local organizations as Better Business Bureaus serve educational roles in their communities, as well as corrective roles.

Professional organizations such as the American Public Health Association and the American Dietetic Association have quite active programs for educating the general public regarding nutrition. Nutrition education offers what may be the best hope for combatting quackery and food fads. A constant flow of nutrition information from reliable sources can stem the success of those who prey upon ignorance. For those who use half-truths and slightly twisted scientific facts, the challenge is greater. The public not only must learn nutritional facts but also must become informed enough to identify quackery themselves. The establishment of community nutrition centers also represents an effective source of nutrition education. Another highly successful approach is the use of nutrition columns in newspapers. Unfortunately, quackery and faddism are also able to utilize the press for their own nutritional claims.

One thing that remains certain is that the battle against nutrition misinformation will continue. New products will regularly surface in the marketplace, and new claims will be made for them. The growing national interest in nutrition should prove helpful in the long run, though that interest also generates consumers for faddism. In the final assessment, profit will remain a significant motivator for faddism and quackery. Nutrition education can make the most long-lasting inroads into such practices.

WHERE CAN I FIND RELIABLE INFORMATION?
With the maze of advertising surrounding food fads, and with cases of downright food quackery included in that advertising, where can the consumer turn for nutrition information? Fortunately there is a growing number of good sources, some of which have come into being to try to offset the misinformation that is available. Probably the least utilized sources of nutritional information are the professional sources. These include university nutrition departments and related disciplines, medical research institutions, health professionals, government information offices, and the food industry itself. These sources simply have not attracted the attention of consumers, who tend to rely upon popular

information sources. In defense of consumer choices, though, there are some reasons why professional sources are not popular (Frank, 1982; Guthrie, 1983; Todhunter, 1973).

Research Results

Because of strict regulations regarding the use of human subjects, many research studies must rely upon animals for experimental investigations. Also, research studies tend to focus on very technical methods. Results are not easily translated into practical directions for consumers. Consumers may have little faith that the nutritional results obtained with rats will necessarily hold true for them; moreover, such research results usually appear in professional journals. Consumers do not typically read such publications and additionally find their technical language difficult to understand.

Government Sources

Government information publications have improved to the point where they are more informative for the typical reader, but most consumers do not know how to obtain these publications. Further, governmental publications still lack the flair that characterizes popular sources.

Recent budget cuts have added a price tag to most of those previously free items. This further alienates interested consumers.

Health Professionals

Physicians are in an ideal position to give advice regarding nutritional matters, but many are not trained in nutrition. Further, consumers are reluctant to take on the costs that would likely result from seeking information from their physicians.

Food Industry

Consumers tend to mistrust food industry publications, thinking them biased. Consumers assume that the food industry is motivated strictly by profit and that such publications are designed to stimulate sales.

Nonprofessional Sources

For the foregoing reasons, professional sources do not prove nearly as popular as newspapers, magazines, television, radio, and word of mouth. Popular sources are easily found, entertaining, and understandable. Though advertisements are rarely untruthful, they certainly do not provide balanced viewpoints. Thus, the consumer's task becomes one of evaluating the information obtained.

HOW CAN I EVALUATE NUTRITION INFORMATION?

As a consumer, you can take several steps in evaluating food and nutrition claims. The first of these involves determining the promoter's intent. The second step involves determining whether the claim flows logically. The final step focuses on the research upon which the claim is based.

Determine whether the promoter is biased. Among the clues to watch for are seductive advertising, unrealistic claims, emotional appeals, and attempts to intimidate you. What kind of publication does the advertisement appear in? Is it credible?

Be attuned to certain natural laws. For example, is it likely that a promoter has discovered a cure for a disease when that cure has eluded researchers for years? Similarly, certain changes take time. If a promoter promises sudden and dramatic change, be suspicious. Watch for the use of words like "may," "probably," or "seems to," and phrases such as "it appears" and "it is thought." These are clues that the advertisement is protecting itself.

More complex techniques involve the use of "buzz words" like "power," "energy," "new," and "improved." Such words cast a product in favorable light, but look beyond them to determine whether there is justification for the use of such favorable terms.

Has the promoter cited research to support such claims as "new" or "improved"? Has an authority been cited? What are the authority's credentials? Are any data provided? Are the facts recent? It is also important to determine whether the research was conducted with humans or animals. The nature of the research design also proves helpful to the consumer. Researchers who conduct experiments in which human subjects are actually tested to determine the effect of certain treatments typically use one of three research designs: single-blind studies, double-blind studies, and anecdotal records.

Single-blind studies utilize two groups in the experimental study, an experimental group and a control group. If, for example, a supplement is being tested to determine side effects, the experimental group will receive the actual product being tested, while the control group will be receiving an identically appearing product that will have no effect. This "pretend product" is called a **placebo**.

Single-blind studies have one potential drawback in that those conducting the study know who constitutes the experimental group. There is, therefore, a tendency to see in the experimental group the results hoped for in the study.

In a *double-blind study*, a third party selects who receives the product being tested and who receives the placebo. Those conducting the research do not know which is which and can therefore be more objective about their findings.

When a researcher draws conclusions based upon testimonials from individuals, those brief accounts are called *anecdotal records*. They are of limited benefit, since no one can be sure of the cause and effect relationships. For example, assume that you have frequent headaches and are told that prune juice cures them. You drink prune juice, and the headaches disappear. Did prune juice cause the change? Could there have been other intervening variables? Could you have been influenced by the "placebo effect"—the tendency to feel better because you expect to feel better?

For the foregoing reasons, anecdotal records are of limited value. However, anecdotes often catch the attention of researchers and point to areas in need of formal research. As a consumer, you should be aware that a personal testimony, even one from a popular individual, can be of limited value and does not necessarily reflect a product's worth.

Newspapers and magazines frequently refer to another type of study that gets significant attention. For example, a newspaper article carries the following statement: A study done by a certain individual or group shows that Americans who drink more than five cups of coffee daily are likely to have stomach ulcers. Usually, the article refers to a type of study that the public has very little knowledge of, an *epidemiological* or population study.

In an epidemiological study, the researchers scientifically assemble two groups of patients; for example, five hundred in each. All patients in one group have stomach ulcers, with none in the other group. By carefully questioning the patients, the researchers discover that nearly 70 percent of those who have ulcers drink more than five cups of coffee daily, while in the other group only 40 percent do so. By evaluating just that much information scientifically—that is, statistically—the researchers come to the conclusion about coffee and ulcers. Note that there is no direct proof of a cause and effect relationship. Rather, a scientific "observation" has been made, one that can however, influence consumer behavior and decisions.

IS THIS SAFE?

In the last decade, it seems that everybody has been worried about food safety. For example, one frequently asked question is: Is this preservative safe? Although Chapter 26 discusses this topic in great detail, it will help if certain premises are stated here.

Actually, there are two basic principles to remember about the safety of anything we eat. First, the safety of a food substance or chemical is relative. There is no such thing as absolute safety. There is a risk element with every bite we take. However, the risk varies. What is important is the risk:benefit ratio. That is, will the benefit surpass the risk or vice versa? We may go so far as to state that it is a matter of trade-off. That is, when we use some chemicals in food, we are exchanging some benefits for a certain element of risk. The degree of risk will of course be judged by experts. Second, when we refer to safety, we indirectly mean harm. Again, it is important to remember that some dangers are measurable and can be studied, whereas others are difficult to measure and study. For example, losing hair, bleeding, and birth defects are measurable harm in humans. Behavior changes (such as depression, irritability, tiredness), shorter lifespan, and human cancer are very difficult to measure and define. Under such circumstances, it is easy to prove whether a food substance causes bleeding, but its ability to shorten lifespan by a few years can be a difficult claim to prove. As a result, when we talk about food safety, we must bear in mind that safety is relative and that harm can be difficult to assess.

The Human Body: A Complex Marvel

Your body is truly a complex marvel, one unequaled in the world. We are drawn to try to understand its complex operation, a field of study called *physiology* (Guyton, 1981). That study involves us in a myriad of intriguing bodily functions ranging from the chemical and electrical reactions within our cells to the movements accomplished by means of our musculoskeletal (muscle and bone) structure.

Consider the various systems and organizational units that we comprise. The most visible is our skin, which separates our inner world from the outer world. Beneath that lies our musculoskeletal system, which enables us to move both our entire body and individual parts of that body. Within that greater structure our respiratory system enables us to take in the oxygen upon which our lives depend and to release carbon dioxide back into the air. Our digestive or gastrointestinal system brings nutrients into us to sustain our lives. The cardiovascular system distributes those nutrients among body parts. Our hormonal (endocrine) system regulates numerous body processes by sending chemical messages through the blood. Our endocrine glands secrete those chemicals. For example, when a mother nurses, the hormone prolactin stimulates the breast tissues to make more milk. Our reproductive system provides a mechanism whereby we can replicate ourselves. Our nervous system transmits messages throughout the body, controlling motor functions. The urinary system helps remove fluid and eliminates dissolved substances. This system in turn forms part of the larger excretory system, which has as its main organ the kidneys; the excretory system works with our skin to regulate body temperature. Our whole process of heat production via metabolism comes under control through cell cooperation, blood vessel contraction and dilatation, sweating, urination, and fluid balance.

As remarkable as each of these major systems is, the greatest marvel is that each operates continuously and essentially automatically. We do have some choices, such as when to move our arms and legs, but most choices are made automatically to preserve the harmony with which our systems function. That functional harmony is called *homeostasis*. The word literally means that we stay the same, stay in balance, within the process of constant change. So, our life forces flow.

Through the maintenance of homeostasis we maintain not only our well-being but also our survival. If homeostasis is briefly disturbed, we experience sickness. If one of our major systems becomes totally dysfunctional, we die. A remarkable aspect of homeostasis is that it exists not only for our entire body but also for each of the cells within us. The impressiveness of our cellular life begins to become clear when we realize that we are composed of some *one hundred trillion cells*. Each is constantly receiving nutrients, undergoing chemical change, reacting to stimuli. Because cells are minute, cellular homeostasis is a delicate balance.

Our bodies live in a world of gases, but our inner world is a world of liquids. Some 60 percent of your body is composed of fluids (see Chapter 13). Two thirds of that fluid content exists inside the cells and is called *intracellular fluid*. The remainder, *extracellular fluid*, forms the environment within which our cells live.

Two activities of our body are of special significance in the study of nutrition. The first is the storage function of our bodies, and the second is the circulatory system.

HOW ARE NUTRIENTS STORED—AND WHY?

As you will encounter when you learn about such specific nutrients as vitamins, minerals, carbohydrate, protein, and fat, many excess nutrients are placed in storage in your body. The primary purpose for such storage is to provide for future energy need.

The sugars from carbohydrate are stored in the form of glycogen, which can then be converted to blood sugar as needed for energy. Sugars can also be stored as fats. Fatty acids—components of fat we eat—are stored with protein in a form called lipoproteins. Of course, fatty acids are also stored in our body fat.

The liver can store glycogen for about a six-hour reserve. This is why our bodies can function between meals, since that reserve energy can be drawn upon after meal energy is fully absorbed. The fat cells hold fat that is in storage, and that energy supply can sustain us for days or weeks should ingested energy not be available.

In addition to liver storage and lipoprotein storage, protein is stored as an energy source in the blood. Calcium and other minerals are stored in our bones. The storage process is thus a system in its own right, one that deserves mention here just as does our gastrointestinal system or our circulatory system—a system we will now explore by means of a guided tour.

A GUIDED TOUR OF THE BLOODSTREAM

I am a drop of blood. Follow me on my tour through your body. We'll begin our journey in your lungs where I have stopped by the lungs' alveoli to pick up some oxygen needed by some individual cells and some groups of cells that work together for common purposes. We call those cell groups organs.

The tour I am taking you on is not a long one. I make the complete circuit, we call it the circulatory system, at least once each minute. When you are really active, I make the circuit five times per minute. Your heart propels me with two pumps. One of them sends me through the lungs, and the other sends me through the rest of the system, a process called systemic circulation.

Even with my load of oxygen I have room for more, so I pass through the gastrointestinal tract. Here I pick up dissolved nutrients like vitamins, minerals, amino acids (protein), carbohydrates, and fatty acids. The cells need these too. I don't get all my nutrients there, though. Some of them I pick up in the liver, where they've been undergoing some additional refining. Also, sometimes you aren't eating the nutrients that the cells need at a particular time, but we are prepared for that because we store essential nutrients for such emergencies.

I carry the products necessary for energy to the cells by way of the capillaries. I do much of my trading in the capillaries, since the extracellular fluid surrounding the capillaries picks up nutrients from me in exchange for some things not needed there, like carbon dioxide. The

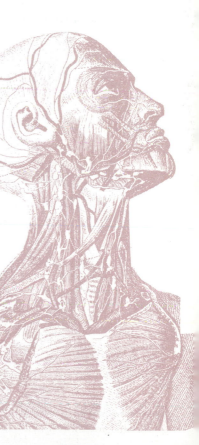

cells are right beside the capillaries, so the exchange is quick and efficient and helps me keep on that one-minute schedule I mentioned.

When you are really active and burning up energy quickly, the glucose, or blood sugar, really flows through here. Of course, I get good help when I'm on a five-trips-per-minute run. The heart's pumping action really raises the arterial pressure. The brain is involved in that one, since the vasomotor center tells the heart and blood vessels to speed things up. When you are burning energy rapidly, the carbon dioxide output is tremendous, as is the need for oxygen, so the lungs are really busy. I speed up to them with carbon dioxide and trade for some more oxygen.

The liver stays busy during the high-energy times, too, since that's where we store glycogen, or "human starch," for conversion into glucose. The pancreas sends out a load of insulin to signal the need. Actually, you can't imagine how many things we have going at once. For example, when we need to speed up, the arteries have receptors that tell the brain, via transmitters, of the need. The brain uses transmitters to tell the heart and blood vessels, and the heart and vessels are the effectors that get the job done. Sometimes almost everybody gets involved.

For example, when we are regulating glucose, or blood sugar, the receptors in the pancreas are the *islets of Langerhans*. They get the insulin moving. Insulin becomes the transmitter of the message, and the membranes of every cell in your body become the effectors by transporting glucose from extracellular fluid to intracellular fluid. Insulin is just one of the chemical messages I carry from the endocrine glands. Through me, chemicals tell the cells to slow metabolism if the body temperature is too high. They can also alert repair crews if there is an injury or an invasion of pathogens that threatens illness.

So here I am, one of the means by which your body maintains homeostasis. These processes I've been describing are called homeostatic mechanisms. They respond to changes in the internal environment by means of adaptive responses. We haven't always been this quick, though. When you were young we weren't too good at things yet, but we went through some developmental processes and really got our act together. We know our time is limited, though. Out there at the other end of the life system is a thing called aging processes. They are going to slow us up a bit.

Your part in all this is to use that musculoskeletal system to bring in good nutrients. You also rely on your brain to help in that regard, since it can tell you about good choices for a balanced diet and healthful nutrition. If anything goes wrong, we'll let you know because we'll develop symptoms that are characteristic of the problem. For example, my role in the bloodstream can get fouled up because of a nutrient need. If that happens, I may show signs of anemia. Or, I may get too much cholesterol. If I do, it will stick to the sides of the blood vessels, and blood pressure will rise because of the tight squeeze I'll be faced with on my one-minute run. If that occurs on a high-speed run, you'll probably even face a little pain. Unfortunately, that may be the only way we can communicate with you.

Whatever you do, don't let me and too many others like me get away. If you bleed, get it stopped quickly. If you don't, there won't be enough of me to enable the heart to pump effectively. Then the arterial pressure will decrease, sending even less of me to the heart. This can become a vicious cycle—one leading to death. Of course, we have a control mechanism, coagulation, that will try to solve the problem, but we may need your help to guarantee survival, the whole purpose of the homeostasis I already mentioned.

Your body is one fantastic piece of equipment, one that you fuel by your nutritional efforts. In forthcoming chapters we will look at the nutrients you obtain from food, the stages of life and how they relate to nutritional need, and the special efforts you need to make regarding certain clinical conditions. What you have encountered in this chapter is an overview of the major tools and premises involved in the study of human nutrition.

STUDY QUESTIONS

1. Use different references to provide five other definitions for *nutrition*.

2. Select five of the basic nutrition concepts and give practical examples of each.

3. Different countries have different food guides. Make up a new food guide and provide the rationale behind the choices you made.

4. Conduct a small survey of your friends to determine whether they are eating as recommended by the U.S.D.A.

5. Select five food and nutrition articles from five popular magazines. Read them carefully and determine whether the information presented is valid.

6. Talk to several teachers of nutrition and several teachers of physiology. Then list ten similarities between nutrition and physiology.

REFERENCES

Frank, R. C. "Information Resources for Food and Human Nutrition." *J. Amer. Diet. Assoc.* 80 (1982): 344.

Guthrie, H. A. *Introductory Nutrition.* 5th ed. St. Louis: C.V. Mosby, 1983.

Guyton, A. G. *Textbook of Medical Physiology.* 6th ed. Philadelphia: Saunders, 1981.

Herbert, V. *Nutrition Cultism: Facts and Fictions.* Philadelphia: George F. Stickley, 1980.

Herbert, V. "Will Questionable Nutrition Overwhelm Nutrition Science?" Am. J. Clin. Nutr. 34 (1981): 284.

Herbert, V., and S. Barrett. *Vitamins and "Health Foods": The Great American Hustle.* Philadelphia: George F. Stickley, 1981.

Todhunter, E. N. "Food Habits: Food Faddism and Nutrition." *World Rev. Nutr. Diet.* 16 (1973): 287.

Nutrition Basics

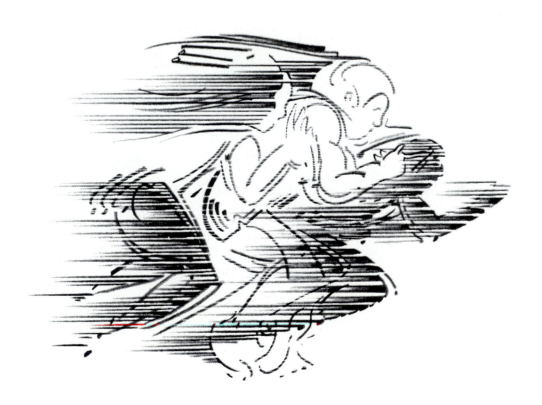

3

ENERGY:

THE POWER TO DO WORK

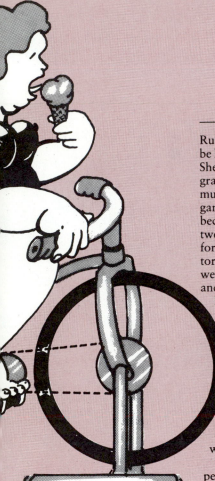

Ruth's DIET COLLAPSES WHEN SHE SNACKS FOR EXERCISE ENERGY

Ruth had lost enough weight to be half-way to her ideal weight. She then began an exercise program to firm up her skin and muscles. Once the exercise began, she stopped losing weight because she was snacking between meals to gain more energy for exercising. How would doctors advise Ruth to balance her weight loss, her exercise need, and her available energy?

Doctor Number 1 would advise Ruth to continue exercising but to eliminate the snacks. He would prescribe appetite-depressing medication, encourage her to visualize herself at goal weight, and have her come to the office daily for injections so he would have an opportunity to reinforce her weight loss.

Doctor Number 2 would suspect that the exercise program is causing hypoglycemic attacks. He would order a glucose tolerance test and would make no further recommendations until Ruth's test results are evaluated.

Doctor Number 3 would see the problem as an educational need. He would counsel Ruth to realize that exercise does not increase appetite, that she has rationalized her snacking. Then he would introduce her to calculating calories in relation to exercise cost, showing her how she can exercise and continue her weight loss.

We do not know the final outcome of Ruth's case, but the case illustrates the fundamental principle of energy balance. We need energy to survive, to work, and to exercise. We eat to get this energy. However, there must be a good balance between the energy we consume and the energy we expend.

Measuring Energy

We move; we think; we breathe; we replenish our cells. Some of these actions are voluntary and some are involuntary, but they all have in common the need for energy. Traditionally, energy is defined as the capacity to do work. In that definition, "work" does not specifically refer to jobs and careers; rather, it refers to bodily functions. Energy fuels us, and we draw energy from the food we eat.

Since energy is a subject within the field of nutrition, our concerns become understanding how to measure it, knowing how to obtain it, and knowing how to avoid excess energy, that is, excess caloric intake.

CALORIE OR "JOULE"

Though you may not have previously made the connection, calories are the measurement of energy. A **calorie** is the amount of heat energy necessary to raise the temperature of one gram of water from 15°C to 16°C. Many nutritionists currently prefer to work with a larger unit, the kilocalorie (= 1,000 calories). You should become familiar with the forms and abbreviations of these terms:

calorie: cal

kilocalorie: kcal, Kilocalorie, Kcal, Calorie, cal

Although the kilocalorie is the preferred unit of measurement, many nutritionists simply refer to it as "calorie" or "cal" instead of "Calorie" or "Cal." This practice is convenient and traditional.

There is an alternative measurement for energy, one based on mechanical energy rather than heat energy. The basic unit in that system, the joule, deals with the force needed to move an object. One thousand joules equal a Joule; and one Joule is the amount of mechanical energy required when a force of 1 newton (N) moves 1 kilogram (kg) a distance of 1 meter (m). Should you wish to convert calories to joules, multiply calorie units by 4.18, the equivalency factor.

SOURCES OF FOOD ENERGY

Primarily, we receive our food energy from the basic nutrients—protein, carbohydrate, and fat. Energy can also be derived from alcohol. The percentages of total energy received from each source will vary from person to person, and from country to country.

In the United States, we find that about 10 percent to 15 percent total daily caloric intake derives from protein, 50 percent to 60 percent from carbohydrate, 35 percent to 45 percent from fat, and a range of from 0 percent to 50 percent from alcohol. Note that, though alcohol is not a nutrient since it is not a nourishing substance found in foods, it does contain calories, as well as vitamins in the case of beer. Some individuals consume significant amounts of alcohol, usually at the expense of nutrient intakes (Windham et al., 1983).

As discussed in Chapter 6, some nutritionists are concerned that Americans obtain too many of their calories from fats. The focus of that concern is the heart itself and the threat of heart disease. Definitive evidence regarding a cause-and-effect relationship between fat and heart disease has not been established, since fat utilization depends upon a number of complex factors.

MEASURING TECHNIQUES

Although scientific advances have brought detailed insights to many previously mysterious nutritional processes, certain processes remain difficult to pin down. For example, scientists determine how much energy people consume by analyzing the caloric content of the different foods they eat. This process is complicated by differences in the ways

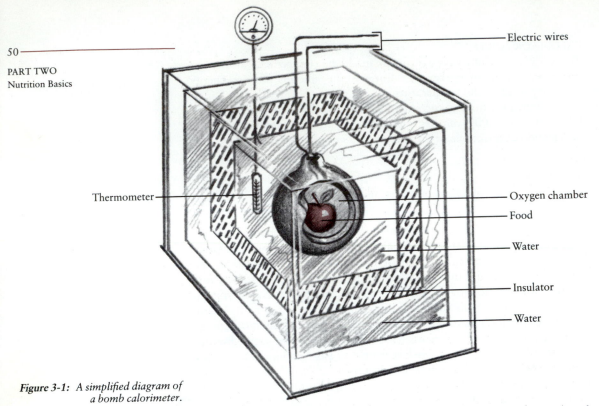

Electric wires

Oxygen chamber

Food

Water

Insulator

Water

Thermometer

Figure 3-1: *A simplified diagram of*
a bomb calorimeter.

laboratory devices and human bodies release and use the energy stored in foods (Horton, 1983).

In laboratory analysis to determine food energy, the food sample is oxidized (burned) by placing the sample in a bomb calorimeter (see Figure 3-1). A spark ignites the food sample in the presence of oxygen and a catalyst, such as platinum. The heat energy (caloric content) of the food sample can then be measured by the rise in water temperature. Chemically, the heat release depends upon the relative content of carbon and oxygen in the food sample. The chemical transformation is easily explained in an equation form:

Carbohydrate + oxygen $\rightarrow$ **Heat energy + water + carbon dioxide**
(protein or fat)

A process similar to that of the bomb calorimeter occurs in our bodies, especially in the liver and in muscle. The big difference between our bodies and the bomb calorimeter is that our bodies derive less energy than the machine would measure. Three reasons account for the difference. First, part of the ingested food is digested and absorbed from the intestine, part eliminated as fecal waste, and the remainder retained as residue in the bowel. Second, some of the food energy is expended on the processing of the food itself—on ingestion, digestion, and absorption. Third, part of the absorbed food ingredients is not used up for energy. Instead, it is lost in various ways—for example, by passage into urine or as a byproduct in the body.

Table 3-1
Energy Values of Food and Alcohol

| SUBSTANCE (1 g) | ENERGY CONTENT | | |
| | IN BOMB CALORIMETER | IN HUMAN BODY | |
	kcal	kcal	kJ*
Protein	5.65	4	17
Carbohydrate	4.1	4	17
Fat	9.45	9	38
Alcohol (ethanol)	7.1	7	29

*The numbers are rounded for easy reference.

The mathematical differences between our utilization of food energy and the potential energy that is scientifically measurable are presented in Table 3-1. As the table indicates, one gram of ingested protein or carbohydrate will provide 4 kcal of energy. One gram of fats will provide 9 kcal.

By using these approximate energy values, the energy content of a food sample can be determined from the protein, carbohydrate, and fat content of the food. By either laboratory analysis or use of food composition tables (see Chapters 2 and 15), each of these three nutrients is identified in grams. Multiplying the grams by four or nine yields the kcal total. Table 3-2 gives the caloric content of some common foods.

Table 3-2
The Caloric Contents of Some Common American Foods

FOOD ITEM	SERVING SIZE	kcal
Cheese, natural blue	1 oz	100
Milk, fluid, whole	1 c	150
Egg, scrambled in butter, milk added	1	95
Butter	1 pat	35
Beef, rib roast, lean and fat	3 oz	375
Salmon, pink, canned, solids and liquid	3 oz	120
Banana	1	100
Raisins, seedless	1 c	420
Bread, French, enriched	1 sl	100
Rice, white, cooked, long-grain	1 c	225
Beans, lima, dry, cooked, drained	1 c	260
Peas, split, dry, cooked	1 c	230
Honey, strained or extracted	1 T	65
Sugar, white, granulated	1 T	45
Broccoli, raw, cooked, drained	1 stalk	45
Potato, baked	1	145
Vegetables, mixed, frozen, cooked	1 c	115
Beer	12 fl oz	150
Cola beverage	12 fl oz	145
Yeast, brewer's, dry	1 T	25

SOURCE: Adapted from *Nutritive Value of Foods*, Home and Garden Bulletin No. 72 (Washington, D.C.: U.S. Department of Agriculture, 1981).

How Much Energy Do We Need?

Our energy need is a daily calculation, composed of the sum of the energy we need for resting periods and the energy we need for physical activities. We can make this calculation in either of two ways, direct calorimetry or indirect calorimetry (Horton, 1983).

LET US ESTIMATE THE ENERGY WE SPEND

In direct calorimetry, an individual's energy use is measured in much the same way that food sample energy content is determined. The individual is placed in a chamber (see Figure 3-2) that is specially insulated and equipped to detect any slight rise in temperature due to heat released by the person. This rise is usually gauged by the temperature change in water circulating around the chamber or by an electrical device wired to the walls.

In the direct calorimetry method, the amount of heat released by the person indicates the approximate energy expenditure. This information is usually accompanied by a measurement of the amount of oxygen consumed and carbon dioxide released before and after the experiment. These additional data give a general idea of what kinds of fuel the body is burning. A formula exists for this measurement, called the *respiratory quotient* (RQ):

RQ = amount of carbon dioxide released/amount of oxygen consumed

This method will determine the type of fuel being burned by your body. If the RQ equals 1.0, carbohydrate is being utilized. Fat utilization yields an RQ of 0.71, and protein 0.81. If your body burns a mixture of the three nutrients, an RQ of 0.8 to 0.85 will result.

Indirect calorimetry involves a simple measurement of oxygen consumed and is a less expensive method of measuring energy expenditure. By fitting an individual with a respirometer, pure oxygen can be inhaled, and carbon dioxide is exhaled into a separate container. Such a closed-circuit system yields a precise measure of oxygen consumed. In an open-circuit system, oxygen available in a sealed room is measured before and after a person spends a definite period in the room. In both methods, energy spent is calculated by the formula that one liter (L) of oxygen utilized equals 4.82 kcal of energy released.

WHEN THE BODY IDLES

When your body is at rest, the energy utilized to maintain your basic bodily functions is known as your **basal metabolic rate** (BMR) (Goodhart and Shils, 1980). Following the analogy that energy fuels us, the BMR is the body idling. Among the basic bodily functions maintained in that state are heart beat, brain activity, respiration, and muscular and nervous coordination. Note, however, that food digestion and absorption are excluded.

Basal metabolic rate differs among individuals. The calculation is made 12 hours after eating and requires complete physical and mental rest, freedom from worry and emotional excitement, and normal health.

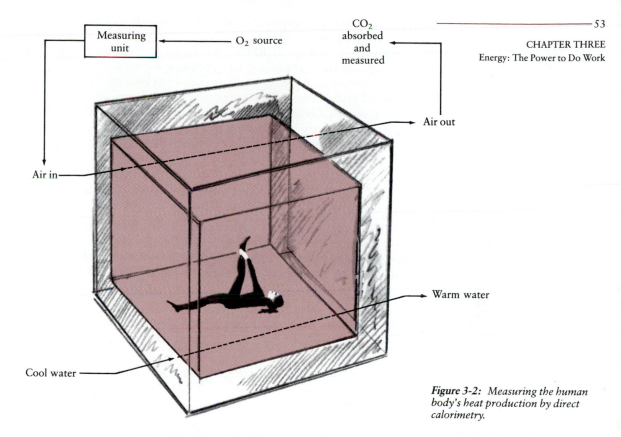

Measuring
unit ← O₂ source

CO_2 absorbed and measured

Air out

Air in

Warm water

Cool water

Figure 3-2: *Measuring the human body's heat production by direct calorimetry.*

The measurement typically occurs with the individual lying down in a room controlled for humidity and temperature.

After eating, the basal metabolic rate increases by from 5 percent to 30 percent. The increase is known as **specific dynamic action** and is illustrated in Table 3-3. The physiological and biochemical reason for this increase, which is complicated and not fully understood, will not be further explored here. If you are interested in this topic, consult the references provided at the end of this book. Though the range can be large, the average meal increases the BMR by about 10 percent within 5

Table 3-3
Effect of Specific Dynamic Action of Food on BMR

STATUS OF BASAL METABOLISM	HYPOTHETICAL VALUE OF BASAL METABOLISM (kcal)	INCREASE OVER NORMAL (%)
After an overnight fast (i.e., normal basal metabolism)	1,500	0
Within 7 hr after eating a meal	1,575–1,950	5–30

hours of eating. The increase ranges from 0 percent to 5 percent by 24 hours after eating.

Though the change in BMR after eating is not fully understood, ingesting, digesting, absorbing, and oxidizing (burning) foods accounts for a portion of the increase. Protein is known to increase BMR, and it is suspected that amino acids, components of protein, stimulate body metabolism (see Chapter 7). Further, the breaking down of the amino acids (a process called *deamination*) is suspected to be an energy-consuming process. The formation of protein byproducts such as urea and uric acid is also energy consuming.

While the basal metabolic rate of an "average" adult is about 1 kcal per kg of body weight per hour, various factors create considerable variations in the BMRs of individuals. These factors are summarized here.

Age. The BMR of a person varies from birth through adulthood, as shown in Table 3-4. The fluctuation is the same for males and females, unless pregnancy and lactation are involved. After the age of 21, growth-related energy requirements decrease.

Pregnancy. The BMR of a woman increases throughout pregnancy, with the highest value at the end of pregnancy. The average rise is about 20 percent. This increase is the direct result of high metabolic activity of the fetus, placenta, and maternal tissues.

Undernourishment. When a person is undernourished, as in starvation, the BMR decreases and may remain lowered until the body is replenished. This drop results from the body's response to a reduction in caloric intake.

Body composition. Muscle mass has a higher metabolism than body fat. A person with high muscle mass will have a higher BMR than a person of equivalent weight who has a higher proportion of body fat.

Sexual difference. Because females have less muscle and more body fat, their BMR is about 5 percent lower than that of males.

Hormones. Thyroid hormones have important effects on body metabolism. A person with hypothyroidism, and thus less body thyroid hormones, will have a decreased BMR; a person with hyperthyroidism typically has a higher BMR. Hypothyroidism may be remedied by an oral dose of thyroid extract. Surgical removal of part of the thyroid may be indicated for a person with hyperthyroidism, though the common practice is to use radioactive iodine. Adrenal hormones also affect BMR. The adrenals are small glands located at the top of the kidneys. When stimulated, as in fright or excitement, they secrete epinephrine (adrenaline), causing a temporary but intense increase in BMR.

Body temperature. When body temperature rises, as in fever, the BMR increases. For each degree Fahrenheit rise, the BMR increases by 7 percent.

Environmental temperature. The BMR also responds to changes in environmental temperature. As the ambient temperature increases, the normal BMR of a person increases. As the ambient temperature decreases, the body BMR initially decreases. Without warming devices

Table 3-4
Changes in BMR with Age

AGE RANGE (YR)	BMR
0–2	Increases
2–puberty	Drops
Puberty–20	Rises slowly
21–old age	Falls

AGE (YR)	AVERAGE BMR (kcal/m²/h)*
6	53
20	41
60	34

*Basal metabolic rate is more accurately reflected in the kilocalories needed per square meter of body surface area per hour than in kilocalories needed per kilogram body weight per hour.

such as clothes or a heater, the process of shivering takes over and the BMR goes up. Since this process cannot continue indefinitely, some warming remedies must eventually be available.

ENERGY AND PHYSICAL ACTIVITY

Studies have confirmed that about one third of our time is spent on keeping our body functioning, that is, on basal metabolism. About 10 to 15 hours of a person's daily life are spent on activities such as driving, sports, walking, or daily routines. In this section we will examine the relationship between our energy expenditure and physical activities (Katch and McArdle, 1983).

Running versus Swimming: Energy Cost

Researchers have been interested in comparing energy expenditure in different athletic activities. Using modern devices, scientists who study human performance can calculate the oxygen consumed by a steady pace for various activities during specified time periods. The formula of 1 liter of oxygen consumed equaling nearly 5 kcal of energy enables the calculation of total energy used (see earlier discussion) for both BMR and the activity. When BMR energy, based upon the athlete's size and age, is substracted from the total, the difference is the energy cost of the activity.

In the case of running, assume consumption of oxygen has been measured as 85 liters over a half-hour period, for a total energy expenditure of 425 kcal. If 30 kcal is required by BMR, the running activity utilized the difference, 395 kcal.

The total energy cost calculation for a swimmer of the same age and weight over the time period would be approximately 400 kcal. After subtracting the BMR energy cost of 30 kcal, the swimming cost would be 370 kcal.

In the preceding examples, the energy cost for the activity itself is called the *net energy cost*. The net energy cost is greater for running than it is for swimming. Net energy costs can, however, fluctuate according to the intensity of performance. Remember that the foregoing examples are based upon steady pace; if jogging or treading water are measured, the net energy cost is lower.

Net energy costs can be approximated by measuring oxygen consumption at intervals, but costs are more difficult to calculate for sports or activities for which intensity varies. For example, energy expenditure in a basketball game can vary significantly between being at the free throw line and racing down the court. In such varying-intensity activities, oxygen consumption must be measured more frequently than in a steady-pace activity. For steady-pace activities, we know that oxygen consumption increases at the start of the exercise and then levels off and remains relatively constant. A few measurements taken at the start, until the leveling-off point, and very few taken during the level stage, can provide an accurate estimate of steady-pace net energy cost. In extremely strenuous activities, total energy cost can easily be 15 percent higher than would be the case for steady pace in the same activity.

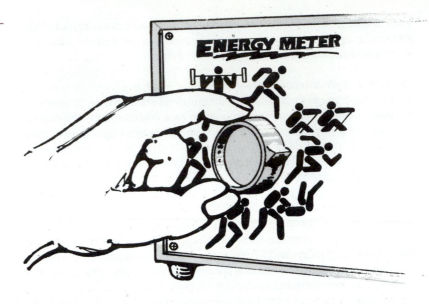

Energy Requirements for Various Sports and Recreational Activities
Just as we saw in the swimming and running examples, net energy costs have been determined for a variety of activities ranging from formal sports to leisure recreational activities. Comparisons between them are interesting and can also be beneficial for purposes of weight control, physical therapy, and fitness training. For example, golfing can be calculated as costing 6 kcal per minute for an average-sized golfer. In the example for running, the cost was over 13 kcal per minute. The golfer must golf over twice as long as the runner runs to expend the same amount of energy.

Such comparisons are, however, very dependent upon body size. Especially in activities where the body's weight must be moved, energy expenditure increases. A heavy individual must expend more energy than a lighter person performing the same activity at the same pace. Once a sufficient number of individuals have had their net energy cost calculated for any activity that requires movement of body weight, it is possible to quite accurately predict energy requirements based upon body weight alone.

Such energy-need estimations based upon body weight cannot, however, be made for activities in which weight-bearing does not occur. For example, rowing and bicycling can be strenuous activities, but they do not have the weight-bearing characteristics of running or walking and cannot be estimated on the basis of body weight. All net energy costs for sports and other recreational activities are, of course, based upon averages. Differences in your skill, fitness, and intensity of performance will produce differences in your energy cost.

Hard Work Uses More Energy
Physical activity adds energy need to that required for maintaining BMR. This extra energy need varies with the activity performed,

body build, and intensity and duration of the activity. Table 3-5 describes the approximate energy cost of various activities for a man who weighs 70 kg.

For convenience, we can divide human activities into four types depending upon energy expenditure: very light, light, moderate, and heavy. Very light activities—including driving a car, painting the inside of a house, and sewing or ironing—increase energy need to 130 percent of BMR. Light activities—waiting on tables, fixing cars, or working on an assembly line—reach 150 percent of BMR. Moderate activities—riding a bicycle, scrubbing the floor or bathtub, or gardening—raise energy need to 175 percent of BMR. Heavy activities—chopping wood, moving a piano, or playing football or basketball—will increase energy need to 200 percent or more of BMR.

When we consider that one third of our day is spent sleeping, and half is spent sitting or standing, we lead rather sedentary lives. The President's Council on Physical Fitness and Sports has determined that walking is the most common exercise for half of American women and one third of American men. Though we note in Chapter 21 that physical fitness is gaining in popularity, it is still safe to say that close to half our population expend little energy beyond the basal metabolic rate.

OUR ENERGY NEED VARIES

Our BMR combines with our physical activity need to yield our total energy need. There are general influences that affect total energy need.

You Need More When You Are Young

The age factor. A high energy requirement exists during infancy and childhood. Both BMR and activity make the need high relative to body size. With maturation, physical activity decreases, so adult need is lower than child need. The BMR also decreases with age.

You Need Less If You Are a Small Person

The body-size factor. Certainly a larger person requires more energy to move or work. The combination of BMR and activity energy for a large person will be greater than that for a smaller person.

All of Us Need More When It Is Cold

The climate factor. Shivering and extra clothing increase basal metabolic requirement. It also seems that a person would need more energy when it is hotter than normal (65°F); however, when it is hotter, people work less. Hence, the total energy need may actually decrease.

A Pregnant or Nursing Mother "Eats for Two"

The child-bearing factor. A woman needs more energy when she is pregnant, because her BMR increases and her body becomes larger. A nursing mother also requires more energy, since part of hers flows to the infant. Chapter 16 addresses these increased needs in greater detail.

Table 3-5

Approximate Energy Cost of Different Forms of Activities for a 70-kg Man*

ACTIVITY	kcal/min
Basketball	9.0–10.0
Boxing	9.0–10.0
Cleaning	4.0– 4.5
Coal mining	6.0– 8.0
Cooking	3.0– 3.5
Dancing	3.5–12.5
Eating	1.0– 2.0
Fishing	4.0– 5.0
Gardening	3.5– 9.0
Horse riding	3.0–10.0
Painting	2.0– 6.0
Piano playing	2.5– 3.0
Running	9.0–21.0
Scrubbing floors	7.0– 8.0
Standing	1.5– 2.0
Swimming	4.0–12.0
Typing, electric	1.5– 2.0
Walking	1.5– 6.0
Writing	2.0– 2.5

*The data in this table have been collected from many sources. Because of large variations among the results of different investigators, ranges of values are used so as to give a general idea of the relationship between types of activity and the energy cost.

Using the foregoing influence factors, certain reference figures can be developed. For example, assuming that a "standard" person is 23 years old and moderately active at 65°F, this person's total energy need would be:

	WEIGHT		DAILY CALORIC NEED (kcal)
	LB	KG	
Man	154	70	2,700
Woman	128	58	2,000

The above reference standards were established by the National Research Council of the National Academy of Sciences in 1980. More information on caloric need is presented in other chapters.

What Is My Most Desirable Weight?

The phrase *ideal* or *desirable body weight* describes a nutritional principle based on the premise that for each person there is an optimal weight for good health. Scientifically, "ideal" is not the same as "desirable," but for discussion purposes we will use them interchangeably in this book. Four methods are used to determine ideal weight: (1) standard tables, (2) the sex-frame-height rule of thumb, (3) standard growth charts for children, and (4) various popular physical measurements.

WE CAN ALWAYS REFER TO A TABLE

The most widely used standard tables of desirable body weight are those issued by the Metropolitan Life Insurance Company, the Society of Actuaries, the Association of Life Insurance Medical Directors of America, the National Academy of Sciences, and the U.S. Public Health Services. Table 3-6 provides two samples of life insurance standard tables.

Although standard tables are frequently used in the United States, they fail to indicate amount of body fat. This omission can be misleading, since excess weight may not be fat but may be fluid, muscle, or bone instead—important distinctions relative to health. Further, some popular tables do not distinguish between average weights and desirable weights. That lack of distinction can be statistically important, since

Table 3-6
Desirable Weights by Height and Body Frame for Adults

	DESIRABLE WEIGHT (LB)		
	SMALL FRAME	MEDIUM FRAME	LARGE FRAME
Man, 5'10" with shoes on 1" heels*	144–154	151–163	158–180
Woman, 5'7" with shoes on 2" heels*	123–136	133–147	143–163

SOURCE: Issued by the Metropolitan Life Insurance Company of New York and derived from the Build and Blood Pressure Survey of 1979 by the Society of Actuaries

Note: The complete tables are located in the appendix.

*Dressed in indoor clothing.

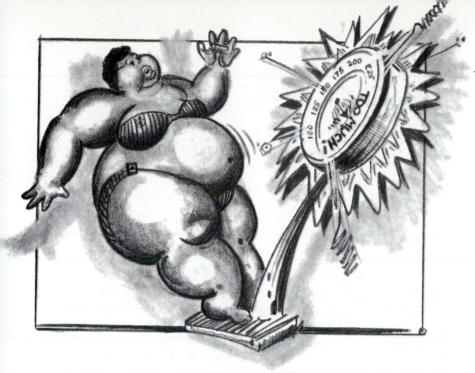
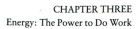

individuals in the extreme body weight ranges are excluded from calculation of averages. Averages can, in effect, penalize individuals over 40, many of whom tend to be overweight. A further drawback to standard tables is their reliance on three body frames—small, medium, and large. Lacking a means to scientifically distinguish among these three choices, the general public must guess. If, for example, a female insurance applicant inaccurately describes herself as small of frame, she penalizes herself.

In addition to guessing, the general public has devised two methods for determining body frame (see Table 3-7).

Table 3-7
Layman's Method to Determine Body Frame

A. Encircle the wrist bone with index finger and thumb.

   If the fingers do not touch or overlap, the body frame is large.

   If the fingers just touch or overlap, the body frame is medium.

   If the fingers overlap, the body frame is small.

B. Measure the circumference of the wrist bone.
   Men
   If the circumference is less than 6 in., the body frame is small.

   If the circumference is 6 to 7 in., the body frame is medium.

   If the circumference is more than 7 in., the body frame is large.

   Women
   If the circumference is less than 6 in., the body frame is small.

   If the circumference is between 6 and 6½ in., the body frame is medium.

   If the circumference is more than 6½ in., the body frame is large.

Table 3-8
Ideal Body Weights Using the Height-Frame Rule

FRAME SIZE	HEIGHT DATA	WEIGHT (LB) MEN	WOMEN
Medium	First 5 feet	106	100
	Each inch above 5 feet	6	5
Large	Each inch above 5 feet	$\frac{110}{100} \times$ weight calculated for medium-frame person	
Small	Each inch above 5 feet	$\frac{90}{100} \times$ weight calculated for medium-frame person	

A RULE OF THUMB HELPS

For many years, calculations based on sex, frame, and height have been used in determining ideal body weight for both men and women. Table 3-8 describes the process. As a rule-of-thumb process, this method approximates ideal body weight and is subject to the same drawbacks as those you encountered with standard tables.

GROWTH OF CHILDREN IS PREDICTABLE

Ideal body weights for infants, children, and adolescents can be ascertained by using standard growth charts (height–weight) such as those of Wetzel, Iowa, Stuart, or the U.S. Public Health Service. Growth charts can be quite helpful in evaluating the growth rate of children. Some of these charts are reproduced in the Appendix. Although these growth charts may have a few technical drawbacks, they are the best tools available for evaluating children's health or growth.

POPULAR WAYS OF MEASURING YOUR "FIGURE"

Various popular methods are used by individuals to determine their own ideal weight. One method, the "pinch test," presumes that if more than one inch of abdominal skin can be pinched, the individual is overweight. The "girth test" is used for males. It presumes that waist and chest circumferences should be about the same. A "ruler test" is also a popular method for determining whether an individual is above ideal weight. A ruler extending from the rib cage to the pubic bone should lie flat when the subject is lying on his/her back. Of course, individuals can also weigh themselves and compare that weight to ideal weight.

Many of the popular methods of estimating ideal weight are also used to determine whether an individual is overweight. You will encounter more about overweight and obesity in Chapter 20.

Exactly How Much Energy We Need Daily

To estimate the daily caloric need for ideal body weight, we can either use a general standard or the sum of basal metabolic need plus activity caloric need discussed earlier in this chapter. The former is less accurate but can be used by everybody. Each method is examined below.

Table 3-9
One Method of Calculating Daily Caloric Needs According to Basal Metabolism and Activity Level

PHYSICAL ACTIVITY	TOTAL CALORIES NEEDED DAILY
Sedentary to light	$\frac{130}{100} \times$ basal caloric need
Moderate	$\frac{150}{100} \times$ basal caloric need
Strenuous	$\frac{175-200}{100} \times$ basal caloric need

WE CAN APPROXIMATE

The 1980 Recommended Daily Dietary Allowances (RDA) (see Chapters 2 and 15) established by the National Academy of Sciences/National Research Council include recommended daily caloric allowances according to sex, age, and height. For example, a 5′ 10″, 154 lb man requires 2,700 kcal/day between the ages of 23 and 50. A 5′ 4″, 120 lb woman requires 2,000 kcal in the same age range. These standards presume moderate physical activity. The Appendix provides more information for RDA data.

For children, either the RDA or the age rule can be used for approximating caloric need. Under the age rule, 1,000 kcal per day is allowed for one year of age, with an additional 100 kcal for each additional year of age. This method proves functional until age 13 for girls and age 16 to 18 for boys.

WE CAN BE SPECIFIC

There are many ways to calculate the caloric need for ideal body weight under the basal metabolism plus activity level method. For example, basal metabolic rate uses a standard of 1 kcal/kg ideal body weight per hour. Using this handy formula, 70 kg × 24 hours × 1 kcal/kg equals 1,680 kcal for an average man, and 58 × 24 × 1 equals 1,392 kcal for an average woman.

Three other methods should be briefly mentioned. Table 3-9 uses BMR multiplied by an activity factor. Table 3-10 uses known caloric need per pound of ideal body weight according to activity level. Finally, Table 3-11 gives the U.S. Department of Agriculture's rule of thumb for the calculation.

Table 3-10
Daily Caloric Needs According to Activity Level and Ideal Body Weight by Using Approximations of Caloric Expenditure per Pound Body Weight

PHYSICAL ACTIVITY	kcal/lb IDEAL BODY WEIGHT
Sedentary	11–12
Light	13–14
Moderate	15–16
Strenuous	18–19

Table 3-11
USDA Rule of Thumb for Calculating Daily Caloric Needs

PHYSICAL ACTIVITY	TOTAL CALORIES NEEDED DAILY*	
	WOMEN	MEN
Sedentary	Ideal body weight × 14	Ideal body weight × 16
Moderate	Ideal body weight × 18	Ideal body weight × 21
Strenuous	Ideal body weight × 22	Ideal body weight × 26

*All ideal body weights expressed in pounds.

The basic problem with all the foregoing methods is the determination of activity level. Since judging activity level can be very subjective, many professionals prefer tables that tie caloric need to specific occupations or work tasks.

Obviously, individual differences make most attempts at devising standards somewhat shaky. What is important, though, is that we realize that there *is* an ideal body weight for us and that there *is* a given caloric need for maintaining good health and performing necessary tasks at that ideal body weight.

Energy Consumption and Expenditure

In the introduction to this chapter, you had an opportunity to see how various doctors would react to Ruth's problem—a problem of energy balance. In Chapter 20, obesity is also addressed in relation to energy balance. If your energy intake—your calorie intake—exceeds the energy you use, you will gain weight. If you are engaged in exercise and lack sufficient calorie intake for the energy cost of the activity, exhaustion results.

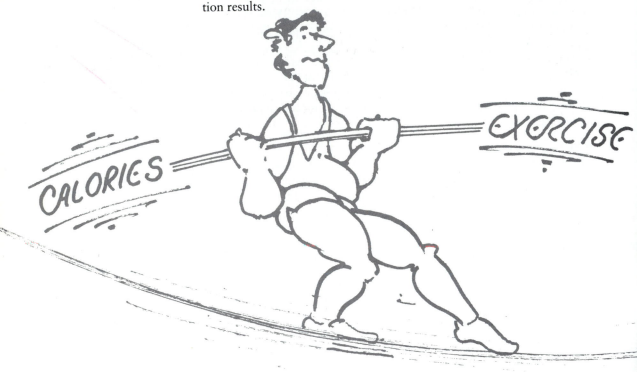

The two preceding energy balance situations are by far the most common, but the issue of energy balance can be even more complex. As in Ruth's case, even with exercise it is possible to have excess energy available. The result will still be excess body weight. For fluctuations in body weight, energy is the fulcrum on which our body balances; it is our equilibrium.

STUDY QUESTIONS

1. What is one calorie? One joule?

2. How is energy in food samples measured in the laboratory? How does this method differ from the actual utilization of food energy in the body? What numerical values are used to account for this difference?

3. Discuss the two methods of determining individual energy expenditure.

4. Define basal metabolic (BMR). What is the average BMR? What variables influence individual differences in BMR? How?

5. How is a person's total energy need calculated?

6. Discuss some drawbacks of standard body weight tables.

7. What are the two basic ways of determining an individual's daily caloric need?

REFERENCES

Goodhart, R. S., and M. E. Shils, eds. *Modern Nutrition in Health and Disease.* 6th ed. Philadelphia: Lea & Febiger, 1980.

Horton, E. S. "Introduction: An Overview of the Assessment and Regulation of Energy Balance in Humans." *Am. J. Clin. Nutr.* 38 (1983): 972.

Katch, F. I., and W. D. McArdle. *Nutrition, Weight Control, and Exercise.* 2nd ed. Philadelphia: Lea & Febiger, 1983.

Windham, C. T., et al. "Alcohol Consumption and Nutrient Density of Diets in the Nationwide Food Consumption Survey." *J.A.M.A.* 82 (1983): 364.

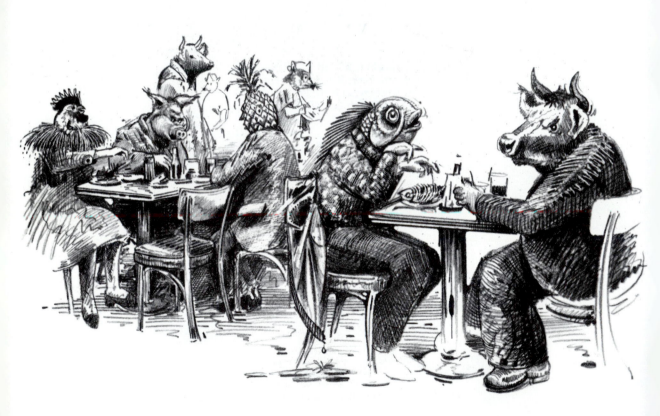

4

BODY

COMPOSITION &

GROWTH:

ARE WE WHAT WE EAT?

COMPARING TWIGS FROM THE BRADEN FAMILY TREE

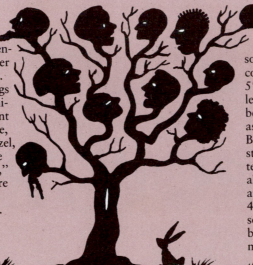

At the family reunion, three generations of Bradens got together for the first time in some years. "It's easy to see that we're twigs from the same tree," said Jennifer, age 20, as she stood in front of the mirror with mother Jane, age 45, and Grandmother Hazel, age 70. "Some of the twigs are weathering better than others," said Jane wryly. "And some are shorter," said Grandmother. "Not by much," said Jennifer. "Let's make some comparisons."

An observer could have made some guesses regarding body composition of the three. At 5' 5" and a member of the college track team, Jennifer could be guessed as the youngest and as having the best muscle tone. But what about upper body strength, hair health, water content, lean body mass, and general nutritional status? Could Jane at 5' 7", or Grandmother, at 5' 4", be as healthy as Jennifer in some respects? The study of body composition provides a means of eliminating guesswork.

Body Composition: Some General Descriptions

As mentioned in Chapter 3, the muscle content of the body is one factor in determining energy need. In addition, our body composition is related to our dietary needs, nutritional status, and growth and development. Scientists use several methods of describing body composition, depending on what they want to emphasize. Most nutritionists prefer to use the following common descriptions as reference points.

1. Functionally and physiologically, we can divide the body into **extracellular** (outside of cells) and **intracellular** (inside of cells) components. The former include bones and extracellular fluids such as blood plasma, lymph, and fluid that bathes cells. The latter include fat and organ cell mass, such as kidney, muscle, heart, and so on. In clinical medicine, this division is probably one of the most important considerations in patient care. It is the major frame of reference in any discussion of fluids, electrolytes (minerals), and body acidity (pH). Chapter 13 provides a brief discussion of this topic.

2. Structurally, we can partition the body into water, fat, and cell mass

solids. Scientists who specialize in developmental nutrition recognize the importance of water, fat, and cell mass distribution in the fetus and in pregnant women (Chapter 16).

3. Metabolically, the ingredients of the body may be separated into two categories: body fat and lean body mass. The **lean body mass,** also known as the "fat-free body" or the "body cell mass," is what is left after the weight of body fat is subtracted from the total body weight. According to one argument, this way of describing body composition works better in theory than in fact, because some fat may be hidden in muscle and bone cells. At any rate, the lean body mass does all the work of keeping the body functioning. This metabolic division of body composition is used extensively in facets of nutritional sciences. We can understand losing weight (Chapter 20) and undernutrition (Chapter 19) much better when we consider the body to be made up of fat and lean body mass. Such comparisons also help us understand stages of growth.

4. Nutritionally or chemically, the body is made up of protein, fat, carbohydrate, water, and ash (minerals). This is an important principle in understanding body metabolism (Chapter 14) and growth (see below and Chapters 16, 17, 18).

These four ways of describing body composition will be explored to varying degrees throughout this book. Although an in-depth analysis is beyond the scope of this book, these descriptions allow some well-known but unrelated observations that have a direct bearing on body composition from a nutritional point of view. They are briefly mentioned below.

When a person's body weight changes, the change may involve body water, body fat, or body cell mass. Muscle cells contain about 75 percent water; red blood cells and cells of the brain, tendons, and connective tissues contain less. Fluids outside body cells (extracellular fluids) contain mainly sodium and chloride; fluids inside the cells (intracellular fluids) contain mainly potassium, phosphates, protein, and organic acids. The electrolytes (minerals) must be balanced both inside and outside the cells and must be kept at a constant physiological equilibrium. This balance must be maintained even when the body is at rest.

In a normal, healthy individual, the total body water usually remains constant. But with **overhydration** (edema) there will usually be a gain in body water and/or a loss in body cell mass relative to total body weight; with **underhydration** (dehydration) there will usually be a loss of body water or a gain in relative body cell mass.

Nutritionally, the carbohydrate content of the body is the most easily depleted because it is the main body fuel. Fat and protein are very difficult to deplete in most people, though there are exceptions. Unlike the average individual, an athlete may lose weight and gain cell mass (muscle) with a decrease in body fat. Under conditions of partial or total starvation, protein and fat will be degraded to provide calories after all available carbohydrate is depleted.

67

CHAPTER FOUR
Body Composition and Growth:
Are We What We Eat?

Table 4-1
Approximate Body Composition of
a 25-Year-Old Male (70 kg) and
Female (58 kg)

BODY COMPONENT	BODY WEIGHT			
	MAN		WOMAN	
	kg	% OF TOTAL	kg	% OF TOTAL
Protein	11.90	17.0	4.93	8.5
Fat	9.45	13.5	12.76	22.0
Carbohydrate	1.05	1.5	0.87	1.5
Water	43.40	62.0	35.96	62.0
Ash (minerals)	4.20	6.0	3.48	6.0
Total	70.00	100.00	58.00	100.00

Table 4-1 indicates the approximate body compositions of a 70 kg (154 lb) man and a 58 kg (127.6 lb) woman by chemical components. These data should be used only as general guides, for individuals vary considerably, and body composition changes with age, conditioning, diet, and disease.

How Body Composition Is Determined

Biologists and medical scientists have tried for many years to devise an acceptable method of directly determining the actual body composition of individuals. Brief descriptions of some available techniques are provided below (Brozek, 1965; Katch and Katch, 1983). Note that one of the oldest techniques, anthropometric measurements, are discussed in a separate section.

CADAVER ANALYSIS
Chemical analysis of dead bodies is the most direct technique of measuring body composition, and it is one of the oldest used. But this method has many disadvantages, such as the limited number of bodies available; the limited availability of bodies of different ages, races, and sex; the formidable task of analyzing the massive amount of fat, protein, and bones; and the need for extensive space, equipment, and training. Most important, the basic differences between a dead body and a live one have been the center of controversy for many years. Obvious complications of using a dead body include the varying causes of death, dehydration, pathological deterioration, damage from accidental death, and the length of time stored in preserving fluid. However, the chemical analysis of a dead body does provide some general ideas of the approximate composition of fat, protein, carbohydrate, and ash in the human body.

BODY DENSITY OR SPECIFIC GRAVITY MEASUREMENT
The body density method derives from the fact that the buoyancy of a body depends on how much fat it has. Basically, Archimedes' principle is used. By weighing a person inside and outside of water and approximat-

ing how much air is trapped in the body, one can obtain certain essential data: body weight in air, body weight in water, volume of water that is equivalent to the volume of the body, and volume of gas or air space within the gastrointestinal and respiratory tracts. This information is then incorporated into a formula from which one can calculate the approximate fat content in the body. In general, the more fat a person has, the lower the specific gravity or density (weight per unit volume).

69

CHAPTER FOUR
Body Composition and Growth:
Are We What We Eat?

POTASSIUM ISOTOPE MEASUREMENT

The mineral element potassium has two natural radioactive *isotopes*, ^{40}K and ^{42}K. One technique of determining body composition directly estimates the amount of body potassium. Radioactive ^{40}K (found in foods as well as in body tissues) occurs in a constant proportion in relation to "natural" potassium and emits gamma radiation measurable by placing the person in a whole-body counter. Since we know the approximate concentration of potassium in the lean body mass, we can estimate lean body mass if we know the relative contents of ^{40}K and "natural" potassium. Another technique, using ^{42}K, called *isotopic dilution*, measures the amount of exchangeable potassium in the body. Again, if total body potassium is known, the lean body mass can be calculated.

After determining a person's lean body mass, one can calculate the amount of fat in his or her body by subtracting the lean body mass from the body weight.

BODY WATER MEASUREMENT

Using the dilution principle, one can also measure the total amount of water in the human body. Water contains hydrogen atoms, which can be replaced by isotopic hydrogen, tritium, or deuterium. This "hot" water can either be injected into body fluid or administered orally. It will dissolve in and penetrate all the available water in the body without itself being metabolized. After a period of stabilization, a small amount of body fluid can be withdrawn and analyzed to determine how much water the body contains. From this information one can calculate the lean body mass. Subtracting the lean body mass from the body weight gives the approximate amount of fat in the body.

Other chemicals such as antipyrine and *n*-acetyl-4-aminopyrine have recently been used in place of radioactive water for this dilution technique.

FAT ANALYSIS AND X-RAY STUDIES

Chemicals such as cyclopropane can penetrate directly into body fat, a sample of which can be analyzed after a period of stabilization to determine how much body fat a person has.

New x-ray techniques permit body fat, bone mass, muscle mass, and so on, to be estimated.

Anthropometric Measurements

Assessment of growth and development by studying **anthropometric** measurements (physical measurements of the human body) provides

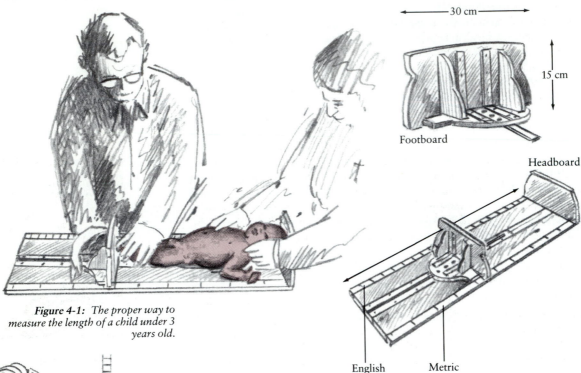

Footboard

Headboard

Figure 4-1: The proper way to measure the length of a child under 3 years old.

English   Metric

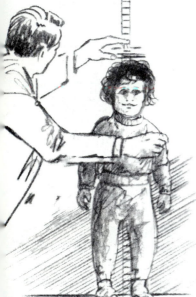

Figure 4-2: The proper way to measure the height of a child older than 3 years.

important information about the nutritional status of infants, children, adolescents, and pregnant women (Centers for Disease Control, 1972; Harries et al., 1983). Standard measurements include weight, height, head circumference, midarm circumference, chest circumference, and skinfold thickness. These data provide developmentally significant ratios, including weight:height; midarm circumference:head circumference; chest circumference:head circumference; and midarm circumference:height. Data obtained over a period of time are especially helpful.

HEIGHT AND WEIGHT MEASUREMENTS
Although height and weight measurements are common, they are usually made improperly. For infants, the body weight should be measured to the nearest ½ oz or 10 g, for children to the nearest ¼ lb or 100 g. Whenever feasible, a beam balance scale should be used, which should be calibrated against reference weight as frequently as possible. Zero alignment must be adjusted at every weighing session. The length of children under 3 years old should be measured with the child lying on its back; standing measurements of height are recommended for older children. Lengths and heights should be measured to the nearest ¼ inch or 1 cm. Figures 4-1 and 4-2 show the proper ways of measuring length

71

CHAPTER FOUR
Body Composition and Growth:
Are We What We Eat?

and height. Head circumference is obtained by using an insertion tape; the measurement is taken as shown in Figure 4-3.

SKINFOLD MEASUREMENTS

During the *Ten-State Nutrition Survey, 1968–1970* (see Chapter 23), the Department of Health and Human Services used the following guidelines for skinfold measurements.

Skinfold measurements appear to be the best single determination of adiposity (degree of fat in body tissues). This measurement reflects the amount of subcutaneous (beneath the skin) fat. Skinfold thickness can be obtained from the subscapular area, abdomen, triceps, and biceps.

The accepted national standard is a pressure of 10 g/mm² on the caliper face. The contact surface should be about 20 to 40 mm². These recommendations are satisfactorily met by the Lange calipers, which are used by most public health workers. The reading of the calipers should be checked daily; small metal blocks for this purpose are available from suppliers of anthropometric tools.

The skinfold measure obtained is the double thickness of the pinched, folded skin plus the subcutaneous adipose tissue. In the approved method of measuring skinfold, a full fold of skin and subcutaneous adipose tissue is pinched between the thumb and forefinger of the left hand, away from the underlying muscle, and held firmly while the measurement is being taken. The calipers are applied to the skinfold about a centimeter from (below or distal and below) the fingers and at the least depth of the fold at which the surfaces of the skin are approximately parallel. The distance of the measuring point from the fingers should be such that the pressure on the fold at this point is exerted by the faces of the caliper rather than by the fingers. The handle of the caliper is then released slowly to permit the full force of the caliper arm pressure. The dial is read to the nearest millimeter. Caliper measurement should be made at least twice to obtain a stable reading. If the skinfold is extremely thick, dial readings should be taken 3 seconds after the caliper pressure is applied for utmost accuracy. The two examples below underscore the importance of carefully attending to the locations of and procedures for skinfold measurements.

The triceps skinfold (Figure 4-4) is measured midway between the shoulder (tip of the *acromion*) and the elbow (tip of the *olecranon*) of the *right* arm, with the crest of the skinfold parallel to the long axis of the arm. The midpoint is critical because of the gradation of subcutaneous fat thickness from elbow to shoulder. With the subject's arm flexed at 90°, the midpoint is located by measuring with a tape and marking with a pencil. The subject's arm should then hang freely when the skinfold measurement is made. Care is necessary to avoid lifting the muscle tissue along with the skinfold on some subjects.

The subscapular skinfold (Figure 4-5) is taken just below the angle of the *right* scapula (with shoulder and arm relaxed), following the natural cleavage of the skin. This is often along a line about 45° from the horizontal extending medially upward.

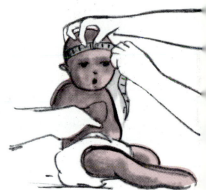

Correct method

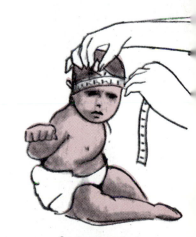

Incorrect method

Figure 4-3: *The proper way to measure head circumference. Tape should be placed level at mid-forehead with overlapping ends.*

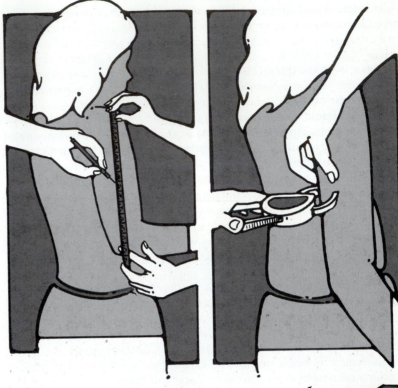

Figure 4-4: *Measuring the triceps skinfold.*

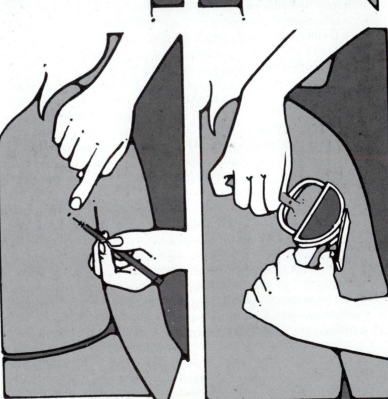

Figure 4-5: *Measuring the subscapular skinfold.*

Growth, Body Composition, and Life Span

In addition to measuring body composition by the foregoing techniques, we can make some general assumptions about how individuals vary in body composition. The relative content of each component varies with age, sex, exercise, dietary intake, disease, and other environmental conditions. We will study body composition and growth during different stages of the life cycle (Pike and Brown, 1984).

73

CHAPTER FOUR
Body Composition and Growth:
Are We What We Eat?

The chemical composition of the human body changes during its entire life cycle. The values presented previously in Table 4-1 apply only to 25-year-olds. It is difficult and unrealistic to provide similar reference approximations for the young and old, since they are extremely variable. However, to provide some general ideas of the changes in water, fat, and lean body mass that occur at different stages of life, a brief analysis is presented below.

FIRST YEAR

You grew more rapidly during the first year of your life than you will at any other time. Birth weight generally doubles in the first 4 months. This weight gain results from both lean body mass growth and the deposition of fat. At birth, fat typically accounts for 10 to 15 percent of body weight. By 1 year of age, fat accounts for one fourth of body weight. At birth, water provides almost three fourths of body weight. By one year of age, approximately 60 percent of body weight is water. Such increases in weight during the first year of life will vary somewhat according to sex.

Boys typically have higher birth weights and greater weight gain during the first year. The nature of gain also differs according to sex, with girls gaining more weight from fat and boys gaining more from lean body mass. Skeletal growth in the first year tends to parallel weight gain, with two thirds of the first year's gain occurring in the first 6 months of life, and the last third in the second 6 months. Bones increase not only in length and width but also in density.

Table 4-2 shows the approximate body composition in newborns and 1-year-olds.

PRESCHOOL YEARS

While an infant will typically increase 25 cm in length during the first year, the second year adds only half that amount. Year 3 can add about 8 cm, and the fourth, fifth, and sixth years will add about 7 cm.

Table 4-2
Approximate Body Composition in
Newborns and 1-Year-olds

| COMPONENT | % OF BODY WEIGHT | |
	NEWBORN	1-YEAR-OLD
Water	74.3	59.1
Fat	11.5	21.9
Ash	2.7	4.7

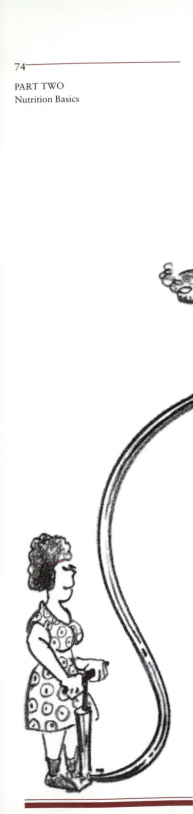

Since head growth primarily occurs before birth, body changes after birth progress toward a more proportional appearance. The child has 90 percent of head growth by age 6, but only 65 to 70 percent of body size. By the end of that sixth year, the child is taller and has longer legs, making the head appear smaller in relation to body size.

Weight gain in the second year is approximately half that of the first year, about 2.5 kg. The next 4 years will average 2 kg per year. During these preschool years, individual differences in growth patterns emerge. These differences can partially be understood genetically.

During the first year, child growth is thought to be primarily influenced by the mother's hormones. Gradually these maternal factors are replaced by the genetic influences of both parents. For example, studies have shown that significant changes in body measurements occur in the first 4 years, suggesting that different control mechanisms are in effect during that period of life than were in effect during gestation or early infancy.

Tooth development can vary. During the second and third years, all twenty deciduous teeth will generally erupt, but individual differences can affect both the timing and order of appearance of teeth. Generally, all eight incisors will have erupted by age 1.

Studies have also found racial differences in childhood growth patterns. For example, black children tend to have lower birth weights than white children, but they grow faster than white children. By 2 years of age, black children are taller and heavier and have less body fat. Some health experts have maintained that these differences are significant enough to warrant different growth standards for blacks and whites, but that issue remains controversial.

During the preschool years, sufficient comparisons between boys and girls are available for studies to confirm true differences in body composition between the sexes. Even when comparing boys and girls of the same age, girls have skinfold measurements some 25 percent thicker, a result of their greater fat content. Differences in caloric intake in relation to energy expenditure also become apparent during the preschool years.

75

CHAPTER FOUR
Body Composition and Growth:
Are We What We Eat?

ELEMENTARY-SCHOOL YEARS

During elementary-school years, the earlier maturation of girls begins to show. By about age 9 or 10, girls pass boys in height and weight. During this age period, individual differences in growth patterns also become more obvious. Racial differences become less pronounced, though black children tend to have longer legs and shorter trunks, resulting in shorter sitting height but taller overall height.

By the end of the elementary-school years, approximately age 11, some 12 percent of girls can be said to have reached the adult stage of their skeletal development. That is, their bones are as dense as they will become. From this age on, boys will continue to grow, owing to their later maturation. For both sexes, leg growth during the preschool years is greater than trunk growth.

Children may gain excessive amounts of weight at any age, and such gains may be gradual or sudden. Long-term studies of children, known as *longitudinal studies*, have shown that children can begin the buildup of excessive adipose or fat tissue while they are infants. That trend will then continue through adolescence and proves difficult to control, even when such intervention techniques as dietary restrictions are utilized. Because of individual metabolic differences, a child's caloric intake in relation to individual need is the only meaningful measurement.

PUBESCENCE AND ADOLESCENCE

During this age span the differences between the sexes and the individual differences within the same sex make generalizations difficult. Generally, it has been found that the extremities reach maximal growth before the trunk. Accordingly, maximum leg and arm length would be attained before maximum trunk length is attained. The skeletal measurements that are the last to reach peak growth are usually trunk length and chest depth.

From about age 13 on, boys become taller and heavier than girls. By age 18, the average boy is 13 cm taller and 12 kg heavier than the average girl. Though both boys and girls experience hormonal changes at the same time, the more rapid growth of girls places them about 2 years ahead of boys in entering puberty. Boys thus have a longer childhood period and enter puberty heavier, taller, and older than girls entering puberty. During puberty boys grow more rapidly than girls. Boys may be as much as 4 years older than girls when growth terminates. In summary then, males are taller and heavier than females at maturity as a result of a longer period of childhood growth, greater gains during growth spurts, and a longer period of adolescence.

Boys develop longer forearms and greater leg lengths during adolescence. The influence of hormones such as testosterone results in muscle mass and shoulder width development in males. Females, owing to the influence of such hormones as estrogen, develop wider hips and more adipose (fat) tissue. The changes of adolescence, including such secondary sex characteristics as facial hair, contribute to significant differences in appearance between males and females.

Another way to observe the differences between boys and girls is to note body fat and muscle. Sex differences in body fat continue throughout the life cycle. In the female, body fat increases continuously until about 3 years of age, when the increase slows down somewhat. During the prepubescent ages of 8 to 13, the female's body fat continues to rise at a much faster rate, reaching a peak shortly after 14. This rise is then followed by a drop in body fat until the age of 16.5, when body fat content again rises steadily.

The pattern of fat deposition in a male is nearly similar to that of a female until about 3 years of age, when there is a plateau or actual loss of body fat until about 7.5 to 8 years. The male prepubescent period of 8 to 12 is characterized by a rise in body fat, though the difference at this time between the male and female body fat is already very great. For example, at the age of 12, the female averages about 25 percent to 30 percent more body fat than the male. In the male, there is another drop in body fat between the ages of 12 and 14, so that by the age of 14.5, the female generally has 70 percent to 80 percent more body fat than the male. After the age of 14, the male's body fat rises until the age of 16.5 to 17, when the body fat starts to drop again.

Body muscle reaches a peak at 8 or 9 years of age, followed by a sharp decline, after which sex differences become apparent. In the male, a second increase occurs between 14 and 16 years, reaching a peak by the 19th year, followed by another decline. In the female, lean body mass continues to decline during adolescence. The muscular appearance in the male during late adolescence is explained by the simultaneous decrease in body fat and rapid rise in lean body mass. The increase in lean body mass in females is slower than in males. In 15-year-olds, it reaches its maximum, about 75 percent of that of a male's maximum. However, as discussed earlier, a female's body fat generally rises between the ages of 8 and 17. She therefore gains fat at the expense of lean body mass, which contains mainly muscle (that is, protein).

If you will recall the significant differences in height, weight, and appearance between members of your own sex during your junior high school years, you will have an idea of how the differences in timing of puberty and adolescence can be significant. Those differences then began to close again as maturity was reached. The age span of pubescence and adolescence contains individuals who have experienced the growth spurt and have slowed in growth, but it also contains individuals who have not begun the growth spurt.

Because of such wide individual variations, chronological age proves an inefficient measure of both physical growth and nutrition need. Scientists and health practitioners thus must rely on other standards, such as maturation age. Girls may begin their growth spurt from age 7 to age 12, though the average is at age 10. Boys will generally be 2 years behind. The maximum growth rate occurs in about the middle of the growth spurt, approximately 2 years after the onset of the spurt. It is at the peak of the growth spurt that nutrient need is greatest. Thus, the highest nutrient need for girls could occur as early as age 10 or as late as age 14, and is as early as 12 or as late as 16 in boys.

The span of the growth spurt can also vary significantly. It may be as short as 5 years in duration, or it may be spread over a period of 12 or 13 years following the onset of puberty.

Given such individual variations during pubescence and adolescence, each child's nutritional needs must be individually evaluated. Nutrient requirements parallel growth patterns.

ADULTHOOD TO OLD AGE

Longitudinal studies have provided data on physical growth from birth to adulthood, but no such studies have continued into old age. Accordingly, what we know about physical growth between adulthood and old age comes from cross-sectional studies (comparing people of different ages, for example). Since the studies are cross-sectional, the data derived from them are of limited usefulness, since their applicability depends on how representative the sample data were.

In the United States, health examination surveys were conducted at intervals between 1960 and 1974 by the National Center for Health Statistics. Those studies showed that our height was increasing for both men and women. They also showed that height decreased with age, perhaps as a result of postural change. While height was found to gradually decrease, weight increased after adulthood. Weight peaks in men at about age 40, but it peaks in women at about age 55.

Fat content at adulthood is about 13 percent of body weight for men at age 25 (see Table 4-1) and about twice that for women. By age 55, men have about one fourth of body weight as fat, while slightly over one third of women's body weight is fat at that age. Fat content proves somewhat difficult to assess, since in older individuals fat also deposits internally, not just as adipose tissue where skinfold measurements are used.

From the age of 25 to 85, a person's body water gradually decreases, both in absolute and relative amounts. This reduction varies from individual to individual, depending on body size and build. However, it has been established that the loss of body water takes place within the intracellular mass. A person "shrinks" somewhat with age because of this loss of body water, and the skin becomes dry from the combined effects of a loss of **turgor** from reduced intracellular fluids and a decrease of oil secretion.

As one ages from 25 to 50, the body shows an average decrease of 0.11 kg of cell mass annually. Since the decrease in body water during old age occurs within the cells, the decrease reflects a definite reduction

77

CHAPTER FOUR
Body Composition and Growth:
Are We What We Eat?

in body cell mass. Since potassium is found predominately within the cells of lean tissue, measuring its concentration gives an estimate of lean body mass. Thus, one documented observation is the progressive decline of total body potassium as one gets older. The average amount of potassium per kilogram of body weight falls steadily during adulthood. But since the amount of potassium per kilogram of lean body mass is higher in the adult than in the newborn infant, less body mass is actually lost than absolute levels of potassium would suggest.

In summary, from the period of 25 years to death, the body changes in a predictable pattern. Body fat continues to increase while body cell mass and water content continue to decrease relative to total body weight. For instance, if a man weighs the same at ages 25 and 65, more of that weight will probably be body fat and less will be lean body mass at 65. This pattern is the same for women, only more so. Women have more body fat and less cell mass and water content than men throughout their life spans.

What is the significance of this change with aging? For one thing, since the lean body mass is the metabolically active part of the body, its continuous decline as one gets older is one major clinical problem with geriatric patients. In addition, since drugs and nutrients are destined for this metabolically active part of the body, the estimation of appropriate drug dosages and nutrient requirements should be based on the quantity of lean body mass rather than total body weight.

Body Composition and the Athlete: Activity versus Inactivity

Many studies have been conducted to compare the physically active to the physically inactive (Haskell et al., 1982; Katch and McArdle, 1983). The most consistent finding is that active persons have a higher body density; that is, their lean body mass is proportionally greater. This finding holds true for both sexes at all ages.

A study of Olympic athletes showed that body fat dropped as lean body mass increased during training. If training stopped, the lean body mass dropped, and body fat increased. Similar results have been found with obese individuals who begin to diet and exercise.

Interesting studies have also been conducted to compare body composition resulting from various sports. Table 4-3 presents physical characteristics and body composition comparisons for athletes in four different sports. Notice that men typically are leaner than women. This occurs not because of better training habits but because of basic differences in the size of fat cells. The leanest women competitors, who may be as low as 10 percent body fat, are typically distance runners.

Running and weight training have been compared for their effects on body composition. Both reduce body fat and increase lean body mass; weight training, however, also increases strength, while running does not. Such studies usually make use of a statistical method of evaluating body build that compares fat-free body weight to height. Studies have also compared contents of minerals such as potassium and calcium.

Table 4-3
Fat Contents of Athletes in Four Types of Sports

ATHLETE	SEX	AGE (YEAR)	HEIGHT (cm)	WEIGHT (kg)	FAT (%)	FAT (kg)	FAT-FREE WEIGHT (kg)
Basketball	F	20	170	63	21	13	50
player	M	25	198	91	10	9	82
Runner	F	30	170	57	15	9	48
	M	25	178	64	5	3	61
Swimmer	F	20	169	64	26	17	47
	M	20	183	80	9	7	73
Shotputter	F	25	168	78	28	22	56
	M	25	188	109	16	18	91

Data have been obtained from a number of investigators and serve as illustration only. All numbers are rounded.

Regardless of the method of comparison, all body composition studies are limited in that we cannot be taken apart to distinguish, for example, between muscle and bone, or between fat and water content. Although we can fairly accurately determine fat content, we cannot precisely know the mix between the nonfat portions of our bodies.

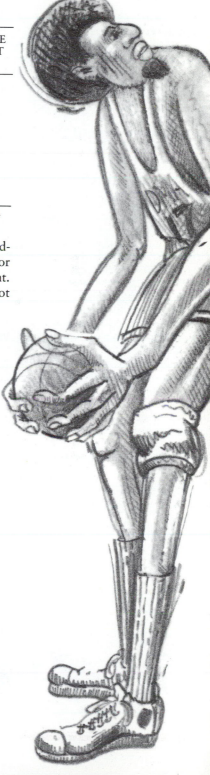

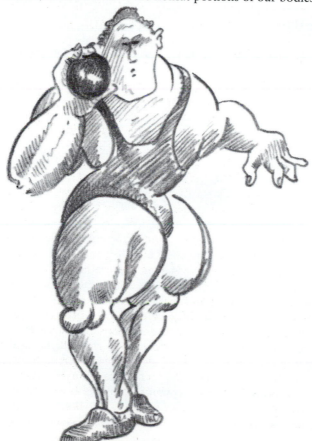

WRESTLING AND FOOD AND WATER RESTRICTION

Wrestling is a sport in which competition is based upon weight classifications (Hursh, 1979). Such weight categories give rise to the habit of attempting to rapidly lose weight just before a competition in order to make "a certain weight division." The practice is strongly opposed by the American Medical Association, especially for age groups still undergoing growth.

Crash diets and dehydration are two techniques used to retain eligibility at weight levels. These practices have very definite risks:

Reduction in muscular strength

Decrease in performance

Lowered plasma and blood volumes

Reduced cardiac (heart) function

Lowered oxygen consumption

Impaired body temperature regulation

Decreased renal (kidney) blood flow

Depletion of liver glycogen storage

Increased loss of electrolytes (minerals)

Studies of wrestlers have shown dehydration at weigh-in and inability to regain losses between weigh-in and competition.

The trends among wrestlers have also been studied. Typically, wrestlers lose 3.1 kg prior to certification and usually gain twice that amount after the season. The after-season gain demonstrates the extent to which wrestlers are competing below ideal body weight. The American Medical Association recommends that body fat not fall below the 7 to 10 percent level, that weight obtained after six-week intensive training be the minimum weight for competition, and that any further weight reduction is an undue hardship on the wrestler. Such reasonable efforts can prevent the risks associated with efforts to force weight below the appropriate level.

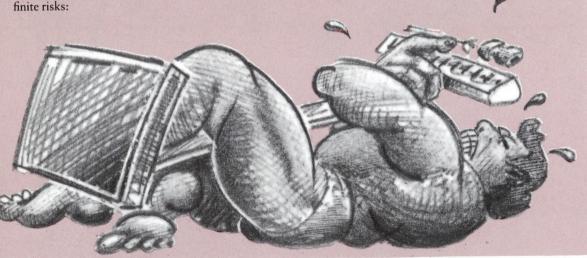

81

CHAPTER FOUR
Body Composition and Growth:
Are We What We Eat?

STUDY QUESTIONS

1. Discuss the four ways of describing body composition and at least four methods of determining the composition of a particular person's body.

2. How do relative amounts of body water, body fat, and lean body mass change as a person ages?

3. What are anthropometric measurements? What do skinfold measurements determine? Do some library research and provide the names of five commercial calipers for skinfold measurements.

4. Explain the different effects of running and weight training on body composition. Do some library research and compare the body compositions of mountain climbers, baseball players, and cyclists.

5. List the current Olympic weight classifications for wrestlers.

6. Write a two-page essay about the changes that occur in body composition from infancy to old age.

REFERENCES

Brozek, J. *Human Body Composition.* Oxford: Pergamon Press, 1965.

Centers for Disease Control. Ten-State Nutrition Survey, 1968–1970. (I.: Historical Development; II.: Demographic Data). USDHEW Pub. No. (HSM) 72–8130. Atlanta: Centers for Disease Control, 1972, pp I-39, I-40.

Harries, A. D., et al. "Assessment of Nutritional Status by Anthropometry: A Comparison of Different Standards of Reference." *Human Nutrition: Clinical Nutrition* 37c (1983): 227.

Haskell, W., et al., eds. *Nutrition and Athletic Performance.* Proceedings of the Conference on Nutritional Determinants in Athletic Performance, San Francisco, September 24–25, 1981. Palo Alto, CA: Bull Publishing, 1982.

Hursh, L. M. "Food and Water Restriction in the Wrestler." *J.A.M.A.* 241 (1979): 915.

Katch, F. I., and V. L. Katch. "Computer Technology to Evaluate Body Composition, Nutrition, and Exercise." *Preventive Medicine* 12 (1983): 619.

Katch, F. I. and W. D. McArdle. *Nutrition, Weight Control, and Exercise.* 2nd ed. Philadelphia: Lea & Febiger, 1983.

Pike, R. L., and M. L. Brown. *Nutrition: An Integrated Approach.* 3d ed. New York: Wiley, 1984.

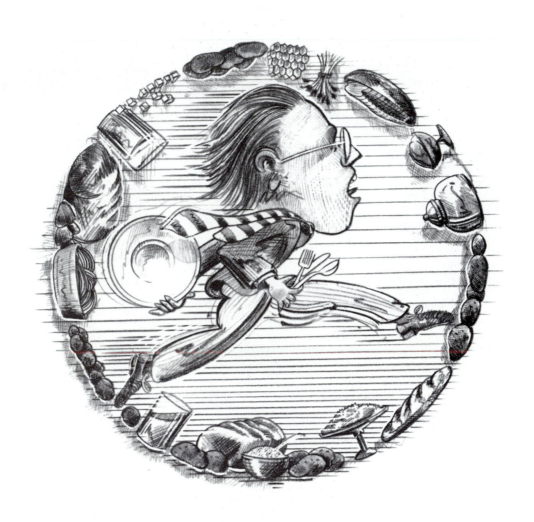

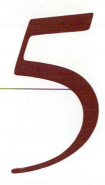

5

CARBOHYDRATES:

SOME CAN SURVIVE WITHOUT THEM

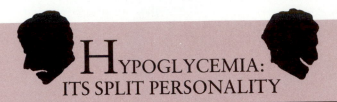

HYPOGLYCEMIA:
ITS SPLIT PERSONALITY

Jeffrey, a college student, reported to his campus health center that he had frequent and burning urination, depression, weakness, thirst, and a craving for sweets. The health center gave Jeffrey a thorough examination, including blood and urine tests. No disease was present, yet he was clearly emotionally unstable and seemed sincere about his symptoms.

The health center then conducted a glucose tolerance test. Half-way through the test, Jeffrey's blood sugar had fallen to the unusually low level of 50 milligrams per 100 milliliters of blood (50mg/dL). This test result was consistent with Jeffrey's symptoms for a diagnosis of hypoglycemia. Hypoglycemia is not a disease but is, rather, a physiological state in which the bloodstream contains too little blood sugar.

Jeffrey was placed on a hypoglycemic diet that prescribed three balanced meals per day, snacks between meals, and an avoidance of refined carbohydrates and sweets. Jeffrey's condition improved dramatically. Within a month his thirst and urination problems stopped. He became more outgoing, he no longer felt depressed, and he received an unexpected benefit as well when his vision significantly improved (Walker, 1975). Jeffrey truly had hypoglycemia. Does that mean that depression, weakness, and a craving for sweets in a person are reliable signs of hypoglycemia? We will look more closely at this question later in our discussion on sugars and diseases.

Carbohydrates Are What We Eat the Most

Carbohydrates are a major source of food energy for most people. At present, Americans obtain approximately half of their energy requirements from carbohydrates. Since carbohydrates are generally an inexpensive source of food energy, the consumption of carbohydrates is inversely related to income. In poorer countries, 80 to 90 percent of people's food energy may come from carbohydrates.

As a whole, the human body derives most of its energy needs from plant carbohydrates, the most abundant organic substances on earth. By means of photosynthesis, all green plants convert carbon dioxide and water, with the assistance of sunlight, into carbohydrates and oxygen. Plant carbohydrates exist in two forms: the woody structure or **cellulose**, and the plant's sugar and starch storages. The relative amounts of sugar and starch stored in plant foods depend on the plant's maturity (as in the ripeness of a fruit) and environmental conditions such as temperature, humidity, acidity, moisture, fertility, contamination, and storage conditions. For example, recall how the sweet taste of fruits changes after a period of storage.

We ingest most of our carbohydrates from sugar and the starch in grains, vegetables, and fruits, though some carbohydrates are also available in milk and dairy products (see Figure 5-1). Whether it comes from a plant or the milk of a dairy animal that has eaten green plants, a carbohydrate is always made up of carbon, hydrogen, and oxygen in the ratio of 1:2:1. Because there are two molecules of hydrogen to one of oxygen, as in water, the term **carbohydrate** literally means "hydrated carbon" (that is, water attached to carbon).

Chemically, there are many different kinds of carbohydrates. Table 5-1 classifies carbohydrates and gives some common examples. The major categories are monosaccharides, oligosaccharides, polysaccharides, and organic acids. **Monosaccharides** are considered to be the simplest carbohydrate molecules, for they cannot be hydrolyzed, or "split," into simpler forms. When a carbohydrate contains many units and each unit is made up of two to ten monosaccharides chemically joined, it is called an **oligosaccharide**. In **polysaccharides**, the repeating units contain hundreds to thousands of monosaccharides. Either in the laboratory or in the intestine, the individual units of oligosaccharides can be hydrolyzed so that all the monosaccharides are released and exist in their free forms.

Organic acids are also carbohydrates, since their carbon, hydrogen, and oxygen units exist in the ratio of 1:2:1. However, most consumers are not aware of this form of carbohydrate. For example, citric acid, tartaric acid, and others are common organic acids occurring in many foods we eat. Though this chapter will not discuss organic acids further, you may find detailed information in standard textbooks on food science.

The most common monosaccharides are six-carbon sugars such as glucose, fructose, galactose, and mannose. Other monosaccharides include five-carbon sugars, six-carbon sugar alcohols, and five-carbon sugar alcohols. The intestine of a healthy person can absorb all of them, though the extent and rate of absorption vary. Monosaccharides also vary in known importance to human health.

Starchy foods such as grains, cereal products, starchy vegetables and fruits

Regular table sugar including that used in pastries, desserts, candies, and beverages. Items such as syrup are included

Milk and other dairy products

60% 30% 10%

Figure 5-1: *Relative contribution of digestible carbohydrates by different food sources in the American diet.*

Table 5-1
Classification and Common Examples of Carbohydrates

MONOSACCHARIDES	POLYSACCHARIDES
6-carbon sugars: glucose, fructose, galactose, mannose	Homopolysaccharides: starch, cellulose, dextrans, glycogen, dextrins, inulin
5-carbon sugars: D-ribose, D-2-deoxyribose, L-arabinose, D-xylose	Heteropolysaccharides: mucopolysaccharides, glycolipids, glycoprotein
6-carbon sugar alcohols: sorbitol, mannitol, dulcitol, inositol	
5-carbon sugar alcohols: xylitol	ORGANIC ACIDS
	Acetic acid, citric acid, tartaric acid, and others
OLIGOSACCHARIDES	
Disaccharides: sucrose, lactose, maltose, trehalose	
Trisaccharides: raffinose	
Tetrasaccharides: stachyose	

Table 5-2
Approximate Contents of Glucose, Fructose, and Sucrose in Selected Fruits and Vegetables*

FOOD ITEM	% OF FRESH WEIGHT		
	GLUCOSE	FRUCTOSE	SUCROSE
Asparagus	1	1.4	0.3
Celery	0.5	0.5	0.4
Onion	2	1.2	0.9
Tomato	1.1	1.4	0.01
Corn	0.35	0.35	2.9
Apple	1.2	6.2	4
Grape	6	6	2
Pear	1	6.5	1.5
Plum	3.2	1.5	4.5
Strawberry	2	2.2	1.5
Lima bean	0.03	0.1	2.5
Cowpea	0.1	0.05	1.6

*These data are the average values obtained from the results of different investigators. The contents of these monosaccharides vary widely in different plant products. This table is intended to serve as a guide only.

Table 5-3
The Relative Sweetening Power of Selected Carbohydrates and Carbohydrate-Rich Foods

CARBOHYDRATE OR FOOD	RELATIVE SWEETENING POWER
Sucrose (table sugar)	100
Fructose	140–170
Honey	120–170
Molasses	110
Glucose	75
Corn syrup	60
Sorbitol	60
Mannitol	50
Galactose	30
Maltose	30
Lactose	15

BLOOD SUGAR: IT'S YOUR SOURCE OF ENERGY

Glucose is the only known six-carbon monosaccharide existing in a fair amount in the human body. It is found mainly in the blood, where it serves as an important and readily available energy fuel. When needed, the glucose in a cell is oxidized (burned) to form water, carbon dioxide, and energy.

Normally, there are about 70 to 100 mg of glucose per 100 ml of blood; a person with this range is considered **normoglycemic. Hyperglycemia** and **hypoglycemia** refer to high and low blood glucose levels, respectively. Diabetes is associated with hyperglycemia; one preliminary test for the disease is confirmation of glucose in the urine. However, ingesting a large amount of certain chemicals such as vitamin C can complicate this method of identification. Since vitamin C is similar to glucose in its *chemical-reducing* property, the vitamin C in the urine may be mistakenly identified as glucose.

Glucose has many other names: D-glucose, fruit sugar, corn sugar, and, commercially, dextrose. It is about 70 percent as sweet as table sugar. Free glucose is found in very few other foods. Some health food stores carry various brands of free glucose commercially prepared from starch. In clinical medicine, dextrose is sometimes used intravenously to feed hospitalized patients.

In table sugar, milk sugar, and starch, glucose occurs as a chemical component in combination with other monosaccharides. Glucose contents of selected foods are shown in Table 5-2. The fascinating topic of blood sugar and health will be discussed later.

For reference, Table 5-3 presents the relative sweetening power of selected carbohydrates and carbohydrate-rich foods.

Fructose, also known as fruit sugar or levulose, is commonly found in many fruits, in honey, and in plant saps. Like glucose (also a fruit sugar), it contains six carbons, but its chemical structure is different. Its fate in the body, however, is fairly similar to that of glucose. Fructose consumed with other foods will eventually be changed to glucose in the liver or broken down into carbon dioxide, water, and energy.

Fructose is one of the two monosaccharides that form the disaccharide sucrose (table sugar). Commercial fructose is intensely sweet—much sweeter than glucose (see Table 5-3). At present, fructose is used extensively in the pharmaceutical industry and is beginning to be used in food processing.

Table 5-2 lists the fructose contents of a number of common food items. Later in this chapter we will discuss the recent health claims for fructose.

SUGAR IN "SUGARLESS" GUM

Sorbitol, the most common six-carbon sugar alcohol, is found naturally in fruits such as apples, cherries, pears, and plums. It tastes sweet, though less so than sucrose or table sugar. Commercially, it is made by chemically adding hydrogen atoms (hydrogenation) to glucose, and it is a major ingredient in many dietetic foods. Since the absorption and utilization of sorbitol in the human body has little effect on blood glucose level, sorbitol is used in the manufacture of "diabetic" jams, marmalade, canned fruits, fruit drinks, chocolate, and other items. However, the body does not absorb sorbitol well, and when the ingested amount exceeds 50 g, diarrhea may result (see Box).

DIARRHEA
AND SUGARLESS GUM

A 29-year-old man who was otherwise healthy had diarrhea of two weeks' duration. Attempting to reduce weight by dieting, he found it difficult to adhere to the diet and resorted to daily intake of dietetic foodstuffs to aid in his dieting and weight reduction. Within a few days, he noted the onset of diarrhea, defined as five to six watery stools per day, associated with abdominal cramps but no other symptoms. His usual bowel habit consisted of formed stools without associated abdominal complaints.

Careful medical studies did not reveal the cause of the diarrhea. However, dietary history disclosed that the patient was consuming the following sugarless foods on a daily basis: two packs of sugarless gum (5 sticks per pack, 1.2 g of sorbitol per stick); two rolls of sugarless mints (11 tablets per roll, 1.4 g of sorbitol per tablet); two dietetic candy bars (5 to 7 g of hexitols per bar); and two dietetic wafers (ranging from 2.8 g of hexitols to 4.4 g of sorbitol per wafer, depending on wafer flavor). The total hexitol ingestion from these products in the patient ranged from 50.9 to 55.1 g/day. Discontinuation of dietetic food intake produced complete cessation of diarrhea and cramps. The patient has since remained free of symptoms.

SOURCE: Adapted from: M. J. R. Ravry, *Journal of the American Medical Association 244* (1980):270. Copyright 1980, American Medical Association.

The other six-carbon alcohols **mannitol** and **dulcitol** occur naturally and can also be prepared commercially; for example, mannitol may be obtained from a certain seaweed. Both substances are used as food additives in food processing (mannitol, for instance, is used in sugarless chewing gum). They are also used occasionally in testing for the normality of kidney clearance.

Inositol occurs naturally in different foods, especially cereal brans. The chemical arrangement of this six-carbon sugar alcohol is cyclic. When the alcohol groups of inositol are chemically attached to "phosphates," a molecule of phytic acid or its salt, phytate, is formed. Phytic acid is found in whole wheat flour and oatmeal and is thought to interfere with the absorption of calcium, iron, and zinc.

Although inositol is suspected to be at least partially essential for mice, its need by humans is doubtful. It has been labeled as a vitamin for humans, but this claim has not been scientifically substantiated. For more information on inositol and phytic acid, refer to Chapters 11 and 12, respectively.

TABLE SUGAR: WHAT'S IN THE SUGAR BOWL?
The most well-known of the oligosaccharides (carbohydrates containing many individual units, each of which is made up of two to ten monosaccharides) are the **disaccharides**. Each of the many units in a disaccharide contains two monosaccharides that are chemically joined. Similarly, trisaccharides and tetrasaccharides contain three and four monosaccharides, respectively.

Probably the most well-known disaccharide is **sucrose**, regular table sugar, sometimes called white or refined sugar. Household sugar is obtained mainly from sugar beets or sugar cane.

Sucrose is made up of many repeating units, each of which is a chemical combination of glucose and fructose. In a laboratory, heat, enzymes, or acids can split each unit into its constituents, glucose and fructose. In the human and animal intestine, sucrose must be degraded to its components by the intestinal enzyme *sucrase* before it is absorbed.

Sucrose is used extensively in cooking and commercial food processing. Pharmaceutically, it is used as an ingredient in the production of tablets because of its sweetness, digestibility, and other properties. One good example is its use in *buccal* (dissolved in the cheek) and *sublingual* (dissolved under the tongue) *tablets,* designed to release the active ingredient over a period of 15 to 30 minutes.

The relationship of table sugar to human health is currently the subject of intense debate in both public and scientific forums. It will be discussed later in this chapter.

MILK SUGAR: NOT IN HIPPOPOTAMUS MILK
The monosaccharides within the disaccharide **lactose** are glucose and galactose. Lactose is also called milk sugar because it is found in the milk of all mammals except the whale and hippopotamus. It is very insoluble in water and not very sweet.

It is well known that lactose can facilitate the absorption of calcium in the human intestine. Since breast milk has more lactose than does homogenized cow's milk, a breast-fed infant is expected to receive more calcium. However, lactose is now added to many commercial infant formulas. At present, lactose is also used in food processing and pharmaceutical preparations.

The enzyme that can digest lactose in the intestine is called **lactase**. Among members of some ethnic groups and under other conditions, the enzyme may disappear anytime from childhood to adulthood. Such individuals develop problems when drinking milk. More is presented later.

Starches: Potatoes, Rice, Bread, and All That Wonderful Pasta

The *polysaccharides* are carbohydrates made up of more than ten monosaccharides. Examples include starch, glycogen, and cellulose.

Starch is a polysaccharide of many units, each of which contains hundreds or thousands of chemically joined glucose molecules. Starch is stored in granules within plant seeds and roots such as grains, cereals, beans, and rice. As the major energy storage of a plant, starch is made up of two types of polysaccharides: **amylose** and **amylopectin.**

About 15 percent to 20 percent of starch is made up of amylose, which consists of many glucose units joined linearly without branching. When starch is put in water and iodine is added, the intense blue color is caused by the water-soluble amylose. Certain varieties of corn and rice do not contain amylose, however.

About 75 percent to 80 percent of starch is made up of *amylopectin*, which is composed of many glucose units joined in branched configurations. If amylopectin is separated from amylose, it produces a brownish violet color when iodine is added. Since amylopectin, which occurs in wheat flour, is insoluble in water, it is responsible for the thickening of gravy when flour is heated in water, fat, and other ingredients.

When starch granules are first obtained from plants, they hardly dissolve in water. Heat produces a solution of starch, which jells on cooling. Starch granules in a vegetable are actually confined within the plant cell walls in clusters. Solubility produced by heating swells the granules and eventually ruptures the cell walls. Cooking therefore increases the digestibility of a starch food; starch that is only semisolible (for instance, because of inadequate preparation) may cause indigestion after a meal.

Within the digestive system, starch is hydrolyzed into simpler carbohydrates such as the disaccharide maltose and eventually into the individual molecules of glucose. The simple process of heating starch at 100°C (the boiling point) can also release the glucose molecules and make it taste slightly sweet. The frying or grilling of starchy food or the malting of barley may release glucose and maltose (malt sugar) from the polysaccharides to produce a mild, sweet flavor.

Glycogen: What Keeps Marathon Runners Off the "Wall"

Glycogen, sometimes called **animal starch**, is the form in which energy is stored in an animal. It occurs in a small amount in the muscles and livers of land animals and in a more significant quantity in shellfish, especially oysters and scallops. Chemical substances similar to glycogen are also found in algae, yeasts, fungi, tapeworm, and golden bantam sweet corn.

Glycogen resembles the amylopectin of starch, though glycogen is more branched. It contains about 30 to 60 thousand glucose molecules with many branches, each of which is made up of 10 to 18 glucose molecules. Glycogen also differs from amylopectin in another respect: It is fairly soluble in water, forming a very attractive opalescent solution. When iodine is added to a glycogen solution, it forms a deep red color. The chemical linkage between the individual glucose molecules is the same as that in starch. The size of a glycogen molecule varies with the animal and its metabolic status. Land animals—such as beef cattle, chickens, lambs, and sheep—do not contain sufficient glycogen to be significant dietary sources of this carbohydrate. During the process of slaughtering, the glycogen in land animals' muscles and livers is so degraded that the meat and fowl sold in the grocery stores contain very little glycogen.

Even though the foods we eat may not be rich in glycogen, we can make this compound from other carbohydrates we eat. In the body, glucose and other monosaccharides are converted to glycogen in the liver and muscles. This stored glycogen is an important and readily available source of glucose. When needed, the glycogen releases glucose, which can be metabolized to form energy and, eventually, carbon dioxide and water. Glycogen is therefore especially important for people undergoing strenuous activity. A detailed discussion of this topic is provided in Chapter 21. Human muscles contain about 5 to 6 oz (150–180 g) of glycogen; the human liver contains 2 to 3 oz (60–90 g). In the digestive system, glycogen can be split by alimentary (digestive) enzymes to form the individual glucose molecules, which can then be absorbed.

In a number of popular cooked shellfish, such as oysters, lobsters, and scallops, the glycogen content is partially responsible for the delicate sweet flavor. For example, about 6 percent of the wet weight of an oyster is made up of glycogen. Heat degradation of glycogen releases glucose, which is sweet.

Do We Need Carbohydrate to Survive?

Current evidence does not indicate that carbohydrate is an essential nutrient for the human body (Anderson, 1982; Hodges, 1966). For instance, two Arctic explorers once survived without any plant carbohydrate food for at least one year by subsisting mainly on animal meat and fat. They did, however, have some body distress such as bowel discomfort, and the amounts of uric acid and acetone in their urine and of triglyceride and cholesterol in their blood were elevated.

Anthropological and medical studies have shown that a number of herdsmen and tribesmen survive well on animal meats and fats without consuming any plant-food carbohydrate. Many Eskimos subsist on little or no carbohydrate, obtaining less than 20 percent of their daily energy requirement from plant carbohydrate. Eskimos eat significant quantities of meat and fat without suffering from any disease directly traceable to the lack of carbohydrate. However, it is currently suspected that

Eskimos actually consume more carbohydrates than most nutritionists have assumed. Because Eskimos frequently eat their meat raw and frozen, they take in more glycogen than a person purchasing meat with a lower glycogen content in a grocery store. The Eskimo practice of preserving a whole seal or bird carcass under an intact whole skin with a thick layer of blubber also permits some proteins to ferment into carbohydrates.

Although normal human adults can seemingly survive without carbohydrates, many nutritionists favor the daily consumption of a minimum quantity. Carbohydrate is the main source of energy fuel for the body, chiefly in the form of glucose. Although fat and protein can provide glucose and thus energy, dietary glucose is obviously the more readily available form. If little or no carbohydrate is consumed, the body derives its energy mainly from protein and fat in the diet or from the body tissues (as in the case of starvation). The process takes place mainly in the liver. When protein is degraded for energy, an important nutrient that could build muscles and bones is wasted. Physiologically, carbohydrate thus "spares" protein.

Excess degradation of fat and protein for energy also results in the formation and accumulation of an undesirable quantity of ketoacids, ketones, acetone, and similar intermediate byproducts. This can create **ketosis**, a condition that can disrupt the acid balance of the body. This does not seem to pose a problem for a normal, healthy, male adult within a certain period of time (e.g., 2 years), as in the case of the two Arctic explorers. However, ketosis is considered harmful to pregnant women. Also, if an excessive amount of body protein is degraded as a result of a lack of carbohydrate, the loss of body tissues and muscles is accompanied by a loss of water and electrolytes such as sodium, calcium, potassium, magnesium, and phosphorus. It is argued that a daily intake of 100 g of carbohydrates will prevent ketosis and conserve water and electrolytes.

Excessive consumption of meat protein and animal fat in lieu of carbohydrates will also raise blood cholesterol and triglyceride levels, predisposing the individual to heart disease, as discussed in Chapter 6. In addition, the increase of uric acid in blood and urine may predispose the person to gout and urinary stones.

Although fat and protein can be degraded for energy, if necessary, carbohydrates may perform some functions that other nutrients cannot. For instance, brain cells and cells of the eye lens and nervous tissues depend specifically on glucose as a main source of energy. Occasionally they may be able to use ketone bodies for this purpose. Under certain conditions, an extremely low blood glucose level may affect the brain and result in drowsiness, coma, and death. Carbohydrates also play a very important role in body metabolic processes, such as the conversion of carbohydrates into protein (amino acids). Certain carbohydrate molecules combine with other chemicals to form specific structural components of cells, tissues, and organs. And the indigestible parts of dietary carbohydrates such as roughage or fiber serve special purposes in the body.

Eating carbohydrates often supplies us with other essential nutrients as well. Apart from table sugar, honey, and syrup, very few foods are made up of carbohydrates alone. Foods such as potatoes, rice, corn, and bread are high-carbohydrate foods, but they also carry other nutrients, such as vitamins, minerals, and minimal amounts of usable, though usually incomplete, protein.

Many population groups and countries have one or more staple foods that are high in carbohydrates, for example, potatoes, rice, plantain. As an agricultural product, plant carbohydrate is a good return on the investment of soil, fertilizers, and labor. It is cheap and sustains many people in undeveloped countries. And carbohydrate-rich foods are practically the only ones that can be stored for a reasonably long period without deterioration.

Finally, the color, flavor, and texture of carbohydrate-rich foods make them attractive and palatable. Many people find it difficult to prepare a complete and attractive meal without carbohydrates, and many find that eating just meat and fat does not satisfy their appetites.

Fiber: Can It Cure All Ills?

Dietary fiber, also known as roughage, used to be considered one of the least important of our food components. It has for years been recognized as a cleansing agent owing to its laxative effect; but recent studies suggest that it may also help protect us against modern ills such as cancer, heart disease, and diabetes (Heaton, 1983; Kritchevsky, 1982). Fiber zealots are now attributing almost mystical powers to the consumption of diets high in fiber or roughage, while more moderate advocates acknowledge its usefulness in the treatment of constipation and the symptomatic relief of diverticular disease of the colon. For various reasons, there remains much we do not know about fiber.

WHAT IS FIBER?

Fiber can be generally defined as the food component that is not digested. More scientifically, it can be described as the cell wall of plants. Cellulose is a polysaccharide made up of many chemically joined glucose molecules. In the past, the term *cellulose* usually referred to dietary fiber, residue, or roughage in general; its content in foods was found by using the "fiber" values given in food composition tables. However, because of renewed interest in dietary fiber, the definition of cellulose has recently been subjected to intense debate. Figure 5-2 provides a description of the tentative terminology used for dietary fiber and other carbohydrates. All terms used will likely be standardized in the near future.

The fiber values given in food composition tables are actually less than true fiber contents. Figure 5-2 lists six other groups of undigestible substances in addition to cellulose: hemicellulose A, hemicellulose B, pectin, lignin, mucilages, and gums. Knowing that foods contain these components still leaves us a long way from knowing how much of each a given food contains.

This measurement difficulty occurs because the official method of measuring fiber, called the *crude fiber method*, involves placing food

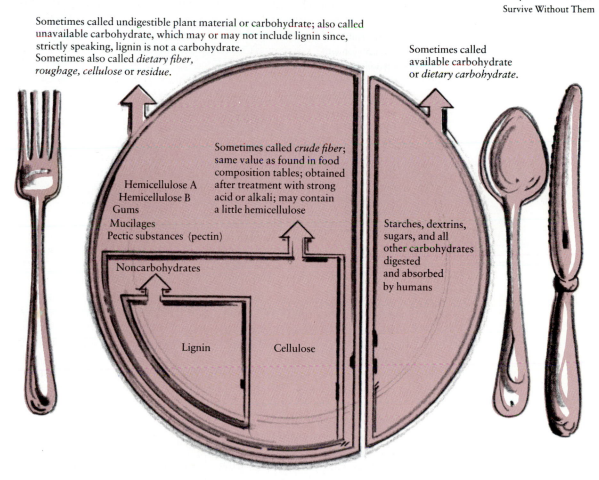

Sometimes called undigestible plant material or carbohydrate; also called unavailable carbohydrate, which may or may not include lignin since, strictly speaking, lignin is not a carbohydrate.
Sometimes also called *dietary fiber*, *roughage*, *cellulose* or *residue*.

Sometimes called available carbohydrate or *dietary carbohydrate*.

Hemicellulose A
Hemicellulose B
Gums
Mucilages
Pectic substances (pectin)

Sometimes called *crude fiber*; same value as found in food composition tables; obtained after treatment with strong acid or alkali; may contain a little hemicellulose

Starches, dextrins, sugars, and all other carbohydrates digested and absorbed by humans

Noncarbohydrates

Lignin   Cellulose

CARBOHYDRATES IN FOOD

residue in both acid and alkali and then measuring what remains, since the remainder is the indigestible portion. The drawback to the crude fiber method is that it does not measure the content of dietary fiber. Estimates suggest that the crude fiber measurement may miss as much as half the cellulose and half the lignin, and well over half the hemicellulose. Crude fiber calculations cannot be converted to dietary fiber calculations because the relationship is not consistent from one foodstuff to another. For example, the dietary fiber in lettuce is three times the crude fiber, whereas the dietary fiber in peanuts or carrots is almost four times the crude fiber (see Table 5-4).

Other methods of measuring dietary fiber include detailed chemical processes and detergent processes, but some of these methods have drawbacks related to differences in chemical content of fiber. What we

Figure 5-2: *Terminology for "dietary" carbohydrates.*

Table 5-4
Dietary Fiber (g/100 g) in Edible Portions of Some Vegetables*

VEGETABLE	TOTAL DIETARY FIBER (g/100 g)
Leafy vegetables	
Broccoli (boiled)	4.0– 4.5
Brussels sprouts (boiled)	2.5– 3.0
Cabbage (boiled)	2.5– 3.0
Cauliflower (boiled)	1.5– 2.0
Lettuce (raw)	1.5– 2.0
Onions (raw)	2.0– 2.5
Legumes	
Beans, baked (canned)	7.0– 7.5
Beans, runner (boiled)	3.0– 3.5
Peas, frozen (raw)	7.5– 8.0
Peas, processed (canned)	7.5– 8.0
Root vegetables	
Carrots (boiled)	3.5– 4.0
Parsnips (raw)	4.5– 5.0
Rutabagas (raw)	2.0– 2.5
Turnips (raw)	2.0– 2.5
Potato	
Main crop (raw)	3.5– 4.0
French fries	3.0– 3.5
Potato chips	11.5–12.0
Canned	2.5– 3.0
Peppers (cooked)	0.5– 1.0
Tomato, fresh	1.0– 1.5
Tomato, canned	0.5– 1.0
Sweet corn, cooked	4.5– 5.0
Sweet corn, canned	5.5– 6.0

*These data are the average ranges obtained from the results of different investigators. The contents of fiber vary widely in different plant products. This table is intended to serve as a guide only.

are left with then is a food component that, owing to difficulty of measurement, prevents determination of our requirements for it!

FIBER MAY BE MORE BENEFICIAL THAN WE THOUGHT

We do know that fiber affects water absorption, that it affects organic compound absorption, that it affects calcium, and that it affects many other chemical and biological processes. Many scientists recommend that we increase our intake of fiber because of its benefits.

Dietary fiber serves various uses in the body. It provides bulk in the diet, thus increasing the satiety value of foods. It maintains good intestinal motility, establishes regular bowel movements, and prevents constipation. The human small bowel does not have the necessary enzymes to digest dietary fiber; fiber is passed on to the large intestine, where it is fermented.

Studies of dietary fiber have concentrated on its cleansing properties. For example, we know that fiber affects the transit time of wastes through the gut by making transit times more normal—2 to 3 days. Individuals with rapid transit can slow that transit by increasing fiber intake, and individuals with slow transit can speed up the transit time by increased fiber intake. For clinical conditions at either extreme, diarrhea or constipation, fiber proves beneficial.

Fiber also affects stool weight, generally by increasing it. For example, the stool weight of vegetarians can be three times that of those eating a low-fiber diet. Cereal fiber, such as bran, significantly increases stool weight. Pectin and other water-soluble fiber have little effect on stool weight. The coarser the fiber, the greater the increase in stool weight.

Diverticular Disease

The term **diverticular diseases** describes a group of specific diseases of the large intestine. A **diverticulum** (plural *diverticula*) is a blind pouch along the length of the colon. *Diverticulosis* refers to the presence of diverticula, and *diverticulitis* is inflammation of the colon due to a perforated diverticulum. Diverticular disease is an all-inclusive term covering one or more of these conditions.

Diverticular disease affects approximately one third of the adult population in the United States. Many patients with the disease are asymptomatic. However, some develop pain, altered bowel habits, bleeding, infection, and perforation. Symptomatic patients complain of occasional pain originating from the lower quadrant of the abdomen. Pain can last for days and ranges from cramps to severe abdominal discomfort. Constipation alternates with diarrhea. After a bowel movement or passing of flatus (gas), symptoms subside temporarily. Some patients have blood and mucus in their stools. Massive hemorrhage may also occur with diverticular diseases.

In the past, a low-residue diet was prescribed for patients with symptoms of diverticular diseases. The treatment was based on the premise that such a regimen minimizes irritation to the intestine and inhibits gas and distention of the bowel. But it has been recently suspected that diverticular disease could develop from a lifetime of consuming low-fiber foods. Within the last decade, some clinicians have successfully managed diverticular diseases by recommending high-fiber diets. Currently, such treatment is advocated in most diet manuals as well as in medical textbooks on intestinal diseases.

To increase dietary fiber, many clinicians now recommend the use of unprocessed bran, a detailed discussion of which is presented later. Since the extent of fiber deficiencies varies, the amounts of bran needed will differ also. Each patient must therefore find by trial and error the correct amount of bran to use. An average of 2 teaspoons of unprocessed bran three times a day (the equivalent of 2 to 3 g of fiber) usually relieves the symptoms of the disease. The dose of bran needed to produce results may be higher for some patients. Most treated patients show decreased diverticulitis, return of normal bowel habits, and a lessening of pain. Patients who cannot tolerate bran should eat a high-fiber diet consisting of commercially available foods. However, many clinicians still advocate the use of a low-residue diet for patients with diverticular diseases in the inflammatory and bleeding stages.

Colon Cancer

Epidemiological studies have found a relationship between low-fiber diet and the incidence of colon cancer. Despite that finding, conclusions prove difficult to draw since not all fibers have the same relationship to the incidence of colon cancer and since other dietary components—fats, for example—have equally strong relationships to the incidence of colon cancer.

Various theories have been suggested as to why fiber might reduce the incidence of colon cancer. One theory is that certain food residues may become carcinogenic over time. Fiber may remove those potentially damaging residues. Fiber can similarly remove strong acids such as bile acids. Fiber also increases transit time, shortening the exposure of the colon to potentially harmful residue.

Cardiovascular Disease

Population studies have shown that populations with high fiber intake tend to have lower cholesterol levels and a low incidence of cardiovascular disease. Both pectin and gums have proved beneficial in reducing blood cholesterol. Other fibers such as corn bran, wheat bran, and cellulose do not, however, reduce cholesterol or triglyceride levels, so the most beneficial fibers in that regard seem to be those that retain water. Their benefit may lie in their ability to increase fecal fat excretion or to increase fecal bile acid excretion.

Patients have been successfully treated with both pectin and gum to reduce the level of lipids (fats) in the blood. Using 15 g of pectin per day, for example, one study reported a decrease of over 10 percent in the blood cholesterol level after 3 weeks. Guar gum has had similar results.

Diabetes

Because high fiber intake has proved closely related to low incidence of diabetes, some diabetics have been treated with fiber. Diets that are high in carbohydrate and fiber, called HCF diets, have especially been beneficial in reducing glucose absorption. Diabetic patients dependent upon insulin injections have had their insulin need cut by one third as a result of HCF diets, possibly because such diets are low in fat.

Some studies suggest, however, that it is not fiber that helps diabetics so much as the weight loss resulting from such diets. The mixed results of studies involving fiber and diabetes lead to the conclusion that drastic increases in fiber intake cannot be recommended. What is recommended is that patients work with their doctors and nutritionists to develop a healthy diet that includes grains, fruits, and vegetables.

RECOMMENDED FIBER INTAKE

We need fiber in our diet to maintain both normal peristaltic action in the intestinal tract and removal of wastes from the tract. Fiber achieves this by absorbing moisture and providing bulk that stimulates emptying of the large intestine. How much is needed for these purposes is not precisely known. One recommendation is daily consumption of 100 mg of fiber per kg of body weight; for the average adult, about 5 to 6 g of fiber per day should be sufficient. This recommended daily allowance is easily met by one serving of whole-grain cereal or bran, two servings of vegetables, and two servings of fruits. Vegetables with long fibers, such as celery and greens, have a laxative effect. Whether cooked or uncooked, fruits and vegetables maintain the same fiber content, for cooking does not reduce the amount of cellulose and hemicellulose.

It is important, though, to emphasize that a high fiber intake is not without potential problems. For one thing, a high fiber intake can interfere with the absorption of certain drugs. Second, ingested fiber can reduce the intestinal tract's ability to digest and absorb food by reducing digestion time and rate of absorption. Third, high amounts of fiber cause continuous mechanical irritation of the mucosal (intestinal) wall. Hence, there is some increased loss (from wear and tear) of mucosal substances. A fourth problem is that whole-grain products contain phytic acids, which may chelate (combine with) trace minerals and decrease their presence in the body. Finally, the large amount of phosphorus in high-fiber foods may create problems for certain individuals, especially patients with kidney problems.

Population studies have shown that dietary fiber intake varies significantly. For example, vegetarians consume twice as much as those eating normal diets. The daily per capita intake in this country approximates 20 g. If you eat whole-grain breads and cereals daily, as well as vegetables and fresh fruits, your dietary fiber intake should be adequate and will likely be in the range of 25 to 50 g per day.

SOURCES OF FIBER

Because of their high water content, fruits and vegetables provide less dietary fiber than grains and nuts; however, the type of fiber also varies: Vegetables rank high in cellulose; fruits rank high in pectin; and grains rank high in hemicellulose. Among the grains, wheat bran has the highest hemicellulose content. The range of total fiber content in selected vegetables and fruits is shown in Tables 5-4 and 5-5, respectively.

Dietary fiber can be found only in plant foods, and refining processes affect its content. For example, whole wheat bread has higher fiber content than white bread. The effect of cooking on fiber content has not been clearly determined.

FIBER SUPPLEMENTS

As consumers have become interested in fiber, fiber supplements have appeared (Hui, 1983). Many are marketed as stool softeners, but their effects vary. For example, bran tablets are quite effective, but purified

Table 5-5
Dietary Fiber (g/100 g Edible Portion) of Some Fruits and Nuts*

FRUIT OR NUT	TOTAL DIETARY FIBER g/100 g
Fruits	
Apple skin	3.5–4.0
Apples, without skin	1.0–1.5
Bananas	1.5–2.0
Cherries, whole	1.0–1.5
Grapefruit, canned	0.0–0.5
Guavas, canned	3.5–4.0
Mandarin oranges, canned	0.0–0.5
Peaches, whole	2.0–2.5
Pears, without skin	2.0–2.5
Pear skin	8.5–9.0
Plums, whole	1.5–2.0
Rhubarb, raw	1.5–2.0
Strawberries (raw)	2.0–2.5
Preserves	
Strawberry jam	1.0–1.5
Marmalade	0.5–1.0
Mincemeat	3.0–3.5
Nuts	
Brazil nuts	7.5–8.0
Peanuts	9.0–9.5
Peanut butter	7.5–8.0

*These data are the average ranges obtained from the results of different investigators. The contents of fiber vary widely in different plant products. This table is intended to serve as a guide only.

cellulose has very little effect as a stool softener. As mentioned earlier, gums and pectin lower blood cholesterol, but bran has little effect on blood cholesterol. Guar gum proves the most effective fiber for treating diabetes.

Bran is the byproduct of the milling of wheat or rice. Bran from wheat contains almost 20 percent indigestible cellulose and is an excellent source of dietary bulk. Unprocessed bran contains about 14 percent fiber, in contrast to the lesser bran or fiber content of such products as 100% Bran (7.5%), All Bran (7%), Bran Buds (7%), and Raisin Bran (3%). Since the fiber in unrefined bran is the important ingredient, natural bran flakes or whole bran should be used, not products such as 40% Bran Flakes or compressed pellets such as All Bran. Bran and other natural-fiber bulk foods do not irritate a healthy intestinal mucosa, and they readily add fiber to the diet.

Types of fiber vary, and so do their effects, so purified fiber generally is not recommended. If you need to increase your fiber intake, it is better to do so by eating more wheat bran, bran muffins, bran cereals, whole-grain breads, nuts, fresh fruits, and vegetables. The increase should be gradual, since you must allow your body to adjust to the increase in fiber. Consuming too much too quickly can result in gas and possibly diarrhea. By gradually increasing the intake, adjustment can usually be achieved within a few days (Hui, 1983).

INTAKE IS DIFFICULT TO GAUGE

An average serving of fruit, vegetables, whole-grain bread, or cereal provides about three g of fiber. With estimates indicating that 25 to 50 g daily should be an appropriate level for maintaining proper laxation without inhibiting the absorption of other nutrients, it is obvious that fiber intake is difficult to determine. It is equally obvious that the average American diet is low in fiber intake.

Because fiber research continues, we may soon see that fiber types and their benefits are more fully understood. Similarly, we can expect that fiber supplements will be improved to assist those whose intake of natural fiber sources is low.

Believe It or Not: Many Chinese Cannot Drink Milk

Milk contains the sugar lactose. Normally, when lactose reaches the small intestine, the enzyme *lactase* digests it to form glucose and galactose. This is necessary because the intestinal system can only absorb monosaccharides such as glucose and galactose and not disaccharides such as lactose. Lactase belongs to a group of enzymes called disaccharidases. Much information has been discovered about the enzyme lactase in the last two decades (Page and Bayless, 1981).

SOME BACKGROUND INFORMATION ON MILK OR LACTOSE INTOLERANCE

Researchers have discovered that in some persons, lactase is either missing or exists in a very small quantity. This causes a problem, since lactose will not be digested.

Lactase deficiency may result from an isolated lack of the enzyme or a generalized deficiency secondary to some intestinal diseases, such as damage to the intestinal walls by a virus or infection. An individual with this enzyme deficiency will display a combination of symptoms such as loud bowel sounds, bloating, flatulence, cramps, and diarrhea if a certain amount of whole milk is ingested. The nonhydrolyzed (undigested) and unabsorbed lactose in milk remains within the space of the gut and creates a high "osmotic load." This draws a large amount of water from the body fluids into the space of the intestine. Bowel distention and discomfort also occur. In addition, the bacteria in the colon metabolize and ferment the lactose to form a large amount of lactic acid, carbon dioxide, butyric acid, and other volatile substances. All of these changes are responsible for the observed symptoms.

Some individuals have normal lactase activity immediately after birth but experience a gradual decline up to the age of 4 or 5. In others, lactase deficiency becomes apparent only during adulthood. Yet some people have normal lactase activity throughout life. Sometimes low lactase activity may be induced during intestinal infection, trauma, pregnancy, and other clinical conditions. Table 5-6 indicates the extent of lactase deficiency among different population groups.

Table 5-6
Lactose Intolerance among Different Population Groups*

POPULATION GROUP	% OF POPULATION WITH LACTOSE INTOLERANCE
Caucasians (U.S.)	2–20
Indians (U.S.)	65–70
Blacks (U.S.)	70–75
Eskimos (North America)	85–90
Orientals (worldwide)	90–100

*Figures derived from reports of a number of investigators. The ranges are approximations and serve only as a general guide.

Scientists have discovered interesting geographical patterns regarding lactase activity in adults. They have found that lactase activity generally only continues into adulthood among Caucasians living in northern and western Europe, or among their descendants living in other parts of the world. Blacks, Orientals, Jews, and American Indians exhibit the normal pattern of decreasing activity in childhood.

Scientists have theorized that humans once experienced decreasing activity of lactase at weaning, just as other mammals do. They further suggest that domestication of animals and consumption of their milk resulted in a mutation that altered the pattern of lactase loss and resulted in the retention of lactase activity into adulthood. Whether or not the theories are correct, an advantage in maintaining lactase activity occurs when food supplies are short. Adults with milk tolerance have better survival capabilities than those who lack milk tolerance.

WHO IS LIKELY TO HAVE LACTOSE INTOLERANCE?
Since milk is the major source of lactose, many individuals who are unable to tolerate fluid milk have lactose intolerance, although the reaction depends on the amount consumed. Many can tolerate a small quantity. Confirmation of lactose intolerance should first include a history of the recurrence of symptoms after drinking milk. A simple test can be used to identify individuals with lactase deficiency. A patient is given 50 grams of lactose orally, and his or her plasma glucose is then measured at intervals of 15, 30, 60, and 120 minutes. Intestinal lactase deficiency should be suspected if blood glucose levels fail to rise above the fasting level by at least 20 mg per 100 mL of blood. If the patient can absorb glucose or galactose normally, the diagnosis is further confirmed. Another technique used in diagnosing lactase deficiency is assaying lactase activity in a tiny sample of small-intestinal tissue (a biopsy specimen). However, most clinicians use only the lactase test. For information on the latest diagnostic technique of breath hydrogen analysis, consult a modern medical textbook.

A NON-MILK DRINKER NEEDS SOME ALTERNATIVES
People who have a lactase deficiency vary considerably in their reactions to milk. Most individuals who have this deficiency react to one quart of

milk. Others may react to as small an amount as one milligram of lactose. Nutritionists are most concerned with reactions to one glass of milk, and it has been found that one glass, especially if consumed with a meal, does not produce adverse symptoms.

Some unusual findings surround lactase deficiency. For example, those with hereditary deficiency may not exhibit symptoms until adulthood, despite loss of the lactase activity in childhood. Why this occurs is not known. Sometimes the symptoms will occur when milk intake is increased for treatment of such problems as peptic ulcers. Increased milk intake among expectant mothers can also cause symptoms to occur.

Nutritional studies indicate that those who have a lactase deficiency tend to experience calcium malabsorption as well. Accordingly, osteoporosis (*osteo* = bone, *porous* = holes) incidence is higher in lactase deficient persons. Since lactase deficiency often occurs in developing countries, the value of milk distribution in those countries has been questioned, though reactions are minimal when milk is taken with a meal.

DIETARY CARE OF A CHILD WITH LACTOSE INTOLERANCE

The treatment for a child with lactose intolerance depends on the severity of the child's reaction to dietary lactose, which can vary from mild to violent (Hui). If a child's condition warrants a lactose-free diet, Table 5-7 should be used in meal planning. However, most young patients benefit from a lactose-restricted diet that excludes only nonfermented

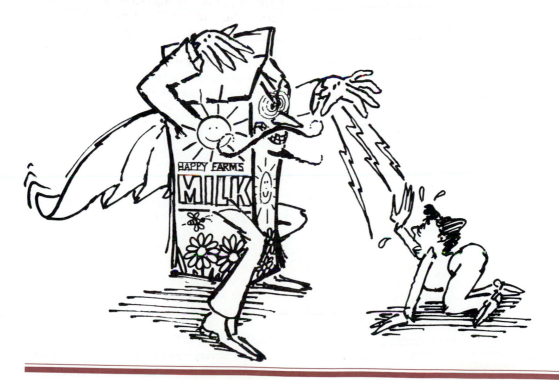

Table 5-7
Foods Permitted and Prohibited in a Lactose-Free Diet

FOOD GROUP	FOODS PERMITTED	FOODS PROHIBITED
Milk, milk products, and equivalents	Milk substitute and nondairy cream excluding those with restricted ingredients; commercial infant and dietetic formulas with lactose-free ingredients*	All forms of milk and milk products (cow's, human, goat milk); examples include yogurt, chocolate milk, cocoa, etc.
Potatoes and equivalents	White and sweet potatoes; rice, noodles, spaghetti, macaroni, pasta	All commercial and homemade potato products made with milk, cheese, butter, and margarine containing milk solids; e.g., dehydrated potato flakes, breaded, creamed, or buttered products; instant mashed potatoes
Breads and equivalents	Any of the following made without milk, milk products, whey, casein, and lactose: breads of any variety, rolls, English muffins, crackers; cooked and dry cereals; flours of all varieties	Pancakes, biscuits, waffles, doughnuts, muffins, and ready-to-use baking mixes; any bread or baked goods made with milk, milk products, whey, casein, or lactose; cereals (hot instant or high protein); e.g., Cream of Rice, Cream of Wheat
Fruits and vegetables	All fresh fruits and fruit juices; all processed (dehydrated, frozen, or canned) fruits and fruit juices containing no excluded ingredients, such as lactose and monosodium glutamate; all vegetables and vegetable products not specifically excluded	All processed fruit and fruit juice (dehydrated, frozen, and canned) products containing any excluded ingredients such as lactose and monosodium glutamate; all vegetables and vegetable products prepared with excluded ingredients; e.g., buttered, creamed, or breaded products; beans (dried, lima, and soy), peas, lentils
Meat and equivalents	Beef, lamb, pork, veal, poultry, fowl, fish; peanut butter and certain cold cuts (check labels for presence of prohibited ingredients); kosher frankfurters; nuts of all varieties	Any meat, fish, or poultry product prepared with a batter, stuffing, or cream sauce; any processed meats prepared with milk, milk products, casein, lactose, or monosodium glutamate; e.g., sausages, nonkosher frankfurters, luncheon meats, etc.; certain shellfish and organ meats if not tolerated
Fats and equivalents	Pure mayonnaise, vegetable oils (e.g., olive and safflower), shortening, lard, bacon fat; kosher margarine (margarine without milk solids or butter added); some cream substitutes (check labels)	Any product not specifically permitted, especially all cream, butter, and margarine with added butter or milk solids; most salad dressings; certain cream substitutes
Soups	All homemade soups prepared with permitted ingredients, such as clear soup or broth; any commercial products prepared without prohibited ingredients such as milk or milk products; e.g., bouillon	All commercial soups containing milk, milk products, lactose, or monosodium glutamate; e.g., chowders and cream soups; most commercial dried soups including dehydrated powder
Sweets	Pure jam, jelly; pure hard candy, jelly beans, lollipops, gumdrops; molasses, honey, syrups, sugars	Any product with milk, milk products, or lactose added, such as caramels, toffee, and milk chocolate

*To be recommended by qualified health professionals.

Table 5-7 (*continued*)

FOOD GROUP	FOODS PERMITTED	FOODS PROHIBITED
Beverages	Cereal beverages; soft drinks; lemonade, limeade; beverages with fruits or added fruit flavors, including punches; tea and coffee (regular, some instant, some decaffeinated)	Malted milk, milk shakes, eggnog; some decaffeinated and instant coffees; any commercial beverages or mixes with prohibited ingredients
Cheese and eggs	Eggs prepared without milk and milk products	All varieties of cheese; eggs prepared with prohibited ingredients
Desserts	All products prepared without milk and milk products, for example, homemade cakes, cookies, and pies; Popsicles, flavored ices with or without fruits, gelatin	Any products made with prohibited ingredients such as ice cream, regular puddings and custards, and all commercial bakery products
Miscellaneous	Pepper, salt, pure spices and seasonings; popcorn prepared with permitted margarine; lemon, vinegar, pickles, olives, mustard, catsup, chili sauce, horseradish; gravies without milk and milk products	Many diabetic and dietetic preparations containing prohibited ingredients; dips for snacks; malted products; Worcestershire sauce, soy sauce; pharmaceutical agents (tablets, powders, and capsules) or packaged products using lactose or glutamate as carriers; most commercially prepared mixes; cream sauces and milk gravies

milk and milk products. Fermented dairy products usually contain less lactose and are tolerated well by many patients. Every patient, young or old, learns from experience what foods can be tolerated. Some patients can drink a small amount of milk over the course of a day. Table 5-8 describes those foods permitted and prohibited in a lactose-restricted diet. For a young child, such a limited diet may not have adequate amounts of some or all of the following nutrients: calcium, iron, and vitamins A, D, E, K, and B_2. Thus, meals must be planned according to the age and physiological status of the patient, and particular attention must be paid to providing the child with his or her RDAs.

"Sugar Is Bad for You"

Although we need a certain level of carbohydrates for optimal health, how carbohydrate intake relates to health and diseases is currently one of the most debated topics in the field of nutrition. Numerous issues are involved (Stare, 1975).

HOW IS SUGAR BAD FOR YOU?

Any bookstore or magazine rack yields examples of the theory that sugar is bad for everybody. Many popular items with high carbohydrate content, such as soft drinks, candies, potato chips, and french fries, are considered to contain only "empty" calories with no nutritive value. Many consumer groups hold such foods responsible for a number of human diseases, especially among children. Although excessive consumption of such foods will make a child lose interest in other, more

Table 5-8
Foods Permitted and Prohibited in a Lactose-Restricted Diet

FOOD GROUP	FOODS PERMITTED	FOODS PROHIBITED
Milk and milk products	Moderate amount of fermented dairy products such as yogurt, buttermilk, acidophilus milk, and sour cream	All nonfermented milk and milk products including whole, skim, and chocolate milk and milk shakes
Potatoes and equivalents	All products not prohibited	All products made with milk or milk products, such as mashed, creamed, and scalloped potatoes, dehydrated potatoes, potato balls and cakes, and other processed potato specialties that contain lactose
Bread and equivalents	All varieties	None unless patient unable to tolerate the small amount of milk used in making bakery products
Fruits and vegetables	All products not prohibited	Any product containing cream, milk, milk products, and lactose; commercial fruit drinks with lactose added; creamed vegetables
Meat and equivalents	All products not prohibited	Meat, fish, and poultry products made with unfermented milk and milk products, such as creamed chicken, Swiss steak, cream sauces, and gravies; any commercially processed meat, fish, or poultry products in which lactose is used as a carrier or extender
Fats	All products not prohibited	All products with cream, milk, milk products, and lactose; all varieties of cream
Soups	All products not prohibited	All commercial and homemade soups prepared with cream, milk, and milk products
Sweets	Any pure candy made without lactose, cream, milk, and milk products; e.g., clear hard candy; jams, jellies; molasses, syrups, honey; sucrose, glucose, fructose, table sugar	Any product made with lactose, cream, milk, and milk products; e.g., chocolate candy
Beverages	All beverages containing no unfermented cream, milk, or milk products; regular coffee, some decaffeinated coffee, some instant coffee, some coffee substitutes; tea, cereal beverages, soft drinks; any commercial drinks made without lactose	All beverages containing unfermented cream, milk, milk products, and lactose
Cheese and eggs	Any fermented cheese or cheese aged with bacteria; eggs prepared without the use of milk and milk products	Any cheese containing unfermented milk and milk products; eggs or omelets prepared with cream, milk, or milk products
Desserts	Any product, especially homemade, prepared without unfermented milk or milk products (cream substitutes may be used); sponge, angel food, and other types of cake; fruit-flavored ices, fruit ices; gelatin, plain puddings (from fruit juice)	Commercial and homemade products containing milk and milk products, such as ice cream, custard, puddings, chocolate cake, and eclairs
Miscellaneous	All products not prohibited	All products containing lactose, cream, milk, and milk products

nutritious items, no scientific evidence indicates that those particular foods cause disease. No evidence demonstrates that sugar interferes with the nutritive value of food or negatively affects an otherwise adequate diet. Our only danger in regard to malnutrition is that some individuals allow sugar to take the place of needed nutrients. In those cases, sugar robs you of vitamins, minerals, and other nutrients.

DOES SUGAR MAKE YOU FAT?

For years, dietary carbohydrates, such as potatoes, rice, spaghetti, sugar, bread, and pastries, have been regarded as foods that make us fat. It is true that excess consumption of such carbohydrate-rich foods will increase fat deposition. However, dietary fat provides nearly twice the calories of carbohydrates per unit of weight. While there are individuals who have a "sweet tooth" and overeat foods containing carbohydrates, the basic problem is not the sugar but the overeating. We know, for example, that many obese people have low sugar intake. They simply take in more calories than they utilize.

For individuals who consume excessive amounts of sweets and starches, decreasing consumption of them will yield weight loss. However, it was not just the sweets that contributed the weight. Rather, the overeating, the excess calories, are to blame. Carbohydrates by themselves do not cause obesity; it is the bad habit of overeating these foods (or any food) that produces the large weight gain.

CAN SUGAR MAKE YOU A DIABETIC?

A basic question that scientific studies have sought to address is whether carbohydrate, sugar, or sucrose can cause diabetes. We know that diabetes tends to occur in adults who are obese. But we also know that certain forms of diabetes are hereditary, or at least the predisposition for diabetes is hereditary. For example, pancreatic cell defect is genetic and predisposes an individual to diabetes. But we also know that not all obese people become diabetic, even if they are obese all their lives.

In those cases where diabetes develops in obese adults, weight loss can eliminate the diabetes—and this has led to the conclusion that excess body fat due to excess calorie intake is related to diabetes. But that relationship exists whether the excess caloric intake comes from protein, fats, or carbohydrates. Once diabetes exists, regardless of whether the patient is or is not obese, overeating will increase blood sugar. Accordingly, treatment of diabetes involves reduction of calories, and that includes reduction of sweets.

We know that hyperglycemia that is not controlled can lead to coronary heart disease and strokes, thickening of capillaries, and various other health conditions. For insulin-dependent diabetics whose diabetes cannot be alleviated, there is no evidence that carbohydrates have a role in causing the diabetes.

DO YOU HAVE HYPOGLYCEMIA?

Hypoglycemia is the opposite condition of diabetes. It can result from too much insulin production in your body since the insulin triggers removal of blood sugar from the blood (Danowski, 1975).

A Condition of Imbalance

The process by which our bodies change carbohydrates to glucose and glucose to energy involves numerous organs, such as the liver, pancreas, pituitary gland, thyroid gland, and adrenal glands. If a malfunction occurs in any of these key organs, excess insulin can result, leading to hypoglycemia. If a key organ is not damaged or otherwise malfunctioning, hypoglycemia can usually be corrected by a high-protein/low-carbohydrate diet, as it was in Jeffrey's case presented at the beginning of this chapter.

The "Trendy" Side of Hypoglycemia

There is, however, another side to hypoglycemia, called the "trendy" side. Hypoglycemia has become a fashionable condition. Doctors specialize in its treatment and patients often specialize in having it. For these reasons, misdiagnosis cannot be thought of as unusual (Walker, 1975).

The symptoms of hypoglycemia can occur from various other causes. For example, neurological diseases, endocrine diseases, and infections can cause sudden weight loss, increasing thirst, frequent urination, and emotional instability. Patients can have blurred or double vision, weakness, profuse sweating, loss of balance, and recurring urinary or vaginal infections—all symptoms that can occur with hypoglycemia.

An example of a case similar to Jeffrey's serves to illustrate the other face of hypoglycemia. A college student had been treated for hypoglycemia, though she had not taken a glucose tolerance test, a blood sugar response to an oral dose of glucose (see Chapter 14).

She had pain in one leg, loss of balance, double vision, frequent urination, recurring urinary and vaginal infections, sudden weight loss, and increasing thirst. When her symptoms persisted despite diet modifications, a glucose tolerance test was administered. The test results were normal.

An alert doctor then noticed an additional symptom, a lack of abdominal reflexes, and administered a different test, which showed abnormal cerebrospinal fluid. The patient was ultimately diagnosed as having multiple sclerosis, not hypoglycemia.

Diagnosis Difficulties

Hypoglycemia's symptoms overlap those of other maladies. Excess insulin can result from several causes. Taken together, these two characteristics can make diagnosis difficult. The problem for physicians becomes confounded when there are patients who seem to want to be diagnosed as hypoglycemic. The confusion for the patient becomes compounded when "sugar doctors" tend to find hypoglycemia among many patients, while more conservative doctors send patients who mention hypoglycemia to a psychiatrist.

It is common knowledge that some individuals can also exhibit ripple effects of fatigue and emotional depression. Studies have shown that such ripple effects can be relieved in some individuals by a low-carbohydrate/high-protein diet. But emphasis on carbohydrates tends to obscure what may be emotional problems that contribute to the symptoms. For example, ripple effects are found to occur in persons who have difficulty coping with school, marriage, job, or finances. Therapy can be most successful when it addresses weight loss and emotional management, rather than carbohydrates or sweets.

As consumer, you must hold tenaciously to the realization that if you have both physical and emotional symptoms, it is not a problem "just in your head." You should seek tests such as the glucose tolerance test to be certain. Similarly, consumers and health practitioners must be certain that treatment for hypoglycemia does not continue on while another cause of the symptoms goes undiagnosed.

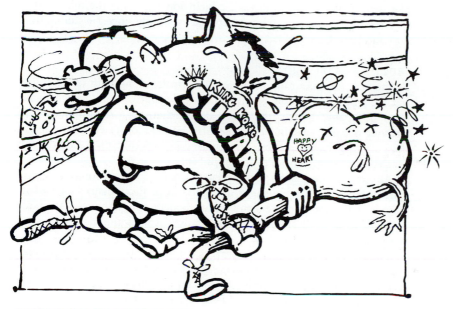

IS SUGAR BAD FOR YOUR HEART?

Both diabetes and obesity due to excess caloric intake predispose an individual to imbalance in blood fat levels. The incidence of certain heart diseases, such as atherosclerosis, increases with diabetes and obesity, regardless of sugar intake. There is, however, a condition known as "hypertriglyceridemia," which results from a person's sensitivity to high carbohydrate (for example, table sugar) intake. This condition is one potential cause of atherosclerosis.

Despite the existence of hypertriglyceridemia, a cause-and-effect relationship to sucrose cannot be established. It is known, for example, that this condition does relate to coronary difficulties; however, the same hypertriglyceridemic effect does not occur in men unless other factors are present, such as smoking or hypertension. In the case of atherosclerosis, as in the case of diabetes, hypoglycemia, and obesity, sucrose intake in moderation cannot be considered a cause.

CAN SUGAR CAUSE HYPERACTIVITY IN A CHILD?

A recent study found that aggressive and restless behavior in hyperactive children was related to their diet. The study addressed carbohydrate:protein ratios and estimated sugar intake. Among normal children, carbohydrate:protein ratios also affected restless behavior. Despite the findings, it cannot be concluded that sugar caused behaviors that were being investigated. For example, active or aggressive children might simply crave sugar.

Some studies have failed to establish behavior changes in children following the administration of sugar, even among children whose parents had identified them as having adverse behavior that appeared to worsen after sweets—yet other studies have found that behavior can worsen after sugar is consumed. Since so few studies have been completed, it is premature to draw a conclusion regarding the relationship between dietary sugar and hyperactivity, especially since the studies thus far conducted have yielded conflicting results.

FRUCTOSE—A DIET AID?

Fructose occurs naturally in honey and fruits, along with other sugar, but the fructose available commercially is produced from refined sugar. Your body absorbs fructose more slowly than glucose and can do so without releasing insulin. Fructose also has less of an effect on dental decay. These characteristics, along with concerns regarding the safety of saccharin, have given rise to the popularity of fructose.

Advertisers have claimed significant benefits for fructose as a natural substitute for both table sugar and saccharin. Proponents boast of its role as a hunger appeaser and of its benefit for diabetics. Available scientific and medical evidence generally suggests the claims are unfounded.

The Food and Drug Administration's findings about fructose indicate that research on fructose has been insufficient to justify the claim that fructose, or any other carbohydrates, can benefit diabetics. The calorie content of fructose is the same as that of sucrose (table sugar), so weight reduction benefits are doubtful, despite fructose having a sweeter taste than sucrose.

The American Diabetes Association has noted that long-term studies of fructose are needed. A 1976 report done for the association by the Federation of American Societies for Experimental Biology found that most diabetologists do not recommend fructose for their patients. In the case of high-fructose corn syrup, many diabetologists warn their patients not to use the product, since most diabetics need to reduce caloric intake and need to lose weight.

Since health professionals are concerned about excessive caloric intake, the increasing industrial use of fructose presents some worries. As producers add sugar to more and more foods, it becomes increasingly difficult for consumers to control their sugar/caloric intake. In slightly over 10 years' time, consumer consumption of high-fructose syrups has increased fifteen-fold. Soft drinks are high on the list in using such fructose syrup.

An added health concern regarding fructose and similar sugars is their potential for causing diarrhea. Consumption of 70 to 100 g of fructose in a day can cause diarrhea. While that level of consumption would be unusually high, similar sugars produce the same side effect at lower levels. For example, 10 to 20 g of mannitol, 20 to 30 g of sorbitol, or 30 to 40 g of xylitol can produce diarrhea. We saw early in this chapter, for example, that sugarless gum can cause diarrhea.

In summary then, fructose requires long-term studies before its potential can be understood. The present evidence does not suggest that fructose is vastly superior to sucrose.

STUDY QUESTIONS

1. What are our major sources of carbohydrate? What is the basic chemical composition of all carbohydrates? Which foods provide most of the carbohydrates in the American diet?

2. Define monosaccharide. Describe the main functions and sources of glucose, fructose, galactose, and mannose.

3. Define oligosaccharide. What are the scientific names for table sugar, milk sugar, and malt sugar? What are the two sweetest carbohydrates?

4. What functions does dietary fiber serve in the body? What is the current confusion regarding the amount of fiber or roughage we ingest?

5. Conduct a survey among your friends to obtain their answers to the following questions:
   a. How is sugar bad for you?
   b. Do you have hypoglycemia?
   c. Can sugar cause hyperactivity in a child?

6. Plan a diet for a ten-year-old who suffers from lactose intolerance. Check with your teacher or a knowledgeable health professional to determine the diet's nutritional adequacy.

REFERENCES

Anderson, T. A. "Recent Trends in Carbohydrate Consumption." *Ann. Rev. Nutr.* 2 (1982): 113.

Danowski, T. S., et al. "Hypoglycemia." *World Rev. Nutr. Dietet.* 22 (1975): 288.

Heaton, K. W. "Dietary Fiber in Perspective." *Human Nutrition: Clinical Nutrition* 37c (1983): 151.

Hodges, R. E. "Present Knowledge of Carbohydrates." *Nutr. Rev.* 24 (1966): 65.

Hui, Y. H. *Human Nutrition and Diet Therapy.* Monterey, CA: Wadsworth, 1983.

Kritchevsky, D. "Dietary Fiber and Disease." *Bull. N.Y. Acad. Sci.* 58 (1982): 230.

Page, D. M., and T. M. Bayless, eds. *Lactose Digestion: Clinical and Nutritional Implications.* Baltimore: Johns Hopkins University Press, 1981.

Stare, E. J. "Sugar in the Diet of Man." *World Rev. Nutr. Dietet.* 22 (1975): 237.

Walker, S. III. "Sugar Doctors and Hypoglycemia." *Psychology Today* 9 (July 1975): 68.

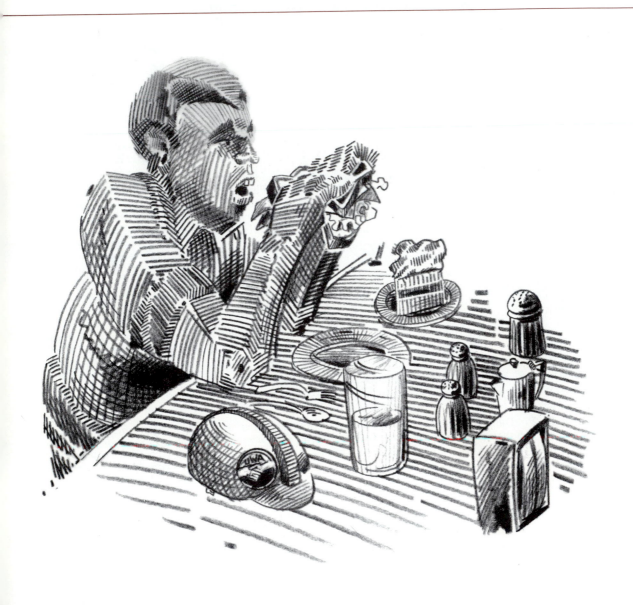

FATS:

A CAUSE OF HEART DISEASES?

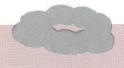

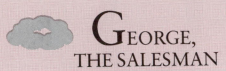

GEORGE, THE SALESMAN

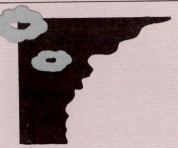

George, a 63-year-old salesman on the verge of retirement, smoked two packs of cigarettes a day and was 20 pounds over-weight. Despite the loss of a parent to heart disease, George had experienced no *cardiovascular* difficulties and no serious illness in over 15 years.

George's eating habits reflected his "heartland" up-bringing. He ate robust meals of red meat, baked potatoes, gravy, dairy products, and pastries.

A company-sponsored blood pressure checkup and blood lipid analysis revealed normal blood pressure, but elevated levels of serum cholesterol and triglycerides. George wisely con-sulted his own physician, whose further lipid determinations con-firmed the earlier findings and suggested blood glucose testing, which subsequently helped rule out diabetes.

The physician determined that weight loss should yield the de-sired reduction of serum lipid levels and arranged for George to visit a dietitian. Two months later, George's low-calorie diet showed positive results. He had experienced a 5-pound weight loss and a measurable reduction in both serum cholesterol and triglyceride levels. The doctor concluded that continued weight loss would restore George's serum lipid profile to normal and recommended that George stop smoking and get more exer-cise.

Fat in Our Diet: How Much Is Too Much?

If, like George, you have a high blood cholesterol level, you may have a greater chance of having a heart attack. If you smoke, your risk also increases. Further, a major dietary risk factor is reflected in a high blood cholesterol level. The variations in our diets and in our individual metabolism complicate such issues, however. Some of us can eat signifi-cant amounts of food containing beef fats and cholesterol with no accompanying increase in our blood levels. Others of us are not so fortunate. Thus, any understanding of fats and health involves the realization that controversy exists. Not all the answers are in.

Fats in our diet have occupied the attention of nutritional scientists for several years. Despite research efforts, many questions remain un-answered. Scientists know that, like carbohydrates and proteins, fats are made up of carbon, hydrogen, and oxygen. However, fat provides more than twice as many calories per molecule because it has a lower ratio of oxygen to carbon and hydrogen. People are understandably concerned about fats and oils since most people realize that "oil and water don't mix"—and water is the primary ingredient of our bodies. The answers to that concern lie in body chemistry, as we shall see.

Though some foods, such as butter and oils, are almost pure fat, the fats in most foods coexist with other nutrients and dietary factors such as protein, carbohydrate, vitamins, and fiber. Vegetable oils and meat are our major sources of fat. This fat may be visible, as in marbled meat, or hidden, as in cheese, nuts, and bakery products. Table 6-1 shows the fat content of typical foods. You should refer to the Appendix for the fat level of other foods.

Although fat's role in health and disease generates controversy, many nutritionists agree that we eat either too much fat or too much of the wrong type of fat. In this chapter, we will examine why we need fats, what fats are, and how the fats we eat affect our health. As we proceed with the discussion, you should relate some of the information to the situation of our salesman, George.

Why Do We Need Fats?

Although excessive fat intake may contribute to health problems, we need some fat in our diet; fat is an essential nutrient that serves a number of important functions. First, fats carry essential nutrients such as fatty acids and fat-soluble vitamins (A, D, E, and K).

Second, fats are concentrated sources of energy. Providing 9 kcal per gram, fat has over twice the energy supply of carbohydrate or protein.

Table 6-1
Fat Content of Representative Foods

FOOD	SERVING SIZE	FAT (g)
Cottage cheese, creamed, large curd	1 c	10
Milk, whole	1 c	8
Ice cream, regular	1 c	14
Eggs, whole	1	6
Butter	1 T	12
Mayonnaise, regular	1 T	6
Fish sticks, breaded, cooked	1 fish stick	3
Ground beef, lean	3 oz	10
Chicken breast, fried	2.8 oz	5
White bread, enriched	1 sl	3
Rice, enriched	1 c	trace
Almonds, shelled	1 c	70
Peanut butter	1 T	8
Honey	1 T	0
Green beans, cooked	1 c	trace
Carrots, cooked	1 c	trace
Tomato, raw	1	trace
Apple, raw	1	1
Grapefruit, raw	½	trace
Beer	12 fl oz	0
Chocolate, baking	1 oz	15
Soup, cream of mushroom	1 c	10

SOURCE: Adapted from *Nutritive Value of Foods*, Home and Garden Bulletin No. 72 (Washington, D.C.: U.S. Department of Agriculture, 1981).

Although glucose serves as the direct source of energy for most of our organs, the resting muscles and the heart can metabolize fatty acids (components of fat) for energy. Stored body fat is a prominent source of energy, one especially necessary in enabling you to cope with periods of illness or starvation.

Third, fat guards us against cold and injury. The fat our bodies store acts as insulation, protecting us from cold temperatures. As cushioning for vital organs such as heart, kidneys, and ovaries, and as padding for stress sites such as soles of the feet and palms, stored fat protects against injury.

A fourth important function of fat surfaces in its biochemical interrelationship with carbohydrate and protein. The unique metabolism of fatty acids enables fat to be converted to protein. The conversion of fat to glucose can decrease the body's demand upon carbohydrate. In essence then, fat can take some of the demand off protein and carbohydrate, can literally and figuratively take the "heat" off them. You will find a more thorough discussion of body-fat metabolism in relationship to protein and carbohydrate in Chapter 14.

Fifth, fats increase the **satiety** value of foods, that satisfying feeling of being full. It may be that fats accomplish this by causing a prolonged distention of the stomach after eating.

Finally, fats raise the desirability of food by providing aroma and enhancing taste. Many of us like the smooth richness of fatty foods such as beef fats and bakery products because they enhance the palatability and attractiveness of food.

What Are Fats Made Of?

Once you understand some key terms, you will be better able to appreciate the chemical nature of fats, the digestion of fats, and the unique role of fats in our bodies. The chemical term for *fats* is **lipids**. In chemistry, lipids are classified into three types: simple, compound, and derived. Simple lipids include **fatty acids** (containing only carbon, hydrogen, and oxygen) and **glycerides** (fatty acids and the chemical glycerol linked in a special form called **esters**). Compound lipids include **phospholipids** (compounds of fatty acids and phosphoric acid with a nitrogenous base) and **lipoproteins** (lipids combined with protein). Derived lipids include **sterols** (such as cholesterol and steroid hormones) and vitamin D, a **fat-soluble vitamin**. You will encounter these basic terms throughout this chapter.

FATTY ACIDS AND TRIGLYCERIDES

A fatty acid, the basic chemical unit in fat, is composed of a linear chain of carbon atoms with attached hydrogen atoms. The length and structure of fatty acids vary. Fatty acids can be visualized as a chain in which each link is a carbon atom and each link has a "spike" jutting from each side. Each spike is a hydrogen atom. One end of the chain, a carboxyl group, is acidic (able to donate or give up hydrogen ions) and contains oxygen. The other end is a methyl group, a carbon atom surrounded by three hydrogen atoms. The number of carbon atoms in the chain and the

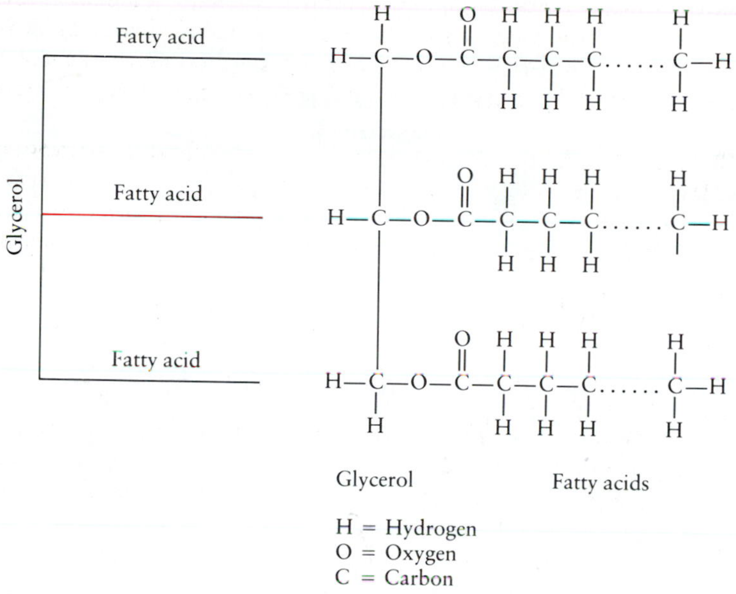

Fatty acid

$$H-\overset{\overset{\displaystyle H}{|}}{C}-O-\overset{\overset{\displaystyle O}{\|}}{C}-\overset{\overset{\displaystyle H}{|}}{\underset{\underset{\displaystyle H}{|}}{C}}-\overset{\overset{\displaystyle H}{|}}{\underset{\underset{\displaystyle H}{|}}{C}}-\overset{\overset{\displaystyle H}{|}}{\underset{\underset{\displaystyle H}{|}}{C}}\ldots\ldots\overset{\overset{\displaystyle H}{|}}{\underset{\underset{\displaystyle H}{|}}{C}}-H$$

Glycerol

Fatty acid

$$H-\overset{|}{C}-O-\overset{\overset{\displaystyle O}{\|}}{C}-\overset{\overset{\displaystyle H}{|}}{\underset{\underset{\displaystyle H}{|}}{C}}-\overset{\overset{\displaystyle H}{|}}{\underset{\underset{\displaystyle H}{|}}{C}}-\overset{\overset{\displaystyle H}{|}}{\underset{\underset{\displaystyle H}{|}}{C}}\ldots\ldots\overset{\overset{\displaystyle H}{|}}{\underset{|}{C}}-H$$

Fatty acid

$$H-\overset{\overset{\displaystyle }{|}}{\underset{\underset{\displaystyle H}{|}}{C}}-O-\overset{\overset{\displaystyle O}{\|}}{C}-\overset{\overset{\displaystyle H}{|}}{\underset{\underset{\displaystyle H}{|}}{C}}-\overset{\overset{\displaystyle H}{|}}{\underset{\underset{\displaystyle H}{|}}{C}}-\overset{\overset{\displaystyle H}{|}}{\underset{\underset{\displaystyle H}{|}}{C}}\ldots\ldots\overset{\overset{\displaystyle H}{|}}{\underset{\underset{\displaystyle H}{|}}{C}}-H$$

Glycerol   Fatty acids

H = Hydrogen
O = Oxygen
C = Carbon

Figure 6-1: The chemical structure of fatty acids and a triglyceride (. . . indicates varying number of carbon atoms).

number of hydrogen atoms that chain can hold regulate the characteristics of each fatty acid, from hardness to liquidity, and from water insolubility to water solubility. See Figure 6-1.

Visible fats or oils, such as beef fat, lard, or corn oil, are mostly triglycerides, with a small amount of di- and monoglycerides. A **triglyceride**, sometimes called a neutral fat, is made up of glycerol and three fatty acids. (Two molecules of fatty acids yield a diglyceride and one yields a monoglyceride.) Also see Figure 6-1.

Glycerol is a neutral substance, whereas fatty acid is highly active. Hence, the characteristics of the fatty acids determine the chemical property of simple fat. Fatty acid characteristics, as mentioned earlier in this section, are dictated by the presence of long-chain or short-chain fats, as well as "saturatedness" or "unsaturatedness." These factors in turn result in hardness or liquidity at room temperature. Most important, these characteristics help determine the ease of fat absorption in our bodies.

SATURATED VERSUS UNSATURATED FATTY ACIDS

Saturation and unsaturation are terms that describe the chemical structure of fatty acids. If all chemical linkages of a carbon atom "saturate," then each carbon atom, except for those at the ends of the chain, has two hydrogen atoms attached to it. These were earlier referred to as "spikes." Two hydrogen atom attachments constitute the maximum possible for each carbon atom, so the chain is "saturated." When saturated, one or more pairs of adjacent carbon atoms may form a double, rather than a single, bond between each other, resulting in a pair of carbon atoms sharing a single hydrogen atom. If a double bond occurs in more than one place in the chain, the resulting fatty acid is called a

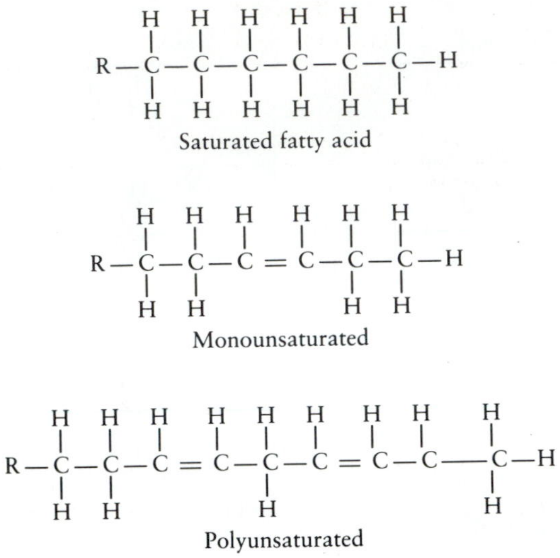

Figure 6-2: Structures of saturated, monounsaturated, and polyunsaturated fatty acids. (R indicates the remainder of the molecule.)

polyunsaturated fatty acid (PUFA). Those with only one double bond are sometimes called **monounsaturated fatty acids.** See Figure 6-2.

Table 6-2 lists the most common fatty acids. Approximately 40 fatty acids are believed to occur naturally, with a range of 2 to 24 carbon atoms. Most have an even number of carbon atoms, though fish and bacteria are among the few organisms with an odd number.

Why Are Some Fats Solid, Some Liquid?

We all know how difficult it is to butter toast with very firm butter. The nature of the fats we eat partly results from their chemical characteristics, which are determined by their fatty-acid components. Glycerides (fats) with more short-chain or unsaturated fatty acids will be soft fats or oils and will be liquid at room temperature. We say they have a low melting point. Fats with long-chain fatty acids are hard fats and thus are solid at room temperature; they have a high melting point. Short-chain fatty acids are fairly soluble in water, unlike those with longer chains.

Lipids containing mostly oleic, linoleic, and other unsaturated fatty acids will be liquid at room temperature. The oil on the surface of an orange or the oil from corn typifies this group. Fats containing mostly palmitic and stearic saturated fatty acids are solid at room temperature—for example, the fat around a pork chop. See Table 6-2. Fats that melt at temperatures above 50°C (122°F) are not so easily utilized by the body.

Oxidation (an interaction between oxygen in air and any other chemical component) occurs more readily in unsaturated fatty acids than in saturated ones. Thus, cooked fats or oils with a higher content of unsaturated fatty acids have a greater tendency to become rancid (from oxidation). Short- or medium-chain fatty acids are also easier to absorb. Similarly, given a like number of carbon atoms, polyunsaturated fats are absorbed more efficiently than saturated ones. These observations en-

Table 6-2
Common Fatty Acids

NAME	NO. OF CARBONS	NO. OF DOUBLE BONDS
SATURATED FATTY ACIDS		
Butyric acid	4	
Caproic acid	6	
Caprylic acid	8	
Capric acid	10	
Lauric acid	12	
Myristic acid	14	
Palmitic acid	16	
Stearic acid	18	
Arachidic acid	20	
Behenic acid	22	
MONOUNSATURATED FATTY ACIDS		
Palmitoleic acid	16	1
Oleic acid	18	1
Erucic acid	22	1
POLYUNSATURATED FATTY ACIDS		
Linoleic acid	18	2
Linolenic acid	18	3
Arachidonic acid	20	4

able us to understand why ordinary fats can be solid or liquid, why some fats become rancid faster than others, and why absorption of fatty acids by our bodies is varied.

Important Components of Dietary and Body Fats

As mentioned earlier, fats are made up of many components. The health roles of four of these have been increasingly in the news: essential fatty acids, cholesterol, phospholipids, and lipoproteins. The following will help you better understand these substances and their effects on our well-being.

ESSENTIAL FATTY ACIDS
Though the human body can manufacture or synthesize a few polyunsaturated fatty acids, it is unable to make two important ones—linoleic acid and linolenic acid (both having 18 carbons as seen in Table 6-2). These are, therefore, called **essential fatty acids** since they must be obtained from our diets. The body also needs arachidonic acid (20 carbons), but our bodies can synthesize this substance from available linoleic acid if vitamin B_6 is present. Hence, linoleic acid can be said to be doubly essential.

Physiologically, essential fatty acids have important and specific functions: (1) regulating cholesterol metabolism, including transportation, storage, and excretion; (2) permitting cell membranes to function properly; and (3) serving as basic ingredients for body synthesis of a number of hormonelike substances.

As early as 1929, researchers found that when deprived of PUFA (linoleic acid in particular) rats develop skin and kidney lesions. Other animals such as mice, dogs, pigs, calves, poultry, and insects are susceptible to essential fatty acid deficiency, but to a lesser extent. In general, linoleic acid can cure all deficiency symptoms, though linolenic and arachidonic acid are also useful in partial treatment.

In humans, infants can develop essential fatty acid deficiency if they are fed nonfat milk for a long period. The classic fatty acid deficiency symptom in an infant is **eczematous dermatitis,** which responds to linoleic and/or arachidonic acid therapy. In deficiency cases, skin lesions develop as essential fatty acids in the blood decrease. Such deficiency is much less common in adults because the adult body stores a large amount of fats. Figure 6-3 shows deficiency symptoms in an adult after a prolonged period of intravenous feeding without fat (therefore, without essential fatty acids). The symptoms are relieved by administering linoleic acid orally, topically, or intravenously. Any vegetable oil containing an adequate level of linoleic acid is effective for topical (rub-on) application.

The question of our need for dietary fat is more properly the question of our need for essential fatty acids. Scientists have successfully calculated this need in fairly accurate ranges. Experimentally induced deficiency symptoms in infants disappear when the infants are fed over 1.3 percent of their total calories as linoleic acid. Estimates indicate that a 3 percent to 4 percent intake of dietary calories from linoleic acid prevents deficiency. Linoleic acid in breast milk accounts for 6 percent to 9 percent of the caloric content. Although these numbers are routinely converted to weight (g, oz, etc.) of fatty acids in research and clinical

Figure 6-3: Relief of dermal symptoms of essential fatty acid deficiency that had been induced by fat-free intravenous feeding of fat emulsion.
SOURCE: M. C. Riella, et al. Ann. Int. Med. 8 (1975): 786.

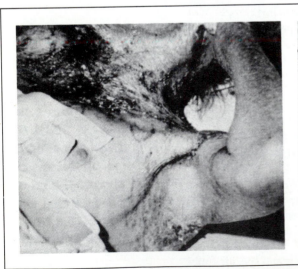
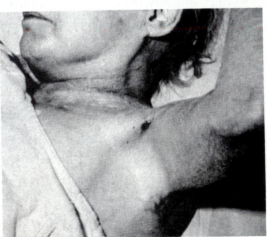

care, percentages are more readily understood. Studies have shown that the younger the person, the greater the essential fatty acid requirement. High intake of saturated fatty acids and cholesterol also increases the requirement.

The standard American diet easily satisfies the adult requirement of 1 percent to 2 percent calories from linoleic acid. The typical American diet has 25 percent to 50 percent calories as fat, and this will provide 5 percent to 10 percent calories from linoleic acid. The U.S. Department of Agriculture estimates that 6 percent of total dietary energy as linoleic acid is available per person per day in our food supply. About 10 percent of dietary fat is linoleic acid, and a diet with 15 to 25 g of the appropriate fatty acids meets the essential fatty acid requirement.

The fatty acids we most commonly consume are linoleic and oleic acids (both unsaturated) and stearic and palmitic acids (both saturated). An estimated 90 percent of the daily fatty acids consumed consists of the foregoing four acids, ranging from palmitic acid, which contributes 10 percent to 15 percent to oleic acid, which contributes 30 percent or more.

Our two major sources of fatty acids are animal fats and plant oils. Plant oils tend to be unsaturated, and animal fats tend to be saturated. Table 6-3 gives an analysis of the amounts and ratios of saturated and unsaturated fatty acids in common foods.

While the average American receives an adequate amount of linoleic acid or PUFAs, the quantity of unsaturated fats ingested in relation to saturated fats creates controversy. Some scientists hold that we eat too much saturated fats, and they recommend that we consume more unsaturated fatty acids by using more vegetable seed oils. Other scientists believe that there is insufficient evidence to support such conclusions. We will discuss these issues more fully in the section on fats and health.

As we have seen earlier, most oils of land plant seeds contain relatively more linoleic acid than do animal fats. Nevertheless, these vegetable oils contain mostly oleic and palmitic acids, followed by linoleic acid; most seed oils also contain some linolenic acid. Olive and coconut oils are exceptions. Olive oil has little linoleic acid but a large amount of oleic acid, while coconut oil contains little linoleic or oleic acid but a large amount of short-chain, saturated fatty acids. Vegetable oils contain practically no arachidonic acid (recall that it is easily synthesized from linoleic acid in our bodies).

Sometimes our cooking procedures require additional considerations. For example, neither solid or liquid fats nor oils are suitable for certain baking processes, preparing certain dishes, or spreading cheeses, sauces, or the like on bread or crackers. The food industry has developed "hydrogenated" fats and oils for these purposes. **Hydrogenation** is a process whereby oils with a large concentration of unsaturated fatty acids can be turned into a fat with a texture ranging from soft to hard. The actual chemical change involves saturating the unsaturated bonds with hydrogen. Technology enables partial or complete hydrogenation so the final product can be of any texture desired. Hydrogenation additionally reduces the potential for oils to oxidize and become rancid,

Table 6-3
Fat Content and Major Fatty Acid Composition of Selected Foods

FOOD	TOTAL FAT (%)	FATTY ACID* SATURATED (%)†	UNSATURATED OLEIC (%)	LINOLEIC (%)	P/S‡
Salad and cooking oils					
Safflower	100	10	13	74	7.4/1.0
Sunflower	100	11	14	70	6.4/1.0
Corn	100	13	26	55	4.2/1.0
Cottonseed	100	23	17	54	2.3/1.0
Soybean§	100	14	25	50	3.6/1.0
Sesame	100	14	38	42	3.0/1.0
Soybean, special processed	100	11	29	31	2.8/1.0
Peanut	100	18	47	29	1.6/1.0
Olive	100	11	76	7	0.6/1.0
Coconut	100	80	5	1	0.2/1.0
Margarine, first ingredient on label‖					
Safflower oil (liquid)—tub	80	11	18	48	4.4/1.0
Soybean oil (liquid)—tub¶	80	15	31	33	2.2/1.0
Butter	81	46	27	2	0.4/1.0
Animal fats					
Poultry	100	30	40	20	0.67/1.0
Beef, lamb, pork	100	45	44	2–6	0.04–0.13/1.0
Fish, raw					
Salmon	9	2	2	4	2.0/1.0
Mackerel	13	5	3	4	0.8/1.0
Herring, Pacific	13	4	2	3	0.75/1.0
Tuna	5	2	1	2	1.0/1.0
Nuts					
Walnuts, English	64	4	10	40	10.0/1
Walnuts, black	60	4	21	28	7.0/1
Brazil	67	13	32	17	1.3/1
Peanuts or peanut butter	51	9	25	14	1.6/1
Egg yolk	31	10	13	2	0.2/1
Avocado	16	3	7	2	0.67/1

SOURCE: Adapted from *Fats in Food and Diet*, U.S. Department of Agriculture Information Bulletin No. 361.

*Total is not expected to equal total fat.

†Includes fatty acids with chains containing from 8 to 18 carbon atoms.

‡P/S = Linoleic acid content/saturated fatty acid content.

§Suitable as salad oil.

‖Mean values of selected samples, which may vary with brand name and date of manufacture. Includes small amounts of monounsaturated and diunsaturated fatty acids that are not oleic or linoleic.

¶Linoleic acid includes higher polyunsaturated fatty acids.

so the oils may be safely stored, even at room temperature. Three familiar hydrogenated products are shortening, margarine, and cheese spreads.

As discussed later, heart patients advised to increase polyunsaturated fat intake can utilize partially hydrogenated margarines, which may contain up to 50 percent PUFA. Hydrogenated oil can be made from corn, soybean, cottonseed, safflower, peanut, or olive oil. This hydrogenation can improve flavor, inhibit rancidity, and prevent separation.

Characteristics of animal fats vary, depending on whether the animal lived on land or in water, and their differences in chemical composition have ignited debate among nutritionists. Many land animal fats contain 16 to 24 carbon-atom fatty acids, predominately oleic and palmitic acids. These animal fats are hard, since 20 percent to 30 percent of the fatty acids are saturated palmitic acids. Harder fats from cattle and other ruminants have more saturated stearic acid rather than unsaturated oleic acid. Milk fats such as butter differ from all other land animal fats by containing some fatty acids with only 4 to 12 carbons (butyric and myristic acid).

Freshwater animal fats vary in saturation. Fatty acids typically contain 16-, 18-, 20-, and 22-carbon atoms. Palmitic acid is most common, accounting for 10 percent to 18 percent of the fatty acids in these foods. Saltwater animal fats, with 20 to 22 carbons and up to six double bonds, are polyunsaturated. Fish that live in both fresh and saltwater, such as salmon, have the fatty acid characteristics of marine animals.

Nutritionists debate whether animal fat or fish oil offers greater benefit to us. Only one point in such debates is certain. If a doctor wants a patient to avoid red meat because of its high saturated fat content, greater intake of poultry and fish should be recommended.

CHOLESTEROL

Another type of fat occurring in both plants and animals is sterols. Although scientists believe that the human body does not absorb plant sterols to any significant extent, animal sterols hold the spotlight in a spirited debate. At the center of this controversy rests the animal sterol **cholesterol** and its possible relationship to heart disease. Table 6-4 identifies the cholesterol content of selected foods. Figure 6-4 shows cholesterol structure.

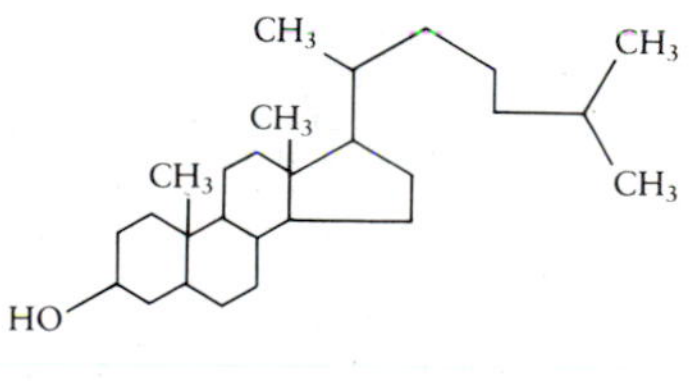

Figure 6-4: *Cholesterol structure. (Each angular position where lines meet is occupied by a carbon atom.)*

Cholesterol concentrates in our bile (stored in the gallbladder) and nerves and is a fat, waxy substance. Some of the cholesterol in our blood and tissue is synthesized by the intestinal mucosa (lining) and the liver, and some is supplied by the diet. Since we can make cholesterol, our diet need not contain it, especially since we make two or three times more than we consume (the average Western diet contains 500 to 1000 mg/day, while the body makes 1 to 3 g/day).

Cholesterol does perform a number of important functions. It is a basic building block from which bile salts, vitamin D, and sex hormones are formed. Cholesterol facilitates the absorption of fatty acids by forming esters with the acids (fatty acids + cholesterol = esters). Cholesterol esters then transport fatty acids in the blood.

Table 6-4
Cholesterol Content of Selected Foods

FOOD	AMOUNT	CHOLESTEROL (MG)
Milk, skim, fluid or reconstituted	1 c	5
Cottage cheese, uncreamed	½ c	7
Lard	1 T	12
Cream, light table	1 fl oz	20
Cottage cheese, creamed	½ c	24
Cream, half and half	¼ c	26
Ice cream, regular, approximately 10% fat	½ c	27
Cheese, cheddar	1 oz	28
Milk, whole	1 c	34
Butter	1 T	35
Oysters, salmon; cooked	3 oz	40
Clams, halibut, tuna; cooked	3 oz	55
Chicken, turkey; light meat, cooked	3 oz	67
Beef, pork, lobster; chicken, turkey, dark meat; cooked	3 oz	75
Lamb, veal, crab; cooked	3 oz	85
Shrimp, cooked	3 oz	130
Heart, beef, cooked	3 oz	230
Egg	1 yolk or 1 egg	250
Liver (beef, calf, hog, lamb), cooked	3 oz	370
Kidney, cooked	3 oz	680
Brains, raw	3 oz	1,700 +

SOURCE: Adapted from Feeley, R. M., et al., "Cholesterol Content of Foods." *J Amer. Dietet. Assoc.* 61 (1972):134.

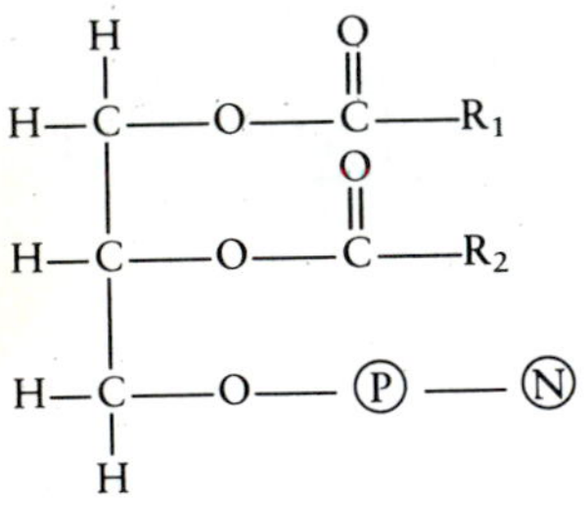

R_1, R_2 = fatty acids

P = Phosphate group, PO_3^-

N = a special compound usually containing nitrogen.
If N = choline, then the phospholipid is a lecithin.

Figure 6-5: Phospholipid structure.

Increasing numbers of health professionals believe that reduction of dietary cholesterol decreases the risk of heart diseases. The concern lies with elevated levels of cholesterol in the blood, yet the relationship between ingested cholesterol and cholesterol levels in blood remains unclear. This will be further explored at the end of this chapter.

PHOSPHOLIPIDS

Phospholipids contain glycerol, fatty acids, and phosphorus (a derived lipid), as shown in Figure 6-5. This class of fats primarily serves as a structural component of cell membranes. Since they can mix with fat-soluble as well as water-soluble ingredients, phospholipids provide for both mixing and transporting, especially in helping both fat- and water-soluble substances to cross membrane barriers. This is such a vital bodily function that, even in starvation, phospholipids are not broken down to serve as an energy source.

Virtually all foods contain phospholipids, since they occur in all cell membranes, yet we do not need them in our diet, because we can synthesize them from components. Ingested phospholipids are **hydro-**

lyzed (split up) in the small intestine, primarily into glycerol, fatty acids, and phosphates.

Phospholipids have commercial importance for use in combining fat and water ingredients to prevent separation, as in mayonnaise. One phospholipid, lecithin, has been championed as preventing heart disease by reducing blood cholesterol levels. These claims have made lecithin a familiar product in health food stores. You will understand why these claims are unfounded if you remember that lecithin is broken down into its component parts in the small intestine.

LIPOPROTEINS

Lipoprotein, containing a component of fat and a component of protein, is a derived lipid. The fat component can be fatty acids, cholesterol, glycerides, and/or phospholipids. See Figure 6-6. Lipoproteins are hydrolyzed to components, just as are phospholipids, and cannot be absorbed intact. Also as in the case of phospholipids, they can be synthesized. This occurs in the liver and in the intestinal walls. Lipoproteins also serve a vital transport function in transporting fat and protein in our circulation. It is currently speculated that, for both men and women, lipoprotein is important in reducing the risk of heart disease. This will be explored further in this chapter.

How the Body Utilizes Fats

While an understanding of the chemistry of fats is necessary in making distinctions among fatty acids and their functions in our bodies, what happens to fat during digestion, absorption, transportation, and excretion proves central to health considerations. Although details of body utilization of fats are presented in Chapter 14, we'll summarize briefly here.

All ingested fats are digested to varying extents in the intestinal system, resulting in their components being released and absorbed. In sum, the digestion of glycerides (mono, di, tri), phospholipids, and lipoproteins results in the formation of fatty acids, glycerols, nitrogenous and phosphorus compounds, and a small amount of glycerides. Cholesterol remains intact and will be absorbed as such.

After absorption and recirculation, glycerides, fatty acids, glycerols, cholesterol, and phospholipids are eventually combined with proteins to form different types of lipoproteins that can permit fatty substances to be transported freely in a "water" medium, the blood. The various fatty components within the lipoproteins vary in quantity. Two especially noteworthy lipoprotein types are low-density lipoproteins (LDLs) and high-density lipoproteins (HDLs). Both carry cholesterol and other fatty components. Popular interest has focused on the role of these two lipoproteins in heart disease, and that role will be explained further in this chapter.

Fats and Health

The relationship between health and dietary fats is complex and remains one of the hottest nutritional issues. We know that individual need in

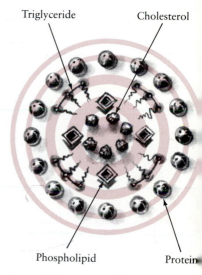

Triglyceride   Cholesterol

Phospholipid   Protein

Figure 6-6: Structure of lipoprotein.

relation to intake causes variations. We especially know that unresolved issues concerning saturated and unsaturated fats, cholesterol, and risk of heart disease all serve to cloud the main issue, but the importance of preventing heart disease demands our attention.

CARDIOVASCULAR DISEASES

Cardiovascular disorders affect the heart and the circulation. The incidence of heart disease has reached epidemic proportions in industrialized societies. In the United States, for instance, heart disease is still the number one killer, despite recent declines in mortality rates from heart-related disorders.

In a healthy person, the insides of the blood vessels are wide and clear, permitting blood to pass easily. If the process of **atherosclerosis** has started, the walls of a blood vessel may become thickened by deposited lipid materials. This is the process of **plaque formation** (see Figure 6-7). Blood then moves through a narrower passage, and its rate of flow slows. As the plaque deposition increases, the ensuing blockage may completely stop the blood flow. If this occurs in a coronary (heart) artery, the heart muscle cells die from lack of oxygen. In industrialized societies, atherosclerotic coronary artery disease leads death statistics. In the United States, estimates hold that 150,000 to 200,000 people under 65 years old die from this disease annually. Also, occlusion of the blood vessels can occur in the brain (stroke), feet and hands (gangrene), and the major abdominal artery (aneurysm). The progression of these disorders is illustrated in Figure 6-8.

Figure 6-7: Cross sections of coronary arteries showing blockage by fatty substances. (a) Near-complete blockage by deposits (plaque). (b) Normal coronary artery. (c) Hardened deposits severely narrow vessel. (d) Deposits in inner lining. Area in brackets is a small platelet thrombus.
SOURCE: *W. C. Roberts, et al. Am. J. Cardiol. 31 (1973): 55.*

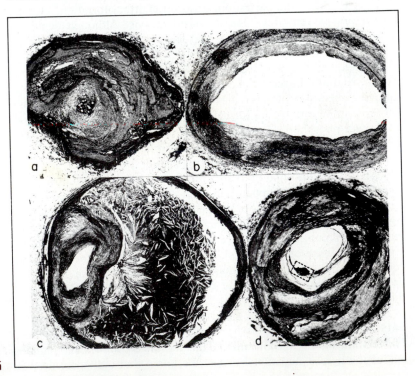

Figure 6-8: *Clinical disorders resulting from the atherosclerotic process.*

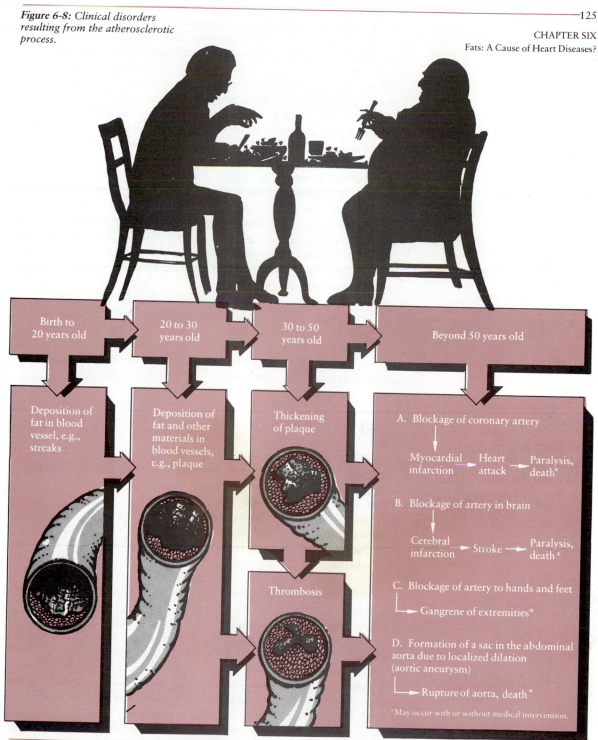

Birth to 20 years old

20 to 30 years old

30 to 50 years old

Beyond 50 years old

Deposition of fat in blood vessel, e.g., streaks

Deposition of fat and other materials in blood vessels, e.g., plaque

Thickening of plaque

Thrombosis

A. Blockage of coronary artery

Myocardial infarction → Heart attack → Paralysis, death*

B. Blockage of artery in brain

Cerebral infarction → Stroke → Paralysis, death *

C. Blockage of artery to hands and feet

⌐→ Gangrene of extremities*

D. Formation of a sac in the abdominal aorta due to localized dilation (aortic aneurysm)

⌐→ Rupture of aorta, death*

*May occur with or without medical intervention.

RISK FACTORS AND PREVENTIVE MEASURES

Cardiovascular experts have identified clues we can follow for the prevention of heart diseases (Kritchevsky, 1983; Rapaport, 1980). These clues are known as risk factors—traits and habits that signal increased risk of heart disease. You will recall the example of George at the beginning of this chapter. George exhibited several risk factors that marked him as a heart attack candidate.

Smoking constitutes an important risk factor. The more a person smokes, the greater the chance of a heart attack. Similarly, smokers have a greater heart attack incidence rate than nonsmokers.

High blood pressure (hypertension) causes the heart to work harder, increasing the likelihood of heart attack. Also, high blood pressure accelerates atherosclerosis. As the walls thicken, the flow of blood constricts, causing even more work for the heart muscle.

In George's case high blood cholesterol is a risk factor. Scientists who believe that high serum cholesterol is a major factor in atherosclerosis use medical data to support their contention. Several important correlations have been found between high serum cholesterol and the development of atherosclerosis:

1. Since the major lipid in plaque is cholesterol, it is assumed that the logical source of the substance is the blood.
2. Many patients with coronary heart disease, especially those identified at an early age, have high levels of blood cholesterol.
3. Many, but not all, patients with a high serum cholesterol level related to hereditary factors develop heart disease early.
4. Studies of selected populations have shown that the risk of having heart disease is directly related to the level of serum cholesterol (the higher the level, the higher the risk).
5. Countries with populations having a higher serum level of cholesterol have high mortality rates from heart diseases. Conversely, countries with a low mortality rate from heart disease have populations with low levels of serum cholesterol.
6. Finally, many human disorders such as diabetes mellitus, renal failure, and hypothyroidism are associated with a high serum level of cholesterol. The rate of heart diseases among such patients is also higher.

It must be emphasized that there are exceptions to most of the positive associations described above.

Animal studies have already shown that reduction of blood cholesterol brings corresponding reduction of atherosclerosis. Many nutritionists agree on one approach. From a dietary standpoint, reducing intake of dairy products and fatty meat reduces the intake of cholesterol. If blood cholesterol is elevated, using poultry, fish, lean meat, and cottage cheese as sources of protein and using vegetable oils will reduce the risk of coronary heart disease from the cholesterol risk factor.

A relationship between dietary fat, serum cholesterol, and coronary heart disease is suggested by the following observations, although exceptions exist for each of them. First, in many population groups where the intake of fat is low, serum cholesterol and the incidence of heart disease are also low, and vice versa. Second, the saturatedness of fat plays a role. A high consumption of saturated fats relates to a high serum cholesterol level and high incidence of heart disease. A high intake of polyunsaturated fats relates to a low serum cholesterol level and low incidence of heart disease. Monounsaturated fats have no effect on serum cholesterol level. In addition, twice the amount of dietary polyunsaturated fats is needed to restore serum cholesterol to normal after being raised by a specific amount of ingested saturated fats.

For many years *high* blood levels of certain fat-related chemicals, such as cholesterol and triglycerides, have been considered bad for the heart. In the last decade, nutritional scientists have been speculating that an *elevated* serum level of one particular chemical substance may be good for us—**high-density lipoprotein** (HDL). Recent research suggests that this substance may protect us from heart and circulatory diseases. However, because of the scarcity of available information, the following discussion of such findings must be considered tentative.

Most of the cholesterol in the blood is transported by two major carriers. About 80 percent is transported by low-density lipoproteins (LDLs), while the rest is carried by HDLs. Physiologically, LDLs carry cholesterol and deposit it in the blood vessels, causing plaque and ultimately heart disease to develop. Conversely, HDLs seem to remove deposited cholesterol and carry it away to the liver for excretion through the bile (by way of the gallbladder). Some researchers claim that we have two types of cholesterol circulating in the blood. The type carried by LDLs seems to be undesirable, whereas that carried by HDLs is beneficial. Of course, the body contains only one chemical type of cholesterol. However, an increased serum level of HDLs is a good clinical sign. Recently, additional epidemiological (population group) studies have confirmed that a high serum level of HDL is associated with a low risk of cardiovascular disease.

If high blood levels of HDL are beneficial, is it possible to induce this condition in individuals to reduce their risk of heart disease? If individuals born with a high blood HDL level are excluded from consideration, some current but tentative observations are as follows (Hartung, et al., 1983; Horwitz, 1975; Medical World News, 1979; Vessby, et al., 1982):

1. Females have higher blood HDL levels than males.
2. The more cigarettes one smokes, the lower the HDL blood level.
3. The more exercise (running in particular) one does, the higher the blood HDL level.
4. Moderate alcohol drinking increases the blood HDL level.
5. Obesity often produces higher blood HDL levels, and weight reduction often produces low blood HDL levels.
6. Lower blood pressure reduces the blood HDL level.
7. There is at present no information on the effect of diet on blood HDL levels.

Given the inconclusiveness of the above observations, it will certainly be some time before a specific strategy is available for raising blood HDL levels, assuming that a higher level is good for us.

Excess weight is a risk factor, but not directly. Rather, excess weight contributes to other risk factors such as high blood pressure and elevated cholesterol levels. Excess weight can also make blood sugar levels higher.

High blood sugar is the condition commonly associated with diabetes. Although the risk factor has been widely recognized as a health problem, fewer of us realize that over 80 percent of all diabetics will die from some form of premature cardiovascular disease, usually heart attack.

Other risk factors include a sedentary way of life, family history of heart disease (as in George's case), and age. Males have more heart attacks than females. We can do nothing about maleness, age, and family history, but there appear to be some risk factors we can affect.

Since studies have shown that the presence of each risk factor increases the overall risk two- to threefold, many health experts promote risk factor intervention. As discussed in Chapter 2, the U.S. Senate Dietary Goals recommend a reduced intake of cholesterol, total fat, and saturated fats and an increased intake of unsaturated fats. The recommendations encourage us to lower blood pressure, lose weight, stop smoking, and to exercise more. All such suggestions are expected to reduce our chances of heart attack. We should intervene in defense of ourselves. (For information on menu planning, see Chapter 15.)

SHOULD CHILDREN BE SCREENED FOR LIPID LEVELS?
Some experts feel that children should be screened for abnormal lipid profiles (Rapaport). They theorize that atherosclerosis begins in child-

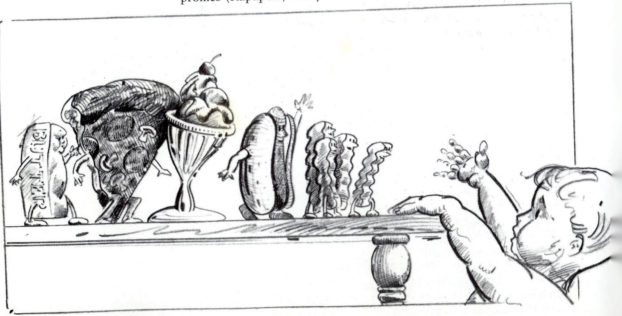

hood, and they know that children in the United States have higher cholesterol levels than children in other countries where the incidence of atherosclerosis and coronary heart disease is much lower. These experts also agree that high blood levels of fats (lipids) result from disease, drug and nutritional excesses, and other environmental influences that are subject to intervention.

Another group of experts cautions that screening is costly, time consuming, impractical, and of less importance than other public health issues. They note that no clinical evidence has substantiated that high blood lipids in childhood lead to atherosclerosis and coronary heart disease in adults.

Other clinicians support screening of children from families with a history of heart disease. This risk factor intervention represents an obvious middle-of-the-road approach to the screening controversy.

The screening process involves analyzing blood cholesterol and triglyceride levels. If a complete blood analysis is warranted, total plasma cholesterol, triglyceride, and lipoprotein undergo evaluation. As seen earlier, low-density lipoprotein carries cholesterol and deposits it in the blood vessels, so a high blood level of low-density lipoprotein represents increased risk of coronary heart disease. A high blood level of high-density lipoprotein assumes the risk is lower.

The screening controversy goes further, however. If lipid levels are elevated, a physician must determine whether the condition is genetic or acquired (from an environmental source, for example). This necessitates testing of urine blood sugar, thyroid functions, liver function, and so on. Further, dietary intervention for such children draws mixed reactions. Although reduction of cholesterol may decrease the risk of heart disease, sustained low fat intake can result in deficiency of essential nutrients normally found in fat. Animal studies have shown that long-term feeding of polyunsaturated fats can delay nervous system development. This would be unfavorable to a child's development.

Diet is only one factor in the prevention of coronary heart disease and atherosclerosis. Therapeutic drugs and exercise play significant roles. Yet all these factors prove difficult to implement with children. Only with concerted effort by all involved—patient, parents, doctors, dietitians, nutritionists—can preventive measures have a chance of being effective.

COOKING AND STORAGE OF FATS

Food preparation often involves frying with fats and oils. Temperature control is important, as too high a temperature causes fat to smoke and produce **acrolin**, a byproduct toxic to animals if they are fed large doses. Too high a temperature also yields unpleasant flavor caused by the resultant hydrocarbon. Otherwise, frying does not reduce the nutritional value of fats and oils.

Storage of fats also requires special care to avoid oxidation and the resulting rancidity. In addition to becoming rancid, fat can also lose important vitamins, such as A and E, during oxidation. Refrigeration can retard the oxidation process.

The food industry has various techniques for retarding oxidation, primarily vacuum or nitrogen packaging and adding antioxidants. Propyl gallate, BHT (butylated hydroxytoluene), and BHA (butylated hydroxyanisole) have been successfully used as antioxidants, though health controversy surrounds the use of both BHT and BHA (see Chapter 25). Some foods naturally contain antioxidants, such as vitamin E in wheat germ.

INDIVIDUAL VARIATIONS

Any discussion of nutrition must recognize individual differences. For example, eating too much fat can result in obesity or perhaps even heart disease, yet not everyone who eats large amounts of fat suffers those problems. Part of such individual differences may be the result of varying processes in the hormonal system, since the thyroid, adrenal, and pituitary glands, and the pancreas and ovaries all produce hormones and influence fat utilization. Exercise increases oxygen in tissues, improves circulation, relieves stress, and generally improves metabolism. Our activity level thus affects our ability to utilize fat. Similarly, our emotional state and lifestyle can affect fat utilization.

Because metabolism slows with aging, we utilize fat less efficiently as we grow older. Certain body tissues become less active, and our enzyme mechanisms become decreasingly able to handle the foods we ingest. Our dietary habits formed throughout our lives and our nutritional status also influence fat utilization. Some of us may have specific diseases that interfere with otherwise normal bodily functions. For example, cardiovascular weaknesses are exacerbated by fat intake.

FATS ARE AFFECTED BY OTHER FOODS YOU EAT

Fat utilization is subject not only to individual body differences but also to overall dietary differences. Calcium, magnesium, chromium, zinc, vanadium, niacin, biotin, pantothenic acid, vitamin B_6, and vitamin E all serve important functions in fat utilization. We do not know how these effects are accomplished, nor to what extent. Theory holds that requirement is relative, not absolute. If, for example, polyunsaturated oil intake increases, the need for vitamin E increases.

The kind of carbohydrate in the diet has been proved to affect fat metabolism. Studies with both humans and laboratory animals have demonstrated elevated blood lipid levels in correlation with high sucrose intake. Some investigators believe the tissue changes related to high sucrose ingestion are not the same as those associated with atherosclerosis.

UNANSWERED QUESTIONS

Although nutritional scientists continue to find clues to the relationship between health and fats, major questions remain unanswered. We know little of the body's processes in handling dietary fats or synthesizing fats. We do not sufficiently understand how emotions, lifestyle, and other diet elements affect fat metabolism. Finally, no one can articulate upper and lower limits of polyunsaturated fats, cholesterol, and total fats in our diets.

While the U.S. Senate has, through the issuance of "Dietary Goals," demonstrated a commitment to improving our health, we have seen that much remains to be learned. For example, some scientists will remain unconvinced until children with high risk factors have been monitored through adulthood. Such longitudinal studies remain to be performed. Similarly, while significant gains have been made in understanding the chemical and biological processes that occur in our bodies, we have seen that many of the unanswered questions are pivotal issues. The most important understanding we have is that, if we find ourselves in a situation such as George's, there are positive steps we can take to improve our health.

STUDY QUESTIONS

1. How are fats chemically similar to carbohydrates and proteins? How do they differ chemically and calorically?

2. Discuss at least four important functions of fats in the body.

3. What is fatty acid? Distinguish between saturated and unsaturated fatty acids. In general, which kind is found mostly in animal fats? In plant oils? Discuss some exceptions to these generalizations.

4. Which fatty acids are considered essential? What are their functions? Discuss the symptoms of essential fatty acid deficiency. Which four fatty acids are most common in the American diet.

5. What is hydrogenation?

6. What are the origins and functions of body cholesterol?

7. Define phospholipids and lipoproteins.

8. How can cooking and storage affect the nutritional value of fats?

9. In what ways do individuals vary in the ability to use fats? How do intakes of other nutrients affect the body's use of fats?

REFERENCES

Hartung, G. H., et al. "Effect of Alcohol Intake on High-Density Lipoprotein Cholesterol Levels in Runners and Inactive Men." *J.A.M.A.* 249 (1983): 747.

Horwitz, L. D. "Alcohol and Heart Disease." *J.A.M.A.* 232 (1975): 959.

Kritchevsky, D. "Diet and Atherosclerosis: Everything Counts." *Cereal Foods World* 28 (1983): 415.

Medical World News. "A Tot of Booze a Day May Keep a Heart Attack Away." *Medical World News* 20 (December 1979): 37.

Rapaport, E., ed. *Current Controversies in Cardiovascular Disease.* Philadelphia: Saunders, 1980.

Vessby, B., et al. "Reduction of Low-Density and High-Density Lipoprotein Cholesterol by Fat-Modified Diets: A Survey of Recent Findings." *Human Nutrition: Clinical Nutrition* 36c (1982): 203.

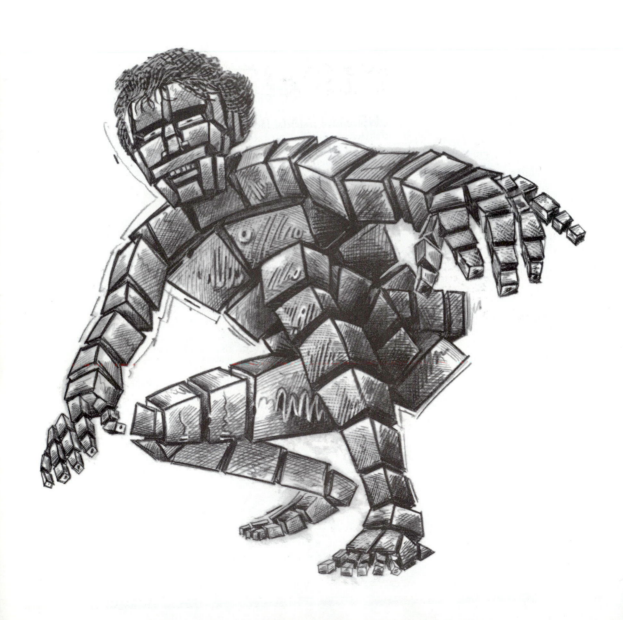

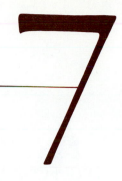

Proteins:

OUR BUILDING BLOCKS

A
CURE FOR PROSTATE TROUBLE:

A
PROTEIN
FORMULA

On June 14, 1982 the United States Postal Service determined that Nutrition Headquarters, Inc., and their agents were engaged in conducting a scheme for obtaining money through the mails by means of false representations in violation of 39 U.S. Code 3005 with respect to the sale of the product Manotex (PS Docket No. 12/156; G.C. 233-81-F).

Court evidence confirmed that Manotex was composed of three nonessential amino acids (components of protein food such as meat, cheese, and so on). Each six-grain capsule contained glutamin acid, alanine, and glycine. The company claimed that the formula would relieve symptoms of benign pro static hypertrophy (enlargement of the prostate gland) "regardless of the cause, nature or extent of the condition."

The condition of enlarged prostate gland is frequent in males over the age of 50. The symptoms of obstruction of urinary flow vary; thus, the natural history of the disease and its symptoms is variable.

The amino acids found in Manotex are widely present in food typically consumed in the United States and will not relieve the symptoms of benign prostatic hypertrophy. Therefore, Nutrition Headquarters' representations as to the effectiveness of Manotex for this purpose were found to be false.

The United States Postal Service will intercept any mail directed to the company. The therapeutic claim for amino acids in the cure of prostate disorder is common. Other commercial products under litigation include Urex, Prostex, and Prostall.

MANOTEX

A scientific formula of pure food substances for relieving the symptoms of Benign Prostatic Hypertrophy.

. . . before using Manotex for the relief of symptoms due to Benign Prostatic Hypertrophy, such as frequency, nocturia (getting up nights), abnormal retention, and dribbling. . . .

Manotex is only effective in relieving the symptoms of Benign Prostatic Hypertrophy.

. . . the exact reasons why Manotex often furnishes welcome relief to many men suffering from the distresses of this ailment are not known.

SOURCE: An advertisement run by Nutrition Headquarters, Inc. (104 West Jackson St., Carbondale, IL 62901)

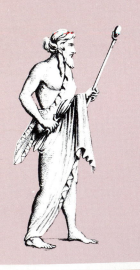

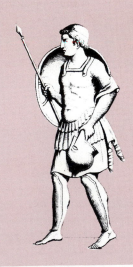

Synonymous with Power

You may have come to think of protein as a power nutrient. We associate protein with muscle development, and most of us know that athletes consume protein-rich foods as a dietary practice. The word "protein" derives from the Greek word *protos*, meaning primary, or in first place. All living substances—plants, animals, even viruses—contain protein.

Our bodies are approximately one-fifth protein. Table 7-1 shows how that protein is distributed. Our protein content constantly undergoes change, almost in the way water changes when you view a river from a single location. As you look at a river, the water you see moves downstream, to be replaced by other water. So, too, our body protein constantly undergoes change. Although we can synthesize, or manufacture, protein within our bodies, certain substances necessary to that process can be obtained only from food. An understanding of protein's composition involves an understanding of amino acids, the components of protein.

Amino Acids Are Numerous

The body contains many types of protein, and each protein substance may contain many chains of molecules. Each chain of molecules is composed of individual units called **amino acids**. There are 20 to 25 amino acids that occur naturally. These protein substances all contain hydrogen, carbon, oxygen, and nitrogen. Some additionally contain iron, sulfur, phosphorus, and zinc and/or copper.

If we consider the biochemistry of protein, we find that the amino acids can be divided into those that our bodies can synthesize (**nonessential amino acids**) and those that must be obtained from our diet (**essential amino acids**). The distinction can be somewhat misleading, however. For normal protein metabolism, the ten essential amino acids must be present in our bodies in the proper amounts, and in the right proportion to the nonessential amino acids, which serve as nitrogen sources.

Table 7-2 lists the amino acids. You will notice that two are presented as essential for children only. The essentiality of these two has been questioned by scientists.

To fully appreciate the importance of amino acids, you should also understand that nonessential amino acids are not solely manufactured by our bodies. They can be obtained from our diets as well but are classified as nonessential simply because they *can* be manufactured in our bodies. Cystine and tyrosine can be manufactured from only methionine and phenylalanine, respectively, two essential amino acids.

Protein substances vary in form, size, and content. If an amino acid occurs singly, it is known as a **free amino acid**. A unit of two amino acids is referred to as a **dipeptide**, three, a **tripeptide**. If as many as fifty to one hundred amino acids are chemically joined as a unit, they are called **polypeptides**. Larger groupings are simply called proteins. When we ingest the more complex protein units, digestive enzymes break them down into free amino acids (a process called hydrolysis) prior to absorption.

Table 7-1
Distribution of Protein in the Body*

TISSUE	% OF BODY PROTEIN (APPROX.)
Blood proteins (albumin and hemoglobin)	10
Fat cells of adipose tissues	3–4
Body skin	9–9.5
Bones	18–19
Muscles	46–47

*The values have been obtained from different investigators and are presented in ranges to emphasize their variability in human bodies.

Table 7-2
Amino Acids Occurring in Nature

ESSENTIAL FOR ADULTS AND INFANTS	ESSENTIAL FOR INFANTS ONLY	NONESSENTIAL	QUESTIONABLE†
Isoleucine	Arginine*	Alanine	Hydroxyproline
Leucine	Histidine*	Asparagine	Norleucine
Lysine		Aspartic acid	Thyroxine
Methionine		Cysteine	
Phenylalanine		Cystine	
Threonine		Glutamic acid	
Tryptophan		Glutamine	
Valine		Glycine	
		Proline	
		Serine	
		Tyrosine	

*Preliminary evidence suggests that histidine is also an essential amino acid for adults. Some scientists question the essentiality of arginine.

†These substances are sometimes called amino acids.

Nitrogen Is a Partner

Protein differs chemically from fat and carbohydrate in that it contains nitrogen in addition to oxygen, carbon, and hydrogen. Owing to this fact, scientists can analyze the protein content of food or human tissue by determining nitrogen content. This measurement process works for the more complex protein substances but does not measure the smaller amounts of nitrogen found in free amino acids or in such nonprotein substances as ammonia and nucleic acids (components of chromosomes.) Table 7-3 summarizes the contributions of both protein and nonprotein nitrogen sources.

Analysis of nitrogen content has shown that milk is 15 percent nitrogen; cereal is 17 percent; and nuts are 18 percent. Once the nitrogen weight of a food is known, multiplying by the conversion factor of 6.15 will yield the amount of protein. For example, if a food contained 2 g of nitrogen, it would contain 2 × 6.15 or 12.3 g of protein. Table 7-4 presents the protein content of some common foods.

Table 7-3
Functional Contributions by Different Sources of Nitrogen to the Human Body

NITROGEN SOURCE	FUNCTIONAL CONTRIBUTION
Essential amino acids (protein and nonprotein substances)	Most needed by the human body both quantitatively and qualitatively.
Nonessential amino acids (protein and nonprotein substances)	Needed by the human body in quantity. No specific need for any of the particular amino acids.
Other nonprotein substances	Because the body can make them, they are not needed for any specific function. However, when present in a normal and nonpathological condition, they may facilitate different aspects of body metabolism.

Table 7-4
Protein Content of Some Common American Foods

FOOD PRODUCT	SERVING SIZE	PROTEIN (g)
Cheese, natural, cheddar	1 oz	7
Milk, whole, 3.3% fat	1 c	28
Ice cream, regular, hardened	1 c	5
Egg, cooked in any form	1	6
Butter	1 T	trace
Beef, ground, lean, broiled	3 oz	18
Tuna, canned in oil, drained	3 oz	24
Apple	1	trace
Grapefruit	½	1
Bread, white, enriched	1 sl	2
Breakfast cereal, hot, cooked (oatmeal or rolled oats)	1 c	5
Spaghetti, tomato sauce with cheese	1 c	6
Beans, cooked, drained	1 c	15
Peanut butter	1 T	4
Walnuts, English, chopped	1 c	18
Cabbage, raw, shredded	1 c	1
Corn, canned, cream style	1 c	5
Potatoes, cooked, baked (2/lb)	1	4
Beer	12 fl oz	1
Gelatin, dry	7 oz	6
Yeast, brewer's, dry	1 T	3

SOURCE: Adapted from *Nutritive Value of Foods*, Home and Garden Bulletin No. 72 (Washington, D.C.: U.S. Department of Agriculture, 1981).

Protein: A Building Block in the Body

Although our bodies use protein for many purposes, you can best understand its importance by considering how many body components have protein as part of their structure. Enzymes are protein. Hormones, chromosomes, and antibodies all have protein as a structural component. When you consider that enzymes metabolize oxygen and release carbon dioxide, protein's importance becomes clear: It is vital to life processes. Such blood substances as hemoglobin and albumin are plasma proteins. Since antibodies are proteins, protein plays a significant role in infection, a role that is one of the most studied aspects of human nutrition. In our chromosomes, protein is included in a nucleoprotein. Genetically important nucleic acids such as DNA (deoxyribonucleic acid) and RNA (ribonucleic acid) direct the types of protein to be made by the body and predetermine the pattern of amino acids in each protein molecule.

In a child, the absence of protein will terminate growth. This occurs because the second major body function of proteins is the growth, repair, and maintenance of most body structures.

Protein functions in body metabolism. In enzyme form, protein catalyzes many biological and chemical reactions. It also participates in many of these reactions.

The fluid and acid-base balance of our bodies depends upon protein. In maintaining body fluid balance, protein controls osmotic pressure between body compartments (see Chapter 13). If protein deficiency exists, blood volume decreases as fluid moves from blood vessels into interstitial space, and the person becomes swollen with water, a condition known as *edema*. Protein functions in the acid-base balance by serving as a buffer system.

The general public's concept of protein as synonymous with power derives from protein's function as an energy source. If protein is completely oxidized, each gram yields 4 kilocalories (see Chapters 3 and 21).

Protein also has a special role in detoxifying the body. Many detoxification processes are performed by enzymes, which are protein. If protein intake is inadequate, our capability of detoxifying foreign substances that have been ingested is impaired.

Vital to Our Health

Despite the importance of protein to our nutrition, experts do not agree about the exact amount of protein our bodies require. Table 7-5 does, however, provide recommended dietary allowances, which represent an approximation of the need for different age groups. Our minimum need can also be stated in terms of our need for essential amino acids. Table 7-6 presents these needs.

Scientists treat protein need on an individual basis. For children, protein need can be measured in relation to growth, which entails height and weight changes. Based upon this estimation, if height and weight changes are within normal parameters, it is assumed that protein intake is adequate.

For adults, measurement of protein intake adequacy generally depends upon a technique known as **nitrogen balance study**. Measurement of nitrogen intake is compared to measurement of nitrogen loss (urine,

Table 7-5

1980 Recommended Dietary Allowance (RDA) for Protein for Different Age Groups and During Pregnancy and Lacation

AGE (YEARS) OR CONDITION	RDA (g PROTEIN/DAY)
0.0–0.5	Body weight (kg) × 2.2
0.5–1.0	Body weight (kg) × 2.0
1–3	23
4–6	30
7–10	34
11–14, male	45
15–51+, male	56
11–18, female	46
19–51+, female	44
Pregnancy	+30
Lactation	+20

feces, perspiration, skin sloughing, hair loss, and menstruation). If intake exceeds loss, a positive nitrogen balance exists. If intake and loss are equal, **nitrogen equilibrium** exists. Table 7-7 provides some examples of nitrogen balance studies. Table 7-8 shows some examples of different types of nitrogen balance.

Measurement of protein adequacy via nitrogen balance studies has some obvious weaknesses. For example, we have noted that nitrogen content cannot be exactly equated to protein content. Also, a nitrogen balance study would ideally need to be conducted over a period of time so that various body states (eating, sleeping, resting, exercising) could be included in nitrogen utilization.

Table 7-6
Estimated Amino Acid Requirements of Man

AMINO ACID	REQUIREMENT, mg/kg BODY WEIGHT/DAY			AMINO ACID PATTERN FOR HIGH-QUALITY PROTEINS, mg/g OF PROTEIN*
	INFANT (4–6 MONTHS)	CHILD (10–12 YEARS)	ADULT	
Histidine	33	?	?	17
Isoleucine	83	28	12	42
Leucine	135	42	16	70
Lysine	99	44	12	51
Total *S*-containing amino acids (methionine and cystine)	49	22	10	26
Total aromatic amino acids (phenylalanine and tyrosine)	141	22	16	73
Threonine	68	28	8	35
Tryptophan	21	4	3	11
Valine	92	25	14	48

SOURCE: *Recommended Dietary Allowances* (Washington, D.C.: Food and Nutrition Board, National Research Council, National Academy of Sciences, 1980).
Note: The essentiality of arginine is undetermined.
*2 g/kg/day of protein of the quality listed will meet the amino acid needs of infants.

Table 7-7
Hypothetical Examples of Nitrogen Balance in the Human after Ingesting 90–95 g Protein

NITROGEN STATUS	EXAMPLES				
	1	2	3	4	5
Nitrogen ingested (g)	15	15	15	15	15
Nitrogen in feces (g)	1.5	2.0	1.5	1.5	1.8
Nitrogen in urine (g)	10	16	13.8	13.5	13.0
Nitrogen retained by body (g)	3.5	0	0	0	0.2
Total nitrogen lost by body (g)	0	3.0	0.3	0	0
Nitrogen balance	Positive	Negative	Equilibrium	Equilibrium	Equilibrium

Note: All values are approximations.

Table 7-8
Some Common Examples for the Different Types of Nitrogen Balance

NITROGEN BALANCE	MOST LIKELY SITUATION	REMARK
Positive	Growing child	Growth and development
	Pregnant woman	
	Person recovering from an illness	
	Person's diet changed from low to high protein	
Negative	Person receiving surgery or crush injury	Body wasting
	Person suffering starvation	
	Person immobilized	
	Person receiving a low fat and carbohydrate diet	
	Person's diet changed from high to low protein	
	Elderly person*	
In equilibrium	A normal, healthy adult 21–40 years old†	Maintenance; repair of body
	Subject in a human nitrogen balance experiment	

*This is not necessarily true in all elderly individuals.
†This is theoretically true and the exact age limit is not yet defined.

What nitrogen balance studies have shown is that individual differences exist, which means that individual protein need varies. A number of factors determine these variations (Porter and Rolls, 1973).

1. *Body size.* For two healthy, nonathletic persons of different body size, the need for protein per unit of body weight will be fairly similar. The total protein need of the larger person will therefore be greater.
2. *Age.* During the growing years, protein need per unit of body weight is two to three times higher than during the adult years. The increased need for protein stabilizes during puberty. The need for protein during old age is about the same as that for a 25-year-old adult, although some clinical evidence indicates that old people tend to retain nitrogen less efficiently. The possibility that an older person may therefore need to eat more protein than a younger adult is controversial, however.
3. *Sex.* For a man and woman of the same age and weight, the male's requirement for protein per unit of weight is slightly higher. This condition is reflected by the greater body fat and lesser muscle mass in the woman, because protein is essential for maintenance of the muscle or lean body mass. However, in practice, the requirement of 0.8 g of protein per kg body weight applies to both adult men and women.
4. *Nutritional status.* Starvation, wasting, undernutrition, weight loss, and any form of substandard nutrition increase a person's protein need.
5. *Pregnancy and lactation.* A pregnant woman needs more protein for the developing fetus, increased hemoglobin formation, and other physiological adjustments. A nursing mother requires more protein

to make milk protein. See Table 7-5 and Chapter 16 for more information.

6. *Climate*. Low ambient temperature means that the body will need more energy, not more protein. By contrast, high ambient temperature may cause sweating, and excess perspiration means that a significant amount of nitrogen (that is, protein) will be lost. In this case, more dietary protein is needed.

7. *Activity*. Unless it causes profuse sweating, heavy physical activity does not require additional protein, though the need for calories is higher. However, a person who is inactive over a prolonged period—as in lengthy confinement to bed—may require more protein to repair atrophied muscle mass.

8. *Conditioning*. Conditioning may affect body protein requirement in different ways. If a person is provided with a subnormal amount of essential amino acids (as in semistarvation), the body may adjust to the lower supply and eventually decrease the protein requirement for maintenance, repairs, and life processes. On the other hand, when a person starts athletic training, such as in football or weight lifting, an increased amount of protein is needed to build up the muscles for constant repairs, maintenance, and development. However, an *established* athlete needs only a normal amount of protein for repairs and maintenance, and any additional amount will not provide extra benefits.

9. *Dietary components*. If people have access only to low-quality protein, their quantitative need for such protein sources will be very high. The relative amount of carbohydrate and fat in the diet is also very important in protein requirements. If these nutrients are present in subnormal amounts, the body will have to divert part of the ingested protein as an energy source, and some other body functions will suffer.

10. *Emotional stability*. Preliminary evidence indicates that stresses such as fear, anxiety, and depression may predispose the body to excrete more nitrogen, thus increasing body protein need. This increased need may be the result of changes in body hormonal profile.

11. *Diseases*. Illness generally increases the need for protein for a number of reasons. Any form of physical injury that involves tissue loss obviously requires protein replacement. Since the susceptibility to infection is increased during illness, more protein is needed for manufacturing antibodies, and some special diseases such as cancer call for additional protein intake. Body temperature commonly increases during illness with two effects: Increased basal metabolism may increase the need for protein for repairs, and insensible loss due to perspiration will increase nitrogen loss.

Certain nonspecific hormonal responses in the body during illness may increase the need for protein. For example, the increased synthesis and release of adrenal hormones during sickness may increase breakdown of body muscle mass, which in turn increases protein need. Bed confinement, fractures, and other forms of illness may immobilize the patient, forcing the muscles to atrophy. An increase in body protein is needed for their regeneration. Finally, a person with parasites will suffer a great disadvantage, since many parasites such as worms can consume so much of the protein ingested by the patient that he or she may be "starving in times of plenty."

What Is a Quality Protein?

The quantity of our protein intake is of no greater importance than its quality. Nutritional experts have three methods for determining protein quality.

One method relies upon an analysis of biological value. Here we must determine whether the protein contains the essential amino acids in the necessary proportions. If the essential amino acids are present in the correct proportions, a minimum of nitrogen will be utilized after ingestion. If, for example, the biological value of a protein product is 70 percent, then 70 percent of the protein eaten is retained by the body. Table 7-9 shows the biological value of a number of protein foods. The table does not take into consideration the differences in digestibility of the food products.

A second method of evaluating protein quality known as **net protein utilization** does take digestibility into account (see Table 7-9). If you compare the biological values to the net protein utilization, you will see how digestibility varies.

A third method of protein quality evaluation, the simplest method, is called **protein efficiency ratio**. This method requires no chemical analysis and was developed by feeding a specific amount of protein food to a group of animals for a specific period and then measuring growth. Table 7-9 also includes this measurement.

What, then, is a good-quality protein? A good-quality protein is one in which the eight to ten essential amino acids exist in a proportion that reflects our minimal needs. Such a protein is usually made up of half essential and half nonessential amino acids. Most animal protein (with the exception of the animal byproduct gelatin, which lacks the amino

Table 7-9
Biological Value, Net Protein Utilization, and Protein Efficiency Ratio of Various Food Products*

FOOD CATEGORY	EXAMPLE	BIOLOGICAL VALUE (%)	NET PROTEIN UTILIZATION (%)	PROTEIN EFFICIENCY RATIO (USING RATS)
Meat and equivalent	Beef	70–75	70–75	2.1–2.5
	Fish	80–85	80–85	3.3–3.7
Dairy products	Milk	80–85	80–85	2.8–3.4
Egg	Egg	90–95	90–95	3.7–4.1
Grains	Whole wheat	60–65	55–60	1.5–2.0
Beans	Soybeans	70–75	65–70	2.1–2.5
Nuts	Peanuts	50–55	45–50	1.4–1.8

*These data have been obtained from the results of a number of investigators. Because of highly variable results, ranges are provided to serve as a general guide only.

acids tryptophan and lysine) is therefore good-quality protein. When fed
to animals, animal products support growth and maintenance. Such a
protein usually has a high biological value. By contrast, most vegetables
such as wheat (low in the amino acid lysine) and corn (low in amino
acids lysine and tryptophan) will not support growth or maintenance of
an animal when fed as the only protein source. Terms used for this
contrast in both scientific and lay literature are *good* versus *bad, complete* versus *incomplete, high* versus *low biological value* and *high* versus
low-quality protein.

The term **incomplete protein** usually refers to a protein in which one
or more of the eight to ten essential amino acids exist in low or deficient
quantity. Eating such proteins may cause nutritional inadequacies, especially in children. If a protein is grossly deficient in one or more of the
amino acids, a child who has no better source of protein may suffer in
body maintenance, repairs, life processes, and growth. However, if the
lack or deficiency is not too severe, life processes, body repairs, and
maintenance will be normal, though growth may be arrested. Sometimes, the deficient or missing amino acids in vegetable proteins are
known as **limiting amino acids**, for their low content limits or determines the extent to which other essential amino acids can be used. Table
7-10 indicates the different categories of vegetable proteins and the
amino acid(s) that are most likely to be low or deficient in them.

Because Americans eat a lot of animal proteins, protein deficiency in
the United States is insignificant compared with that in many undeveloped countries. However, insufficient protein intake occurs among
many low-income individuals, especially elderly and ethnic populations.
And the increasing trend toward vegetarianism has caused concern
among health professionals, since many vegetable proteins lack certain
essential amino acids. However, under certain circumstances, we can
obtain an acceptable intake of essential amino acids from vegetable
products. This is discussed below.

Vegetarianism

Within the last decade, many young people in this country have adopted
nontraditional lifestyles with nontraditional food choices. Vegetarianism
has become quite common, especially among college students.

The reasons for adopting a vegetarian diet are many, including
health, ethics, economics, politics, ecology, religion, metaphysical be-

Table 7-10
Limiting Amino Acids in Categories of Vegetable Protein Foods

CATEGORY	LIMITING AMINO ACID(S)
Most grain products	Lysine, threonine (sometimes tryptophan)
Most legumes or pulses	Methionine, tryptophan
Nuts and oil seeds	Lysine
Green leafy vegetables	Methionine
Leaves and grasses	Methionine

liefs, and lately, current fads. The overall category of vegetarianism includes various dietary practices, some nutritionally sound and others not. Anthropological, epidemiological, experimental, and clinical studies have indicated that a person can enjoy good health while on a vegetarian diet, whether practiced for a short or long period, although certain vegetarian practices may promote nutritional inadequacies.

DIETARY ADEQUACY

There are three major types of vegetarians: (1) individuals whose diets contain no flesh (meat, poultry, or fish), called **lacto-ovo-vegetarians**; (2) individuals whose diets contain no flesh or milk and milk products, called **ovo-vegetarians**; (3) and individuals whose diets contain no flesh, milk and milk products, or eggs, called strict or pure vegetarians or **vegans** (Anderson, 1982).

Individuals who consume dairy products with or without eggs can receive nearly the same nutrient intake as those who eat animal flesh. This diet can support the young. However, a strict vegetarian, or vegan, must exercise care and comply with certain guidelines to assure a sound diet.

The average body weight of vegetarian adults and children is below reference standards (see Chapter 20). This is because they eat fewer calories and have a low fat deposition. There are no data to indicate whether their daily activities are reduced or whether the lighter body weight poses any problem. Clinical records indicate that heart disease, gout, and diabetes are positively correlated with a higher body weight among those living in the western hemisphere. Does that mean that vegetarians have a better chance of survival? On the other hand, an underweight person is more susceptible to infection, delayed recovery

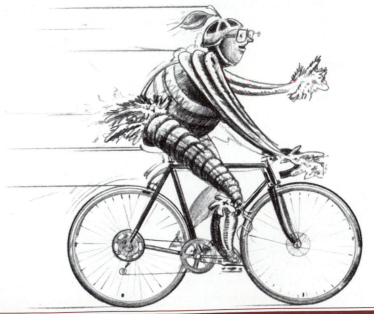

from trauma such as a car accident, and anemia with easy fatigue. Does this mean that vegetarians have a reduced chance of survival? Neither question can be answered from existing data.

If vegetarians eat an adequate quantity of foods, their intake of iron is equal to or higher than that of those who eat flesh. However, there are two points to be noted. First, iron from animal sources is better absorbed than iron from vegetable sources. Second, most vegetarians do not eat an adequate amount of foods, and iron deficiency is not uncommon among them. Nevertheless, its occurrence is not necessarily higher than that for nonvegetarians.

Vitamin B_{12} deficiency has been identified in strict vegetarians, since the nutrient occurs only in animal products. However, its deficiency can be easily prevented by a chemical supplement or an intake of plant foods fortified with vitamin B_{12}, such as soy or nut "milks." Such products are now widely available. It should be noted that symptoms of vitamin B_{12} deficiency may not appear, depending on many circumstances, including masking of the deficiency by a large intake of folic acid from products such as green vegetables and grains (see Chapter 9).

SPECIFIC NUTRIENT CONSIDERATIONS

The nutrient that requires the most consideration in a vegetarian diet is protein. Most animal proteins are complete proteins with the exception of gelatin, which is low in lysine and tryptophan. By contrast, most vegetable proteins are incomplete proteins (low in one or more essential amino acids), with nuts most resembling a complete or animal protein (see Table 7-10).

Because of the world's unequal distribution of animal proteins, scientists have proposed many ways to improve the protein quality of vegetable products. One common method is to add the deficient or limiting amino acids; for instance, lysine may be added to rice. A second method is to combine two or more appropriate vegetable products so that the missing or low amino acids will be mutually supplemented. There are various names for this practice, including **complementary proteins** and **protein supplementation**. For example, wheat, which is low in lysine, may be combined with corn, which is low in tryptophan. In the last decade many strict vegetarians have learned to obtain the proper amount of complete proteins by eating any of the following combinations: grains and legumes (including nuts), legumes (including nuts) and seeds, and grains and seeds. If these foods are eaten separately, the same desired effect can be achieved if the interval between them is less than 2 or 3 hours.

A third method of improving protein quality in a vegetarian diet is to supplement a vegetable protein with a small amount of an animal product. For instance, wheat, low in lysine, may be supplemented with a small amount of milk powder. In addition to using complementary vegetable proteins, lacto-ovo-vegetarians use the following combinations to obtain their share of complete proteins: grains and dairy products, legumes (including nuts) and dairy products, and seeds and dairy products.

Table 7-11
Examples of Different Groups of Vegetable Products

GRAINS	LEGUMES OR PULSES	NUTS AND OILSEEDS	GREEN LEAFY VEGETABLES
Whole rice	Black beans	Sunflower seeds	Brussels sprouts
Whole wheat	Cowpeas (blackeye)	Sesame seeds	Kale
Millet	Mung beans	Sesame meal	Collards
Wheat gliadin	Broad beans	Black walnuts	Asparagus
Whole oats	Kidney beans	Brazil nuts	Turnip greens
Barley	Lima beans	Cashew nuts	Cauliflower
Whole rye	Navy beans		Mustard greens
Corn	White beans		White potatoes
	Various peas		Okra
	Chickpeas (garbanzos)		
	Lentils		
	Green peas		
	Soybeans		
	Peanuts		
	Peanut butter		

Vegetarians must carefully consider the amount of foods they consume. Table 7-11 provides examples of various vegetable products. Those such as grains and potatoes are bulky and have a high satiety value. However, to obtain adequate calories and other nutrients, a large quantity of food has to be consumed. In some cases, part of the protein ingested is metabolized to give calories, thus reducing the nitrogen source and increasing the risk of protein deficiency. To increase protein intake, vegetarians must eat more legumes, or pulses.

The risk of nutrient deficiency among vegetarians cannot be overemphasized. The risk of calories, protein, vitamin, and mineral deficiencies is increased if people depend excessively on one cereal or confine themselves to a small selection of foods. The three micronutrients that may pose special problems are calcium and vitamins B_2 and B_{12}. Ordinarily, calcium and B_2 are obtained mainly from milk, while B_{12} is obtained entirely from animal products.

FOOD GUIDES FOR VEGETARIANS
An adequate diet can be planned without using foods shunned by vegetarians. The major contributions of vegetable products are shown in Table 7-12. Table 7-13 summarizes the four food groups for lacto-ovo-vegetarians; Table 7-14 describes the four food groups for a strict vegetarian. Information for planning menus using these food guides is discussed in Chapters 2 and 15. Table 7-15 gives a sample menu for a strict vegetarian.

As in the foundation diet discussed in Chapters 1 and 15, there are many miscellaneous food items not indicated in Tables 7-13 and 7-14. These foods include sugar and other sweeteners; table fats, other fats, and oils, including salad dressings; and unenriched refined breads, cere-

Table 7-12
Nutrient Contributions of Vegetable Products

FOOD GROUPS	NUTRIENT CHARACTERISTICS
Legumes and pulses (beans, peas, lentils), nuts, nutlike seeds	They provide, among all vegetable products, high-quality protein in good quantity. Soybean formulas that have been fortified are included in this category. The major nutrients provided are iron, niacin, vitamins B_1 and B_2, and others. Nuts and nutlike seeds provide fat, which tends to be low in a vegetarian diet.
Whole-grain or enriched cereals and breads	They provide calories, protein, iron, and some of the B vitamins.
Vegetables and fruits	They provide rich amounts of vitamins and minerals, especially vitamin C. There is a wide selection of this food group. Dark green and leafy vegetables help to supply an adequate amount of calcium and riboflavin, both of which will be lacking if the patient does not drink milk. They also provide roughage or fiber, which promotes motility and the general health of the gastrointestinal tract.

Table 7-13
Food Groups for Lacto-ovo-vegetarians

FOOD GROUPS	MAJOR PRODUCTS	DAILY SERVINGS
Meat equivalents	Legumes, pulses, nuts; textured vegetable proteins (soy meat analogues and other formulated plant protein products and spun soy isolates)	≥ 2
Milk and dairy products	Milk, eggs, cheese, yogurt, many other milk products	≥ 2
Breads and cereal	All varieties	4–6
Fruits and vegetables	All varieties	Vegetables: 3 Fruits: 1–3

Table 7-14
Food Groups for Strict Vegetarians

FOOD GROUPS	MAJOR PRODUCTS	DAILY SERVINGS
Meat equivalents	Legumes, pulses, nuts; textured vegetable proteins (soy meat analogues and other formulated plant protein products and spun soy isolates)	≥ 2
Milk equivalents	Soybean milk, preferably fortified with calcium, vitamins B_2 and B_{12} (if not fortified, supplements, especially vitamin B_{12}, may be necessary)*	≥ 2
Fruits and vegetables	All varieties	Vegetables: 4 Fruit: 1–4†

*Nut milks are nutritionally inadequate, especially for infants.
†Including a source of vitamin C.

Table 7-15
Sample Menu Plan for a Strict Vegetarian Diet

BREAKFAST	LUNCH	DINNER
Orange, 1	Split pea soup, 2 c	Soybeans, 1 c
Bulgur, 1 c	Peanut butter sandwich	Brown rice, cooked, 1 c
Brewer's yeast, 1 T	Peanut butter, 2 T	Fried in oil, 2 T
Wheat-soy bread,	Whole wheat bread, 2 sl	Chestnuts, 2 T
toasted, 1 sl	Honey, 1 T	Sesame seeds, 2 T
Honey, 1 T	Fruit-sunflower seed	Collards, 1 c
	salad	Pear, medium, 1
Snack	Apple, medium, ½	Snacks, ¼ c
Shelled almonds	Banana, medium, ½	
	Sunflower seeds, ¼ c	
	Lettuce, leaf, 1	
	Snack	
	Peach, medium, 1	

SOURCE: Raper, N. R., and Hill, M. M. "Vegetarian Diets." *Nutrition Program News* (July–August, 1973).

als, flours, and meals. Often these are ingredients in a recipe or are added to other foods during preparation or at the table. Although a number of these foods provide some protein, minerals, vitamins, or essential fatty acids, their main contribution is often food energy (calories).

To assure an adequate intake of nutrients, vegetarians should be careful to follow certain guidelines. They should use a wide selection of foods based on the food groups and not limit their diets to a small number of items. An adequate amount of foods should be eaten to provide the caloric requirements and some spare protein; one way of doing this is to increase the amount consumed from each food group. Only a minimal amount of nutrient-light, calorie-dense foods such as candy, soft drinks, sugars, jams, and jellies should be eaten. However, if a person is unable to maintain weight on a vegetarian diet, sugars and fats are needed to provide calories. If dairy products are not consumed, good sources of calcium and vitamin B_2 are dark green, leafy vegetables such as dandelion, kale, mustard greens, turnip greens, and collards; green vegetables such as cabbage, spinach, broccoli, and brussels sprouts; legumes such as soybeans; nuts such as almonds; and dried fruits.

The following three special requirements are important for a vegetarian:

1. Include 2 c of legumes daily to meet calcium and iron requirements.
2. Include 1 c of dark greens daily to meet iron requirements for women.
3. Include at least 1 T fat daily for proper absorption of vitamins.

The use of nutrient supplements may also be necessary.

The pregnant vegetarian provides a special challenge for the nutrition professional, for the diet must meet nutrient needs of mother and fetus without infringing upon the mother's deeply held beliefs (National Research Council, 1982). Especially challenging is the vegan diet, because strict practitioners may refuse nutrient supplements. The vegan dieter is especially at risk of deficiency in iron, calcium, vitamin B_{12}, and vitamin D. If dietary sources are unacceptable, supplemental tablets are necessary. Iodized salt and fluoride also prove necessary. For the lacto-ovo dieter, if sufficient milk and eggs are consumed, supplements necessary generally include iron, iodized salt, and fluoride.

Typically, vegetarians not only promote the avoidance of certain foods but also the avoidance of other practices, such as smoking, taking illicit drugs, or drinking alcoholic beverages. The goal of ingesting only natural foods can, however, lead to avoidance of prescription drugs and even avoidance of traditional health practitioners, such as doctors.

One concern regarding vegetarian dieting during pregnancy is the need for adequate weight gain. Deliberate fasting must also be discouraged. Food guides are available that emphasize food combinations that will yield adequate protein. Such combinations as peanuts with wheat, corn, oats, or rice, and corn or rice with beans are included. Soy flour with wheat or corn and breads and cereals with legumes provide beneficial combinations.

Calcium need places a dietary emphasis on leafy green vegetables, nuts (almonds or filberts), and legumes. Vitamin D need requires a supplement, as does iron. The need for zinc has been established. If high sources, such as oysters, are refused, emphasis must be placed on wheat germ, nuts, dried beans, and whole-grain products. For the vegan diet, vitamin B_{12} must be obtained through a supplement or through a fortified product, such as soy products with B_{12} added.

These realizations demonstrate that vegetarians require special assistance during pregnancy. Part of the need for that special assistance relates to the fact that most nutritional information available for pregnancy is prepared for women who eat both plant and animal products. Vegetarians cannot generally benefit from the information typically available.

HOSPITALIZED VEGETARIANS

Most vegetarians need simple advice on menu planning to achieve a balanced and nutritionally adequate diet. Some are extreme in their habits. Some suffer because of a prolonged adherence to a diet that is nutritionally unsound. The extreme practice of eating only a few food items can produce scurvy, anemia, low blood calcium and protein, body wasting, and kidney malfunction. Iron and zinc deficiencies have been documented. A vegetarian may be hospitalized for nutrient deficiencies, which vary with patient nutrient requirement, food choices, and length of time on the diet.

Two major considerations in caring for vegetarian patients are familiarity with the patient's background and identification of those at nutritional risk. It is also important to determine how the patient handles social interaction. The following questions should be used in evaluating the patient's background:

1. How long have you been a vegetarian? What kind?
2. Do you practice vegetarianism with a group?
3. What are your food choices? (A vegetarian belonging to a group tends to have a wider selection of foods.)
4. What is your ethical and philosophical attitude?
5. What is your diet history?

Because the vegetarian prefers an alternative eating pattern and sometimes even an alternative lifestyle, some hospital staffs may have difficulty accepting the preferences of a hospitalized vegetarian. Therefore, individuals caring for vegetarian patients must make an effort to understand and respect their food choices. Otherwise, the health professional's chief goal of a speedy recovery for the sick may not be achieved.

Protein Supplements and Related Products

While protein proves essential to our nutritional health, it is not the power source that most people believe. No evidence demonstrates that athletes require any more protein than the average person of the same age and size, nor does evidence support the popular belief that protein improves physical performance. The following evaluate some popular claims in the therapeutic values of protein and related products (Dubick and Rucker, 1983).

MUSCLE BUILDING
Despite the evidence, protein continues to be popular among athletes for muscle building. Some nutritionists have advocated that young athletes who are still growing should have diets slightly higher in protein than would otherwise be normal. They recommend a daily intake of about 1.5 g per kg of body weight. Such increases do not, however, require supplements. They can be achieved through the increased food intake that naturally occurs as the result of increased energy expenditure.

Athletes must bear in mind that high-protein diets increase the body's water need. Hence, the higher water content may hinder performance. The high protein intake can overwork the kidneys and liver while depriving the body of its use of carbohydrate, a more efficient energy fuel.

LIQUID PROTEIN DIET
Despite such facts, protein supplements are widely available for various purposes. For example, liquid protein has been promoted for weight reduction programs in which the liquid protein serves as the only energy source in the diet. Numerous deaths have resulted from this weight reduction practice, and dieters have reported other adverse side effects.

The danger in liquid protein diets cannot be overstated. Especially for those who use such products, whether liquid or powder, while concurrently attempting weight loss, the risk of death looms large. The Food and Drug Administration requires a warning label because of numerous confirmed deaths due to use of these products. While the precise cause of death remains unknown, all who have died as a result of taking such supplements have suffered from heart failure. Also see Chapter 20.

GELATIN AND GLYCINE

Gelatin and glycine have been promoted as "ergogenic" foods—foods that improve human performance. Evidence fails to support these claims. Glycine is a major component of gelatin and is a precursor of phosphocreatine, which functions in muscle contraction. Gelatin itself contains only small amounts of most essential amino acids and provides little benefit as a single food.

Positive effects in some patients have been achieved in the administration of gelatin for damaged fingernails (Rosenberg and Osler, 1955; Tyson, 1950). In cases where no dietary deficiency or disease affecting the nails could be found, yet the nails were fragile, peeled and had fissures, 70 g of gelatin taken daily in water or fruit juice resulted in the nails' returning to normal condition in about 3 months.

STARCH BLOCKERS AND GLUCOMANNON

Promotion of starch blockers has been a cause for concern among health professionals. A glycoprotein derived from kidney beans, the primary ingredient of starch blockers, inhibits the enzyme that functions in the digestion of carbohydrate. Promoters claim that starch blockers present an effective aid to weight control (see Chapter 20).

Health professionals are concerned because starch blockers have significant side effects, including stomach cramps, nausea, diarrhea, and vomiting, and could especially be hazardous for diabetics.

A product similarly promoted is glucomannon, which is extracted from konjac root. The product supposedly moves food through the

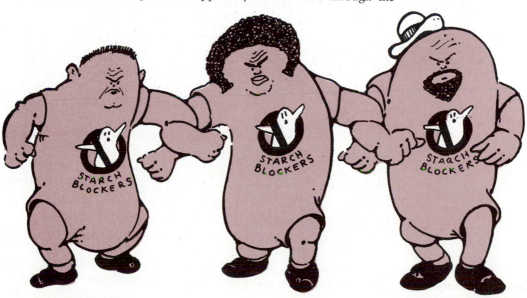

gastrointestinal tract more quickly, thereby preventing weight gain. Promoters claim it has been used successfully in the Orient for centuries.

LYSINE

Lysine is an essential amino acid that has proved effective in treating cold sores resulting from herpes simplex. Lysine is undergoing additional study since it has proved effective in treatment, though it is not a cure. The long-term effects of lysine are unknown.

Studies have also shown that lysine can be effective in some patients in preventing the recurrence of the lesions that characterize genital herpes. The effectiveness of lysine lies in its ability to depress another amino acid, arginine, which is essential to reproduction of the herpes virus. Arginine is found in chocolate and nuts, so patients avoid those foods while orally taking about 1,000 mg daily until they are lesion-free for about half a year. At the first sign of the stinging sensation that signals an attack, resuming the oral lysine can terminate the attack. For those who already have lesions, lysine can relieve the pain in one day and can accelerate healing.

ASPARTAME

Aspartame is a combination of two amino acids, aspartic acid and phenylalanine. It is receiving interest as a nutritional sweetener that may be of some benefit in weight control. The brand name for this product is NutraSweet. Aspartame also has the same food value—four calories to the gram—as regular sugar, so its main appeal to calorie-conscious Americans lies in the fact that it is about 180 times sweeter than ordinary table sugar. A teaspoon of sugar has 18 calories; aspartame would provide only one-tenth of a calorie for the same amount of sweetness in a teaspoon of sugar. Although saccharin is ten times sweeter than aspartame, one of aspartame's appeals is that it has no bitter aftertaste. Aspartame is now available for sale in grocery stores and is being used in soft drinks.

TRYPTOPHAN

Tryptophan is an essential amino acid that functions as an essential ingredient for the brain neurotransmitter serotonin (see Chapter 1). Tryptophan has been promoted as a natural sedative, and it has been used with insomniacs. Megadoses are, however, required, and the long-term effects are unknown.

Doses of 1 to 15 g of tryptophan have enabled people to fall asleep more easily. Tryptophan in 2-g doses taken three times daily has also proved effective in curbing depression. In Great Britain the product is marketed as an antidepressant. Although tryptophan may cause nausea, no serious side effects have been found.

PROTEIN ENZYMES

Various protein enzymes are promoted as aids to digestion or cures for indigestion. Among them are pepsin, papain (from papayas), and pancreatic enzymes. Evidence suggests that such claims are doubtful, given the ability of stomach acid to inactivate such enzymes.

A protein product that is promoted as helpful in cancer prevention is superoxide dismutase. As with other protein products given orally, digestion would prevent the product from remaining intact. Research does, however, continue into the possibility that the drug form of copper-zinc superoxide dimutase may be beneficial in treating arthritis when administered by ingestion.

Most protein supplements have in common the need for further research into long-term effects. One of the concerns in that regard is that taking one amino acid may interfere with the balance with others, owing to the unique amino acid balance discussed earlier.

STUDY QUESTIONS

1. What are the four major elements found in all proteins?

2. Define: amino acid, essential amino acid, and nonessential amino acid. Why is regular consumption of nonessential amino acids important?

3. What are free amino acids? How are they involved in the digestion and absorption of proteins?

4. Why is nitrogen content used as an indicator of protein level in food? How is nitrogen level equated mathematically to protein level? What is the drawback of this method?

5. Discuss at least five important functions of protein.

6. When we talk of protein need, we imply three important premises. What are they?

7. Define nitrogen balance study, positive nitrogen balance, negative nitrogen balance, and nitrogen equilibrium. Give an example of each.

8. Discuss at least eight factors involved in determining individual need for protein.

9. What are the three most common methods of determining the quality of proteins? Which kinds of foods are considered complete proteins? Incomplete proteins? What are complementary protein foods?

10. Do some library research and make a list of health advantages claimed for vegetarians.

REFERENCES

Anderson, J. J. B., ed. *Nutrition and Vegetarianism.* Chapel Hill, NC: University of North Carolina Press, 1982.

Dubick, M. A., and R. B. Rucker. "Dietary Supplements and Health Aids: A Critical Evaluation," Part II: Micronutrients and Fiber. *J. Nutr. Educ.* 15 (1983): 88.

National Research Council. *Alternative Dietary Practices and Nutritional Abuse in Pregnancy.* Washington, D.C.: National Academy of Sciences, 1982.

Porter, J. W. G., and B. A. Rolls. *Proteins in Human Nutrition.* New York: Academic Press, 1973.

Rosenberg, S., and K. A. Osler. "Gelatin in the Treatment of Brittle Nails." *Connecticut State Med. J.* 19 (1955): 171.

Tyson, T. L. "The Effect of Gelatin on Fragile Fingernails." *J. Invest Dermat.* 14 (1950): 323.

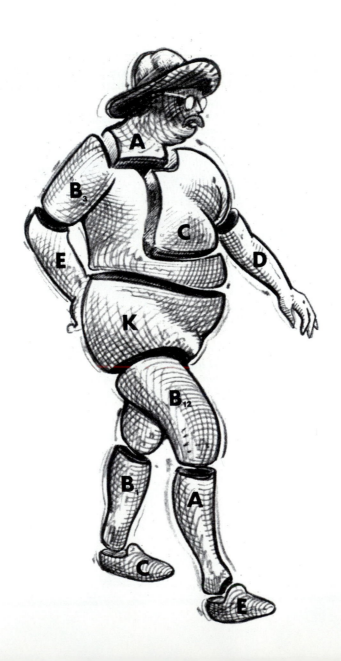

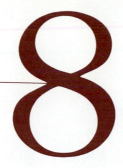

8

Vitamins:

THE SUPPLEMENT QUESTION

Hepatitis From An Overdose Of B Vitamin: A Clinical Report

Sally, who is 23, was admitted to a hospital for severe itching that had persisted for several months, yellowing of skin, dark urine, light stools, and general discomfort and uneasiness. The severe itching, medically identified as pruritus, and the other conditions resulted from jaundice. Sally's history showed she had been taking massive vitamin doses for over two years as treatment for psychological disturbances. The doctors reasoned that the most

likely suspect was nicotinic acid (a B vitamin, see Chapter 9). Sally was consuming 3 grams daily.

A subsequent liver biopsy showed that Sally had acute hepatitis. The administration of nicotinic acid was discontinued. Because of the long history of pruritus, the severe liver condition, and Sally's improvement when nicotinic acid was discontinued, the final determination

was that Sally had a liver disorder resulting from nicotinic acid consumption.

Within the last decade, B vitamins in general and nicotinic acid in particular have received widespread publicity relating to their ability to improve mental conditions when consumed in large doses. The example of Sally is one consequence of this practice. Different investigators have confirmed this trend (Patterson et al., 1983).

Vitamin A Poisoning: Another Case History

Ginger, an 18-year-old woman, complained of tiredness, sore and stiff muscles following exercise, infected finger- and toenails, and dry, cracked skin. Almost two years earlier she had begun taking 300,000 International Units of vitamin A daily (about 90 times the normal requirement) for a skin eruption. Following one month of that therapy, she had continued to take 100,000 to 200,000 units daily, as she found it beneficial for her dry skin.

Ginger had additional problems that included severe headaches, anorexia, and generalized itching that was usually followed by scaling. Her muscle stiffness was so severe that she was unable to walk after bicycle riding. Additionally, her gums had turned bright red.

The physician diagnosed chronic vitamin A intoxication, and Ginger's use of the vitamin was terminated. Within three

months, all symptoms disappeared. She was placed on a low-vitamin A diet with high protein and low fat content (Muenter et al., 1971).

Vitamin A abuse is fairly common. This is partly related to the claim that vitamin A is beneficial for acne and other skin problems. In spite of demonstrated poisoning, many individuals still self-prescribe large doses of vitamin A, which is available without a prescription.

Vitamins: Important to Life

All of us know the word *vitamins*. We attach significant importance to **vitamins**, and we all know they are good for us. Although vitamins, like carbohydrates, proteins, and fats, are organic compounds, vitamins are required by our bodies in much smaller quantities. We know little about the biochemical functions of vitamins, but we do know they serve as coenzymes, a protein substance that facilitates important biological reactions essential to life. Our bodies can manufacture three of the thirteen known vitamins, but the amounts produced vary depending upon circumstances. Because of their importance to life, all thirteen vitamins are considered essential nutrients and must be supplied to our bodies as needed.

Let Us Classify the Vitamins

WATER-COMPATIBLE AND OIL-COMPATIBLE

Individual vitamins have different biochemical functions and perform different essential tasks for our lives. They also differ in chemical structure, but they can be divided into two major classes on the basis of their solubility. These groupings are shown in Table 8-1. If soluble in water, the vitamin is classified as water-soluble. If not soluble in water and soluble only in an organic medium, such as fat or oil, the vitamin is classified as fat-soluble. The major characteristics of water-soluble vitamins can be found in Table 8-2, while those of the fat-soluble vitamins appear in Table 8-3. We will study the individual vitamins in detail in Chapters 9 and 10.

Table 8-1
A General Comparison of Water- and Fat-Soluble Vitamins

CRITERIA	VITAMINS	
	WATER-SOLUBLE	FAT-SOLUBLE
Medium in which soluble	Aqueous, such as water	Nonpolar, organic, such as oil, fat, or ether
Number known to be essential to man	9	4
Number human body can synthesize if precursors are provided	1	2
Body storage capacity	Minimal	High
Body handling of excess intake	Mainly excreted; low toxicity to body	Optimal amount stored, rest excreted; toxicity to body high for two vitamins
Means of body disposal	Urine	Bile; if conjugated, urine
Urgency of dietary intake	At short intervals, e.g., daily	At longer intervals, e.g., weekly or monthly
Rapidity of symptom appearance if deficient	Fast	Slow
Chemical constituents	C, H, and O; S, N, and Co in some vitamins	C, H, and O only

Table 8-2
Major Characteristics of Water-Soluble Vitamins*

VITAMIN	HUMAN DEFICIENCY SYMPTOMS	MAJOR FUNCTIONS	FOOD SOURCES	RDA† ESTAB-LISHED	REMARKS
Vitamin C	Scurvy: loose teeth, bleeding gums, painful joints, bruising, skin hemorrhage.	Healing wounds, collagen formation, utilization of other nutrients, body metabolism.	Citrus fruits, strawberries, cantaloupes, kale, broccoli, sweet peppers, parsley, turnip greens, potatoes.	Yes	Undesirable effects from excess dose. Very unstable substance.
Vitamin B_1	Beriberi: fatigue, mental depression, poor appetite, polyneuritis, decreased muscle tone.	As coenzyme. Metabolism of carbohydrate, fat, and protein.	Pork, liver and other organ meats, grain (whole or enriched), nuts, legumes, milk, eggs.	Yes	Unstable in food processing.
Vitamin B_2	Cheilosis: cracked lips, scaly skin, burning/itching eyes. Glossitis: smooth, red, sore tongue, with atrophy.	As coenzyme. Metabolism of fat, carbohydrate, and protein.	Liver, milk, meat, eggs, enriched cereal products, green leafy vegetables.	Yes	Very susceptible to UV or visible rays of sunlight.
Vitamin B_6	In infants: convulsion, irritability. In adults: microcytic hypochromic anemia, irritability, skin lesions, and other nonspecific signs.	As coenzyme. Metabolism of protein.	Pork, beef, liver, bananas, ham, egg yolks.	Yes	Pharmacological dose occasionally relieves morning sickness.
Niacin	Pellagra (the 4 D's): dermatitis, diarrhea, dementia, death. Also sore mouth, delirium, darkened teeth and skin. Hyperpigmentation.	As a coenzyme in the metabolism of fat, carbohydrate, and protein.	Meat, fish, liver, poultry, dark green leafy vegetables, whole or enriched grain products.	Yes	May be synthesized from tryptophan in body.
Folic acid	Megaloblastic anemia.	Formation of nucleic acids (DNA, RNA). Metabolism of methyl (CH_3) groups. Rapid turnover of cells, e.g., red blood cells.	Pork, liver and other organ meats, peanuts, green leafy vegetables, yeast, orange juice.	Yes	Deficiency probably most prevalent in Western societies.
Vitamin B_{12}	Megaloblastic anemia; neurodegeneration.	Same as above.	Animal products: meat, poultry, fish, eggs, etc. Not found in edible plant products.	Yes	Pernicious anemia infers a lack of the intrinsic factor (see text).

Table 8-2 (*continued*)

VITAMIN	HUMAN DEFICIENCY SYMPTOMS	MAJOR FUNCTIONS	FOOD SOURCES	RDA† ESTAB-LISHED	REMARKS
Pantothenic acid	Nonspecific symptoms: weight loss, irritability, intestinal disturbances, nervous disorders, burning sensation of feet.	As a coenzyme in the metabolism of fat, protein, and carbohydrate.	Widespread in nature. Meat, poultry, fish, grains, some fruits and vegetables.	No	Sensitive to dry heat.
Biotin	In infants: dermatitis. In adults: anorexia, nausea, muscle pain, depression, anemia, dermatitis, and other nonspecific symptoms.	As a coenzyme in metabolism of fat, carbohydrate, and protein.	Organ meats (liver, kidney), egg yolk, milk, cheese.	No	Antagonist, avidin, found in egg white.

*Only an overview is provided. For details and explanations, consult the sections on the individual vitamins in text.
†RDA = Recommended Dietary Allowance, established by the National Research Council of the National Academy of Sciences.

Table 8-3
Major Characteristics of Fat-Soluble Vitamins*

VITAMIN	HUMAN DEFICIENCY SYMPTOMS	MAJOR FUNCTIONS	FOOD SOURCES	RDA† ESTAB-LISHED	REMARKS
Vitamin A	Eye: night blindness, Bitot's spot, partial and total blindness. Skin: dryness, scaliness, hardening and epithelial changes (affecting body surface), mucosa along respiratory, gastrointestinal, and genitourinary tracts.	In the eye: synthesis of rhodopsin, visual pigment. In the epithelium: differentiation. In the bones and teeth: proper development.	Carotene: dark green and yellow leafy vegetables. Dark yellow fruits. Vitamin A: liver, butter, whole milk and other fortified dairy products.	Yes	Large doses may be toxic.
Vitamin D	Infancy and childhood: rickets. Adults: osteomalacia.	Calcium metabolism, especially its absorption from the intestine and mobilization from bones.	Fish, especially liver and oil; liver and fortified whole milk.	Yes	Large doses may be toxic.
Vitamin E	Uncommon in adults. Infants (especially premature): RBC susceptibility to hemolysis.	Not known. An antioxidant in food industry.	Wheat germ, vegetable oils, nuts, legumes, green leafy vegetables.	Yes	Therapeutic effects of large doses not substantiated.
Vitamin K	Prolonged blood-clotting time. Hemorrhage. Delayed wound healings.	Responsible for prothrombin synthesis in liver.	Dark green leafy vegetables; alfalfa.	No	Synthesized by intestinal bacteria.

*Only an overview is provided. For details and explanations, consult the sections on the individual vitamins in text.
†RDA = Recommended Dietary Allowance, established by the National Research Council of the National Academy of Sciences.

INGESTED OR MANUFACTURED IN OUR BODIES

Within the two major classifications of vitamins, further distinction can be made based on whether our bodies can or cannot manufacture or synthesize a vitamin from other ingested ingredients. Three vitamins—A, D, and niacin (another name for nicotinic acid)—can be synthesized by the body, depending upon the availability of the appropriate ingredients. In the process of vitamin synthesis, the ingredient necessary to the conversion process is called a **precursor** or **provitamin**.

Carotene is the precursor of vitamin A, while 7-dehydrocholesterol (a body byproduct formed under the skin with the help of sunlight) and tryptophan (a chemical normally present in meat, cheese, etc.) serve as precursor for Vitamin D and niacin, respectively. When vitamins A, D, and niacin are obtained from our diet, and are thus in a form where conversion is not necessary, they are called **preformed vitamins**.

A process related to conversion, **activation** refers to the metabolic process whereby certain vitamins are ingested in an inactive form and require chemical or biological action before their benefit to our bodies can be realized. Two vitamins require activation: Vitamin D undergoes activation in the liver; folic acid is activated in body cells.

IMPORTANT ROLE IN MEDICINE: CHEMOTHERAPY

Vitamin antagonists, also known as *antivitamins*, *antimetabolites*, or *pseudovitamins*, hold a unique relationship to vitamins. We encounter vitamin antagonists under two different circumstances. They may exist naturally in some of the foods we eat, or they are manufactured by drug companies for specific usages. Though they may or may not be chemically related to their vitamin counterpart, vitamin antagonists can affect the action of vitamins in two adverse ways, by either destroying or displacing the vitamin.

If vitamin antagonists are either ingested or are already present in the body, the vitamins either are rendered ineffective or are pushed out of their proper place in a cell or other body structure. To have this effect, antagonists must be present in a large quantity, known as a *pharmacological dose*. The inability of our tissues, cells, and organs to distinguish between vitamins and antagonists allows both to participate in the bodily processes of metabolism, transport, and storage. If the antagonist's molecules outnumber the vitamins, the vitamin is ousted. Once the antagonist gains occupancy, it proves difficult to displace.

Since antagonists can displace or destroy vitamins, they can cause vitamin deficiency. And because antagonists exist in foods, too much of a food that contains antagonists can directly lead to illness. Fortunately, most vitamin antagonists can themselves be destroyed by heat, and our cooking processes thus destroy most of them. Food sources for vitamin antagonists include egg white, fish, and certain vegetables.

On the positive side, such antivitamins, because of their destructive or displacement nature, can be used to clinical advantage. Such clinical use constitutes a form of chemotherapy and generally utilizes synthetic (man-made) antagonists. When it is necessary to create a vitamin deficiency for experimental purposes, antivitamins can be helpful, especially if the desired deficiency is of a vitamin widespread in foods or one synthesized in the body. Much of our knowledge about deficiency symptoms from certain vitamins has been gained through the use of this unique group of chemicals. A second clinical use, the purest case of chemotherapy, involves the use of antagonists in large doses to treat such disorders as blood clots, cancer, psoriasis, and tuberculosis. The theory behind such treatments is that the antivitamins deprive the unhealthy cells of the vitamins they need for survival. Since such treatment can also deprive healthy cells and organs of the same vitamin, the treatment must be carefully evaluated.

How Do I Know I Have a Deficiency?

Some of us may need to take vitamin supplements to correct an existing deficiency. Others take them to prevent future deficiency. The latter case is generally considered unrealistic and may lead to nutrient imbalances. But the practice is acceptable under certain circumstances, which will be discussed later in this chapter.

The difficulty with determining deficiency lies in the many variables that affect daily vitamin requirements. Human vitamin deficiency typically occurs as a consequence of inadequate intake, malabsorption resulting from conditions such as a lack of bile salts, or increased need resulting from stress, drugs, or excess excretion.

While the causes of vitamin deficiency can be quite complex, a combination of methods makes it possible to diagnose deficiency. First, *clinical manifestations* permit deficiency diagnosis, since certain vitamin deficiencies result in certain specific symptoms. Second, *blood and urine analyses* enable the clinician to determine that the blood and/or urine contains changes indicative of vitamin deficiency. Third, and most popular, *large doses of the vitamin can be administered.* If deficiency exists, normal blood and urine levels will typically not be attained even with the presence of the large dose. This method is not foolproof, however. Certain metabolites or body byproducts may increase with deficiency and decrease with large doses, further complicating the diagnostic process. For such reasons, a combination of diagnostic methods proves necessary.

Vitamins in Food: Our Major Sources

Under normal circumstances, we ingest vitamins from numerous food sources and additionally synthesize small amounts in the body. Our ability to reach daily requirement levels depends upon the foods we eat, how well our bodies synthesize, and how great our needs are. These variables can be complex. For example, many vitamins occur in food in both active and inactive forms. When we ingest a vitamin in its active form, the substance is immediately useful to body functions. A vitamin in inactive form is not. Food processing may release the inactive form. Since our knowledge of active and inactive vitamin forms is limited, our best information on vitamin content in food composition tables may ultimately require revision. Similarly, the quantity of vitamins retained in commercially processed foods varies by type of food, processing techniques, and storage methods. Even fresh foods vary in vitamin content.

Besides the variations in vitamin content of foods, our own bodies vary in their ability to absorb and synthesize. For example, the bacteria in our large intestine, the colon, can manufacture small amounts of certain vitamins. The extent of such synthesis depends on the type and number of bacteria, so the contribution of this source of vitamin varies with the person. Also, drugs such as antibiotics can kill some of the bacteria, thus reducing the amount of vitamin from this source. In addition, some of the vitamins released by these bacteria may not be absorbed, since they may be unable to reach the small intestine, where the absorption takes place.

Natural versus Synthetic: A Controversy

A somewhat controversial distinction has been made between "natural" and "synthetic" vitamins. Naturalness implies that the vitamin can be or has been obtained from a natural source, such as food. Thus, even if the vitamin has been extracted from food before ingestion, it is labeled "natural." Vitamin C from rose hips, B vitamins from liver, and fat-soluble vitamins from fish oil qualify as *natural* under that definition. Vitamins obtained from bacteria or synthesized in a laboratory are considered *synthetic*. There are certain chemical differences between some natural and synthetic vitamins, though the differences are quite subtle.

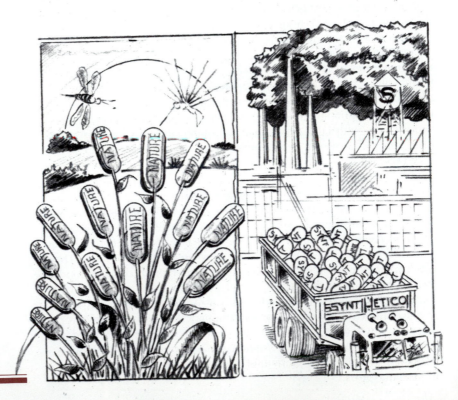

HOW ARE VITAMINS MANUFACTURED?

Many commercial vitamin supplements were prepared from natural, edible sources during the 1940s and 1950s. Since that method of preparation can be prohibitively costly, many of the modern vitamin supplements have been prepared from bacteria which can manufacture vitamins to various extents in their bodies. Many laymen and some scientists maintain that natural vitamins are superior to those produced by either bacteria or laboratory method.

The controversy mentioned earlier surfaces when naturalness is examined. For example, if one pound of fresh liver is dried, 18 mg of vitamin B_2 (in addition to other nutrients in the liver, see Chapter 9) will be present, an amount equal to an adult's requirement for two weeks. A bottle containing a four-month supply of B_2 would contain four pounds of powder. The cost of the liver and the quantity of powder necessary are unrealistic. If the powder is ground, soaked in water, and the mixture filtered, vitamin crystals can be obtained from the liquid by drying or vaporization. The Food and Drug Administration considers such products synthetic rather than natural. Further, there is increasing evidence that vitamins produced from bacteria are added to products labeled natural to increase the vitamin powder's potency. Such processes blur the distinction between synthetic and natural, and create moral and legal issues as well.

ARE SYNTHETIC VITAMINS LESS EFFECTIVE?

Do natural and synthetic vitamins differ in chemical structure, biological activities, and clinical responses? Chemically, the natural and synthetic forms of *most* vitamins are similar, although some are not. To use the best-known examples, vitamins C and E extracted from foods are chemically different from those obtained from bacteria or laboratory methods. The difference is caused by **stereoisomerisms**, or the presence of stereoisomers (that is, compounds with the same structural formula but different in spatial arrangement). However, this difference is rendered insignificant in modern pharmaceutical practices if the biological activity or function of vitamins is considered.

The potency described on the label of a synthetic vitamin supplement accurately reflects the tablet's contents, although the synthetic supplement may weigh more than an equivalent potency of the vitamin found in a natural food source. Numerous studies have, however, confirmed that clinical reactions are similar to both synthetic and natural vitamins. Our bodies cannot tell them apart and do not need to do so.

To Supplement or Not to Supplement: What Is the Fuss About?

Users of vitamin supplements should realize that tablets contain only a small amount of vitamin. The bulk of the tablet contains such inert material as beeswax, paraffin, chalk, shellac, sugar, gelatin, and starch. The amount of inert material varies from supplement to supplement, but when you ingest a great many tablets you are ingesting large quantities of inert materials.

The practice of ingesting large doses of vitamins to prevent or cure disease is currently a source of considerable dispute (Marshall, 1983). Ingesting large quantities of *any* chemical compound is potentially hazardous—and vitamins are chemical compounds. It's a good idea to consider the benefits versus the risks.

The crux of the question regarding vitamin supplements is whether we need to take them at all. Let us look at some examples.

Studies have determined that over one third of athletic coaches recommend vitamin supplementation. B-complex vitamins are especially popular because of their role in energy-release processes. Yet most nutritionists agree that excess B vitamins will not produce extra energy for athletes. The main reason for the nutritionists' position is that athletes obtain sufficient vitamin levels from the foods necessary to supply their heavy caloric demand.

Vitamin supplementation will not replace the need for a balanced diet; our bodies require other nutrients besides vitamins. There are, however, situations in which vitamin supplementation is not only appropriate but also recommended.

Of course, we need vitamin supplements when deficiency exists. A teenage girl anxious to keep her figure trim will diet frequently. If she is not convinced to eat enough food in a varied assortment, she will need a vitamin supplement. Surveys in the past decade have indicated that many poor American children—for example, blacks and native Americans—may suffer vitamin deficiency; lack of money prevents their having a balanced diet. They will need some vitamin supplement, especially at the beginning of treatment, if they are rehabilitated. Eventually, they still need a good diet. Low-income elderly, the infirm, and those recovering from surgery often require supplements.

Infants form a group that has good justification for receiving vitamin supplements. Some are born with low blood vitamins because of the nutritional status of the mother. Some are premature. A milk diet alone does not provide all the needed vitamins. Most infants receive some form of supplements until they are able to eat some solid table foods. Chapter 17 provides a more detailed discussion of the types and amounts of vitamin supplement needed.

Pregnant and nursing mothers generally require some types of vitamin supplements, though the extent varies. Here are some special situations for which a vitamin supplement is especially important:

A nursing mother unable to eat the large amount of food needed to make an adequate amount of milk

A pregnant woman unable to keep down her food because of nausea and vomiting

Some pregnant and nursing mothers who are strict vegetarians

One group of Americans with the greatest problem of vitamin lack is alcoholics. Many of them are so deficient in vitamins from a lack of food or from the direct effect of alcohol that a major part of alcoholic rehabilitation is the use of vitamin supplementation. It is common knowledge among health professionals that some drugs, such as alcohol, have a devastating effect on the vitamin status of some individuals. The drugs may be prescription, over-the-counter, or illicit. These cases require vitamin supplements. Unfortunately, the vitamin lack in this group of individuals is usually undetected.

Perhaps the essence of the supplement controversy can be summed up this way: There are occasions when pills are necessary, but pills are not food.

MEGAVITAMIN THERAPY AND MENTAL ILLNESS: THE THEORY

When vitamin dosages occur at the levels necessary for effective maintenance of bodily processes, the dosage is a *physiological* dosage. A recent trend promotes massive vitamin dosages, ten or more times than the RDAs, as a means of preventing or curing disease. In such situations vitamins are used as drugs, and the dosage level is *pharmacological*. The treatment of disease through massive vitamin dosage, a controversial practice, is called **megavitamin therapy**.

Especially enthusiastic about megavitamin therapy is a group of therapists known as **orthomolecular psychiatrists** (Hawkins and Pauling, 1973). Orthomolecular psychiatrists particularly promote megavitamin therapy as a cure for schizophrenia, but claims have been made for effectiveness in the treatment of mental retardation, senility, hypersensitivity, depression, alcoholism, autism, and learning disabilities. Megavitamin therapy practitioners have formed the Huxley Institute for Biosocial Research and the American Schizophrenia Association. Practitioners also have their own publication, the *Journal of Orthomolecular Psychiatry*. The orthomolecular psychiatrists are at odds with the American Psychiatric Association, which has reviewed their data in regard to schizophrenia and found that the evidence does not warrant the conclusion that megavitamin therapy is effective in alleviating schizophrenia (American Psychiatry Association, 1973).

Primary among the vitamins used in megavitamin therapy for schizophrenia is niacin. Additionally, the therapy utilizes vitamin C and vitamin B_6. Coupled with the administration of massive vitamin doses are more traditional schizophrenia treatment techniques including electroconvulsion therapy, antihypoglycemic diet, and psychotropic drugs (phenothiazines).

Megavitamin therapists theorize that mental illness may result from a low concentration in the brain of one or more specific vitamins. These orthomolecular psychiatrists have also pointed to a recurring relationship between schizophrenia and both hypoglycemia and cerebral (brain) allergy. In the case of both hypoglycemia and food allergies affecting the brain, megavitamin practitioners theorize that megavitamin therapy can be beneficial in treating the resultant schizophrenia, though these circumstances prove the most resistant to therapy.

Megavitamin therapists use two tests to diagnose schizophrenia. The first is a self-administered perceptual test that its proponents claim can yield test scores that detect schizophrenia. The second test measures urinary levels of kryptopyrrole, a body metabolite or byproduct that megavitamin proponents claim is excreted in excessive amounts by schizophrenics. Neither test has been adopted by medical practitioners or clinicians other than those embracing orthomolecular psychiatry.

The psychiatric establishment characterizes orthomolecular psychiatry as a counterculture. Proponents of megavitamin therapy for mental disorders claim that their treatment is so successful that its results cannot be disputed.

VITAMIN C: THE CURE-ALL VITAMIN

Perhaps no vitamin has been used so extensively as a supplement as has vitamin C (ascorbic acid). Since the discovery that ascorbic acid from citrus fruits was the key to the prevention of scurvy, the claims for the vitamin have proliferated (Counsell and Horning, 1982). Many of these claims derive from experiences with scurvy, since the clinical manifestations of the disease are numerous and far-reaching. It seems only logical that, if vitamin C deficiency can result in hemorrhage, fatigue, tooth loss, anemia, fever, convulsions, bone breakdown, skin disorders, ingrown hairs, shock, and death, vitamin C supplement should benefit our bodies in many ways in addition to curing scurvy.

Despite our lack of knowledge about the precise biochemical function of ascorbic acid, it is known to serve as a reducing agent that facilitates the benefit to our bodies of other nutrients such as folic acid (a B vitamin). Vitamin C functions as a cofactor or facilitator relative to the absorption of essential amino acids (components of protein, see Chapter 7). Laboratory evidence indicates ascorbic acid's importance to certain immunologic functions. Vitamin C plays a role in wound healing both in animals and humans. Some proponents have claimed it increases longevity and controls mental dysfunctions such as schizophrenia.

Colds

Once nutritional theories become popular, even misguided enthusiasm can be difficult to change. In the early seventies, a ground swell of support developed for the concept that large doses of vitamin C can prevent the common cold. It was further suggested that massive doses (10 g/day) could terminate a cold even after the appearance of symptoms.

One scientist, Dr. Linus Pauling, theorized that evolutionary processes may have reduced our capacity for vitamin C and that the human diet may at one time have involved ascorbic acid levels as great as fifty times the presently recommended levels. At that level, ascorbic acid intake would more closely approximate the level of intake of chimpanzees, on a weight-for-weight basis.

Dr. Pauling reported studies that statistically demonstrated that vitamin C resulted in fewer cold symptoms. Several investigations have criticized the methods involved in those studies, and other investigators have undertaken studies that failed to produce clinically significant results, but testing has continued. It has, for example, been theorized that vitamin C might function as a mild antihistamine, one capable of decreasing symptoms without affecting the cold itself. Though many theories have been tested, results have been conflicting, leading a signifi-

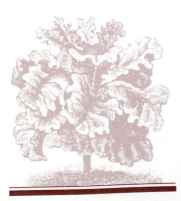

cant number of competent researchers to conclude that vitamin C has no preventive or curative effect on the common cold.

Cancer

Vitamin C is experiencing increasing popularity as a potential cancer treatment. Such treatment involves megadose therapy and has its theoretical basis in anecdotal findings and in successful animal studies.

Experiments with animals have shown that megadoses of antioxidants such as selenium are effective in reducing cancer susceptibility. Since vitamin C and vitamin A possess antioxidant capabilities as reducing agents, it has been theorized that vitamin C can be an effective, or at least a potentially effective, cancer treatment. Suggested benefits include the possibility that ascorbic acid may bring us protection from various physical and chemical carcinogens (cancer-causing chemicals) by reducing their biological activity. It has also been suggested that ascorbic acid's ability to activate the immune system should be logically expected to slow the growth of tumor cells. Further, since vitamin C is known to stimulate the formation of collagen (fibrous connective tissue), such fibrous tissue could theoretically surround and constrain tumor cells.

Although every clinician, physician, and patient hopes that such hypotheses prove true, no clinical trial has yet been conducted to verify these hypotheses. Some studies have failed to reach unequivocal conclusions, and long-term clinical trials are continuing.

LET US LOOK AT THE CLAIMS

Though vitamin C has received considerable attention due to the claims for its benefits, virtually every vitamin has had special claims made on its behalf. Given that three fourths of the American population believes that taking extra vitamins will increase energy levels and given that one in every five of us believes that such diseases as cancer and arthritis occur due to vitamin deficiency, vitamin claims, beyond the elimination of vitamin deficiency symptoms, are a significant nutrition subject. Table 8-4 presents some of the more common claims made for the recognized vitamins (Dubick and Rucker, 1982; Rudman and Williams, 1983).

Table 8-4
Health Claims Made for Selected Vitamins

VITAMIN	SOME HEALTH CLAIMS MADE FOR IT
Water-soluble vitamins	
Vitamin B_1	Part of the B vitamin complex, which, when consumed in large doses, can
	Give a person "energy"
	Protect a person from cancer
	Permit better pregnancy
	Prevent respiratory diseases
Vitamin B_2	As for vitamin B_1

continued on page 168

Table 8-4 (*continued*)

VITAMIN	SOME HEALTH CLAIMS MADE FOR IT
Water-soluble vitamins	
Vitamin B_6	As for vitamin B_1, plus
	Treat schizophrenia
	Treat autism
	Treat neuroses
Niacin	As for vitamin B_1, plus
	Treat schizophrenia
	Dilate blood vessels (hence reducing risk of heart disease)
Folic acid	As for vitamin B_1, plus
	Treat schizophrenia
	Treat hyperactivity
	Treat learning disorders
Vitamin B_{12}	As for vitamin B_1, plus
	Instantly energize
	Treat infectious hepatitis
	Treat multiple sclerosis
	Enhance appetite
	Enhance growth
	Retard aging process
Pantothenic acid	As for vitamin B_1, plus
	Treat personality disorders
	Treat psychoses and neuroses
	Treat learning disorders and dyslexia
Biotin	As for vitamin B_1
Fat-soluble vitamins	
Vitamin A	Prevent and treat cancer
	Treat acne and other skin problems
	Benefits pregnant women
Vitamin D	Build stronger bones
	Treat postmenopausal osteoporosis (bone porousness)
	Benefit pregnant women
Vitamin E	Prevent, reduce, or cure:
	Heart disease
	Muscle weakness
	Cancer
	Baldness
	Ulcers
	Arthritis
	Diabetes
	Skin disorders
	Increase virility and sexual endurance
Vitamin K	Very few claims, most of which are clinical technicalities

Since vitamin C has already been addressed, the other twelve vitamins are listed here with their claims, and they are presented in the order in which you will encounter them in further detail in Chapters 9 and 10.

Obviously, many of the claims are so far-ranging that they instantly invite skepticism among even the most hopeful. Beyond that concern though, lie the very real risks of toxicity.

POTENTIAL HARM FROM OVERDOSAGE

Since vitamins are generally required by our bodies in small quantities, excess supplementation must be carefully watched to avoid toxicity. Such concerns become even more important when promoters champion the use of megadoses as cure-alls for many of the problems that have plagued the human species—aging and cancer, for example—with little or no medical change despite significant research efforts.

Table 8-5
Toxicity Symptoms for Selected Vitamins

VITAMIN	TOXICITY FROM OVERDOSAGE
Water-soluble vitamins	
Vitamin C	Diarrhea
	Nausea, cramps
	Formation of excess oxalic acid in body
	Acidification of urine
	Interference with the use of therapeutic drugs
	Conditioning to a higher requirement both in infants and adults
	Intestinal obstruction
	False positive urine diabetic test
Niacin	Skin burning, flushing, and itching
	Nausea, vomiting, diarrhea
	Liver and eye damage
Vitamin B_{12}	Allergic shock, especially when vitamin is injected
Fat-soluble vitamins	
Vitamin A	Liver damage
	Hair loss
	Bone damage
	Potential birth defects
Vitamin D	Severe high blood calcium
	Brain damage
	Heart damage
	Potential birth defects
Vitamin E	Cramps, diarrhea
	Dizziness, blurred vision, headaches
	Increased serum triglycerides in women (see Chapter 6)
	Decreased serum thyroid hormone in men and women
Vitamin K	Formation of blood clots
	Jaundice in infants

Table 8-5 presents the toxicity symptoms resulting from overdoses of certain vitamins (Herbert and Barrett, 1981; Marshall, 1983). No meaningful information on toxicity is available for those vitamins not mentioned.

Given the severe toxic reactions that can result from excessive doses of certain vitamins, particularly fat-soluble vitamins, those using vitamin supplements are best advised to do so under clinical direction. Certainly the risks of toxicity recommend application of the common adage "all things in moderation."

THE GOVERNMENT TAKES A STAND: TWO CASES
Because of limited resources, the federal government cannot stop all interstate sale of vitamin supplements that carry exaggerated claims and can cause substantial consumer loss in money. But when the amount of money involved is large and many complaints have been brought against certain companies, the United States Postal Service (USPS) is usually the

CLAIMS FOR ATHENA PRODUCTS: GOODBYE TO AGING

ATHENA

Nutrition for Women

50 Tablets

Directions: Take one or two tablets daily as a dietary supplement.

Contents: Each Tablet Contains:

		% RDA
B₂	200 mg.	11,765
Folic Acid	800 mcg.	200
B₆	200 mg.	10,000
B₁₂	1000 mcg.	16,667
Iron	30 mg.	167

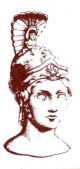

Athena Products, Ltd., with many addresses in Georgia, e.g., Box P.O. Box 81371, Atlanta, GA 30366. The Postal Service Docket Numbers are 10-130 and 10-131 (August 11, 1981).

• Docket No. 10-130: Sale of the product ATHENA NUTRITION FOR WOMEN.

• Docket No. 10-131: Sale of the product META-E.

Both products contain high doses of vitamins.

Athena Nutrition for Women
a. Athena Nutrition for Women retards the aging process. (See "c" below.)
b. Athena Nutrition for Women is effective in the prevention of such conditions as:
   1. fatigue
   2. facial pallor
   3. brittle, dull fingernails
   4. figure-distorting bloating and water retention
   5. hormone imbalance
   6. dry, cracked lips (See "c" below.)
c. Athena Nutrition for Women is effective for:
   1. improving the appearance of hair, skin and nails.
   2. reducing hair loss and thinning.

"Athena contains these nutrients in large enough doses to assure they will help resolve deficiency symptoms. The unique formula can prevent such problems as fatigue, facial pallor and brittle, dull fingernails. In addition, Athena helps improve the appearance of hair, skin and nails, and reduces the hair loss and thinning that accompanies growing older. Then too, Athena aids in the prevention of figure-distorting bloating and water retention, hormone imbalance, and the dry, cracked lips that plague all women as they age.

"No other supplement contains all of the health protecting, age retarding benefits that are found in the exclusive Athena formula."

agency that intervenes, because misuse of the mailing system is involved.

The following boxes provide two typical cases that involved the USPS. In both cases, the defendants were found to be conducting a scheme for obtaining money through the mails by means of false representations in violation of 39 U.S. Code 3005 with respect to the sale of products containing vitamin supplements in large doses and purporting to have special therapeutic clinical effects that were found to be false by the Postal Service. As a result, the postmaster was instructed to hold all defendants' mail relating to the sale of such products or programs.

The accompanying boxes contain (1) Claims and contents of the Athena Products case; (2) Claims of the Maga Research case.

META

NATURAL VITAMIN E
WITH WHEAT GERM OIL
AND LECITHIN

50 CAPSULES

Directions: One or two capsules daily as a dietary supplement or as directed by a physician.

Contents: Each capsule contains:

Vitamin E*	400 I.U.**
Wheat Germ Oil	100 mg.***
Lecithin	100 mg.***

*d-alpha Tocopheryl Acetate from natural sources.
**1333% of U.S. Recommended Daily Allowance
***Need in human nutrition not established.

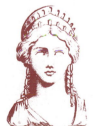

META-E

a. Meta E helps your body's cells utilize oxygen more efficiently so that the aging process is slowed down inside and out.
(See "d" below.)

b. Meta E breaks down fats and cholesterol in blood vessels.
(See "d" below.)

c. Vitamin E, by improving hormone production, has a healthy effect on sexuality and potency.
(See "d" below.)

d. Meta E will effectively:
  1. promote the lungs' self-cleaning mechanism.
  2. bolster the body's immunity response to bacteria and infections.
  3. protect skin fron environmental pollution.

"Meta E is a powerful, nutritional supplement made up of vitamin E and its natural partner lecithin. Vitamin E is one of nature's most dynamic and versatile life support systems. It helps your body's cells utilize oxygen more efficiently so that the aging process is slowed down inside and out. Vitamin E soothes, moisturizes and protects your skin from environmental pollution. And, vitamin E is also vital to proper heart and lung functioning—it actually promotes the lungs' self-cleaning mechanism. Plus, researchers have recently found that vitamin E speeds healing, reduces scarring and bolsters the body's immunity response to bacteria and infections. It has also been shown that by improving hormone production in men and women, vitamin E has a healthy effect on sexuality and potency.

"Lecithin works closely with vitamin E to fight internal pollution. It breaks down fats and cholesterol in your blood vessels, thereby relieving the strain on your heart and arteries."

CLAIMS OF MAGA RESEARCH, LTD.: A BIGGER BUST

Maga Technique Program Maga Research, Ltd., P.O. Box 667, Lynbrook, NY 11563. The Postal Service Docket Number was 12/101 (February 22, 1982). This company sold a special program through the mail. Part of the program contained capsules with large doses of vitamins.

(a) The MAGA TECHNIQUE program will cause a substantial increase in the size of the female user's breasts in a short period of time.

The advertisement, in the form of an article, begins, "Thousands of women, young and old, may be shopping for larger bras this season thanks to a Doctor's newly tested and proven breast enlargement technique." After a week on the program a woman often will "actually see a 1″ to 3″ improvement. Her breasts stand out more prominently, her cleavage is already beginning to make male eyes pop, and likely she's ready to start shopping for new bras. But that's only the beginning . . ."

(b) The MAGA TECHNIQUE program will cause a dramatically visible change in the female user's bust almost immediately.

(c) Any woman will achieve a dramatic new bustline in just one week by using the MAGA TECHNIQUE program.

(d) The MAGA TECHNIQUE program will often produce a 1 to 3 inch increase in the female user's bustline measurement in one week.

(e) The DI-AMATHENE capsules are an integral and essential part of the MAGA TECHNIQUE program and make a material contribution to the promised results.

"After the initial consultation a woman is given the Maga Technique program. Di-Amathene capsules and all, to use in the privacy of her own home. From there, it's up to her. She can follow the program and take 3 capsules daily for 'nutritional insurance' and dramatically visible changes in her bust start to take place almost immediately!"

"Now for the best news of all. The complete Maga Technique program, Di-Amathene vitamin supplement and all, *is* available by mail to women who want the same results but who can't visit the Maga Research clinic. Is this the exact same package which women receive at the clinic? The answer is 'Yes!'"

(f) The breast and bustline improvement claims enumerated in subparagraphs (a) through (e) above have been substantiated by competent medical and clinical tests.

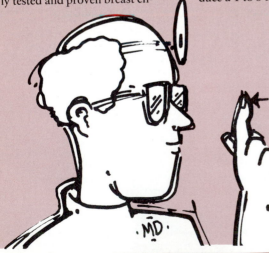
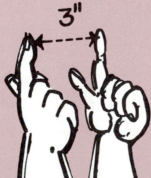

A FINAL CAUTION

Because the importance of vitamins is generally acknowledged, the temptation is to think that more is better. Businesses are built around that belief, at considerable expense to consumers. We have seen that claims are often exaggerated, and frequently unfounded. In the final analysis, there is no substitute for a balanced diet and regular medical checkup.

STUDY QUESTIONS

1. What is a vitamin? How do vitamins differ from other organic compounds?

2. Which vitamins can be synthesized by the body? Which ones must be activated by the body before they can perform their major biological functions?

3. What is a vitamin antagonist? What harm can it cause? How are vitamin antagonists used clinically?

4. What is misleading about the distinction between natural and synthetic vitamin supplements?

5. What three methods are used in diagnosing vitamin deficiency?

6. Make a list of claims about the "goodness" of natural vitamins. Can you challenge their validity? Support your arguments.

7. Do some library research to describe another postal violation by individuals purveying vitamin products with unsubstantiated claims.

REFERENCES

American Psychiatry Association, Task Force on Vitamin Therapy in Psychiatry. *Megavitamins and Orthomolecular Therapy in Psychiatry.* Washington, D.C.: American Psychiatry Association, 1973.

Counsell, J. N., and D. H. Horning. *Vitamin C (Ascorbic Acid).* Englewood, N.J.: Applied Science Publishers, 1982.

Dubick, M. A., and R. B. Rucker. "Dietary Supplements and Health Aids: A Critical Evaluation." Part 1: Vitamins and Minerals. *J. Nutr. Educ.* 15 (1982): 47.

Hawkins, D., and L. Pauling. *Orthomolecular Psychiatry: Treatment of Schizophrenia,* San Francisco: Freeman, 1973.

Herbert, V., and S. Barrett. *Vitamins and "Health Foods": The Great American Hustle.* Philadelphia: George F. Stickley, 1981.

Marshall, C. W. *Vitamins and Minerals: Help or Harm?* Philadelphia: George F. Stickley, 1983.

Muenter, M.D., et al. "Chronic Vitamin A Intoxication in Adults: Hepatic, Neurological, and Dermatologic Complications." *Am. J. Med.* 50 (1971): 129.

Patterson, D. J., et al. "Niacin Hepatitis." *Southern Med. J.* 76 (1983):240.

Rudman, D., and P. J. Williams. "Megadose Vitamins: Use and Misuse." *N. Engl. J. Med.* 309 (1983): 488.

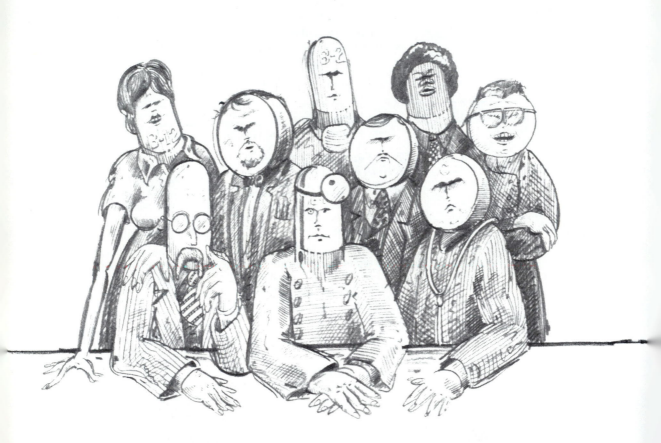

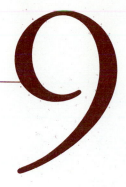

9

WATER-SOLUBLE VITAMINS:

WILL THEY CURE DISEASES?

JERRY PRESENTED A BAFFLING CASE

When he was 10, Jerry underwent treatment for lymphocytic leukemia. His treatment consisted of chemotherapy. He then developed leukemia of the central nervous system, which was also treated with drugs.

Four months later, Jerry's central nervous system leukemia seemed to reappear. This time he did not respond to the drug treatment and was then given radiotherapy.

Two years later, while in remission, he was readmitted to the hospital for a possible relapse. Owing to severe dental problems that made solid foods difficult to chew, he had been on a diet of mashed potatoes, bread, and soft drinks for 3 months. When admitted to the hospital, Jerry had headaches, vomiting, and anorexia.

Five days after admission, his symptoms began to worsen dramatically. He became disoriented, had memory lapses, was very sleepy, and could no longer perform simple mathematical calculations. Neither drug therapy nor radiotherapy had any effect on the symptoms. Jerry's symptoms worsened, and he developed "bilateral sixth nerve paralysis."

Doctors were not able to determine the exact cause of the paralysis. Because of Jerry's poor dietary history, a high dose of thiamine (vitamin B_1) was given on a trial basis. Minimal mental improvement occurred in the first hour.

Within 16 hours of thiamine treatment, definite improvement was obvious. Within a day and a half, Jerry was oriented, and the paralysis began to dissipate.

The doctors concluded that the treatment for leukemia had aggravated a marginal dietary inadequacy, a problem made worse by the vomiting induced by chemotherapy (Shah and Wolff). Jerry was diagnosed as having Wernicke's encephalopathy, a syndrome ascribed to thiamine deficiency. Wernicke's syndrome can lead to death if adequate treatment is not administered early in its development.

Potential Lifesavers?

Thiamine (vitamin B_1) is one of the water-soluble vitamins. Although each vitamin is a unique **organic compound** having its own biochemical and physiological functions and its own chemical structure, vitamins are conveniently classified into two groups, water-soluble and fat-soluble, as discussed in Chapter 8. Of the thirteen known vitamins, nine belong to the water-soluble group: vitamins C, B_1, B_2, B_6, niacin, folic acid, vitamin B_{12}, pantothenic acid, and biotin. The familiar term vitamin B complex usually includes all known water-soluble vitamins other than vitamin C. In Jerry's case, thiamine saved a life. Clinical reports have confirmed that practically all water-soluble vitamins can play a similar critical role under various circumstances.

Vitamin C (Ascorbic Acid)

Vitamin C (ascorbic acid) was discovered and isolated in 1932, though its importance had been known long before in relation to scurvy among

British sailors who lacked access to citrus fruits. Vitamin C was synthesized in 1934. Our bodies cannot store large amounts of vitamin C, so blood levels of the vitamin reflect recent intake and are measurements of the white crystal L-ascorbic acid, the chemically active form of vitamin C. Storage occurs in the *adrenal cortex* and generally is sufficient for 90 days. If no vitamin C is ingested in that period, scurvy symptoms develop. Excess vitamin C is excreted in the urine.

GENERAL CHARACTERISTICS

Vitamin C is the most active reducing agent in living substances and therefore plays an important role in the body's nutritional processes. Its acidity maintains iron in ferrous form, increasing iron absorption. Vitamin C similarly facilitates calcium absorption and thus enables adequate calcification of our teeth and bones. It serves an essential role in converting folic acid from its inactive to active form. Vitamin C's necessity in synthesizing two of the neurotransmitters that transmit nerve impulses between cells is such that the deficiency of those two neurotransmitters results in fatigue and weakness characteristic of vitamin C deficiency.

A major role of vitamin C occurs in relation to cellular connective tissue. **Collagen** is an insoluble protein within connective tissue and is found in skin, cartilage, tendons, ligaments, bones, teeth, and blood vessels. Vitamin C enables synthesizing of two major amino acids in collagen, and collagen holds cells and tissues together in an organized manner. When vitamin C is not present for this major role in collagen synthesis, **scurvy** results.

Table 9-1 presents the 1980 RDAs of vitamin C for different age groups. When vitamin C is deficient, the symptoms of scurvy directly follow. They include fragile blood vessels that rupture easily, resulting in diffuse tissue bleeding, pinpoint (petechial) hemorrhage, and bleeding in the joints and gums. Since collagen is a primary part of our skin, wound healing is adversely affected by vitamin C deficiency, leading many clinicians to recommend 100 to 300 mg of vitamin C both before and after an operation. Individuals with scurvy, especially children, develop bone fractures and malformations, since bones contain collagen, and the vitamin C deficiency adversely affects collagen synthesis.

Table 9-1
1980 RDAs for Vitamin C

POPULATION GROUP	VITAMIN C RDA (mg)
Infants	
0–12 months	35
Children	
1–10	45
11–14 years	50
Males and females	
15 + years	60
Pregnancy	+ 20
Lactation	+ 40

INFANTILE SCURVY

A dramatic reduction in the incidence of scurvy in infants can be attributed to development of fortified commercial formulas for infants. Though maternal deficiency can affect breast milk, vitamin C deficiency is uncommon in breast-fed infants. Infants truly at risk are those fed only pasteurized milk and receiving no vitamin C supplement. Current belief holds that an expectant mother's excessive intake of vitamin C can precondition the child to a higher than normal need for vitamin C, thus creating the likelihood of scurvy even if the child's subsequent intake is normal. A child can develop scurvy in 3 to 12 months of inadequate dietary intake. Symptoms can be reversed by the administration of 25 mg of vitamin C four times per day.

Table 9-2
Vitamin C Deficiency and Symptoms of Scurvy (One Study)

DAYS ON DEFICIENT DIET	URINARY VITAMIN C LEVEL	EXTENT OF SCURVY SYMPTOMS*
29	0	Petechial or pinpoint hemorrhage
90	0	Most of the known symptoms from mild to severe

*In this study, symptoms are reversed when patient is given 6.5, 66.5, or 130 mg of vitamin C.

ADULT SCURVY

Scurvy rarely occurs in adults except among chronic alcoholics, mental patients, and individuals who avoid fruits and vegetables. After dietary depletion, it takes 3 to 7 months for an adult to develop scurvy. Table 9-2 presents the results of an experimental study regarding scurvy symptoms.

Early scurvy symptoms in adults include appetite loss, fatigue, irritability, muscle and joint pain, weight loss, and skin lesions on torso and extremities. The victim coughs frequently and becomes feverish. More advanced symptoms include those discussed earlier, and death can occur from internal hemorrhage. Adult scurvy is treated with 250 mg of vitamin C four times daily for 1 to 2 weeks, followed by a dosage of 50 to 100 mg at the same frequency until healing occurs. Figures 9-1, 9-2, and 9-3 depict scurvy symptoms.

FOOD SOURCES OF VITAMIN C

The finest sources of vitamin C are citrus fruits, tomatoes, and green vegetables. Though potatoes and root vegetables are low in vitamin C, they constitute important sources in our diets because we consume such large amounts of them. (The vitamin C content of representative foods is found in the Appendix.)

Although certain foods are high in vitamin C content, the vitamin is highly unstable, and its benefit is easily lost. For example, cooking destroys 50 to 90 percent of the vitamin C in foods. Since the vitamin is water-soluble, it can be leached by water. It is sensitive to air, heat, and light, and is therefore easily oxidized. The longer that fruits are allowed to ripen, the higher their vitamin C content. Refrigerated storage, high humidity, and minimal air movement preserve the content.

COMMERCIAL USE

In the United States, tons of vitamin C are manufactured daily for use as a nutrient supplement and as a food additive. Used as a color stabilizer in fruit cocktail, as a dough conditioner in white flour, as a preservative in jams and jellies, as a supplement to fruit juices, and as a color and flavor preservative in beer and wine, vitamin C finds its way into our diet through many commercial routes.

Figure 9-1: Healed scorbutic rosary in a boy who had had scurvy off and on since infancy. The sharp edges of the ribs are easily visible. SOURCE: R. W. Viller. "Effect of Ascorbic Acid in Man." In The Vitamins: Chemistry, Physiology, Pathology, Methods, W. H. Sebrell and R. S. Harris, eds. New York: Academic Press, 1967, p. 468. Used with permission of Academic Press.

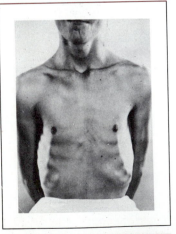

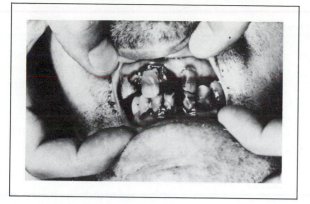

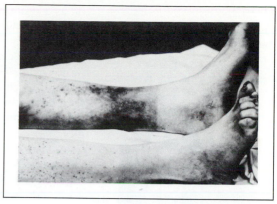

WHAT ABOUT THOSE HIGH DOSES?

Since so many people ascribe to the unproven belief that vitamin C should be supplemented whenever possible to avert colds, any discussion of vitamin C must address the risk of excessive intake (Basu and Schorah). First, large dosages can condition us to needing abnormally high amounts of vitamin C. Sudden reduction can then precipitate scurvy. Second, large doses of vitamin C can negatively affect other therapeutic drugs. For example, large doses can offset the effect of anticoagulants. Third, vitamin C tablets contain other ingredients, such as sodium. Excessive sodium is thought to be related to high blood pressure. Finally, large doses of vitamin C can cause diarrhea, which results in a loss of nutrients.

Vitamin B₁ (Thiamine)

Originally called thiamin or thiamine, vitamin B_1 was discovered in 1921, isolated in 1926, and created synthetically in 1936.

GENERAL CHARACTERISTICS

A white, crystalline substance, thiamine is highly subject to oxidation and high temperatures. It is essential to metabolism, especially the metabolism of carbohydrate. It also serves an essential function in the nerve cell membranes for transmitting high-frequency impulses.

Our need for vitamin B_1 depends on our calorie intake. The greater our consumption of carbohydrate, the greater our thiamine need. (The RDAs for this vitamin can be found in the Appendix.) Excess intake does not present the dangers that excess vitamin C intake does, although intravenous dosage can cause allergic reaction. Absorption can reach the level of 2 to 5 mg per day, primarily in the duodenum. Little of the vitamin is stored, but what is stored is located in the heart and brain tissues. Excessive intake is excreted in the urine.

DEFICIENCY CAN BE FATAL

Thiamine deficiency can occur if intake is too low, or if carbohydrate intake is so high that all the thiamine ingested is utilized in metabolic processes. Deficiency can also occur if triggered by folic acid deficiency

Figure 9-2 (Left): Gingivitis (inflammation of the gums) in a patient with severe scurvy. SOURCE: R. W. Viller "Effect of Ascorbic Acid in Man." In The Vitamins: Chemistry, Physiology, Pathology, Methods, W. H. Sebrell and R. S. Harris, eds. New York: Academic Press, 1967, pp. 465-466. Used with permission of Academic Press.

Figure 9-3 (Right): Bruising (ecchymosis and petechiae pinpoint bleeding in patient with vitamin C deficiency. SOURCE: S. Driezen. Geriatrics 29 (1974): 97. By permission.

and as a result of stresses such as alcoholism, anorexia, vomiting, and drug therapy. Of these last four conditions, Jerry had all but alcoholism.

If deficiency is moderate to severe, **beriberi** results. "Beriberi," literally meaning "I can't; I can't," brings extreme weakness. In the absence of B_1, pyruvate (lactate), a byproduct of carbohydrate metabolism, accumulates in the body, damaging the central nervous system, the heart, the circulation, and the alimentary tract.

Beriberi commonly occurs in Oriental countries where large quantities of refined rice are consumed, since the B_1 content is lost when rice husks are discarded. The problem is severe enough so that in the Philippines, for example, beriberi ranks as the fourth or fifth leading cause of death. Other practices such as low caloric intake, consumption of raw fish, and chewing of tea leaves further aggravate B_1 deficiency. Both raw fish and tea leaves contain a thiamine antagonist (see Chapter 8), thiaminase, which is destroyed by cooking. Vitamin B_1 deficiency occurs in 20 to 30 percent of the United States population, most commonly among alcoholics and among dieters who drastically reduce carbohydrate and fat intake.

ADULT BERIBERI

In adults, beriberi initially results in weak extremities, depression, irritability, disordered thinking, loss of appetite, tiredness, nausea, vomiting, and constipation. Rapid heartbeat, loss of motor coordination, and numbness of legs characterize beriberi victims.

In an advanced stage, beriberi is of two types. Patients with *wet beriberi* exhibit facial and lower body edema (swelling). In some patients the heart swells as it attempts to deliver more thiamine to the body's tissues. Breathing difficulties may occur. Death can result from circulatory shock and cardiac failure. *Dry beriberi* resembles degenerative nerve disease. The victim cannot walk properly, becomes emaciated, and lacks muscular control. Victims cannot rise after squatting because they cannot control their muscles—a symptom used to diagnose dry beriberi in the Orient. If the victim is not treated, immobility and death by infection result. Figure 9-4 depicts beriberi edema.

Vitamin B_1 deficiency in alcoholics and in pregnant women experiencing excessive vomiting results in neurological problems, termed **Wernicke-Korsokoff syndrome**, or Wernicke's syndrome. Characteristics include loss of memory, mental deterioration, abnormal perception, and loss of eye control. Without treatment, sudden heart failure occurs. Table 9-3 shows the relationship between brain thiamine and symptoms.

To avoid irreversible brain damage, thiamine deficiency must be treated quickly. Intramuscular doses of up to 100 mg may be given three or four times per day in severe cases, with dosages tapering off to oral therapy of 5 to 10 mg. Treatment often includes other B vitamins as well. Yeast, rice husk, liver extract, or wheat germ can be given as well.

INFANTILE BERIBERI

In children under 6 months of age, thiamine deficiency disease is called *infantile beriberi*. Though rare in the United States, infantile beriberi

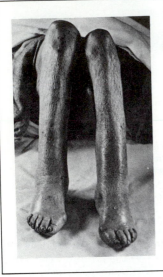

Figure 9-4: *Wet beriberi with edema of the legs.*
SOURCE: *S. Dreizen. Geriatrics 29 (1974): 97. By permission.*

Table 9-3
Relationship Between Neurological Symptoms of Beriberi and Brain Level of Thiamine

BERIBERI SYMPTOM	BRAIN LEVEL OF THIAMINE (% OF NORMAL)
None	50
Slow and steady gait	30
Severe disturbance of posture equilibrium	20

commonly occurs in developing countries, especially among breast-fed children. Cow's milk contains twice the thiamine of mother's milk. If the nursing mother is B_1 deficient, her blood may contain methyl glyoxal, a metabolic byproduct of thiamine deficiency that does not harm the mother but is toxic to the infant.

The infant beriberi victim becomes pale and restless, is unable to sleep, and has a poor appetite. If the disease is severe, the victim has a rapid heartbeat, breathing difficulty, and cyanosis (blueness of the face). Edema, diarrhea, muscle wasting, and crying weakness are characteristic. The disease generally strikes between the ages of 2 months and 6 months and can go from initial symptoms to death in two days. Treatment can have equally dramatic results, as it did in Jerry's case. A dose of 2.5 mg of B_1 can reverse the symptoms in a few hours. In cases of severe heart failure, convulsions, and coma, intravenous doses of 25 to 50 mg may be followed by intramuscular injections.

FOOD SOURCES OF THIAMINE

Whole and enriched grains, pork, and legumes constitute the richest sources of thiamine, though beef, eggs, milk, liver, kidney, fish, green vegetables, and some fruits are also relatively good sources. (The thiamine content of representative foods is found in the Appendix.) Table 9-4 presents the contribution of thiamine in the American diet. In 1941, the United States began mandatory enrichment of bread and flour, and that program has undoubtedly prevented thiamine deficiency in many individuals, especially alcoholics. Although foods such as dried brewer's yeast and wheat germ are thiamine rich, they cannot be considered primary sources because such small quantities are consumed by most people.

Cooking processes such as boiling and stirring destroy thiamine by exposing it to oxygen. The soaking of grains and other dried legumes similarly eliminates thiamine, unless the water is reused. Thiamine is additionally sensitive to heat and alkalinity. Baking soda, used to preserve the green color of vegetables, destroys both vitamin B_1 and vitamin C, and the use of sulfite as a preservative also destroys thiamine.

Vitamin B_2 (Riboflavin)

Also known as riboflavin, vitamin B_2 was discovered in 1932, isolated one year later, and synthesized three years later.

GENERAL CHARACTERISTICS

Although the yellow-orange crystals of vitamin B_2 are stable to heat, acid, and oxidation, the vitamin is highly sensitive to the ultraviolet rays of sunlight. The vitamin is absorbed through the mucosa (lining) of the small intestine and is stored in small amounts in the liver and kidneys. Large doses are nontoxic, and 60 percent of the amount ingested is absorbed when in the presence of food.

Riboflavin makes many biological reactions possible in our bodies. Metabolically, it enables energy metabolism, transformation of folic acid to its coenzyme (a process involved in DNA regulation and protein

Table 9-4
Approximate Contribution of Thiamine to the American Diet by Different Categories of Food

FOOD GROUP	% OF DAILY THIAMINE INTAKE
Cereal products	30–40
Meat, poultry, fish	25–35
Fruits, vegetables	15–25
Dairy products	5–10
Dry beans, peas, nuts	5–10
Eggs	0– 5

Table 9-5
1980 RDAs for Riboflavin

POPULATION GROUP	RIBOFLAVIN RDA (mg)
Infants	
0–6 months	0.4
6–12 months	0.6
Children	
1–3 years	0.8
7–10 years	1.4
11–14 years	
Male	1.6
Female	1.3
Adolescents (15–18 years)	
Male	1.7
Female	1.3
Adults	
Male	
19–22 years	1.7
23–50 years	1.6
50 + years	1.4
Female	
19–22 years	1.3
23 + years	1.2
Pregnancy	+ 0.3
Lactation	+ 0.5

Table 9-6
Approximate Contribution of Vitamin B_2 to the American Diet by Different Categories of Food

FOOD GROUP	% OF DAILY RIBOFLAVIN INTAKE
Dairy products	40–45
Meat, poultry, fish, eggs	25–35
Cereal products	10–20
Fruits, vegetables	5–15
Dry beans, peas, nuts	0– 5

synthesis), degradation of fatty acids, glycogen formation, and production of red blood cells in bone marrow. It facilitates the transfer of hydrogen atoms. It is also a component to the respiratory chain.

DEFICIENCY DOES NOT CAUSE A DISEASE

Table 9-5 presents the 1980 RDAs for riboflavin. Riboflavin deficiency occurs primarily in underdeveloped countries. In the United States, adolescent girls, chronic alcoholics, and the elderly are often subnormal in riboflavin intake. Deficiency often occurs in combination with niacin deficiency.

Riboflavin deficiency results from inadequate intake, intestinal malabsorption, and clinical stresses such as burns, surgery, trauma, tuberculosis, rheumatic fever, cancer, and starvation. Deficiency does not result in a specific disease, as do vitamin C and B_1 deficiency.

Deficiency symptoms include depression, hysteria, personality changes, weakness, and general malaise. Two specific symptoms are **cheilosis** (crusted cracks at the corners of the mouth) and **glossitis** (smooth, red tongue with surface swelling). Some victims exhibit greasy, scaly, dry skin. The skin changes will occur at the base of the nose, corners and edges of the eyes, ear folds, chin, and genital and groin areas. Eye complaints have included swelling, discharges, inflammation, and ulceration; however, these conditions also occur with other B vitamin deficiencies. Treatment with 5 mg two to three times per day will eliminate symptoms in two weeks or less.

FOOD SOURCES OF RIBOFLAVIN

Riboflavin occurs in muscle meats, liver, kidney, heart, milk, eggs, leafy and yellow vegetables, and enriched cereals and bread. Only a few foods, such as sugar and fats, are low in vitamin B_2. Cooking vegetables can deplete 10 to 40 percent of the vitamin, and the loss increases if the vegetable is cut into small pieces or cooking is prolonged. Although milk is a primary source of the vitamin in our diet, 50 to 80 percent of the B_2 content can be lost if milk is exposed to sunlight for 4 to 6 hours.

Table 9-6 provides the contribution by various food categories. (The riboflavin content of some representative foods is found in the Appendix.) The vitamin can be synthesized by the bacteria in the large intestine, but absorption is not high.

Vitamin B_6 (Pyridoxine)

Vitamin B_6, sometimes called **pyridoxine**, was discovered in 1934, isolated four years later, and synthesized in 1939.

GENERAL CHARACTERISTICS

It is unstable to alkali, ultraviolet light, and oxidation but stable to heat and acid. As Table 9-7 shows, B_6 occurs in three forms in food, each of which has a coenzyme in our body. The body stores very little vitamin B_6, a relatively nontoxic substance, though a few toxicity cases have been reported when dosage exceeded 300 mg per day.

The vitamin serves as a coenzyme in various metabolic processes. In the degradation of amino acids, it serves a role in protein metabolism. It is involved in the production of antibodies necessary to healing processes. It also serves in the degradation of glycogen.

DEFICIENCY IS RARE

Since we require only small amounts of vitamin B_6, and it is widely available, B_6 deficiency is rare. (The RDAs as established in 1980 are found in the Appendix.) Deficiency occurred in the 1950s in infants fed sterilized commercial milk formula. A genetic defect can also result in infant deficiency. Some adult anemia will respond to B_6 treatment, as will the infant deficiencies.

Chronic alcoholism, hypothyroidism, and high-protein diet can increase our need for vitamin B_6. Inadequate intake, clinical stresses, and intestinal malabsorption can lead to deficiency. Oral contraceptives, which contain estrogen, increase the need for B_6. Medications such as penicillamine, used to treat rheumatoid arthritis, and isonicotinic acid hydrazide (INH), used to treat tuberculosis, also increase the need—or cause deficiency in the case of INH, an antagonist to B_6.

Table 9-7
Three Chemical Forms of Vitamin B_6

NAME OF VITAMIN IN FOOD AND BLOOD	NAME OF COENZYME IN BODY
Pyridoxine	Pyridoxal phosphate
Pyridoxamine	Pyridoxamine phosphate
Pyridoxal	Pyridoxal phosphate

A TREATMENT FOR PREMENSTRUAL SYMPTOMS?

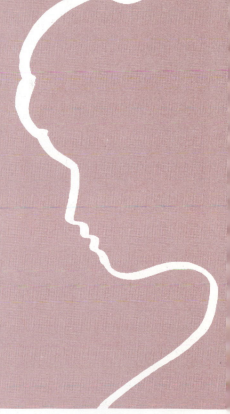

Thirty-year-old Marianne was almost unable to walk when she sought medical attention. For two years she had been taking vitamin B_6 in order to gain relief from premenstrual edema. She increased her dosage from 500 mg to 5 g per day after the first year.

At first, Marianne noticed a tingling sensation in her neck, legs, and feet. Shortly after, she experienced unsteadiness when walking, especially when crossing a room in the dark. She also had difficulty handling small objects. By the time of her examination, she could not walk with her eyes closed and could only walk with them open if she used a cane.

The examination showed sensory nervous system malfunctioning in both her upper and lower limbs. Marianne failed to react properly to such standard tests as temperature, pinprick, vibration, touch, and joint position. After two months of not taking the vitamin, both her gait and sensation began to improve. After seven months of abstinence, she felt close to normal. She was able to walk without a cane, though peripheral sensory nervous system difficulties proved slower to recover (Schaumburg et al.).

Findings in Marianne's and similar cases demonstrate that megavitamin therapy with B_6 should be discouraged. Studies have clearly shown that excessive, long-term B_6 use is unsafe.

Table 9-8

Approximate Contribution of Vitamin B$_6$ to the American Diet by Different Categories of Food

FOOD GROUP	% OF VITAMIN B$_6$ INTAKE
Meat, eggs	45–55
Fruits and vegetables	25–35
Dairy products	5–15
Cereal products	5–10
Dry peas, beans	0– 5

Deficiency symptoms in infants include convulsions, irritability, and abnormal brain waves (as seen in electroencephalograms). Anemia may also occur. In adults, symptoms of weakness, walking difficulty, nervousness, insomnia, and irritability are characteristic. Owing to the vitamin's role in antibody production, skin grafts heal slowly if there is B$_6$ deficiency. Skin lesions similar to those described in B$_2$ deficiency also occur. Since B$_6$ deficiency increases the excretion of oxalate and citrate (acids that bind with calcium and prevent its absorption), the risk of kidney stones increases.

Treatment of 10 to 50 mg per day of vitamin B$_6$ will reverse most deficiency symptoms, though 50 to 100 mg are necessary to eliminate the deficiency caused by INH clinical therapy in treating tuberculosis.

FOOD SOURCES OF VITAMIN B$_6$

Since it is widespread in nature, vitamin B$_6$ is easily obtained. Muscle meats, liver, kidney, egg yolk, corn, and whole grain cereals are good sources. Milk and vegetables have low B$_6$ content, yet vegetables provide a significant amount of our B$_6$ because the vitamin is stable in food storage and food processing. For example, only 20 to 30 percent of B$_6$ is lost in freezing vegetables, whereas 90 percent is lost when grain undergoes milling. Table 9-8 shows the B$_6$ contribution by food category. (The content of representative foods is found in the Appendix.)

PHARMACOLOGICAL DOSES

Pyridoxine is clinically administered for various purposes. For example, 50 mg of B$_6$ can relieve morning sickness in pregnant women. In lozenge form, 1 to 5 mg two to four times daily can reduce dental caries, especially in children and pregnant women. Some types of dermatitis have responded to topical application of vitamin B$_6$. It is additionally prescribed as a treatment for recurring kidney stones (as affected by the chemical "oxalic acid").

Niacin

Though the substance generally known as **niacin** has been known chemically since 1867, it was not discovered as a vitamin and isolated until 1936.

GENERAL CHARACTERISTICS

A white substance, niacin exhibits moderate stability to heat, light, acid, oxidation, and alkalinity, so little is lost during food processing, especially if liquid used in cooking is not discarded.

The vitamin occurs in the forms of niacin (nicotinic acid) and **niacinamide** (nicotinamide), associated with plant products and animal products, respectively. Since both chemicals have similar biological effects, the term niacin conveniently refers to both.

Niacin is required by all living cells and participates in many important body processes such as formation of DNA (chromosome substances) and coenzymes (special protein substances) and the release of energy from nutrient metabolism.

Niacin is readily absorbed by our bodies, so very little of the substance itself is stored. Excess is excreted in the urine. Niacin has the distinction of being the only water-soluble vitamin that can be even partially manufactured by the body. In 1945, scientists discovered that the essential amino acid (see Chapter 7) **tryptophan** can be converted to niacin if vitamins B_1, B_2, and B_6 are additionally present. About 60 units of tryptophan can be converted to one unit of niacin, and tryptophan accounts for approximately 60 to 70 percent of the niacin we metabolize. The primary use of tryptophan is for protein formation. The unique transformation process of tryptophan to niacin explains why milk, low in niacin content, can alleviate niacin deficiency in infants. Milk is high in tryptophan. Because tryptophan is of such importance as a source of niacin, the term *niacin equivalent* is used as a common unit to describe the combination of niacin already in food and niacin from tryptophan.

THE CAUSE OF PELLAGRA

Pellagra, literally rough skin, directly results from niacin deficiency. The disease was common in the southern United States in the early 1900s, causing numerous deaths among prisoners, blacks, and the poor. Where corn still serves as the major cereal, the disease remains; countries such as Rumania, Yugoslavia, and portions of Egypt, India, and Africa experience high incidence of pellagra because corn has a low content of both tryptophan and free niacin. Niacin in rice and corn exists in two forms, one free and the other bound (to a special substance called *niacinogen*). Unlike the free form, bound niacin is unavailable to the body. Bound niacin can, however, be released in the presence of alkali, explaining why such countries as Mexico, Guatemala, and other Central and South American countries have low pellagra incidence despite high corn consumption. The lime used in tortilla dough liberates the bound niacin.

The pellagra outbreaks in the United States in the early 1900s resulted from a dietary lack of niacin. Now the disease rarely occurs in America unless associated with diabetes, alcoholism, cancer, liver cirrhosis, and other clinical disorders. (The 1980 RDAs for niacin are found in the Appendix.)

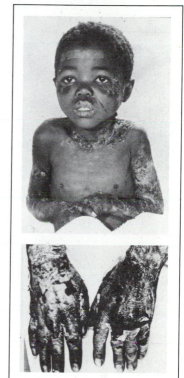

Figure 9-5: Pellagra dermatitis. Note symmetrical symptoms in both patients. SOURCE: (Top) Courtesy J. G. Prinsloo; (Bottom) S. Dreizen. Geriatrics 29 (1974): 97. By permission.

THE "FOUR D's"

The so-called four D's—dermatitis, diarrhea, depression or dementia, and death—if untreated, are the classic clinical manifestations of pellagra. The early symptoms of the disease include loss of appetite, weakness, irritability, depression, numbness, insomnia, and various gastrointestinal problems. The disease also affects the genitourinary tract in some patients. Skin lesions and mental deterioration are the generalized symptoms. Figure 9-5 depicts symptoms of dermatitis.

Skin lesions begin like a sunburn, progressing to blisters, followed soon by infection. The lesions occur on the backs of hands, forearms, face, neck, front of the legs, and feet. Lesions also appear in skin folds, which are subject to friction. Dermatitis outbreaks are symmetrical; that is, they occur on both hands, both feet, and both sides of the face.

Body surfaces with mucous membranes develop specific problems as a result of pellagra. The tongue swells and becomes red and sore (**glossitis**). The pain of chewing and swallowing prevents eating, and even the drinking of fluid brings pain. Oral infection occurs often and can extend to the intestinal system. The pain associated with eating causes weight loss because nutrient intake is deficient. If the genitourinary tract becomes infected, pain will accompany urination. Cessation of menstruation can occur in female victims of pellagra.

The symptoms that affect the central nervous system vary. Some patients experience mild irritability. Others advance to delirium, coma, and death. Generally, the patient's behavior is characterized by lethargy, apathy, stupor, fear, manic depression, and even hyperactivity. Treatment for pellagra is easily accomplished. For acute cases, 300 to 500 mg per day of niacinamide are prescribed. Intramuscular doses are given to patients who have pain when swallowing. Once the patient can swallow and acute symptoms are alleviated, 100 to 300 mg of oral niacinamide daily, in doses of 50 to 100 mg at a time, are continued until all symptoms disappear. Pureed vegetables, strained cereals, eggs, and milk prove beneficial, and skim milk powder provides additional tryptophan. As improvement occurs, fruits, vegetables, and lean meat can be included.

FOOD SOURCES OF NIACIN
When considering food sources for niacin, sources of tryptophan must also be taken into account. Table 9-9 identifies food sources for both. Table 9-10 presents dietary contribution of niacin. (The niacin content of representative foods appears in the Appendix.) Peanuts, chicken, and liver are high sources. Milk, eggs, cheese, and sweets are low sources.

PHARMACOLOGICAL DOSES
Niacin has for years served as a clinical treatment for lowering blood cholesterol and triglyceride levels in heart patients. Dosage ranges from 0.25 to 4.0 g daily. Side effects vary but typically involve gastrointestinal

Table 9-9
Food Sources for Niacin and Tryptophan

CHARACTERISTIC	FOOD
Rich in niacin	Meat (especially lean and organ meats); poultry; fish; yeasts, peanut butter
Fair content of niacin	Enriched whole-grain products (bread, cereal), especially cereal bran and germs; potatoes; some green vegetables
Low in niacin	Unenriched, refined white flour, cornmeal, grits
Low in niacin, high in tryptophan	Milk; eggs; most animal products except gelatin
High in niacin and tryptophan	Legumes (beans, peas); nuts; peanuts

disorders and vision disturbances; however, these problems do not occur with niacinamide, only with nicotinic acid.

Folic Acid

Folic acid was discovered, isolated, and synthesized in 1945. Its most common forms (see Table 9-11) include folate, folic acid, and folacin.

GENERAL CHARACTERISTICS

The yellow crystals of folic acid are rapidly destroyed in neutral or alkaline solutions, so folic acid can be easily lost in food preparation.

Folic acid is readily absorbed, primarily in the upper intestine, and absorption is facilitated by vitamin C. Although RDAs for folic acid conservatively assume a 25 percent absorption rate, 30 percent to 50 percent of ingested food folate and 70 to 80 percent of chemical supplement are absorbed. Figure 9-6 summarizes the chemical processes that folic acid undergoes during absorption. Storage occurs in the liver, and the amount that can be stored will generally last 4 to 5 months before deficiency symptoms appear. Absorption can be decreased by alcohol, oral contraceptives, and anticonvulsants.

Folic acid's roles in our bodies are diverse. It serves an important role in the synthesis of DNA, together with vitamin B_{12}. It is essential for

Table 9-10
Approximate Contribution of Niacin to the American Diet by Different Categories of Food

FOOD GROUP	% OF DAILY NIACIN INTAKE
Meat, poultry, fish, eggs	40–50
Cereal products, raisins, coffee	35–40
Fruits, vegetables	15–20
Dairy products	0– 5

Table 9-11
Different Forms of Folic Acid

FORM	CONSTITUENTS
Pteroic acid	Pterin and paramino-benzoic acid
Folate	Pteroic acid with 1, 3, or 7 units of glutamic acid
Folic acid	Pteroic acid with 1 unit of glutamic acid
Folacin	Tetrahydrofolic acid

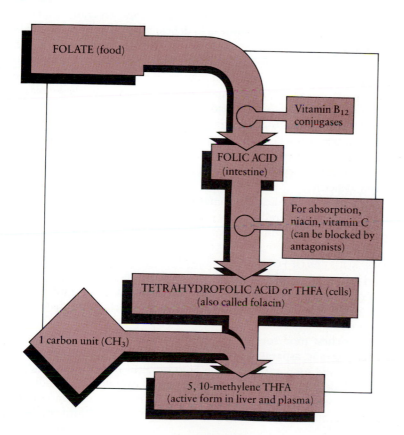

Figure 9-6: *Absorption and activation of folate.*

Table 9-12
1980 RDAs for Folacin for Different Age Groups and During Pregnancy and Lactation

POPULATION GROUP	FOLACIN RDA (μ)
Infants	
0–6 months	30
6–12 months	45
Children	
1–3 years	100
7–10 years	200
Adolescents and adults (11 + years)	400
Pregnancy	+400
Lactation	+100

rapid cell division and therefore is of special importance during pregnancy and other stressful clinical conditions. Red blood cell maturation depends upon folic acid, as do numerous chemical reactions that involve carbon transfer in our bodies.

DEFICIENCY AFFECTS OUR BLOOD

The classic symptom of folic acid deficiency is macrocytic and megaloblastic anemia. In **megaloblastosis** the red blood cells in bone marrow fail to mature. Folic acid deficiency also results in diarrhea, weight loss, sore tongue, and fainting (syncope). Cardiac enlargement and congestive heart failure can occur.

Folic acid deficiency occurs throughout the world for varying reasons, and many consider it the most common vitamin deficiency. The RDAs shown in Table 9-12 are greater than the 200 to 250 mg of folic acid in the typical American diet, so inadequate dietary intake is a primary cause of deficiency. When stored folic acid has been used up, megaloblastic anemia occurs. The condition can develop in an infant in 2 months. Because of the rapid cell division needs in pregnant women, infants, and adolescents, those groups are especially vulnerable.

In poor countries, 20 to 30 percent of the population suffer folic acid deficiency and constitute over half of all hospital admissions. In all countries, the poor and the aged have high deficiency incidence. Affected infants and children in poor countries generally experience malabsorption, intensifying folic acid deficiency, and anemia. Most alcoholics suffer the deficiency, since they are prone to imbalanced diets, liver failure, excess excretion, and metabolic disturbance. Rheumatoid arthritis, parasitic infection, and scurvy increase susceptibility to deficiency. Treatment of diseases such as sickle cell anemia, leukemia, and psoriasis often leads to folic acid deficiency because folic acid antagonists are used in treating these diseases.

Diagnosis of the deficiency usually occurs via analysis of the blood. Abnormally large red blood cells, called *megaloblasts*, are a common indicator, as is the presence of metabolites that are known to accumulate during deficiency.

Patients with folic acid deficiency respond rapidly to treatment. Doses of 5 mg daily generally restore health within a few days. Appetite returns, and the blood profile normalizes.

FOOD SOURCES OF FOLIC ACID

Food folate occurs in two forms, free and conjugated. Conjugated folic acid requires digestion by the enzyme **conjugase** in the intestine to yield free folate. Naturally free folates are easily digested and make up 25 percent of the folates in food.

The richest food sources are green leafy vegetables such as spinach and beet greens, asparagus, liver, kidney, yeast, and wheat germ. Orange juice is a fine source, because the ascorbic acid protects the folic acid. Beef, whole grain cereals, nuts, lima beans, cantaloupes, lemons, and bananas are also good sources. Yeast used in making bread increases the folic acid content, but baking the bread destroys one third of the content. Table 9-13 shows the contribution of folic acid by food category. (The folacin content of representative foods can be found in the Appendix.)

CLINICAL APPLICATIONS

The primary clinical use of folic acid is to correct deficiency, but the vitamin is also helpful in treating *tropical sprue*, a disease of unknown cause characterized by weakness, intestinal disorders, and anemia. Folic acid therapy proves necessary to offset the effects of folic acid antagonists used in the treatment of other diseases. It is also beneficial in treating various forms of anemia, especially those that fail to respond to vitamin B_{12} therapy.

Vitamin B_{12} (Cobalamin)

Vitamin B_{12}, generally called **cobalamin**, was discovered and isolated in 1940 but was not developed synthetically until 1973. In crystal form it is bright red, earning the nickname of the "red vitamin."

GENERAL CHARACTERISTICS

In our bodies, B_{12} is generally combined with a protein molecule, making it difficult for our kidneys to excrete B_{12}. Storage occurs in the liver, and enough can be stored to last 5 to 7 years without any additional intake.

The absorption of vitamin B_{12} differs from that of all other water-soluble vitamins in that it requires the presence of **intrinsic factors**, a mucoprotein (protein and carbohydrate) secreted with gastric juice. If the intrinsic factor is lacking, absorption is virtually eliminated, requiring intramuscular administration. Absorption varies inversely to ingestion, with 60 to 80 percent being absorbed when 0.5 microgram is ingested and only 5 to 15 percent absorption occurring with an intake of 16 micrograms. Absorption can increase during pregnancy.

Vitamin B_{12} serves a major role in cell metabolism, tissue growth and maintenance of the central nervous system. In both cell metabolism and tissue growth, the vitamin functions in the formation of DNA. Its role in the central nervous system is less well understood. One theory holds that vitamin B_{12} deficiency results in an inadequate supply of glucose to the nerve cells. Another theory holds that deficiency results in inadequate sheathing of nerve cells.

DEFICIENCY AFFECTS OUR BLOOD

Like folic acid deficiency, vitamin B_{12} deficiency results in formation of megaloblasts. If the anemia is due to deficiency of intrinsic factors rather than lack of B_{12}, it is known as **pernicious anemia**.

Dietary deficiency is uncommon in America, except among strict vegetarians. Defective intestinal absorption causes deficiency to occur, as does intestinal infection with worms or other parasites. Pernicious anemia has been found to be an inherited trait among northern Europeans, particularly among women and children. Surgical reduction of stomach size also leads to deficiency.

Table 9-13

Approximate Contribution of Folic Acid to the American Diet by Different Categories of Food

FOOD GROUP	% of DAILY FOLIC ACID INTAKE
Fruits, vegetables	40–45
Meat, fish, poultry, eggs	20–25
Dry beans, peas, nuts	15–20
Cereal products	10–15
Dairy products	0– 5
Fats, oils	0– 1

Table 9-14
**Approximate Contribution
of Vitamin B$_{12}$
to the American Diet
by Different Categories
of Foods**

FOOD GROUP	% OF DAILY VITAMIN B$_{12}$ INTAKE
Meat, eggs	75–80
Dairy products	20–25
Cereal products	0– 5

Symptoms also include glossitis, tiredness, headaches, breathing difficulties, and low-grade fever. In cases involving pernicious anemia, lemon-yellow pallor and hyperpigmentation occur. If vitamin B$_{12}$ deficiency becomes prolonged, the spinal cord and peripheral nerves degenerate. Sensation loss occurs in the hands and feet. Spasms, abnormal tendon reflexes, and mood changes can result.

Deficiency treatment generally involves intravenous administration of 50 to 100 micrograms three times per week. Although general relief occurs in a few days, it can take several months for blood profiles to return to normal. If pernicious anemia is involved, vitamin B$_{12}$ administration may have to be permanent. If nerve damage has occurred, treatment may take a year or more.

Diagnosis involves dietary history, clinical manifestations, blood and urinary profile, and the *Schilling test*, which involves administration and tracing of radioactive vitamin B$_{12}$.

FOOD SOURCES OF VITAMIN B$_{12}$

The best sources of vitamin B$_{12}$ are chicken, pork, beef, liver, kidney, eggs, whole milk, and fresh shrimp and oysters. Edible plant foods do not contain vitamin B$_{12}$; this is why vegetarians may suffer deficiencies. Table 9-14 lists approximate contributions by food category.

RDAs for vitamin B$_{12}$ are quite low. The average American diet contains from 10 to 20 times the recommended requirement. (Content in representative foods can be found in the Appendix.)

Pantothenic Acid

Named from the Greek word *pantos*, meaning "everywhere," **pantothenic acid** is widely distributed in nature. It was discovered in 1933, isolated in 1938, and synthesized in 1940. Though it was once known as vitamin B$_3$, that name has been dropped.

GENERAL CHARACTERISTICS

Pantothenic acid is essential to nutrient metabolism. In our bodies it combines with a sulfur-containing substance and with phosphates to form *coenzyme A* (CoA), which is important in metabolism of fat, protein, and carbohydrate. Coenzyme A participates in the citric acid cycle and promotes the release of energy, and CoA is therefore essential to all cells, but especially to high-activity organs such as the brain, heart, liver, kidneys, and adrenal glands.

DEFICIENCY NOT FROM NATURAL CAUSES

No incidence confirms pantothenic acid deficiency as a result of natural causes. Following World War II, American prisoners released from Japanese prisons complained of "electric feet syndrome," a condition of burning feet accompanied by tingling sensations and numbness. Pantothenic acid relieved the symptoms, but cause and effect could not be established. That symptom and other general, nonspecific symptoms of fatigue, insomnia, nausea, and intestinal disturbances have been experimentally induced in humans. Table 9-15 lists specific symptoms of deficiency that occur in animals.

Table 9-15
Symptoms of Pantothenic Acid Deficiency in Animals

ANIMALS	SYMPTOMS
Chicks	Dermatitis around eyes, "spectacle eyes," lesion of thymus gland, spinal cord degeneration, fatty liver
Ducks	Anemia
Rats	Growth failure, whiskers covered with reddish pigment porphyrin, adrenal gland hemorrhage, graying of hair (in black rats)
Pigs	Changes in the sensory system

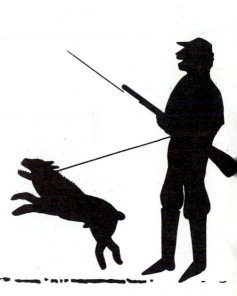

FOOD SOURCES OF PANTOTHENIC ACID

Current belief holds that we require 5 to 10 mg of pantothenic acid per day. We typically consume twice that much from organ meats, fish, egg yolk, wheat bran, and fresh vegetables. Of the amount we consume, about half is absorbed. We additionally obtain the vitamin from skim milk, molasses, lean beef, and sweet potatoes.

Since pantothenic acid is water-soluble, it can be leached from foods. It decomposes in acid or alkaline media. Normal cooking processes destroy little of the vitamin, but dry-heat cooking is quite destructive. The milling of grain results in 50 percent loss.

CLINICAL USAGE

Following surgery, large doses of pantothenic acid are used to relieve intestinal paralysis (paralytic ileus), since the vitamin apparently stimulates gastrointestinal activity. Doses of up to 10 to 20 g can, however, cause diarrhea.

Biotin

Biotin, a widely distributed white crystal, was isolated in 1935 and synthesized in 1942. The vitamin occurs in food in both the free form and bound with protein. Free biotin is formed in plants and is water-soluble. The bound form occurs in animal products and is fat-soluble.

GENERAL CHARACTERISTICS

In our bodies we find biotin as a coenzyme that plays a major role in adding a carbon unit to other chemicals, a process called *carbon dioxide fixation*. It participates in the oxidation of fatty acids and carbohydrates, in the conversion of tryptophan to niacin, and in the *phosphorylation* of glucose (see Chapter 14).

DEFICIENCY RESULTS IN "RAW EGG WHITE INJURY"

Though spontaneous deficiency is uncommon, some cases have been documented. The deficiency has been called the "raw egg white injury," since raw egg whites contain **avidin**, an antagonist that prevents biotin absorption.

Resulting symptoms are characterized by scaly dermatitis and include loss of appetite, nausea, muscle pain, depression, increased skin sensitivity, and raised blood cholesterol. The injection of 150 to 300 micrograms (μg) of biotin per day reverses the symptoms in 3 to 4 days. Nutritional biotin deficiency in infants under 6 months of age causes seborrheic dermatitis. A daily dose of 5 mg via injection or intravenous feeding promptly relieves the condition.

FOOD SOURCES OF BIOTIN

Our typical American diet contains 100 to 300 μg of biotin, a more than adequate amount for a healthy adult. Biotin occurs with other B vitamins, so good food sources include organ meats, egg yolk, milk, and yeast. Fair amounts of biotin occur in legumes, nuts, chocolate, and cauliflower. Cow's milk contains about ten times as much biotin as breast milk. Diet does not affect the biotin content in a woman's breast milk.

Biotin exhibits stability to heat, but it is unstable to alkali and oxidation and can be leached by water.

Intestinal bacteria synthesize biotin and add to our daily supply. Antibiotics such as sulfonamides and oxytetracycline inhibit bacterial activity and therefore have the potential for causing biotin deficiency.

Summing Up

Our question for this chapter addressed whether or not water-soluble vitamins can cure disease. We saw that thiamine administration saved Jerry's life. Perhaps the one discovery we have made in regard to our basic question is that there is a definite link between vitamins and disease. We found several diseases related directly to vitamin deficiencies—diseases such as scurvy, beriberi, and pellagra. Do vitamins cure them? Yes, they do, but, more important, they *prevent* them. Thiamine saved Jerry's life, but if he had not been thiamine deficient, his life would not have been endangered by the deficiency. Such chicken-and-egg distinctions can be confusing, however. What we most need to remember is that vitamins are essential nutrients for our bodies.

STUDY QUESTIONS

1. Describe the functions of vitamin C and symptoms of its deficiency. Discuss the loss of vitamin C in the handling and cooking of foods. What risks have been associated with a high intake of vitamin C?

2. What condition is associated with moderate to severe vitamin B_1 deficiency? In what groups of people has this condition been found?

3. Discuss some reasons why riboflavin deficiency may be difficult to diagnose.

4. What factors may cause vitamin B_6 deficiency? What are the nonspecific symptoms of B_6 deficiency?

5. What is the relationship of tryptophan to niacin?

6. What deficiency disease is classically characterized by the 4 D's? Describe the 4 D's.

7. Which B vitamins are involved in anemia? What is pernicious anemia?

8. Is pantothenic acid deficiency common? Why?

REFERENCES

Basu, T. K., and C. J. Schorah. *Vitamin C in Health and Disease.* Westport, Conn.: Avi, 1982.

Schaumburg, H., et al. "Sensory Neuropathy from Pyridoxine Abuse: A New Megavitamin Syndrome." *N. Engl. J. Med.* 309 (1983): 445.

Shah, N., and J. A. Wolff. "Thiamine Deficiency: Probable Wernicke's Encephalopathy Successfully Treated in a Child with Acute Lymphocytic Leukemia." *Pediatrics* 51 (1973): 750.

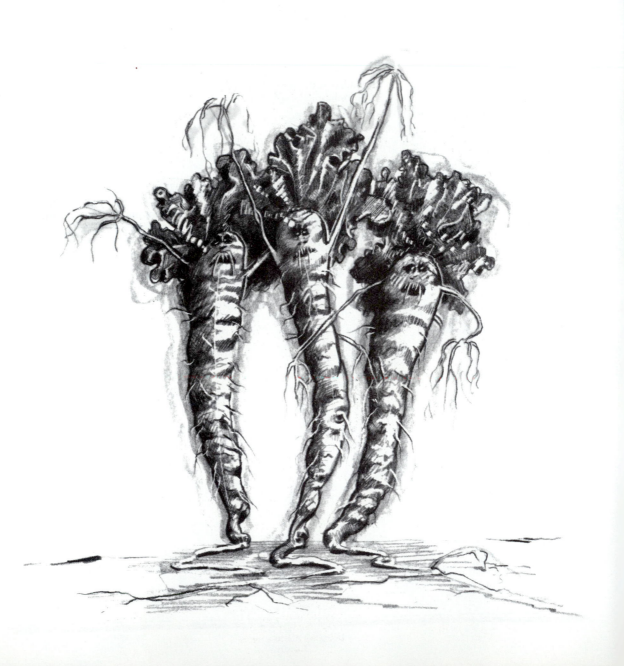

10

FAT-SOLUBLE VITAMINS:

POTENTIAL TOXICITY

A CASE OF CHRONIC VITAMIN A INTOXICATION

Though chronic vitamin A intoxication is uncommon, it can have profound effects—effects that can be mistaken for other vitamin imbalance. For example, an Australian woman in her forties was admitted to a hospital for suspected vitamin B deficiency. She was generally disoriented and confused, had large sheets of skin peeling from her palms, and showed swelling in the face and ankles. Her nails were whitish and brittle; her lips had splits in them; her tongue was smooth; and she bled from her gums.

The hospital staff began treatment with thiamine, and several of her symptoms showed significant improvement. Her general appearance brightened; gum bleeding stopped; lip splitting stopped; and her skin returned to normal. Despite these improvements, her ankles remained swollen, and her hair began to fall out so quickly that she was almost bald after 7 days in the hospital.

The hospital staff learned that she had been taking vitamin A three times a day for 10 years.

Each tablet was thought to contain 30,000 International Units (IU). She additionally drank three to four pints of carrot juice daily. The hospital immediately ceased all medication except thyroxine, one common treatment for vitamin A intoxication. All the patient's symptoms then improved, and she was discharged after 3 weeks' hospitalization. The patient vowed to never take vitamin A again (Teo et al.). (See Figure 10-4.)

This case of chronic vitamin poisoning is one example of abusing the fat-soluble vitamins.

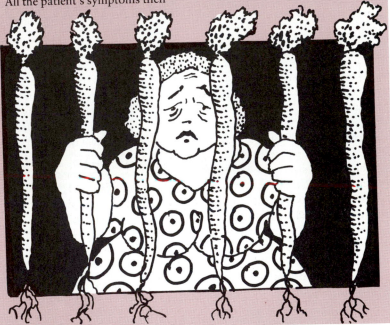

Four of the thirteen known vitamins belong to the group called fat-soluble vitamins. These four compose a special class because they are soluble in organic media such as chloroform and oil. Of the four fat-soluble vitamins, A, D, E, and K, two (A and D) can be synthesized by our bodies, if the **precursors** or **provitamins** are present (see Chapter 8).

The fat-soluble vitamins are similar in chemical composition, body storage capacity, urgency of dietary intake, and rapidity of symptom appearance if deficient, but they differ significantly in function, sources, and other characteristics.

Vitamin A

Although vitamin A was discovered in 1915, it was not until 1937 that scientists succeeded in extracting (isolating) it from food. Chemists synthesized the chemical in the laboratory in 1946.

CHARACTERISTICS AND FACTS

In nature vitamin A occurs in three chemical forms: retinol (vitamin A alcohol), retinal (vitamin A aldehyde), and retinoic acid (vitamin A acid). The first two forms are found in both foods and our bodies and have equal biological activity or function. Retinol and retinal are known as *preformed vitamin A* in animal products, but the body can synthesize retinol and retinal from a precursor, β-**carotene** (also called *provitamin A*), which occurs in plant products. Retinoic acid is a *metabolite* or biological byproduct found primarily in the body, and it has less biological activity.

Physically, vitamin A appears colorless to pale yellow and is soluble in fat and fat solvents. As we saw in Chapter 6, fats are subject to rancidity from oxidation, a process that destroys vitamin A at high temperatures.

FOUND IN YELLOW VEGETABLES

Food sources for vitamin A include sources of carotene (β-carotene), the precursor or the basic ingredient from which the body can manufacture vitamin A within the intestinal wall. Also called *carotenoid pigment* owing to its orange and yellow coloration, carotene occurs in carrots, peaches, sweet potatoes, and other yellow-colored vegetables and fruits. Chlorophyll's green color conceals carotene in green, leafy vegetables, but chlorophyll itself does not contain vitamin A. The body's ability to convert carotene to vitamin A is highly inefficient. Table 10-1 compares the efficiency of conversion in the laboratory versus the body. From one fourth to one third of ingested carotene is converted to vitamin A in our bodies. Half of that comes from leafy vegetables and the balance from carrots and other root vegetables. Storage of carotene occurs in the adrenal glands and in fat, and carotene that is not converted is either absorbed in the circulatory system or excreted.

Table 10-1
Conversion of β-Carotene to Vitamin A

	INITIAL AMOUNT OF β-CAROTENE	EXPECTED AMOUNT OF VITAMIN A FORMED
Laboratory	2 units	4 units
Human intestinal mucosal walls	2 units	1 unit

Table 10-2
Approximate Contribution of Vitamin A to the American Diet by Different Categories of Foods

FOOD GROUP	% of DAILY VITAMIN A INTAKE
Fruits, vegetables	50–55
Meat, poultry, fish, eggs	25–30
Dairy products	10–15
Fats, oils	5–10

Table 10-3
Vitamin A Content of Different Types of Liver

LIVER TYPE*	IU VITAMIN A	μg RE†
Calf	1,900	576
Beef	45,450	13,773
Pork	12,000	3,637
Lamb	43,000	1,303
Chicken	27,000	8,182

*90-g (3-oz) portion.
†Retinol equivalent.

Preformed vitamin A occurs in animal organs (kidney and liver), egg yolk, and butter cream. Table 10-2 lists the contribution of vitamin A by category of food. (The vitamin A content of representative foods is found in the Appendix.) Since animal liver is a major source of dietary vitamin A, Table 10-3 presents its content in different types of liver. Carrots, beet greens, and canned apricots are also good sources.

Special internationally adopted units for measuring vitamin A and carotene are shown below:

$$1 \text{ retinol equivalent (RE)} = 1 \text{ microgram (μg) retinol}$$
$$= 6 \text{ microgram β-carotene}$$

DEFICIENCY CHARACTERISTICS

Functionally, vitamin A is essential in the formation of **rhodopsin** (the substance responsible for night vision), bone growth, and development of the nervous system. Vitamin A is also associated with metabolism in cell membranes and in structure of cell membranes. In animals, vitamin A is essential for reproduction.

Vitamin A deficiency rarely occurs in Western countries, where vitamin A is abundant in the diet. It can also be stored in the body. (The 1980 RDAs for vitamin A are found in the Appendix.) Given that an adult liver can store 500,000 IU, body storage can provide years of vitamin A supply. Deficiency commonly occurs in Central and South America, Asia, and Africa. When deficiency occurs in western countries, it generally results from a low-fat diet or a specific clinical problem (for example, fat malabsorption, jaundice, gallbladder disease, intestinal mucosal disorders, liver cirrhosis, cancer, tuberculosis, pneumonia, or infection).

Vitamin A deficiency in children can cause loss of both taste and smell. The deficiency can also retard growth and cause abnormal bones and teeth. Similar effects are produced in animals. The most common symptoms of human deficiency are, however, disorders of the eye and epithelium (skin or related structure).

Eye Symptoms

Eye symptoms resulting from vitamin A deficiency occur in varying degrees, depending on how severe the deficiency is. Night blindness (*nyctalopia*) develops when a reduction of vitamin A supplied to the eyes leads to an insufficiency of rhodopsin, which enables us to see in dim light. Prolonged deficiency can result in structural changes of the retina. Those suffering from night blindness find they cannot adjust to darkened rooms such as theaters and cannot adjust to darkness after having been blinded by bright lights, for example, in night driving (see Figure 10-1). Dryness of the *conjunctiva* (the delicate membrane that lines the eyelids) is symptomatic of vitamin A deficiency. This dryness (*xerosis*) occurs at the thickened and wrinkled corners of the eye, and the transparent structures of the eye are made opaque by milky droplets in the eyes. If the condition is severe, the patient develops xerophthalmia. Dryness of the cornea leads to loss of light-reflecting ability and plugged tear ducts.

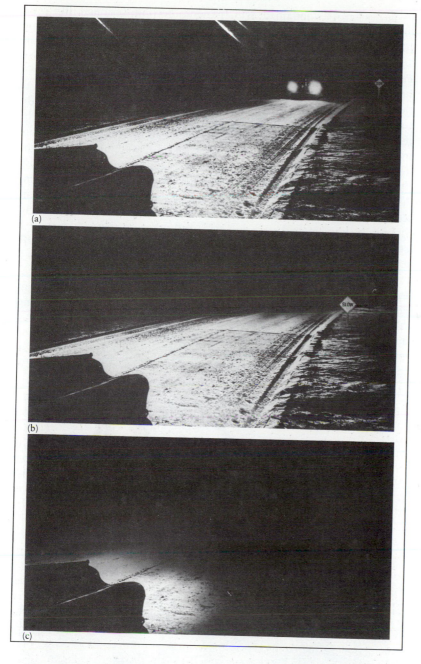

Figure 10-1: Night blindness, loss of visual acuity in dim light following exposure to bright light, is a useful and early diagnostic sign of vitamin A deficiency. Both the normal individual and the vitamin A-deficient subject see the headlights of an approaching car (a). After the car has passed, the normal individual sees a wide stretch of road (b), whereas the vitamin A-deficient subject can barely see a few feet ahead and cannot see the road sign at all (c). SOURCE: Courtesy of the Upjohn Company.

The presence of *Bitot's spots*, triangular spots of aluminum coloring on the outside edge of the center of the eye (in the white near the iris), is believed by some clinicians to be the result of vitamin A deficiency.

Keratomalacia is the softening and subsequent destruction of the cornea. As damage progresses, the iris collapses and is expelled. The eyes hemorrhage and scar over, preventing the entrance of light. In addition to having grossly inflamed eyes, patients become seriously ill. Total blindness occurs in the advanced stages of vitamin A deficiency. Figure 10-2 shows eye lesions of keratomalacia.

Problems with Skin and Related Organs (Epithelial Breakdown)
In addition to causing eye conditions, vitamin A deficiency also affects the *epithelial cells*; that is, cells covering internal organs and body surfaces. Vitamin A ensures the proper functioning of epithelial cells. In its absence, **keratinization**, the horny degeneration of skin and mucous membranes, develops. The skin dries, cracks, and becomes rough. Thickening at the base of hair follicles (folliculosis) results in a bumpy, "toad" skin, especially on the shoulders and buttocks of children. Although vitamin A relieves the symptoms in most patients, the skin lesions probably result from a combination of deficiencies including vitamin A, linoleic acid, ascorbic acid, and other nutrients. Figure 10-3 presents classic symptoms of skin lesions associated with vitamin A deficiency.

In addition to skin symptoms, mucous membranes that line respiratory, gastrointestinal, and genitourinary tracts sustain damage from vitamin A deficiency. In the respiratory tract, the loss of special lining cells called *cilia* increases susceptibility to sore throat, sinus problems, and similar respiratory problems. In the gastrointestinal tract, diarrhea and malabsorption can occur. Urination pain and infection characterize the consequences for the genitourinary tract.

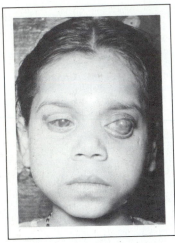

Figure 10-2: *Blindness in one eye caused by keratomalacia.*
SOURCE: *G. Venkataswamy.* Israel J. Med. Sci. 8 (1972): 1190.

Figure 10-3: *Classic skin lesions of follicular hyperkeratosis due to vitamin A deficiency. The lesions are distinguishable from gooseflesh since they do not disappear when the skin is rubbed.*
SOURCE: *S. Dreizen.* Geriatrics 29 (1974): 97. By permission.

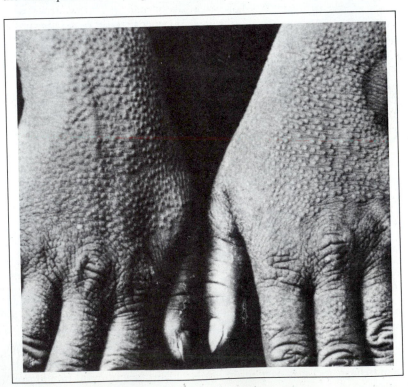

Table 10-4
Vitamin A Therapy for Children with Xerophthalmia and Keratomalacia

DAY	VITAMIN A SOURCE	DOSE OF VITAMIN A*	ROUTE
1	Palmitate (aqueous dispersible vitamin A)	100,300 IU (= 30,000 µg retinol)	Parenteral
2–6	Same as above	50,000 IU	Oral, twice daily
7 and on	Cod liver oil	10,000 IU*	Oral, once daily

*30 mL oil gives 25,000 IU vitamin A or 7,500 µg retinol.

DIAGNOSIS AND TREATMENT

The easiest way to diagnose vitamin A deficiency is through the night vision symptoms we discussed earlier. Blood tests can also suggest deficiency by measuring either vitamin A levels or carotene levels.

Treatment generally includes an oral dose of 30,000 IU. This will correct mild deficiency, but severe cases require much higher dosage levels. The therapy for vitamin-A deficient children is presented in Table 10-4. Supportive therapy for adults and children includes antibiotics and a nutritious diet emphasizing calories, protein, and vitamin A.

TOO MUCH VITAMIN A IS DANGEROUS

Numerous cases of vitamin A overdose have demonstrated its toxicity. Table 10-5 sets out the characteristics of vitamin A poisoning. For adults, more than 20,000 IU of vitamin A per day for one to two months is hazardous. A single dose 200 times the RDA has caused acute toxicity. Our earlier case history illustrates chronic vitamin A intoxication.

Some of the earliest known cases of vitamin A poisoning involved individuals eating the livers of large animals such as polar bears and seals. Following World War II, vitamin A poisoning in children resulted from mothers giving cod liver oil to their children, despite dietary vitamin A being sufficient. Vitamin A poisoning has also occurred among individuals who thought it could cure acne and among those who

Table 10-5
Characteristics of Vitamin A Toxicity

POPULATION GROUP	DOCUMENTED HARMFUL DOSES	CLINICAL MANIFESTATIONS
Infants under 6 months old	18,500–25,000 IU/day for 1–3 months.	Scaly dermatitis, weight loss, anorexia, bone pain, bulging head, hydrocephalus, increased intracranial pressure, hyperirritability.
Adults and children	25,000–1,000,000 IU per day or per dose. If under 50,000 IU, poisoning takes effect in a few months. The effect of 1,000,000 IU may be instantaneous.	Sweating, headache, fatigue, anemia, drowsiness, nausea, loss of hair, dry skin, diarrhea, itchiness, rash, irritability, neurological signs, and enlargement of spleen and liver. Mild fever, tender long bones, periosteal elevation shown under X-rays, with calcium deposition. There are also changes in the long bones as seen by X-rays. Fingernails may be brittle. In girls and women, there may be cessation of menstruation with abnormal blood chemistry, e.g., decreased hemoglobin and RBC potassium.

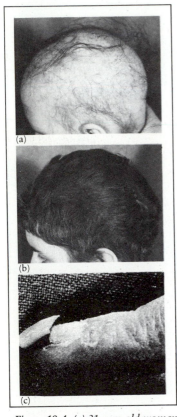

(a)

(b)

(c)

Figure 10-4: (a) 31-year-old woman with hair loss after consuming 75 million equivalents of Vitamin A within 3½ weeks. She believed that the vitamin dose could improve her skin problems. (b) Complete recovery 4½ months after abstinence from the vitamin. (c) Fissured fingernail of 42-year-old woman who had taken about 90,000 International Units of vitamin A daily for at least 10 years. Note: *Original units for vitamin A dosage used.* SOURCE: *(a, b) R. Mausle and H. Zaun.* Fortsche. Med. 90 (1972): 687; (c) S. T. Teo, et al. Med J. Australia 2 (1973): 324. *Copyright © 1973 The Medical Journal of Australia. Reprinted by permission.*

thought it could generally improve health. Figure 10-4 illustrates the clinical effect of vitamin A poisoning.

The only therapy for vitamin A poisoning is to stop ingesting it, from either food or tablets. Except in the most severe cases of toxicity, 72 hours usually enables the excess vitamin A to dissipate.

Excessive carotene ingestion can lead to *hypercarotenemia*. This condition results in yellowish orange skin, especially on the palms, soles of feet, forehead, base of nose, and groin area. The condition usually occurs from excessive ingestion of green, leafy vegetables, carrot juice, tomatoes, citrus fruit, or yellow vegetables.

CLINICAL USAGE

Vitamin A and Cancer

As we have previously seen, vitamin A occurs naturally in three primary forms and also has been synthetically developed. As a group, the natural and synthetic forms of vitamin A are called retinoids, and retinoids show significant promise in the prevention of cancer (Basu). We know that vitamin A is crucial to the health of epithelial cells. What has additionally been found is that retinoids can play an important role after cancer has begun but before it has reached the level of malignant, invasive growth. The retinoids can delay the appearance of tumors, retard tumor growth, and even shrink tumor size. These accomplishments are particular to synthetic retinoids.

The vitamin A we require from our diet serves as a stabilizing force for normal cellular functions, especially the epithelial tissues of skin, kidney, bladder, stomach, intestine, pancreas, bronchi, trachea, testes, prostate, and uterus. Vitamin A deficiency, or prolonged exposure to carcinogens even when there is no deficiency, opens the door to abnormal cellular activity and the initiation of cancer. Synthetic retinoids hold the promise of chemo-prevention and may become available to supplement the effects of natural vitamin A. Presently, synthetic retinoids are in use in animal cancer experiments.

Synthetic retinoids have significant advantages over natural vitamin A. First, natural vitamin A is toxic in large doses. Synthetic retinoids have much lower toxicity and are not stored in the liver as are the natural forms of vitamin A. Natural vitamin A is generally distributed in tissue, whereas synthetic retinoids have been developed to affect specific organs. Because of such advantages, retinoids hold great promise for health.

Vitamin A Acid and Skin Problems

Vitamin A acid, also called *trans*-retinoic acid, has recently received much attention regarding its role in skin care (Pochi).

Tretinoin, a prescription drug containing vitamin A acid, has been found to produce exciting benefits in the treatment of acne. All forms of acne, from the mild to the most severe, have shown dramatic improvement within 12 weeks. Improvement becomes obvious in 6 to 8 weeks of treatment, and nine out of ten patients achieve good to excellent results. These findings have resulted in the recognition of tretinoin as the most effective topical remedy for acne.

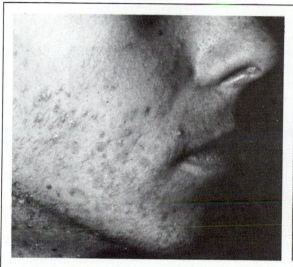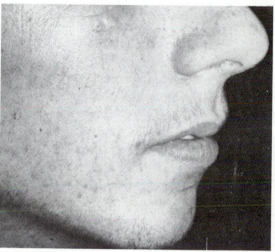

The product is available in medicated pads, cream, and gel. The most effective method of treatment has several important aspects. (1) All patients with acne begin on tretinoin. If the case is mild or the patient's complexion fair, cream is used. If the case is severe, skin is oily, or complexion is dark, saturated pads are used. (2) Patients receive instruction in proper application, which involves a light application 1 hour before retiring. The face must be dry, and care must be taken around the eyes and lips due to the danger of excessive chapping. (3) Patients are advised to wash only with gentle soaps, no more frequently than twice a day. Advice is given on the use of cosmetics, which should be water-based liquids. (4) Patients are cautioned to avoid prolonged sun exposure. If sun exposure cannot be avoided, sunscreens must be used. (5) During weeks two, three, and four, redness and peeling are likely to occur, and the acne may flare. This surfacing of subdural lesions is a positive sign. (6) Finally, the patient visits the doctor every 2 weeks to be certain chapping is not excessive and to watch for allergic reactions. Figure 10-5 illustrates the benefits of tretinoin on acne.

Because large doses of vitamin A acid can harm an unborn child, health authorities do not advise its use during pregnancy.

Figure 10-5: Resolution of acne over 3 months of treatment with vitamin A acid (tretinoin) and benzoyl peroxide.
SOURCE: J. E. Fulton. Postgrad. Med. 52 (1972): 85.

Vitamin D

CHARACTERISTICS AND FACTS

Vitamin D was discovered in 1918, isolated in 1930, and synthesized in 1936. It is found in two forms in food: vitamin D_3 (cholecalciferol) in animal products and vitamin D_2 (ergosterol) in plant products. Vitamin D is popularly called the "sunshine vitamin." The disease resulting from

LYLE HAD BOWED LEGS

Lyle, a 2-year-old black boy, was referred for treatment of bowed legs. The problem had worsened once the patient had begun walking. The child had a good appetite, was otherwise healthy and active, and had received vitamins during the ages of 6 months to 1 year. His height was found to be characteristic of 12- to 18-month-olds, although he was chronologically 2 years old. Laboratory tests showed calcium, phosphate, electrolytes, and amino acids to be normal. Vitamin D deficiency was theorized, because X-rays showed signs of active rickets. After Lyle was given 10,000 units of vitamin D daily, progressive healing resulted.

vitamin D deficiency, **rickets**, has been known for over 60 years, but understandings of the disease are more recent.

IT'S UNDER YOUR SKIN AND RELEASED BY THE SUN

In the presence of sunlight, our bodies manufacture vitamin D from a precursor, metabolite, or body byproduct found under our skin. The ultraviolet (UV) rays of the sun are necessary to this unique process, called **photolytic conversion**. Because UV rays do not penetrate pigment, black people cannot make vitamin D and therefore have a higher risk of rickets. Similarly, infants confined to a hospital are at risk. Many hospitals use mercury-quartz glass in nursery windows so that UV rays can penetrate the glass to offset the risk.

The scarcity of vitamin D in foods makes our dependency on sunlight for photolytic conversion even more important. Of course, this means seasonal variations affect our health, as does geographical location. These variations have produced speculation that sunlight availability has had evolutionary significance on the distribution of the races. Further investigation may confirm these revolutionary theories.

IT CONTROLS BONE GROWTH

Vitamin D's function is to control the calcification of bones by increasing intestinal absorption of calcium and its subsequent deposition in bone. Vitamin D permits 30 to 35 percent absorption of ingested calcium, whereas the rate drops to 10 percent if vitamin D is absent. (The 1980 RDAs for vitamin D are found in the Appendix.)

DAIRY PRODUCTS PROVIDE IT

The most acceptable sources of vitamin D all are animal products—eggs, milk, butter, and cod liver oil. Plant products have very little of the vitamin. The average American diet, even with vitamin-D-rich foods, provides less than the RDA, necessitating fortification of foods, especially milk. Commercial milk has 400 IU added per quart in the homogenization and pasteurization processes. Cod liver oil contains about 340 IU per teaspoon and is a popular vitamin D supplement in European countries, especially for infants and children. Water-soluble vitamin D preparations are available in the United States, thus relieving children from the unpleasant odor of cod liver oil. Supplements can be administered intravenously or orally, with the former method more popular in European countries.

RICKETS: PRIMARILY A CHILD'S DISEASE

As in the case of Lyle, vitamin D deficiency causes rickets, which is a common disease in underdeveloped countries. In Africa, for example, 40 to 60 percent of the children have rickets, and in many parts of the world acute rickets at birth is endemic. A newborn child can suffer from the disease because the mother had inadequate vitamin D or inadequate calcium during pregnancy.

An expectant mother in normal health will give birth to a rickets-free infant, and, with a nominal amount of sunlight, a nursing child will be kept rickets free by a water-soluble analogue of vitamin D that is present in breast milk. Without enough sunlight, vitamin supplementation be-

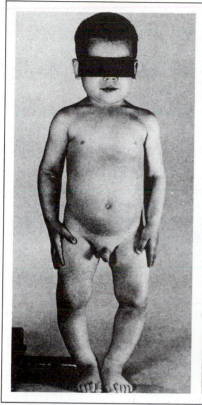
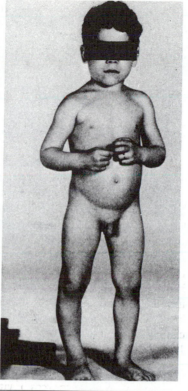

Figure 10-6: Classic signs of rickets. Left: *Bowlegs in a 2½-year-old child with rickets.* Right: *Normal bone development at 4½ years of age after treatment with vitamin D and phosphate.* SOURCE: *C. R. Sriver. Reproduced with permission of* Nutrition Today *magazine, P.O. Box 1829, Anapolis, MD 21404, © September/October 1974.*

comes necessary. If milk is fortified, as in the United States, bottle-fed infants receive sufficient dietary vitamin D.

Other causal factors of vitamin D deficiency include reduction of fat intake, which leads to decreased absorption of the vitamin, and strict vegetarian dietary practices. Both premature infants and elderly people are vulnerable to deficiency as a result of little sunlight and low vitamin D intake. In adults, malabsorption of the vitamin can occur due to a lack of bile salts, stomach bypass surgery, and alcoholism. Since vitamin D absorption occurs in the duodenum and jejunum, it can be adversely affected by such gastrointestinal maladies as steatorrhea (fatty stools) or gallbladder disease. The latter examples are known as *secondary vitamin D deficiency.*

Early symptoms of rickets in children include a drop in serum-ionized calcium levels (hypocalcium), hyperirritability, and convulsions. Since bone mineralization is reduced, skeletal deformities occur. In children, weakened bones and uneven stresses lead not only to skeletal deformities but also to growth retardation. Typically, portions of the skull either protrude or are soft. Swelling occurs at the end of long bones (ankles and wrists), and deformities such as bowed chest or bowleggedness are common. In such children, most any stress causes bone deformity. For example, sitting leads to curvature of the spine. Figure 10-6 shows the classic symptom of rickets—bowlegs.

ADULT DEFICIENCY

Adult rickets mainly occurs in the form of **osteomalacia**, a bone softening resulting from impaired mineralization. Insufficient vitamin D intake
is not usually the sole cause of the disease. Instead chronic steatorrhea
contributes to the deficiency by dissipating both vitamin D and insoluble
calcium salts that are needed for its absorption. **Osteoporosis**, also a
bone disease, is partially associated with vitamin D and calcium metabolism, as well as with minerals (see Chapter 12).

In adults, bone softening occurs at the points where muscles attach to
bones. Severe pain results. Muscular weakness is a common complaint.
As the bones bend, the patient is only able to walk in a waddling gait.
The resulting symptoms, collectively known as **tetany**, include hyperirritability, confusion, cramps, muscle twitching, and convulsions.

Treatment for rickets involves vitamin D therapy. Children receive
1200 IU per day, and healing becomes evident in X-rays in about 3
weeks. Severe cases may require 5000 IU per day for twice that long.
Adult treatment ranges from 5000 to 20,000 IU per day, or more, plus
calcium therapy.

VITAMIN D INTOXICATION

As we saw with vitamin A, vitamin D intoxication is possible. Table 10-6
lists the range of toxic doses. The symptoms resulting from vitamin D
intoxication are rather specific.

In children, growth retardation, weight loss, loss of appetite, "failure
to thrive," and nausea are characteristic. In adults, symptoms include
abnormal calcium metabolism, kidney malfunction, vomiting, nausea,
constipation, and hypertension. Severe toxicity produces severe hypercalcemia, calcium deposition in blood vessels and joints, drowsiness,
and coma.

Treatment for vitamin D poisoning necessitates correction of fluid
and electrolyte (mineral) imbalance. Cortisone is given continuously
until the serum calcium level returns to normal.

Vitamin E

CHARACTERISTICS AND FACTS

Discovered in 1922, vitamin E is called **tocopherol**, Greek for "to bear
offspring." The vitamin was isolated in 1936 and synthesized the follow-

Table 10-6
Doses and Duration for Vitamin D Intoxication

POPULATION GROUP	DOSE AND DURATION FOR INTOXICATION	REMARKS
Adults	100,000 IU vitamin D for weeks or months	——
Infants	10,000–30,000 IU vitamin D per day	Some infants show hypersensitivity to vitamin D at low doses of 1,000 IU/day.
Children	2,500–60,000 IU/day for 1–4 months	Some cases of poisoning: 10,000 IU/day for 4 months to 200,000 IU/day for 2 weeks.

ing year. Vitamin E has been called the "antisterility factor," owing to the discovery that its deficiency causes permanent sterility in male experimental animals and reproductive difficulty in female animals. Surprisingly, however, no evidence corroborates similar deficiency reactions in humans.

In fact, vitamin E's role in human nutrition remains relatively unknown. Its deficiency cannot be produced in humans under experimental conditions, although spontaneous vitamin E deficiency has been identified under limited circumstances. Research continues on vitamin E.

The forms of vitamin E are many, but *alpha*-tocopherol (α-tocopherol) is the most biologically active. Fat-soluble vitamins require the presence of bile salts for absorption and are best absorbed when fat is present. Water-soluble preparations of vitamin E now exist as well.

Our bodies absorb 20 to 30 percent of ingested vitamin E, and absorption decreases as intake increases. The major storage sites include muscles, liver, and fat, with additional storage in the adrenals, heart, testes, and uterus. Excess vitamin E undergoes conjugation in the liver and excretion via bile or urine.

IMPORTANCE AS A BIOLOGICAL CHEMICAL
Vitamin E serves important chemical and biochemical functions in several ways. First, as an antioxidant it protects fat, vitamins A and C, and polyunsaturated fats from oxidation. Since one theory links the cause of

Vitamin E and Leg Cramps

Nocturnal leg cramping troubles many people. It occurs almost twice as frequently among women, especially those over age 50. When scientists and medical practitioners seek specific cures for a problem, they sometimes use a direct clinical trial of a certain treatment. In the case of nocturnal leg cramps, 125 patients, who were suffering from the condition to the extent they considered the cramps a problem, were treated with vitamin E.

Those conducting the vitamin E treatment program carefully recorded age and sex of patients; frequency, duration, and severity of cramping; dosage of vitamin E; and treatment results. Of the 125 patients, 103 experienced complete or almost complete control of the condition. Another 13 had the condition alleviated in the 75 to 90 percent range. Seven patients had the cramping reduced to 50 to 75 percent of what they had been experiencing. Only two patients received little benefit. The administration of vitamin E proved most effective when 300 to 400 IU daily was given.

Since the patients responded quickly and the condition was significantly alleviated, the results of the direct treatment of leg cramping with vitamin E demonstrated that the treatment is effective. The researchers who did the clinical trial concluded that vitamin E can almost be considered the specific treatment for nocturnal leg cramps (Ayres and Mihan).

This trial is an example of the occasional positive benefits of vitamin E we observe in medical literature.

PREMATURE AND ANEMIC

A black male infant weighing 4 pounds at birth had low hemoglobin (blood pigment) and hematocrit values and showed mild signs of other clinical problems common to premature infants. For the first 6 weeks, weight gain was normal on a standard formula. Although overall clinical conditions rapidly improved, the child became progressively more anemic. In his eighth week, he was started on an oral dose of 100 IU per day of vitamin E. The anemia was fully reversed by the tenth week.

Table 10-7
Approximate Contribution of Vitamin E to the American Diet by Different Categories of Foods

FOOD GROUP	% of DAILY VITAMIN E INTAKE
Fats, oils: butter, margarine, shortenings and fats from meat, chicken, fish	60–70
Fruits and vegetables (especially green leafy vegetables)	10–15
Cereal products	5–10

aging to cellular oxidation, speculation surrounds vitamin E's role in the aging process. Second, vitamin E assists **cellular respiration**, the process by which glucose and fatty acids combine with oxygen to yield energy, water, and carbon dioxide (see Chapter 14). Third, vitamin E is necessary for synthesis of other essential body substances. For example, the manufacture of vitamin C in some animals that are food sources for humans requires vitamin E. Fourth, vitamin E enables synthesis of *heme*, a component of hemoglobin. Finally, vitamin E helps maintain the integrity of red-cell membranes, preventing **hemolysis** (liberation of heme into the plasma).

DEFICIENCY IS RARE

The daily requirement for vitamin E increases in relation to polyunsaturated fat intake. The newborn depends significantly on vitamin E in milk, since little of the vitamin crosses the placenta during pregnancy. Human milk's vitamin E content is four times that of cow's milk. Premature infants especially require supplementation, since vitamin E deposition in the unborn child primarily occurs in the last 2 months of gestation. The case history described earlier illustrates this clinical problem.

Though clinical disorders such as steatorrhea, gallbladder disease, and malabsorption can lead to vitamin E deficiency, it is relatively uncommon in otherwise healthy adults. In adults, a symptom of deficiency will be increased destruction of red blood cells. In premature infants, anemia, edema, skin lesions, and increased platelet count will also result. Cystic fibrosis in children is frequently associated with vitamin E deficiency. Deficiency is treated with 30 to 100 mg of vitamin E per day until all deficiency symptoms clear.

VEGETABLE OILS ARE A GOOD SOURCE

The greatest concentration of vitamin E in food sources occurs in vegetable oils, such as wheat germ oil. The level of vitamin E reflects the amount of polyunsaturated fats present, since vitamin E prevents oxidation. Frying or boiling temperatures can destroy vitamin E content. In grain milling processes, 90 percent of vitamin E is destroyed. Whole grain is high in content but subject to oxidation unless refrigerated. Table 10-7 presents vitamin E sources in the American diet.

TOXICITY RISK IS LOW

Though the risk of toxicity is low, a large dose of vitamin E can interfere with the body's utilization of vitamins A and K. If vitamin E ingestion increases, vitamin A and K ingestion must also increase. A dose of 300 mg of vitamin E may lead to intestinal disturbances. Since vitamin E can be stored in the body in large quantity, especially in the liver and pancreas, it is possible that excessive dosages could accumulate to the point of toxicity, but no cases of this have been documented.

Therapeutic Effects of Vitamin E

UNPROVEN CLAIMS

The Institute of Food Technologists lists the following as unproven claims for the therapeutic effects of vitamin E:

Treatment of painful calves of legs when walking
Treatment of dystrophy in humans
Treatment for virility and sexual endurance
Treatment and prevention of heart disease
Increased physical vigor, strength, and endurance
Retardation of the aging process
Treatment and prevention of cancer

POTENTIAL BENEFITS
The Institute of Food Technologists has concluded that the following includes some potential benefits of the use of therapeutic dosages of vitamin E:

Treatment of hemolytic anemia in premature infants
Treatment of deficiencies caused by malabsorption of fats and oils
Protection against air pollutants

In the medical literature, other physicians and scientists have demonstrated the benefits of therapeutic doses of vitamin E in at least isolated case history reports. For reference purposes, these are listed in the box on page 210.

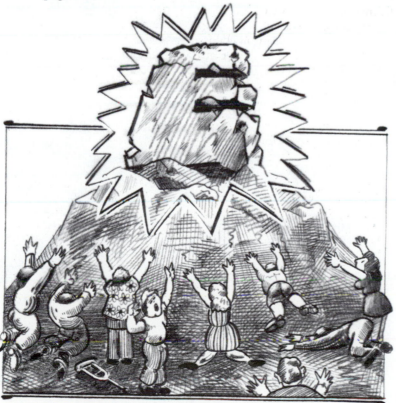

THERAPEUTIC BENEFITS OF VITAMIN E REPORTED BY VARIOUS RESEARCHERS[1]

DISEASE	SUCCESS	DISEASE	SUCCESS
Hemolytic anemia[2]	Definite benefit	Pseudoxanthoma elasticum[2]	Mixed results
Fat malabsorption problems	Definite benefit	Subcorneal pustular dermatosis[2]	One case of good response
Intermittent claudication (calf pain)[2]	Definite benefit	Necrobiosis lipoidica diabeticorum[2]	Mixed results
Epidermolysis bullosa[2]	Mixed results in individual cases	Keratosis follicularis (Darier's disease)[2]	Two cases of good response
Raynaud's phenomenon[2]	Mixed results	Pityriasisi rubra pilaris (PRP)[2]	Mixed results
Systemic sclerosis[2]	Mixed results	Miscellaneous dermatosis (livedo vasculitis, chronic ulcers, benign chronic familial pemphigus)[2]	Some cases of benefit
Morphea[2]	Mixed results		
Yellow nail syndrome[2]	One case of good response		
Cutaneous lesions of lupus erythematosus[2]	Many good responses		
Granuloma[2]	Many good responses	Retrolental fibroplasia[3]	Many good responses
Lichen sclerosis et atrophicus[2]	Mixed results	Bronchopulmonary dysplasia[4]	Many good responses
Porphyria cutanea tarda[2]	Good reponses	Nocturnal leg cramps[5]	Many good responses
		Post-herpes Zoster neuralgia[2]	Some good responses

[1] Most of the clinical problems involve the skin and will not be explained here. Consult a medical reference text for clarification.

[2] Ayres and Mihan, 1975; Rees and Arnold.

[3] Gunby.

[4] Ehrenkranz et al.

[5] Ayres and Mihan, 1974.

Vitamin K

CHARACTERISTICS AND FACTS

Vitamin K was discovered in 1934 and isolated and synthesized in 1939. Although stable to heat and *reducing* agents, it is sensitive to acid, alkali, alcohol, light, and *oxidizing* agents. Various forms appear in Table 10-8, along with usage under varying clinical conditions.

Table 10-8

Table 10-8
Some Characteristics of Vitamin K

NATURAL OR SYNTHETIC*	NAME†	SOLUBILITY	NATURAL ANALOGUE	ROUTES OF ADMINISTRATION	CLINICAL USAGE	SAFETY
Natural (from green plants, e.g., alfalfa)	Vitamin K_1 (phylloquinone)	Fat soluble	None	Oral (not recommended for infants); intravenous or subcutaneous injection	Pregnancy; surgery; countering anticoagulants. (see text)	Acceptable in appropriate doses.
Natural (from bacteria)	Vitamin K_2 (menaquinone)	Fat soluble	None	Same as above	Same as above	Same as above
Synthetic	Menadione (formerly vitamin K_3)	Fat soluble	Menaquinone	Intramuscular or subcutaneous injection	Hemorrhage of infancy and labor; obstructive jaundice	Relatively safe for adults; safe for infants more than a few weeks old if recommended doses are complied with. Effects of large doses in infants: hemolytic anemia, hyperbilirubinemia, kernicterus.
Synthetic	Mephyton Konakion	Water miscible	Phylloquinone	Oral; intramuscular, intravenous, or subcutaneous injection	Newborn infants	Acceptable in appropriate doses.
Synthetic	Mono-Kay	Water miscible	Phylloquinone	Same as above	Same as above	Same as above

*Vitamin K is also located in purified fish meal.

†Other analogues not mentioned are Hykinone, Synkavite, and Kappadione of menaquinone and menadione.

In the normally healthy person, 10 percent of ingested vitamin K undergoes absorption. Jaundice, liver malfunction, and pancreatic disorders interfere with absorption.

NO RDAS ESTABLISHED

We obtain vitamin K from green and yellow vegetables and from bacterial synthesis in the colon. Drugs such as aspirin and antibiotics may inhibit intestinal synthesis. No RDAs have been established for vitamin K, but estimates place the adult daily need at 70 to 140 μg.

VERY IMPORTANT TO BLOOD

The role of vitamin K in blood clotting is highly important. Current research suggests that vitamin K directly or indirectly affects liver synthesis of prothrombin, a vital ingredient for clotting. Anticoagulants used in treating *thrombosis* (blood clots) and *phlebitis* (inflammation of a vein) accomplish their results by interfering with vitamin K's role in prothrombin synthesis. As we would expect, prolonged use leads to vitamin K deficiency and bleeding problems.

DEFICIENCY AFFECTS CLOTTING

Both formula and breast milk are low in vitamin K, explaining why infants have a long blood-clotting time. Breast milk has only one fourth the vitamin K formula, so supplementation is necessary. Infants weaned from milk have other vitamin K problems though, because baby food additives interfere with bacterial synthesis of vitamin K in the intestine. Similarly, children suffering from starvation, malabsorption, diarrhea, cystic fibrosis, or antibiotic exposure will have vitamin K deficiency requiring supplementation.

Bleeding in newborns, occurring due to birth processes, traumatic labor, circumcision, and obstructive jaundice, generally can be managed by vitamin K therapy. Infant hemorrhage studies have shown low thrombin levels, immature livers, inadequate bile salts, few intestinal bacteria, and low vitamin K storage, all factors indicative of vitamin K deficiency.

Deficiency diagnosis involves analysis of blood prothrombin level and clotting time. Avoidance of newborn bleeding involves such techniques as giving vitamin K to the mother just before delivery, and vitamin K therapy for the infant. The latter treatment involves giving *water-*

WILLIAM HAD ABNORMAL BLEEDING

When William, a 9-week-old black child, was admitted to the hospital, he had been bleeding from the mouth and gums for 3 days. Additionally, he had frequent bouts with fever and vomiting. Although William's birth weight had not been abnormally low, nor had he experienced unusual bleeding with circumcision, his mother had recurrent vaginal bleeding during pregnancy. William had previously been hospitalized at 3 weeks of age due to diarrhea.

Hospital examination showed a temperature of 104°F, irritability, and a bulging head. Neurological reactions were, however,

normal. Blood tests showed that various coagulation factors were deficient. A blood transfusion was done, and vitamin K was administered intravenously. Coagulation studies done 10 hours later showed definite improvement. William had a subdural hematoma (bleeding be-

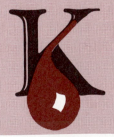

neath the covering of the brain) and mild hydrocephalus (excess fluid within the skull). The hematoma was treated by subdural taps.

Gradual improvement resulted in discharge from the hospital. William was on a normal diet by 7 months and showed normal growth and development at 18 months. William's vitamin K deficiency may have resulted from malabsorption, but this case and others also demonstrate that vitamin K supplement should be given in cases of protracted diarrhea, since diarrhea can also lead to vitamin K deficiency.

miscible vitamin K intravenously, since synthetic vitamin K can cause vomiting if administered orally.

Vitamin K deficiency is uncommon in adults. Low blood prothrombin or long clotting time can be controlled by 2 to 5 mg of vitamin K daily. Synthetic water-soluble vitamin K has been found effective for adults other than pregnant women and is the preferred treatment in cases of malabsorption. If a fat-soluble vitamin compound is administered, bile salts should be given concurrently.

Following surgery of the liver to correct obstructive jaundice, bleeding commonly occurs. Vitamin K before and after surgery can stem the problem. Transfusion is necessary in severe cases but must be followed by vitamin K therapy to guarantee an adequate prothrombin supply.

TOXICITY

Under various conditions, vitamin K in large doses can be toxic. In infants, large doses can cause *hyperbilirubinemia* (a form of jaundice) and hemolytic anemia. In premature infants, the symptoms are exaggerated. Adult tolerance reaches 10 to 40 mg for several weeks before vomiting occurs. Doses of one or more grams can cause increased excretion of albumin and porphyrin.

STUDY QUESTIONS

1. What characteristics do vitamins A, D, E, and K have in common?

2. Summarize the symptoms of vitamin A deficiency.

3. What is the chief function of vitamin D? Which foods contain this vitamin? What condition is created by its deficiency?

4. What is known about the role of vitamin E in human health? What are the richest food sources of this vitamin?

5. Is vitamin K deficiency more common in breast-fed or formula-fed infants? What problem may this deficiency cause?

6. Identify three prescription drugs containing vitamin A acid that were not mentioned in this chapter.

7. Use library resources to locate and describe two clinical cases in which large doses of vitamin E proved beneficial.

8. Summarize the symptoms for overdoses of vitamins A, D, and K.

REFERENCES

Ayres, S., Jr., and R. Mihan. "Nocturnal Leg Cramps (Systremma)." *South. Med. J.* 67 (1974): 1308.

Ayres, S., Jr., and R. Mihan. "Vitamin E and Dermatology." *Cutis* 16 (1975): 1017.

Basu, T. K. "Vitamin A and Cancer of Epithelial Origin." *J. Human Nutr.* 33 (1979): 24.

Ehrenkranz, R. A., et al. "Amelioration of Bronchopulmonary Dysplasia after Vitamin E Administration: A Preliminary Report." *N. Engl. J. Med.* 299 (1978): 564.

Gunby, P. "Trial of Vitamin E Therapy for Retrolental Fibroplasia." *JAMA* 243 (1980): 1021.

Institute of Food Technologists. "Vitamin E." *Food Tech.* 31 (1977): 77.

Pochi, P. E. "Hormones, Retinoids, and Acne." *N. Engl. J. Med.* 308 (1983): 1024.

Rees, R. B., and H. L. Arnold, Jr. "Vitamin E and Thee." *Cutis* 13 (1974): 761.

Teo, S. T., et al. "Chronic Vitamin A Intoxication." *Med. J. Aust.* 2 (1973): 324.

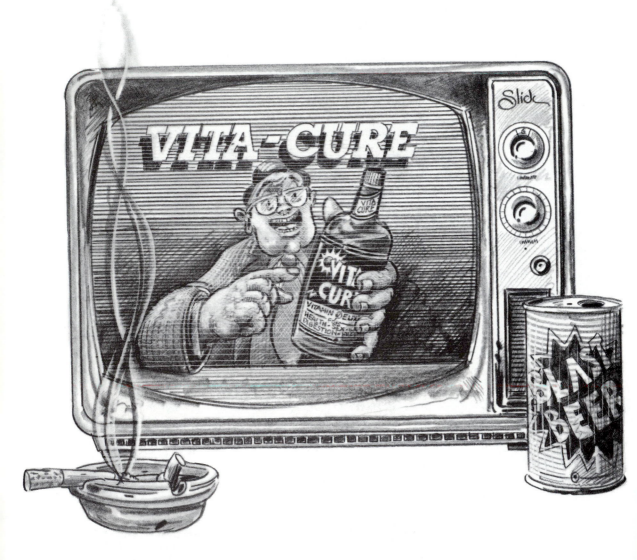

11

SUBSTANCES

Claimed to Be

VITAMINS:

IS LAETRILE A VITAMIN?

Tom
TRIES A RECIPE

Tom, a 35-year-old Southern California stockbroker, bought a one-pound package of raw, dried apricot kernels at a health food store. He had read in a health magazine about an especially healthful milkshake and wanted to try it.

He roasted the apricot kernels at 300° for 10 minutes and used 48 kernels, together with milk and honey, to make a shake for his wife and himself. She consumed only part of hers, disliking the taste. Tom consumed all of his and the remainder of his wife's.

One hour later he developed forceful vomiting, headache, flushing, heavy perspiration, dizziness, and faintness. In a local emergency room, vomiting was induced in both by ipecac. Tom's symptoms rapidly subsided (his wife had no symptoms). The vomitus of both contained fragments of apricot kernels.

Tom was a victim of cyanide poisoning resulting from hydrogen cyanide released from the apricot kernels upon contact with digestive chemicals. Symptoms can develop soon after ingestion and can include Tom's, as well as convulsions, stupor, paralysis, and death, depending on dosage. The minimum number of seeds that can result in cyanide poisoning is not known. Roasting the kernels after crushing them can remove the cyanide—if they are roasted for ten hours (Centers for Disease Control).

Laetrile

Perhaps no health issue has so aroused public sentiment as the laetrile controversy. Laetrile is promoted as a cure for cancer. To the terminally ill who are desperate to find a cure, and to family members who want to do everything possible to save a loved one, the motivation to try any possible cure could not be stronger.

The active ingredient in laetrile is amygdalin, a chemical that was first isolated in 1835. Actually there are two laetriles, amygdalin and prunasin. They are cyanogenic glycosides, found naturally in the kernels of apricot pits, apple seeds, pear seeds, peach pits, plum pits, cherry pits, and in nuts, such as almonds. Amygdalin has been promoted as a cancer cure since the mid-1800s (Dubick and Rucker; Greenberg; Herbert, 1979a; Marshall; Sun).

THE ISSUES
Proponents of laetrile have trade-named it "vitamin B_{17}." Opponents of this claim point out that laetriles are not essential nutritional components, do not promote processes vital to life, have no association with any disease when deficient, and serve no unique physiological function that no other compound can perform. True vitamins (see Chapters 8, 9, and 10) have all the foregoing characteristics. Numerous scientific stud-

ies have failed to confirm any of the essential characteristics of vitamins as being characteristics of laetriles.

The controversy does not, however, stop at the issue of whether or not laetriles are vitamins. Opponents of the industry that promotes laetrile caution that laetrile is dangerous, since it can lead to cyanide poisoning. They cite deaths that have resulted from accidental laetrile ingestion and deaths that have resulted from ingestion of apricot kernels. Death is caused by chemical interaction. When a cyanogenic glycoside (laetrile) comes into contact with hydrolytic enzymes (found in digestive juices and various common foods), the resultant interaction produces hydrogen cyanide (HCN), a deadly poison. Hydrolytic enzymes are found in lettuce, celery, bean sprouts, peaches, alfalfa sprouts, and other popular fruits and vegetables. Laetrile promoters encourage special diets high in fruits and vegetables.

Supporters of laetriles argue that laetriles are not dangerous, because our bodies contain rhodanese (an enzyme) and sulfur, which can detoxify cyanide. Although it is true that our bodies can ameliorate the effects of cyanide poisoning, small amounts must be ingested, *and* levels of rhodanese and sulfur must be adequate. The numerous deaths resulting from general cyanide poisoning demonstrate that the risk is not a good one.

In addition to the danger, another concern of scientists and nutritionists regarding laetriles is that those who rely on them are failing to benefit from scientifically proven and medically accepted anticancer treatments. Certainly, significant progress has been made in the use of both radiation and chemotherapy, as evidenced by the "success" rates achieved with some types of leukemia and certain types of Hodgkin's disease.

One other issue has developed in regard to the laetrile controversy. That issue is a legal one. Does a patient have the right to try whatever cure he or she chooses? This issue has been addressed in various states and in the United States Supreme Court. In the 1979 case *U.S. v. Rutherford*, the U.S. Supreme Court ruled that the U.S. Food and Drug Administration's ban on laetrile as an unlicensed, untested drug whose safety remains unproven is a proper ban. Owing to the FDA's ban, those attempting to market laetrile in the United States have been prosecuted for conspiracy to smuggle.

CURRENT STATUS

Despite mounting scientific evidence that laetriles do not prevent or cure cancer, and are dangerous, the laetrile industry continues to be a thriving business. Patients continue to seek miracle cures that will eliminate what often is a terminal diagnosis. The dynamic leadership of the laetrile business has been characterized by many as conducting cancer quackery with a businesslike enthusiasm unparalleled in health history. The United States Food and Drug Administration has advised every doctor and health professional in America that laetrile is worthless in preventing, treating, or curing cancer and that the substance lacks therapeutic or nutritional value.

217

CHAPTER ELEVEN
Substances Claimed to Be Vitamins:
Is Laetrile a Vitamin?

LOUISE SWALLOWS LAETRILE TABLETS

Louise, a healthy 1-year-old New Jersey girl, accidentally swallowed what was estimated to be four 500-mg laetrile (amygdalin) tablets. The drug was her father's; he was taking it in hopes of curing a cancer.

Approximately 30 minutes after she ate the tablets she became lethargic. Milk caused vomiting, and her parents rushed her to the hospital. By this time she was comatose and in shock and was having difficulty breathing. Her parents reported an overdose of vitamins to the hospital staff.

Immediate treatment included resuscitation efforts via endotracheal intubation and intravenous bicarbonate. Her stomach was also pumped. Two hours later, Louise was transferred by ambulance to a larger hospital. She was still in shock and a coma, with dilated pupils that were unresponsive to light. Her extremities failed to respond to reflex tests. The larger hospital ran a toxicological screen of known vitamins. Results were negative.

Two days later, Louise died. Because her parents believed that laetrile was a vitamin, and therefore stored it with their vitamins, the hospital discovered too late that Louise had cyanide poisoning, not a vitamin overdose. The distinction proved fatal (Braico et al.).

THE AANGAMIK CASE

Case data relating to Bodyscience, Inc., 20 Medford Avenue, Patchoque, New York 11772 (and other addresses)

Product label

AANGAMIK

aangamik 15
Calcium Gluconate
&
N,N-Dimethylglycine
50 mg. Equimolar Mixture
DMG[15]™
100 Tablets

Distributed by:
FoodScience Laboratories
at One Executive Drive
So. Burlington, Vermont 05401

The Original Formula—
First in America DMG[15]™

Suggested use: 3 to 6 tablets daily.

Contents:
Microcrystalline Cellulose (vegetable origin), Dicalcium Phosphate, Calcium Gluconate, N,N-Dimethylglycine, Tricalcium Phosphate

Samples of advertisement claims

With DMG[15], the Supernutrient Pill that can significantly improve your life and give you energy, stamina and endurance at work, at play, or at night with your spouse!

Jaye Robertson says DMG revitalized her dying husband!

"All I can tell you is that it gave my husband new life for four years, and if it could give a dying man life, imagine what it could do for a healthy person."

And, what a night! I was convinced that the sexual enhancing effects that I felt were from the DMG[15] and not just my beautiful companion.

In fact, my husband was feeling so good, our love life was like a perpetual honeymoon.

SCIENTIFIC PROOF!

University tests in Los Angeles and Charleston indicate that DMG may help your body prevent infection and disease as well as speed recovery time.

We read about DMG, a new nutrient called a metabolic enhancer, which could sometimes assist in easing arteriosclerosis by delivering more oxygen to the bloodstream.

. . . how it has helped protect against illness and improve recovery.

These findings suggest that DMG may allow the cells to continue normal functioning even under adverse (low oxygen) conditions. This shows that DMG may benefit athletes who experience pain, muscle cramping, and fatigue; individuals undergoing surgery or suffering from degenerative diseases; and others who require greater oxygen efficiency.

IMPORTANT NOTICE FROM BODYSCIENCE, INC.

This article includes published reports, notarized sworn testimonials, and the opinion of many experts that may not yet be scientific dogma. You see, BodyScience, Inc. is in the forefront of research into alternative methods of increasing your body's natural capabilities. Our goal is to take the latest in nutritional science, biological research, and pharmaceutical knowledge, and combine them to give you freedom of choice and an iron-clad guarantee. If you're not satisfied with how DMG—or any of our products— enhances the quality of your life, just return the unused portion— even the empty bottle or package—for a prompt refund of your purchase price!

Pangamic Acid

Pangamic acid, or pangamate, has been promoted under the trade name "vitamin B_{15}." The promoters of pangamic acid as a vitamin are also promoters of laetrile as a vitamin. As in the case of laetrile, pangamic acid lacks the properties of vitamins (Dubick and Rucker; Herbert, 1979b; Marshall).

Often marketed as calcium pangamate, the product was also initially isolated from apricot kernels and has subsequently been developed by laboratory synthesis. Scientific analysis of the product has shown that its chemical contents vary from product to product. Because evidence fails to confirm pangamic acid as a definite chemical entity that is safe for human use or serves any medical or therapeutic purpose, its distribution is prohibited in Canada.

Promoters of pangamic acid claim it to be effective in treating cancer, asthma, allergies, heart disease, hepatitis, glaucoma, aging, diabetes, alcoholism, and schizophrenia. Other claims include: sexual potentiation, reduction of lactic acid buildup, lowering blood cholesterol levels, normalizing blood-sugar metabolism, and improvement of oxygen utilization. Support for such claims often reference anecdotes from Russia, but no scientific studies confirm the claims.

Scientific evidence states that pangamic acid is not a vitamin, has no proven therapeutic benefit, has no known nutritional worth, lacks standard chemical validity, and may be mutagenic (causing birth defects). The United States Food and Drug Administration has taken a strong stand on "vitamin B_{15}."

What is the current legal status of pangamic acid? The FDA has forced several manufacturers out of business. In 1980, the FDA sought an injunction to prevent major Vermont manufacturers from shipping the substance interstate. The FDA's argument is that the active component of calcium pangamate (N,N-dimethylglycine hydrochloride, frequently referred to as DMG by the manufacturers) has not been proved safe according to FDA standards. Attorneys for manufacturers argue it is a food, not a food additive, and therefore is not subject to proof-of-safety requirements. The FDA's position, that "B_{15}" is an additive for which no evidence of safety exists, makes it illegal to sell it as a dietary supplement and illegal to sell it as a drug.

As indicated in Chapter 8, the United States Postal Service sometimes intervenes in the mail order of such substances. On July 22, 1982, the Postal Service determined that Bodyscience, Inc. (P.S. Docket No. 12/123) was engaging in conducting a scheme or device for obtaining money through the mails by means of false representation in violation of 39 U.S. Code 3005 with respect to the sale of products containing calcium pangamate and purporting to have special therapeutic clinical effects that have been found to be false by the Postal Service. As a result, the postmaster was instructed to hold all defendant's mail relating to the sale of such products. Part of the case presentation is reproduced in the box.

219

CHAPTER ELEVEN
Substances Claimed to Be Vitamins:
Is Laetrile a Vitamin?

FOOD FOR THOUGHT

Dr. Victor Herbert (1979a) has proposed the following four basic scientific canons for evaluating medical information:

1. Does it go beyond "personal observation" to stand the test of scrutiny and criticism by other scientists; that is, is it a study or a story? Is it science or anecdote?

2. Was it compared for effectiveness in controlled studies to other treatments and to suggestibility or to the "doing of nothing"; that is, to a placebo? What is the natural history of the disorder in the absence of therapy? Was the observed result cause and effect, or coincidence due to the natural history of the disorder?

3. Has it proved safe? Safe compared with what? Is the risk justified? What is the risk: benefit ratio? (Note that if there is no benefit, the risk: benefit ratio is infinity, which is not tolerable.)

4. The burden of proof is on those who propose doing or giving something, especially if it involves a remedy or procedure not well established in medical practice.

Choline

Choline is a structural component of lecithin and sphingomyelin. Both substances are a form of fat (Goodhart and Shils). Lecithin transports fat in the body, and sphingomyelin is important to nervous tissues. Choline and **acetyl CoA** (see Chapter 14) produce *acetylcholine*, which transmits impulses at nerve endings.

Since choline is widespread in foods and can be synthesized from glycine (an amino acid, see Chapter 7) in the liver, it has been considered nonessential for the human body and as not meeting the definition of a vitamin.

We obtain 0.5 to 1 g of choline daily from egg yolk, beef, liver, soybeans, whole grains, and fish. Many processed foods contain it as an additive. Neither lecithin nor choline deficiency has been reported in humans. Very high levels of choline consumption have, however, produced side effects including dizziness, nausea, diarrhea, heart disturbances, and a fishy body odor.

Promoters of choline have claimed it beneficial in memory improvement, in treatment of mental disorders, and in the mobilization of fat and cholesterol from the liver. Physicians have reported that its use has been beneficial in the treatment of such conditions as Huntington's chorea, a hereditary twitching that occurs in adults. Some advocates of choline claim it should be classified as a B vitamin.

Advocates of lecithin, the dietary source of choline, claim that lecithin can prevent or cure heart disease and lower blood cholesterol. However, one study of healthy individuals taking lecithin for a month failed to demonstrate any reduction in blood cholesterol levels. Though no human requirement for choline has been established, a committee of the American Academy of Pediatrics has recommended that it be added to infant formula diets at a level equal to its presence in breast milk. This is a significant recommendation, signaling that the encouraging findings regarding choline hold the promise of further discoveries.

Coenzyme Q

Coenzyme Q (CoQ) is fat-soluble and resembles vitamins K and E. The substance is found in nearly all living cells and belongs to a group of chemicals called *ubiquinones*. CoQ functions as an important component in the respiratory chain, assisting the process by which energy is drawn from ingested nutrients and stored as *ATP* (adenosine triphosphate). For more details on this metabolic function, refer to Chapter 14.

Ubiquinone has proved beneficial in therapy for anemia resulting from severe malnutrition. Its deficiency has also been questioned in regard to the presence of heart disease. Clearly, its proven role in oxidation suggests that further research may yield important insights.

Bioflavonoids

Bioflavonoids could be termed the "almost vitamins." In 1936, they were declared essential for humans and, along with hesperidin and rutin, bioflavonoids were claimed to be sources of "vitamin P." This special status was accorded them since red pepper and lemon extracts, substances with high levels of bioflavonoids, could reverse the effects of vitamin C deficiency. Though this claim was subsequently invalidated, as was the existence of vitamin P, bioflavonoids may have pharmacological effects. Their biological functions remain unknown (Dubick).

Bioflavonoids are found in citrus fruits, other fruits, and vegetables. Some claim they prove beneficial to strokes, joint diseases, and respiratory illnesses, but no clinical evidence documents these claims. Bioflavonoids have proved effective in inhibiting *aldose reductase*, an enzyme active in the formation of cataracts associated with diabetes. Bioflavonoids have not been classified as essential.

Inositol

Inositol, the muscle sugar, occurs in high concentrations in both plants and animals (Goodhart and Shils). Inositol is one form of sugar alcohol, the alcohol form of glucose (see Chapter 5). In animals it occurs in phospholipids (see Chapter 6) found in nerve and organ tissues. In grain products, inositol occurs as phytic acid. Too much phytic acid in our diet may interfere with calcium and iron absorption, yet the phytic acid of whole-grain cereals has been shown to be beneficial in the prevention of dental caries (cavities) under experimental conditions. Despite these findings, the function of inositol in our bodies remains unknown. It has proved beneficial in animals in reversing fatty livers and restoring hair loss. It is essential for the action of yeast.

Our bodies can synthesize inositol, though we consume about 1 g each day from meat, milk, vegetables, nuts, fruit, and whole-grain cereals. It occurs in its highest concentration in hair and in heart and skeletal muscle.

Lipoic Acid

Lipoic acid fails to meet the test of essentiality for humans or animals, though some bacteria require it for growth. It participates in many biochemical reactions in the body, but our bodies supply enough lipoic acid for those purposes.

Chemically, lipoic acid exists in five forms, and the chemical is sometimes called thioctic acid, indicating the presence of sulfur. Three of lipoic acid's forms are fat-soluble, one is water-soluble, and one is bound to protein. Although its role in human health remains unknown, in animal studies it regulates plasma lipid formation and stimulates cancer growth. Some suggest it can benefit alcoholics, but documented evidence has not yet supported this claim.

Carnitine

Known as the heart vitamin, and characterized as vitamin B_T, carnitine is a protein present in human tissues, especially the muscles and the liver. In some clinical studies, the administration of carnitine to individuals who regularly experienced heart pain during exercise resulted in a prolonging of the exercise period before heart pain occurred. These test results generated the term "heart vitamin" and demonstrated the possibility that carnitine can permit greater energy expenditure before coronary insufficiency occurs (Goodhart and Shils).

Carnitine has not achieved vitamin status because, despite its success

221

CHAPTER ELEVEN
Substances Claimed to Be Vitamins:
Is Laetrile a Vitamin?

in strengthening the heart, inadequate carnitine in the diet does not result in a deficiency disease. The case history of Paul, an 11-year-old, illustrates carnitine's potential benefits. Paul was a weak child from birth. When he failed to develop proper speech patterns, testing showed he had a hearing loss. By the age of 5, he began experiencing headaches, nausea, and vomiting. By the age of 6 his growth was retarded, and even a slight amount of exercise resulted in breathlessness. He could not run, jump, or hop. After vitamin therapy produced no change and low-fat diets had little effect, carnitine therapy commenced. Paul began to grow and began to develop muscle strength. On the basis of his reaction to carnitine therapy, it was determined that Paul was born with a defect in the normal metabolism of carnitine.

Little is known of the carnitine content in food. Animal products are better sources than plant products. Carnitine research continues, since it is possible that patients who respond to carnitine therapy do not have a dietary deficiency of carnitine but have other metabolic difficulties affecting carnitine utilization. For example, liver synthesis of carnitine may be defective, or carnitine might be transported in the blood in a bound form—a form that the body cannot utilize.

Para-Aminobenzoic Acid (PABA)

Also called PABA or aminobenzoic acid, *para-aminobenzoic acid* was once considered a vitamin, but it is now recognized as a substance that has importance in relation to the body's normal metabolism of folic acid (see Chapter 9). Folic acid and its related compounds are, as a group, known as folacin. Although para-aminobenzoic acid is a vitamin for certain bacteria, it has no known nutritional value for us and does not qualify for vitamin status.

Some have claimed that PABA retards the graying of hair and the development of skin cancer, but these claims have not been scientifically established. It has been proved that PABA interferes with the pharmaceutical effects of sulfa drugs (common antiinfectious medications), so the ingestion of PABA can worsen infection. Para-aminobenzoic acid has proved effective in the prevention of sunburn. Those who have ingested as much as 10 g of PABA have developed nausea, vomiting, fever, and rash.

Because para-aminobenzoic acid can neutralize the effects of sulfa drugs, the product is beneficial to the growth of pathogenic bacteria and additionally isolates them from sulfa therapy.

"Vitamin Q"

Dr. A. J. Quick of the Medical College of Wisconsin has proposed a new term, "hemostatic vitamin." By this he refers to a vitamin similar to vitamins C and K whose deficiency can cause abnormal bleeding. Though C and K stand as the only confirmed vitamins with such effect, Dr. Quick has suggested a third one, "vitamin Q." Found in the phospholipids of soybeans, the proposed vitamin Q (Quick) remains of unknown composition. In case histories, abnormal clotting time has been corrected through dietary supplementation with soybean phospholipids, leading researchers to propose the existence of the vitamin.

223

CHAPTER ELEVEN
Substances Claimed to Be Vitamins:
Is Laetrile a Vitamin?

Vitamin Q does not have formal vitamin status, since its deficiency has not been established in otherwise healthy persons. To achieve official recognition as a vitamin, the substance would have to be required in the diets of healthy individuals to maintain proper blood clotting time. This is the case for vitamin K, but it has not been proved for the proposed vitamin Q. In the meantime, soybean phospholipids continue to serve a therapeutic purpose in abnormal bleeding cases reported by Dr. Quick.

For example, Dr. Quick has reported that the intake of soybean phospholipids (for example, lecithin; see section under choline) was beneficial in controlling his own postoperative bleeding following surgery for an aneurysm (a blood clot formed in the abdominal area). He theorizes that the postoperative bleeding difficulties could have been avoided through a preoperative process involving the ingestion of larger quantities of soybean phospholipids. The initial evidence seems to demonstrate that soybean phospholipids contain a factor (factor Q) that can affect formation and utilization of prothrombin (a protein necessary to the formation of blood clots) and can reduce prolonged bleeding time.

STUDY QUESTIONS

1. Why are certain substances associated with vitamins not labeled as vitamins? What are some of these substances?

2. Using library resources, research and identify five cases of death from laetrile ingestion.

3. What is pangamic acid? What are its claimed therapeutic values?

4. What is choline? List the therapeutic values attributed to this product using library resources.

5. Write an essay on the history of bioflavonoids.

6. Research and describe other products currently claimed to be vitamins.

7. Can you ascertain the current scientific status of "vitamin Q"?

REFERENCES

Braico, K. T., et al. "Laetrile Intoxication: Report of a Fatal Case." N. Engl. J. Med. 300 (1979): 238.

Centers for Disease Control. "Cyanide Poisoning from Ingestion of Apricot Kernels—California." Morbidity and Mortality Weekly Report, December 19, 1975.

Dubick, M. A. "Dietary Supplements and Health Aids— A Critical Evaluation." Part 3. Natural and Miscellaneous Products. J. Nutr. Educ. 15 (1983): 123.

Dubick, M. A., and R. B. Rucker. "Dietary Supplements and Health Aids—A Critical Evaluation." Part 1. Vitamins and Minerals. J. Nutr. Educ. 15 (1982): 47.

Goodhart, R. S., and M. E. Shils, eds. Modern Nutrition in Health and Disease. 6th ed. Philadelphia: Lea & Febiger, 1983.

Greenberg, D. M. "The Vitamin Fraud in Cancer Quackery." West. J. Med. 122 (1975): 345.

Herbert, V. "Laetrile: The Cult of Cyanide-Promoting Poison for Profit." Am. J. Clin. Nutr. 32 (1979a): 1121.

Herbert, V. "Pangamic Acid ('Vitamin B_{15}')." Am. J. Clin. Nutr. 32 (1979b): 1534.

Marshall, C. W. Vitamins and Minerals: Help or Harm? Philadelphia: George F. Strickley, 1983.

Quick, A. J. "Minireview: Vitamin Q." Life Sci. 15 (1975): 1.

Quick, A. J. "Vitamin Q in Control of Bleeding." Wisconsin Med. J. 74 (1975): 585.

Sun, M. "Laetrile Brush Fire is Out, Scientists Hope." Science 212 (1981): 758.

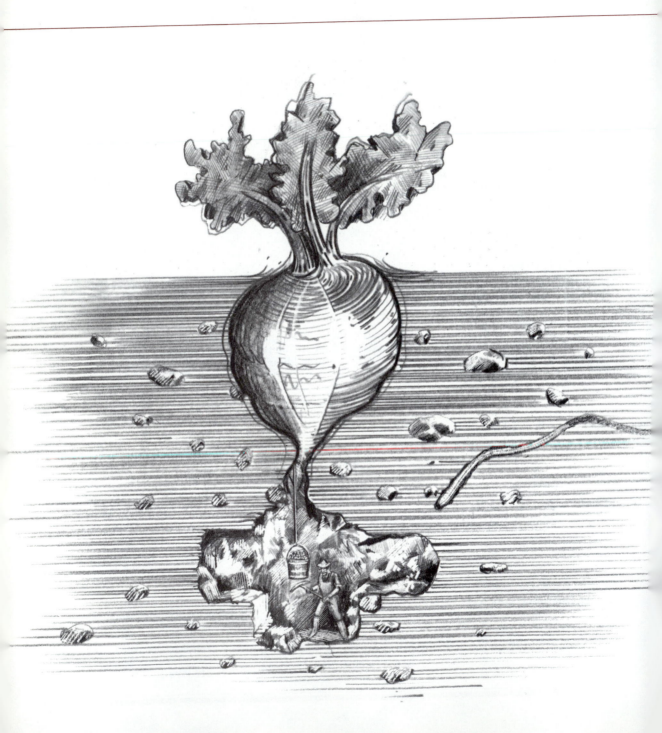

12

Minerals:

IRON DEFICIENCY STILL HAUNTS US

Here is a mineral supplement that "gives you energy to stay young"

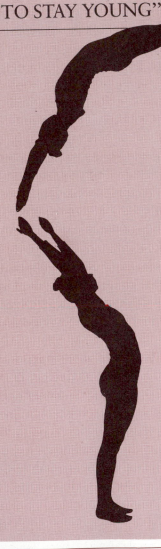

Chromill-GTF can "prevent diabetes"

Unfortunately, as we get older, we tend to absorb less [chromium]. This is further aggravated by the fact that chromium has also become noticeably deficient from our foods. Without sufficient chromium, your body will be deprived of the energy it needs and will be subject to unhealthy fluctuations in blood sugar levels that can lead to hypoglycemia, hyperglycemia and diabetes.

Chromium deficiencies affect many people, but most frequently those in middle age and older. The increasing majority of these deficiencies has led to the discovery that the naturally occurring state of chromium, so vital to blood sugar regulation and energy production, can be duplicated. This is the Glucose Tolerance Factor molecule, or GTF.

Chromill-GTF exactly duplicates the natural chromium GTF molecule and provides you with the most effective and potent source of chromium you can get.

Chromill-GTF will "retard aging"

Sure, it's only natural that we get older. But, who says we have to look and feel older and resign ourselves to less energy and activity. Take Chromill-GTF today. It contains the scientifically developed mineral formulation that will let you, too, recapture the vigor of youth.

With CHROMILL-GTF you'll be participating in all the fun-filled activities you love. Now, there is no reason not to feel as young as you want as long as you want. When you supplement your diet with CHROMILL-GTF, you'll have all the energy you need to stay active, enthusiastic and full of vitality. CHROMILL-GTF gives you energy to stay young.

This material was part of an advertisement run by Athena Products, Ltd. (Box 81371, Atlanta, GA 30366). On August 11, 1981, the United States Postal Service determined that Athena Products, Ltd. and their agents were engaged in conducting a scheme for obtaining money through the mails by means of false representations in violation of 39 U.S. Code 3005 with respect to the sale of the product known as Chromill-GTF (PS Docket No. 10/128). The company was forbidden to use the mail to sell such a product.

Minerals! Perhaps the word makes you think of metals, or of a rock display in a museum. Somehow minerals strike many of us as not belonging in the same general class of nutrients as vitamins, protein, carbohydrate, and other nutrients. It is as if minerals were more removed from our physical bodies, even though they are just as essential to our well-being as the other nutrients are.

In a sense, our conception of minerals is not too far removed from truth. Like metals and gems, minerals are "mined" from the soil, though plants do the mining. When we consume vegetables or meat from animals that have eaten plants, we acquire minerals, which as a group are called **ash.** (The term "ash" dervies from the chemical process by which substances can be burned; the resulting residue, known as ash, contains whatever minerals were in the original substance.)

Our Macro and Micro Mineral Needs

Our need for minerals ranges from those we need in large quantities, known as **macroelements**, to those we need in small quantities, known as **microelements**. Table 12-1 shows how various minerals are classified and our approximate daily need for each type.

You will notice that all the minerals combined account for only 4 percent of our body weight, but despite their small bulk, they serve two vital functions. Minerals serve as structural components of body parts, and they regulate important body processes. Figure 12-1 depicts the distribution of minerals in our body, and Table 12-2 lists the important body parts that contain minerals as structural components.

The body functions in which minerals actively participate include: (1) transmission of electrochemical messages in the nervous system (nerve impulses), (2) control of body acidity, (3) balance of fluids in different parts of the body, (4) digestion, (5) muscle contraction, and (6) other body reactions. The general division of minerals into macroelements and

Table 12-1
Approximate Distribution of Mineral Elements in the Body*

ELEMENTS	% OF BODY WEIGHT	AMOUNT NEEDED IN THE DAILY DIET (mg/DAY/ELEMENT)
Macroelements (calcium, phosphorus, potassium, sodium, sulfur, magnesium, chlorine)	3.2–3.8	100+
Microelements (iron, copper, cobalt, zinc, manganese, iodine, molybdenum, selenium, fluorine, chromium)	less than 0.1	00.5–5

*Although RDAs have not been established for sodium, potassium, chloride, copper, manganese, fluoride, chromium, selenium, and molybdenum, the National Academy of Sciences has estimated the safe and adequate daily dietary intakes of these elements.

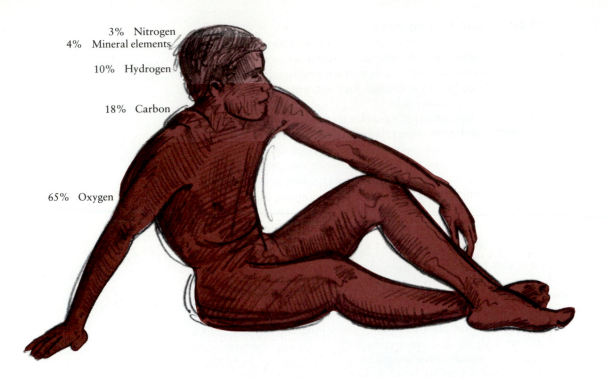

3% Nitrogen
4% Mineral elements

10% Hydrogen

18% Carbon

65% Oxygen

Figure 12-1: Approximate distribution of organic and inorganic (mineral) elements in the body.

Table 12-2

Mineral Elements That Are Components of Important Body Structures

ELEMENT(S)	CHEMICAL SUBSTANCE(S)	BODY STRUCTURES
Calcium, phosphorus, magnesium	Hydroxyapatite	Teeth, bones
Sulfur	Cystine, cysteine, methionine	Protein of skin, hair, nails
Iron	Hemoglobin, myoglobin	Blood components
Iron, copper	Cofactors of enzymes	Enzyme complexes
Iodine	Thyroxine	Hormone of thyroid glands
Cobalt	Cobalamin	Water-soluble vitamin B_{12}

microelements provides a convenient way for us to become more familiar with the role of individual minerals.

Macroelements: The Major Seven

Seven minerals comprise the group of **inorganic** elements, which are required in larger quantities than the organic elements. Of the seven, sodium, calcium, potassium, and magnesium are *basic*, or alkaline, in solution. We obtain these four minerals from fruits and vegetables. Phosphorus, chlorine, and sulfur are *acidic* in solution. We obtain the acidic macroelements from protein foods and cereal products. The effect of acidic or alkaline foods on our urine will be discussed later in this chapter.

Sodium is most familiar to us as sodium chloride, or table salt, but it appears in other foods as well. Although sodium is an important element, we are still unsure how much the body needs of it daily. The body loses about 40 to 220 mg of sodium a day; for example, in perspiration and in the urine and feces (Table 12-3). To provide a safety margin, a daily intake of 500 mg (half a gram) should theoretically satisfy our need. However, we may be consuming 5 to 15 times more than that.

Our Taste for Salt

A rough estimate shows that we eat about 3 to 7 g of sodium a day. The magnitude of this quantity is apparent when you consider that 4 g of sodium is equivalent to the sodium in 2 teaspoons of table salt. However, your actual need for sodium depends on the work you do and the climate you live in, since we can lose a substantial amount of sodium when we perspire. Our personal taste for salt is determined by our childhood eating patterns, family practices, and social and cultural factors.

One of sodium's body functions is to protect against fluid loss by maintaining both water balance and osmotic pressure (see Chapter 13). As an alkaline mineral, sodium also serves in maintaining the body's neutrality (not to become too acidic). Sodium also serves in absorption and transportation of certain nutrients, muscle contraction, electrical transmission in the nervous system, and permeability of cell membranes.

How Much Salt Is Too Much?

A recent study (Miller) indicates the following:

1. Nearly three out of four adults have read or heard about health problems related to sodium or salt.
2. Slightly better than half of the adult population connects high blood pressure with salt consumption.
3. Four out of ten adults are trying to avoid or cut down on salt or sodium.
4. By mid-1982, consumers had a 50 percent better chance of finding salt content on food labels than they did two years earlier.

Because the body stores significant amounts of sodium, and because of our taste for salty foods, sodium deficiency is rare. If, however, need increases at a time when intake decreases, deficiency can result in nausea, apathy, exhaustion, dizziness, intestinal cramping, difficulty in breathing, and vomiting. Such symptoms can be reversed by drinking salt solution. Unless sodium depletion is reversed, dehydration, shock, and death can result.

At the opposite side of the ingestion spectrum, excess sodium intake can be toxic. This condition is even rarer than deficiency, however, since our bodies reject salty food tastes when our sodium content is too high. Excess alkalinity, called **alkalosis**, can result from ingesting too much sodium, a risk with antacid preparations.

Table 12-3
Approximate Daily Loss of Sodium

SOURCE OF LOSS	AMOUNT (mg)
Skin	
Perspiration	15–25
Desquamation (sloughing of skin), hair loss	10–25
Urine	5–40
Stool	10–130
Menstrual fluid	trace
Approximate daily loss of sodium	40–220

Does Salt Cause High Blood Pressure?

Although studies suggest an association between high sodium intake and the onset of hypertension (high blood pressure), a condition that affects an estimated 34 million Americans, it has not been conclusively established that sodium consumption is a major factor in the cause of hypertension (Lecos, 1981; Miller). There are still many scientists who believe that the role of salt in high blood pressure is exaggerated. Perhaps the controversy was best summed up by Harry Schwartz in the publication *ACSH News & Views*: "In summary, many medical experts and policy makers have expressed the view that sodium reduction for everyone can't hurt and might help prevent hypertension in some people."

The evidence is strong enough, however, for most members of the medical and scientific communities to conclude that a substantial portion of the U.S. population, especially those genetically or otherwise predisposed to hypertension, would benefit from a reduction in dietary sodium. The fact is that most people are getting more than enough sodium from the food they eat and the water they drink or by the use of salt in foods they prepare. Sodium is in most foods, either because it occurs naturally or because it was added during the manufacturer's processing or during the preparation of the meal in the home.

Most community water supplies contain varying amounts of sodium because it is naturally present or because it is added by the use of "softeners" in hard water areas. This can mean sodium also is being consumed in coffee, tea, and other beverages prepared from local water supplies. The consumer usually can find out how much sodium is in the water from the local health or water department.

The government's current efforts in regard to sodium have focused on its announced plans to expand its activity in educating consumers about sodium, especially salt intake, and to encourage the food industry to act voluntarily to reduce the sodium in thousands of foods processed and sold in the United States.

Tips for the Salt-Conscious Consumer

Limiting the amount of sodium in one's daily diet is not easy. The sodium-conscious consumer simply must be knowledgeable—and disciplined—about the foods he or she eats (Lecos, 1981; Miller). Limiting sodium intake means working closely with a doctor or a professional dietitian or both to plan a proper diet, especially if sodium restriction is critical in the treatment of high blood pressure or other diseases. It means learning which foods are high and which are low in sodium, and it especially means knowing that cutting down on sodium intake is not just a case of avoiding salt, although regular table salt is the largest single contributor of sodium to the human diet.

The sodium-conscious consumer has other worries, too. Shopping in the supermarket will take longer because food labels and ingredient lists will have to be checked for clues to sodium content—if the information is indeed there. Finding out means knowing how to read a nutrition label and ingredient list. Sometimes, a sodium ingredient is identified by its

HOW DO I CUT DOWN ON SALT?

For the person wishing to cut down on salt, many food options are available (Miller). Indeed, the salt-conscious person (and there now are many of them) can dine for days on processed foods with a minimum of repetition as well as very little sodium.

For breakfast, for example, one can begin with a low-sodium tomato or vegetable juice, move on to cooked or dry low-sodium cereal, including frosted types, and have toast made from no-salt-added bread and spread with unsalted butter or margarine.

Lunch can include a wide variety of soups from some of the nation's major soup and soup mix manufacturers, peanut butter with less than 10 milligrams of sodium per tablespoon, no-salt-added tuna, reduced-salt processed meats, and low-sodium Colby or Swiss-type cheese surrounded by saltine crackers with unsalted tops.

For dinner, there is tomato paste, spaghetti sauce, pasta, a long list of no-salt-added canned vegetables, cottage cheese, turkey breast, bread sticks, condiments such as ketchup and salad dressings, cookies, candies, and frozen desserts, all with little or no salt.

In between these meals, there can be snacking on unsalted peanuts, pretzels, or potato chips. Soda water and bottled water with low sodium content are available for those who like it plain or with a little spirit. Melba toast, pastries, rice cakes and tea crackers are among the other items available for the snacker who wishes to avoid sodium.

The Food and Drug Administration has implemented a sodium program that includes: food labeling requirements, a public education program, and an effort to get food processors to voluntarily label their products as to sodium content.

proper chemical name. At other times a general term is used, such as brine or salt pork.

Of course, we can always turn to commercially available salt substitutes and buy only foods that are labeled clearly as being salt free or low in sodium content. Salt substitutes can be used by the normally healthy person with no apparent ill effect. However, there are problems with these chemicals that we will discuss in the section on potassium.

Does Sea Salt Have Special Properties?

Some promoters insist that sea salt constitutes a more nutritional salt. Analysis has, however, shown that sea salt is chiefly sodium chloride, just like table salt, with small amounts of magnesium and calcium. The typical American diet meets our need for sodium, and nutritionists have not found an advantage for sea salt over ordinary table salt.

HIGH BLOOD PRESSURE, FAINTING, AND POTASSIUM

Like sodium, potassium is an essential mineral for which we do not have an established dietary need. Our normal diet provides 2 to 5 g; however, cooking processes can cause some loss of the potassium that would otherwise be available. (The potassium content of common foods is given in the Appendix.)

Some Background Information

Potassium works with sodium in maintaining fluid distribution and osmotic pressure, in transmitting nerve impulses, in maintaining body neutrality, and in chemical and biological reactions. Whereas calcium stimulates muscle contraction, potassium functions in muscle relaxation. Potassium also serves a special function by regulating the release of insulin into the bloodstream.

The regulation of potassium content in our body involves the kidneys, which can excrete excess potassium. The kidneys cannot, however, conserve potassium. Deficiency can therefore occur, though it is rare except in cases of long-term intravenous feeding and malnutrition.

Too Much or Too Little Can Be Dangerous

Potassium can increase to harmful levels in the blood when the body's normal ability to excrete this mineral is diminished. This condition, called *hyperkalemia*, is frequently a concern for individuals with heart or kidney disorders and may result in the disruption of normal heart function. Such persons require medical supervision to control their intake of potassium (Lecos, 1983).

Besides being found naturally in foods, potassium also reaches the body in other ways: as a nutrient added to foods; in tablets, capsules, or liquids sold in retail outlets; in some prescribed drugs; and in substitutes for table salt. Substitutes for table salt usually have potassium chloride as the main ingredient. The Food and Drug Administration regards salt substitutes as foods for special dietary use and as drugs. As such, the labels on the products must state that the substitutes should be used only on a physician's advice.

Various clinical observations have indicated that individuals who are taking diuretics to reduce body sodium may be losing potassium at the same time. Such patients may develop fainting and other more serious symptoms. However, an increased consumption of fruits, such as grapefruit, and juices such as orange juice, can help prevent the loss.

Another problem is potassium supplements. Misuse has led to several deaths. One involved a young woman on a liquid protein diet who consumed a potassium chloride medication whenever she felt weak or tired. Shortly before her death she took 47 tablets of potassium chloride. In another case, a nursing mother who was following diet advice from a popular health book mixed potassium chloride with her breast milk and fed it to her 2-month-old infant to treat its "colic." The baby died soon after.

WHEN A DOCTOR PRESCRIBES BONE MEAL

Ethel contacted her physician after developing symptoms of weakness. Her physician recommended a calcium supplement, powdered bone meal.

Two years later, Ethel returned to the physician complaining of fatigue, muscular weakness, dizziness, and personality changes. The physician recommended that she increase the bone meal dosage to 50 to 60 g per day, which she did. As her illness progressed over the next several years, she contacted several other doctors. None was able to diagnose her illness.

During the years of her suffering, she lost weight, developed paralysis of her right arm, had to begin using a cane to walk, and had abdominal pain. She complained of a sensation in the bridge of her nose and of a metallic taste in her mouth. Her skin became especially sensitive to sunlight. She was hospitalized for a time owing to a fever. Her blood count showed signs of leukemia, though many of her symptoms were inconsistent with leukemia.

After much personal effort and library research, this patient self-diagnosed the possibility of lead poisoning. With the help of friends, the bone meal she had been taking was analyzed. It was found to be contaminated with lead. Over the six-year period during which she had ingested the bone meal supplement, Ethel had contracted lead poisoning.

Although lead has no biological value and most is excreted in the urine, some lead accumulates in our bones. Estimates placed Ethel's lead accumulation at 500 mg per year. The bone meal she had been ingesting was made from horses at a European glue factory. Since the horses were old, their bones had accumulated lead just as did Ethel's. The resultant bone meal was, therefore, contaminated by lead.

Natural calcium supplement is available in the form of bone meal and in the form of dolomite (pulverized rock). Bone meal, the powder resulting from the grinding of animal bones, became popular because individuals wanted a natural source of such minerals as calcium, magnesium, and phosphorus.

Bone meal promoters claim the product can be beneficial for calming hyperactive children, for preventing leg cramps, and for improving sensitivity to sound. Nutritionists caution that bone meal, especially when made from older animals, carries the risk of lead poisoning due to the lead accumulated by older animals. Ethel's case history illustrates this (Crosby).

Because bone meal is not a food or a drug, it was not under the rigorous control of the Food and Drug Administration, nor had limits been set in regard to heavy metal contaminants. Since Ethel's case occurred, some headway has been made in regulating heavy metal contamination in both foods and supplements.

YES, CALCIUM IS IMPORTANT FOR THE BONES

Of the seven macroelements, you are probably most familiar with calcium. The word instantly makes us think of bones and teeth, where 99 percent of our body's calcium is located. Our bones store calcium, releasing it to the blood as needed.

Calcium's major function involves structure for bones and teeth, but it also aids in the blood's clotting process. Calcium assists in message transmission through our nervous system, in muscle fiber contraction and relaxation, and in heart muscle function.

Calcium Need

Our daily need for calcium has been the subject of debate. Presently, 800 mg daily is recommended for adults, with a higher amount needed for pregnancy or lactation. Milk serves as our chief calcium source, with four times as much found in cow's milk as in human breast milk. Such canned fish as sardines, which contain dissolved bones, also provide an excellent source. Leafy vegetables, whole grains, nuts, and legumes are also high in calcium. (The calcium content of common foods is given in the Appendix.)

Can Unleavened Bread Cause Calcium Deficiency?

Intake proves only the first step in calcium nutrition, for absorption can vary. For example, vitamin D can increase absorption, as can the presence of lactose. Excess fiber or roughage can decrease calcium absorption, as can the use of laxatives. Diarrhea reduces calcium absorption, as does a lack of balance between calcium and phosphorus. When physical activity is inadequate, calcium absorption decreases, a matter of concern for those who are bedridden.

Sometimes, excess consumption of oxalic and phytic acid in the diet can decrease calcium absorption. **Oxalic acid** occurs in some vegetables, such as chard, rhubarb, and spinach. When present in the intestinal tract, oxalic acid can chelate (combine with) calcium and make it unavailable for absorption. Normally, the ingestion of a small quantity of oxalic acid poses no problems. However, the consumption of certain vegetables in considerable excess may interfere with calcium absorption. **Phytic acid**, found in the outer husks of cereals, can complex (combine) with calcium and make it unavailable for absorption. In countries where a large amount of unleavened bread is consumed, there is evidence of calcium deficiency, since the phytic acid in the flour complexes with the calcium. There is less phytic acid in leavened bread because the process of fermentation destroys most of the phytate through the action of the enzyme phytase.

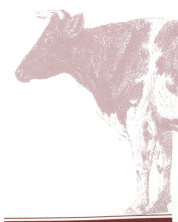

Do Old People Stoop Because They Lack Calcium?

Calcium imbalance accounts for a number of physical disorders. Calcium deficiency can produce rickets in children and osteomalacia in adults. In addition to the bone softening resulting from deficiency, damage to teeth occurs. **Osteoporosis** is a clinical disorder common to older adults in which the body's quantity of bone decreases. One potential sign of osteoporosis is the stooping of an elderly person, especially a woman. This condition is thought to involve not only lifetime calcium deficit but also inactivity, aging, hormonal imbalance, and excess phosphorus consumption. Since it occurs mainly in the elderly population, more details on this common problem are provided in Chapter 18.

Just as the various bone disorders often cannot be attributed solely to calcium deficiency, other calcium problems are often related to other nutrients. For example, **hypocalcemia** (low blood calcium) may be related to defective calcium absorption, even though dietary calcium is adequate. Vitamin D deficiency, magnesium deficiency, or thyroid difficulties can bring about hypocalcemia. **Tetany**, a syndrome caused by decreased "ionizable" calcium, constitutes a clinical emergency requiring prompt treatment. The patient suffers uncontrollable muscular contractions that may lead to seizures, coma, or even death. Calcium gluconate generally serves in the intravenous treatment of tetany.

As in the case of hypocalcemia, which can be related to other factors besides calcium intake, excessive calcium level in the blood (**hypercalcemia**) can result from excess vitamin D intake, thyroidism, or cancer. Symptoms include nausea, vomiting, anorexia, abdominal pain, and mental disorder. Coma and death can follow. Treatment involves rehydration of the patient and reduction of the calcium level by drugs, followed by a calcium-restricted diet.

Thus, we see that calcium serves a vital function in our bodies and that its excess or its deficiency can lead to life-threatening disorders. Yet, because its excessive or deficient state can be related to other conditions, it remains virtually impossible to precisely determine our calcium needs.

Beautiful Teeth Need Calcium and Phosphorus

As we saw previously, calcium is closely related to phosphorus to the extent that a balance between the two is necessary. Our body contains 600 to 700 mg of phosphorus, of which 80 to 90 percent is found in our bones and teeth.

Phosphorus' major functions include: (1) formation and maintenance of bones and teeth; (2) regulation of body neutrality; (3) control of energy storage and release; (4) serving as a structural component of nucleic acid, enzymes, and certain lipids in cell walls; (5) regulation of hormonal activity; and (6) participation in nutrient metabolism.

Phosphorus deficiency is rare since the mineral is widespread in foods. The adult RDA is 800 mg per day, primarily obtained from beef, poultry, and fish. Despite the prevalence of phosphorus, taking large amounts of antacid can prevent its absorption, resulting in anorexia, fatigue, and bone demineralization.

The interrelatedness of calcium and phosphorus begins with their primary function. Both are important to tooth and bone development. Table 12-4 shows the body distribution of each. Bones function in storage and release of both minerals. The absorption of both can be

Table 12-4

Approximate Body Distribution of Calcium and Phosphorus

MINERAL	BONES, TEETH	% OF BODY CONTENT	
		SOFT TISSUES ORGANS	BLOOD, EXTRACELLULAR TISSUES
Calcium	99	Trace	1
Phosphorus	80	19	1

Table 12-5
Ratios of Phosphorus to Calcium Contents of Natural Food Products

FOOD	PHOSPHORUS: CALCIUM RATIO
Meats, poultry, fish	15–20:1
Organ meats, such as liver	25–50:1
Eggs, grains, nuts, dry beans, peas, lentils	3–10:1
Milk, natural cheese, green vegetables	0.1–0.8:1

enhanced by vitamin D, and the blood levels of both are regulated by the hormonal system.

Table 12-5 shows the phosphorus: calcium ratio in some natural, unprocessed foods. Many nutritional experts hold that we need to consume calcium and phosphorus in a one to one ratio. This can prove difficult to attain because phosphorus is more abundant and is also an additive in many processed food products. Table 12-6 shows the calcium:phosphorus ratios in common natural and processed foods. Despite our higher consumption of phosphorus, research has not yet determined whether we consume too much of it.

ALCOHOLICS AND MAGNESIUM

Over one half (10–15 g) of our body's magnesium resides in bone and teeth, and the remainder is bound with phosphate. Magnesium serves in many body functions such as manufacturing of protein, handling of oxygen molecules, muscular relaxation, and numerous chemical and biological reactions.

Table 12-6
Calcium and Phosphorus Content of Representative Foods

FOOD	SERVING SIZE	CALCIUM (mg)	PHOS- PHORUS (mg)
Dairy products			
Milk, whole	1 c	285	227
Milk, skim	1 c	296	233
Meat and equivalents			
Beef, rib roast	3 oz.	8	158
Frankfurter	1	4	76
Luncheon meat	½ lb	25	377
Roast chicken, light meat	½ lb	25	617
Grain and equivalents			
Bread, enriched, white	1 sl	26	28
Rice, white, enriched, cooked	1 c	21	57
Potato, french fried	10 strips	5	39
Fruits			
Grapefruit, medium size	1	16	16
Apple	1	10	15
Figs dried, small	2	40	25
Vegetables			
Beans, green, cooked	½ c	63	46
Corn, sweet, yellow, fresh	½ c	2	75
Peppers, sweet, raw, green, chopped	½ c	5	15
Nuts			
Almonds, roasted	1 oz	67	143
Peanuts, roasted, salted	1 oz	20	115
Miscellaneous			
Shake, vanilla, McDonald's	1	126	105
Soft drink	8 oz	0	500
Pie, baked, sector	1	3	7
Pretzels, thin	10	13	79

SOURCE: Adapted from *Nutritive Value of Foods*, Home and Garden Bulletin No. 72 (Washington, D.C.: U.S. Department of Agriculture, 1981).

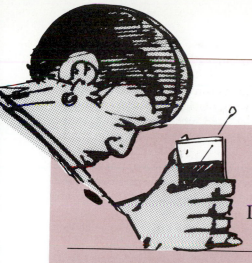

Magnesium DEFICIENCY ALMOST KILLED STEVE

Steve, a 35-year-old black man with a history of alcohol abuse, went to the hospital after two days of cramping in his hands. Shortly after receiving a calcium injection, Steve went into a cardiopulmonary arrest.

When Steve had been resuscitated, the doctors confirmed that he had low blood magnesium. Replacement followed. Before the magnesium could take effect, however, the patient's eyes began to move uncontrollably, both vertically and horizontally. The patient was restless and anxious, and he was disoriented. He also complained of visual hallucinations.

The continual administration of magnesium gradually eliminated his symptoms. After eight days of hospitalization, Steve was discharged. His magnesium deficiency had caused irritability of the central nervous and muscular systems.

Some nutritionists have pointed out that chronic alcoholism, especially in its most severe form, can be considered adult starvation since the alcoholic beverages have replaced caloric values that would otherwise be obtained from nutritious foods. The alcoholic relies on the beverage for sustenance, rather than relying on nutritious foods.

Alcoholics also manifest conditions characteristic of starvation. For example, magnesium depletion occurs in alcoholics because alcohol triggers its loss through the urine. Potassium and phosphate are also depleted in alcoholics. Steve is an example of depletion characteristic of starvation (Smith et al.).

The Importance of Magnesium

An adult RDA of 300 to 350 mg magnesium daily has been established. The mineral is contained in most foods, especially leafy green vegetables, in which it is a control component of chlorophyll. Given its prevalence, the average American diet provides sufficient magnesium. Even though milk is not a good source of magnesium, milk provides adequate magnesium for infants.

Although our consumption of magnesium tends to be high, absorption is subject to many factors. For example, as the amount consumed increases, the amount absorbed decreases. Increased calcium and vitamin D intake decreases magnesium absorption. Phytic and oxalic acids from fruits and vegetables can complex with magnesium, preventing its absorption. When all these dietary factors are considered, less than half the magnesium consumed may be absorbed.

Magnesium deficiency results in characteristic symptoms: (1) tetany similar to that of hypocalcemia; (2) loss of muscular control; (3) nervousness, irritability, and tremors; (4) secondary calcium deficiency; and

(5) changes in the heart, kidneys, and circulation (clinical observations are flushing and other skin changes).

Severe magnesium deficiency is uncommon owing to its storage in bones, but many nutritionists believe our magnesium nutriture is inadequate—in part because both stress and medication can cause deficiency. If either of these conditions exist and calcium or fluoride intake is high, severe deficiency can result.

Conditions such as vomiting and diarrhea cause magnesium to be lost in expelled fluids. Diuretic medications and clinical disorders can cause loss through urine. Alcoholics also tend to be deficient since alcohol interferes with absorption. These conditions, coupled with those previously mentioned, place magnesium high in the list of macroelements likely to be deficient in our bodies.

THE CHEMISTRY OF CHLORIDE

We contain about 100 g of chlorine, most of which occurs in extracellular fluid in the form of chloride. Chlorine maintains fluid balance, body neutrality, mineral distribution, and osmotic pressure. It also facilitates transfer of carbon dioxide from blood to lungs, functions in digestion as part of hydrochloric acid in the stomach, and regulates the functions of enzymes.

INFANT CHLORIDE DEFICIENCY: A LOOPHOLE IN THE LAW OR A FAULT OF THE INDUSTRY?

Since infant formula is often the only food received during the first few months of life, it is a product of vital concern. Although formula ranks below mother's milk in value to an infant, mother's milk is not always available. To meet the need, manufacturers strive to create a safe, nutritious product that will approximate mother's milk as closely as possible.

The Food and Drug Administration carefully monitors the manufacture of formula under the category of foods for special dietary use. Because of a recent formula incident, the FDA also conducts a compliance survey.

The incident that brought renewed interest in the review of formula manufacture involved *chloride* deficiency, which resulted in *metabolic alkalosis*. The problem occurred because a manufacturer stopped adding salt to two soy-based infant formulas. The salt cutback occurred because processors of solid baby foods were also cutting back on salt in response to concerns that salt in baby foods might cause hypertension in later years.

The company recalled the two products that were causing metabolic alkalosis, but the public outcry over the problem caused the FDA to strengthen its review processes. Concern for the health of infants who suffered from metabolic alkalosis remains. The FDA has been encouraged to continue regular monitoring, and manufacturers have been encouraged to strive for even more improvements that will move formulas even closer to mothers's milk (Hopkins).

Currently, the Congress has enacted the new Infant Formula Act, which is expected to remedy the situation.

Our requirement for chlorine is unknown, but dietary deficiency is uncommon because the mineral is present in common table salt and in almost all foods, especially fruits and vegetables. Our kidneys either excrete or reabsorb chloride molecules, depending on its level in our blood. Deficiency generally results only from clinical conditions such as diarrhea, vomiting, alkalosis (opposite to excess acid), or excess perspiration.

SULFUR: WHY BURNING HAIR SMELLS BAD
Though somewhat shrouded in mystery, sulfur is listed with the macroelements since it occurs in our bodies in a larger quantity than do microelements. The mystery surrounding this mineral lies in our not knowing its requirement or its deficiency symptoms.

Despite this lack of knowledge, we know that sulfur is found in every cell in our bodies, in all animal protein, and in hair, skin, and nails. This explains the odor from burning hair and rotten eggs. The sulfur is released as sulfur dioxide. It is found as a component in two amino acids, **methionine** and **cystine**, and is found in nucleic acids. Sulfur also occurs in an inorganic form as sulfite in fruits and vegetables.

In our bodies, sulfur serves six basic functions: (1) storage and release of energy, (2) structural component of nucleic acids and vitamins (thiamine, biotin, pantothenic acid, and lipoic acid), (3) promotion of enzyme reactions, (4) component of body substances for the detoxification process, (5) collagen synthesis, and (6) promotion of blood clotting.

Microelements: Slight but Vital
We should not be misled by the distinction between macroelements and microelements. Even though our bodies contain much less of each microelement than of the macroelements, the microelements are no less important to our nutritional health. The microelements are primarily iron, iodine, zinc, fluorine, copper, and other trace elements.

ALL YOU WANT TO KNOW ABOUT IRON
Iron nutrition has been the subject of significant research and massive health programs, yet deficiency continues to plague many population groups. The prevalence of iron deficiency concerns us because of the two major bodily functions of iron. First, the mineral makes possible the transport of oxygen and carbon dioxide to and from cells. Second, iron regulates important chemical and biological reactions such as vitamin synthesis and synthesis of antibodies.

Iron is found in every living cell, but 70 percent of our entire iron content is in the blood. Most of the remainder of the total 3 to 5 g of iron in our bodies can be found in the liver, spleen, bone marrow, and intestines. Iron generally exists in combination with some form of protein. In blood, for respiration purposes, iron is found in **hemoglobin**. In our blood, for transportation purposes, iron is found in transferrin. In organs, for storage purposes, iron occurs in ferritin. The release and storage capabilities for iron enable constant recycling of the iron within us.

Are You Deficient in Iron?

Each of us requires a certain amount of iron to maintain a normal blood profile. Table 12-7 gives the iron requirements of different population groups. We lose iron each day through body wastes, hair growth, and nail growth. Adults average a loss of 0.7 to 1 mg; in women, menstruation causes an additional 0.5 to 1 mg of loss.

The American diet furnishes 10 to 20 mg of iron daily, with most of it absorbed in the upper portion of the small intestine. Only about 2 to 10 percent of this amount is absorbed daily; however, iron deficiency, pregnancy, and growth all can increase the absorption rate to 50 to 60 percent of the daily intake. Absorption also varies by type of food and by combination of foods. For example, we absorb 30 to 40 percent of the iron in meat, but only 5 to 10 percent of the iron in egg yolk. As we saw with other minerals, both phytic and oxalic acid can decrease absorption. Taking excessive amounts of antacids also reduces absorption.

Since we absorb only a portion of the iron ingested, intake must be high to meet the need level. Liver is an excellent source of iron. Vegetables generally, and potatoes, green leaves, and stalks in particular, are also good sources. Most bread and flour are enriched with iron. Certain specialized foods, such as raisins, oysters, clams, and cocoa, are high in iron but are generally eaten in small quantities.

Although most of us are familiar with the term **anemia**, that condition results from severe deficiency. Prior to reaching the level of anemia, deficiency can result in fatigue and weakness. Pallor, breathing difficulty on exertion, palpitations, and coldness are also common symptoms. Additionally, older persons may experience oral lesions and a condition of the nails known as **koilonychia**. Figure 12-2 depicts these conditions.

Table 12-7
Approximate Iron Requirements of Certain Population Groups

POPULATION GROUP	IRON NEEDED EACH DAY (MG)				
	OBLIGATORY LOSS	LOSS FROM MENSTRUATION	NEED FOR GROWTH	NEED FOR PREGNANCY	TOTAL NEED
Postmenopausal females and adult males	0.7–1.0	0	0	0	0.7–1.0
Menstruating females	0.7–1.0	0.5–1.0	0	0	1.2–2.0
Pregnant females, over 17 years	0.7–1.0	0	0	1.0–2.0	1.7–3.0
12–17-year-old nonpregnant females	0.7–1.0	0.5–1.0	0.4–0.8	0	1.6–2.8
12–17-year-old pregnant females	0.7–1.0	0	0.4–0.8	1.0–2.0	2.1–3.8
0–3-year-olds	0.2–0.3	0	0.3–0.6	0	0.5–0.9
3–10-year-olds	0.3–0.4	0	0.4–0.5	0	0.7–0.9
10–17-year-olds*	0.5–0.8	0	0.1–0.9	0	0.6–1.7
Nursing mothers	0.7–1.0	0–1.0	0.5–1.0†	0	1.2–2.0

*Excluding 12- to 17-year-old females.

†Amount in milk for infant growth.

Iron deficiency can be caused by (1) loss of blood; (2) diarrhea and malabsorption; (3) frequent blood donation; (4) inadequate intake; (5) consumption of nonfood substances (pica); (6) drugs such as antibiotics, laxatives, and aspirin; and (7) vulnerability to deficiency (for example, premature infants are more susceptible).

Treatment of deficiency involves both resolving the cause and restoring the iron level. Although iron exists in several forms, the ferrous form is the most easily absorbed, so treatment usually relies on ferrous sulfate or ferrous gluconate. Satisfactory treatment generally results in a gain of 2 g of hemoglobin per 100 mL of blood, with that gain measurable every three weeks. (The normal hemoglobin level is near 15 g of hemoglobin per 100 mL of blood.) Oral iron dosage is the preferred method, though sometimes intravenous administration is necessary. Injection is the least preferred method of administration because there is danger of anaphylaxis (allergic shock reaction) and death.

Iron Supplementation

Iron supplementation is available without prescription and is most commonly taken in liquid or tablet form. Two forms of iron are available, ferrous and ferric; the ferrous salts are more easily absorbed and occur in different iron salt supplements such as ferrous sulfate, ferrous gluconate, ferrous fumarate, ferrous citrate, and others.

Some 10 to 15 percent of those taking iron supplements will experience side effects. Typical side effects include gastric pain, nausea, diarrhea, heartburn, and constipation. Such problems can be minimized by taking the supplement with food, though the iron is better absorbed on an empty stomach. Table 12-8 shows the quantity of elemental iron contained in various supplements.

Iron Poisoning

Iron toxicity can occur for various reasons, one of which is excess consumption. This may occur accidentally, especially among children ingesting iron supplement tablets without adult supervision, but it can also result from such unusual causes as the use of rusty cooking utensils.

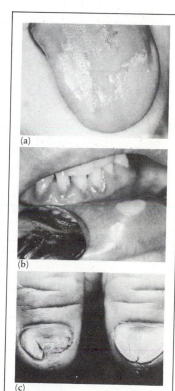

(a)

(b)

(c)

Figure 12-2: Signs of iron deficiency. (a) Patchy depapillation of tongue (latent iron deficiency). (b) Generalized inflammation of the mouth (stomatitis), ulceration, and gingivitis (malabsorption syndrome). (c) Iron deficiency koilonychia.
SOURCE: *(a, b) W. R. Tyldesley. Br. Dent. J. 139 (1975): 232; (c) S. Dreizen. Geriatrics 29 (1974): 97. Reproduced by permission.*

Table 12-8
Quantities of Elemental Iron Contained in Iron Compounds or Supplements

IRON COMPOUND OR SUPPLEMENT	IRON PER TABLET (mg)	NO. OF TABLETS DAILY PER ADULT*
Ferrous sulfate (hydrated or dehydrated)	55–65	4
Ferrous fumarate (small tablet)	65	4
Ferrous gluconate	40	5–6
Ferroglycine sulfate	40	5–6

* To provide 240 mg of iron.

An inherited tendency for excess iron storage, or a clinical disorder that increases absorption, can also result in iron toxicity.

Acute iron poisoning is a dangerous condition, with symptoms of cramps, pains, vomiting, blood-stained black stool, shock, and convulsions. Coma can be followed by death within 24 hours. Treatment necessitates a chemical process called *chelation*, which will prevent the iron's absorption. Administration of sodium bicarbonate and deferoxamine can relieve the condition.

HAVE YOU HEARD OF "GOITER"?
Iodine is an essential element found in the thyroid gland. In combination with the amino acid tyrosine, iodine forms the hormone thyroxine, which regulates basal metabolic rate (see Chapter 3).

Simple Iodine Deficiency
Iodine deficiency results in the condition known as simple **goiter**, a swelling of the thyroid gland in its attempt to produce more thyroxine when blood levels of the hormone are too low. The condition is more common in women than men and occurs more frequently during cold weather, when body metabolism speeds up to maintain body heat.

Since body metabolism regulates body growth and development, iodine deficiency can be especially harmful to infants and children, in whom it can cause the condition known as **cretinism**. Cretinism is characterized by mental and physical retardation and apelike facial features. An expectant mother's iodine deficiency can predispose the infant to goiter and cretinism. Females are additionally susceptible to deficiency during adolescence and menopause. If the deficiency is prolonged, especially during adolescence, sterility may result.

Because the iodine content of the soil varies geographically, iodine deficiency tends to vary geographically. Also, scientists have theorized that areas that were subjected to glacial action, or areas subject to flooding and excessive rainfall, have had iodine leached from the soil. In the United States, for example, iodine deficiency occurs in the Rocky Mountain states and the Great Lakes area. (The latter area has been called the Goiter Belt.) A survey conducted in these areas in 1970 showed that the incidence of deficiency was 5 to 10 percent of the population, despite extensive use of iodized salt. Since iodized salt is used extensively, scientists have theorized that there may be other causes of goiter as well.

When a deficiency or a deficiency condition occurs in a large segment of the population, this condition is said to be *endemic*. In addition to the areas of the United States previously mentioned, goiter is endemic in primitive areas of Central and South America. Figure 12-3 depicts goiter from iodine deficiency.

The RDA for iodine is 100 to 130 micrograms per day. Excellent sources include iodized salt and seafood. If the soil and water content of iodine is high, sufficient intake is obtained from vegetables, milk, eggs, cheese, and water. If 1 to 50 mg of iodine is consumed daily for a prolonged period, toxicity may result.

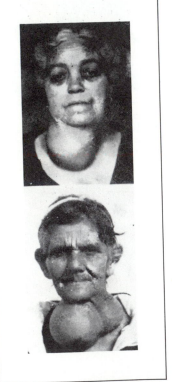

Figure 12-3: Severe endemic goiter in Mendoza Province, Argentina, as seen between 1930 and 1950.
SOURCE: H. Perinetti and L. N. Staneloni. Environ. Res. 3 (1970): 463.

Iodine: First Famine, Now Feast

Iodine is an essential mineral that does not occur naturally in enough foods for us to fulfill our requirement. Accordingly, iodine became an additive to salt. Now, some nutritional experts suggest that our iodine intake may be too great (Taylor).

Studies have shown that our intake averages three to four times the recommended dietary allowances and may be ten times the RDA depending on the amount of milk consumed. It may surprise you to find that it is not salt that leads the list of iodine providers, but dairy products.

Dairy products provide over half the dietary iodine typically consumed. The iodine content is high because iodine is given to dairy cattle, and iodine-containing chemicals called iodophors are used to treat cattle and to clean milk-handling equipment. Grain and cereal products rank high in iodine content, as do sugar and such sugar products as jams, jellies, and candy bars. Much of the iodine content of these latter food products also comes from iodophors used to clean equipment. Additionally, any food products containing milk rank high in iodine content.

Foods using the red food color erythrosine rank high in iodine content since erythrosine is 50 percent iodine. Highly processed convenience foods and fast foods served in restaurants contain large amounts of iodine.

Thus far, the health consequences of excess dietary iodine have not been adverse, perhaps because iodine absorption is not as high as intake. However, it is known that excessive iodine consumption can produce goiter problems, just as iodine deficiency can. It has also been established that excessive iodine intake by expectant mothers can cause goiter in newborns.

Health scientists have noticed an increasing incidence of a disease called *Hashimoto's thyroiditis*. It is suspected that high iodine intake may be contributory. For those suffering from this disease, iodine can disturb hormone synthesis and cause enlargement of the thyroid gland.

Further research into the long-term effects of high iodine intake is definitely needed. Meanwhile, the high levels currently available have caused the Food and Drug Administration to stop approving new iodine compounds for use in foods or food processing. Manufacturers have also been urged to limit their use of iodophors. Dairy farmers and feed manufacturers are being urged to limit their use of iodine supplements. In the meantime, health practitioners will be watching carefully for clinical conditions that may indicate iodine toxicity.

ZINC: DEFICIENCY IS HARD TO DIAGNOSE

We contain about 1.5 to 3 g of zinc, located primarily in our bones, hair, and skin but found throughout the body. The adult RDA is about 15 to 25 mg daily, and the typical American diet provides about 10 to 15 mg per day in utilizable form. Since foods high in zinc content, such as meat and oysters, are generally expensive, low-income people have low zinc intake. (The zinc content of some common foods is given in the Appendix.)

Zinc deficiency proves difficult to diagnose. For example, blood levels fluctuate as a result of tissue utilization, drug usage, infection, pregnancy, and hormonal imbalance. To accurately determine whether deficiency exists, simultaneous analysis of blood, urine, and hair is required. Indications of deficiency have appeared in relation to other disorders of sexual development, growth, and reproductive ability; wound healing and skin health; appetite and sensations of taste and smell.

Recent studies have associated zinc deficiency with arrested sexual development. Adequate zinc intake during the growing years is important for sexual maturation and body development (see box).

Are Zinc Supplements Necessary? Sometimes.
A number of studies have indicated that zinc supplementation may improve growth and sexual development in zinc-deficient children. In Iran, "normal" children with a marginal level of body zinc showed improvements in height, weight, bone growth, and sexual maturation when given zinc supplements, with the boys being more responsive. Before 1975, commercial infant formulas sold in the United States were not supplemented with zinc. In one study, infants on special-formula diets supplemented with zinc showed a slight increment in height and weight compared with nonsupplemented controls. Again, male infants showed a better response.

Zinc supplementation has additionally proved beneficial for promoting wound healing for certain traumas such as burns and surgery and certain types of tissue and skin damage such as leg ulcers.

In addition to aiding wound healing, zinc supplementation has recently been shown to have a beneficial effect on acne. In one study, an

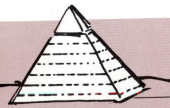

SOME EGYPTIAN BOYS NEVER BECOME MEN

During the last 20 years, health authorities have attributed some forms of adult dwarfism in Egypt and Iran among villagers to zinc and iron deficiency. The patients show deficient zinc levels in their blood, hair, and urine. They develop symptoms such as anemia, liver enlargement, undeveloped genitals, growth retardation, and the absence of other sexual developmental signs such as body hair and deeper voice. The disorder is most common among male adolescents. For example, a 20-year-old man will have the physical and sexual characteristics of a 10-year-old child. Some of these patients have responded to treatment with zinc and iron and showed good recovery.

The deficiency of zinc might have been caused by several factors. First, the unleavened bread eaten by these Middle Eastern people contains a high level of phytate, which can chelate (combine with) zinc and iron, making them unavailable for absorption. Second, frequent infection with *schistosomiasis* (infestation with tropical blood parasites) can increase the zinc and iron excreted in the urine. Third, the practice of pica among these children (eating clay, starch, and other nonfood items) can cause zinc to be complexed (combined with) these ingested substances, rendering it less available for absorption. Fourth, excess perspiration in a hot climate increases the loss of zinc.

oral dose of 135 mg of zinc (as zinc sulfate) resulted in a dramatic decrease of the acne condition within a month. In another study, the simultaneous use of zinc and tetracycline caused a 70 percent decrease in the acne counts. The use of low-dose zinc to reduce perspiration odor has also been suggested.

For patients who have experienced alterations in taste and smell, such as those undergoing chemotherapy and radiotherapy, zinc therapy has restored the sensations to normal.

In some cases, zinc deficiency itself may cause taste and smell alterations, leading people to avoid zinc-rich foods and thereby aggravating the deficiency. In the course of studying hair analyses of 132 apparently normal children, investigators noted a depressed zinc level in eight children. Further examination indicated that these children were below standard in weight and growth. They had not been eating well and had been avoiding meat because of its "bad taste." Supplementation of 0.2 to 0.4 mg of zinc per day per kilogram of body weight improved the taste sensation in three of the patients in three months, and their weight and growth gains improved.

Many patients with sickle cell anemia show retardation of growth and gonadal development as well as poor wound healing. These patients may be suffering from zinc deficiency, since some of them excrete a large amount of zinc in the urine. Their kidneys could be failing to retain the element. Another possibility is that the patients may not be absorbing zinc properly. In a limited number of cases, patients with sickle cell anemia have responded positively to zinc supplementation. At present, intensive research is being conducted to study the relationship between zinc and the disease.

Dietary supplementation of zinc has become popular, and promoters have pointed to impaired sexual development as a reason for supplementation. Americans are not deficient in zinc. No scientific evidence supports similar results for individuals eating a balanced diet, but promoters claim zinc will increase virility and enhance sex drive.

The above information has been discussed in numerous publications (Brewer and Prasad; Karcioglu and Sarper).

YOUR CHILD, TOOTH DECAY, AND FLUORIDATED WATER

Fluorine, more commonly known as fluoride, has received much public attention because of its role in preventing tooth decay, but the essential nature of fluorine has only recently been recognized.

We know that fluoride plays an important role in the formation and maintenance of bones and teeth. During the initial developmental stages of a tooth, body fluoride is incorporated into tooth structure. After a tooth has erupted, fluoride is still important in assisting the ongoing maturation of the outer layer of enamel, for fluoride that is present is incorporated topically into the crystal spaces. In this manner, the tooth is subject to less decay throughout the person's life.

Since the food sources of fluoride are usually inadequate during children's developmental years, the practice of adding fluoride to water is common in many parts of the United States. When children are brought up in areas where the drinking water contains one part per million of fluoride, they have up to 50 percent less tooth decay than children not receiving this benefit. Dietary contribution of fluoride is about 0.3 mg in nonfluoridated areas versus 3.0 mg in fluoridated localities. There is much debate over the safety of water fluoridation, but there is no established scientific evidence that drinking water with one part per million of fluoride is harmful.

In addition to its effect on the teeth, fluoride has been implicated in other clinical roles. Fluoride may also protect against magnesium deficiency, osteoporosis in later life when administered in safe dosages, and certain periodontal diseases, such as jawbone fragility and loss of teeth.

COPPER DEFICIENCY AND COW'S MILK

We contain 100 mg of copper. Our daily need is not known, but it has been estimated that the average American diet provides 2 mg per day, primarily from organ meats such as kidney and liver, shellfish, raisins, and dried legumes.

Since copper functions in maintaining normal blood chemistry, its deficiency in infants can result in abnormal cell development that can yield bone demineralization and death. The administration of copper will reverse clinical manifestation. Some documented cases of copper deficiency in infants include (1) long-term feeding of cow's milk can produce anemia in normal infants, and (2) infants with chronic malnutrition and diarrhea may develop anemia when fed modified cow's milk (formula). Both situations are corrected by the administration of copper and iron simultaneously.

At the opposite end of the content spectrum, copper toxicity produces dizziness, vomiting, and diarrhea. Wilson's disease, a well-known form of toxicity, results in cirrhosis and nerve degeneration.

The Increasing Importance of Trace Minerals

At present, there is much scientific and public interest in other essential trace elements not discussed thus far, especially manganese, chromium, cobalt, molybdenum, and selenium. Table 12-9 provides a brief summary of these five elements. In the following, some health claims for chromium and selenium are briefly presented. More details on these trace minerals may be obtained from references at the end of this chapter.

HEALTH CLAIMS AND CHROMIUM

Chromium appears to be an essential nutrient because of its role in maintaining normal glucose metabolism. One form of chromium, trivalent chromium, has been called the *glucose tolerance factor* (GTF) and has been promoted as a necessary supplement for carbohydrate metabolism, as was presented in the case history at the beginning of this chapter. Chromium deficiency has been correlated with heart disease and with atherosclerosis (see Chapter 6).

Brewer's yeast provides a good source for chromium supplementation, and the element can also be obtained in the form of chromic

Table 12-9
Some Relevant Information on Manganese, Chromium, Cobalt, Molybdenum, and Selenium

MINERAL	FUNCTIONS IN THE BODY	METABOLISM AND DEFICIENCY	FOOD SOURCES	RDA*
Manganese	Component of bone and some enzymes; major role in the intermediate metabolism of carbohydrate; protein synthesis	Not much known	Whole grains, nuts, legumes, fruit and selected vegetables	Not known
Chromium	Suspected to regulate glucose tolerance; associated with enzymes in the intermediate metabolism of carbohydrate and protein synthesis	Not much known	Whole-grain cereals, meat	None
Cobalt	Component of vitamin B_{12}, which plays a major role in body metabolism and physiology (see Chapter 10)	Assumed to be closely related to that of vitamin B_{12}	Associated with vitamin B_{12}	None unless vitamin B_{12} is considered
Molybdenum	Component of xanthine oxidase and flavoprotein, which is very important in body metabolism	Not much known	Whole grains, legumes, organ meats	None
Selenium	Component of enzyme; related to functions of vitamin E and metabolism of fat	Not much known	Grains, meats, vegetables, milk	None

*See footnote to Table 12-1.

chloride. Though research on chromium is still needed, it seems that a significant margin of safety exists for its intake. Care must be taken, however, since other forms of chromium are highly toxic or mutagenic (causing mutation in our genes).

SELENIUM AS A SUPPLEMENT
Selenium functions with vitamin E to protect against oxidant damage in our bodies. Since nutritionists note dietary adequacy of selenium, supplementation has not been recommended. Promoters have, however, claimed that selenium cures cancer, arthritis, sexual dysfunction, heart disease, poor eyesight, skin problems, and aging.

Although selenium has been the subject of animal studies in the United States, no link between its deficiency in humans and any disease has been confirmed. In China, insufficient selenium has, however, been associated with Keshan disease, a heart disease in children. Both toxicity and deficiency have occurred under natural conditions in animals, but much research remains to be done in relationship to humans.

What Makes Your Urine Acidic or Alkaline?
Minerals in different foods influence the acidity of the body. Table 12-10 indicates what these foods are. Certain foods are *acid forming* (acid ash) foods and may produce an acid residue. Such foods can produce acidic urine. The minerals responsible are phosphorus, sulfur, and chlorine. Other foods are *basic forming* (alkaline ash) and may produce an al-

Table 12-10
Substances That Can Influence the Acid-Base Balance of Body Fluids

SUBSTANCE	DIETARY SOURCE	BODY SOURCE
Water	Beverage, food	Metabolism of carbohydrate, protein, and fat
Sodium, potassium, magnesium (base forming)	Most fruits and vegetables	Muscle catabolism
Chlorine (acid forming)	Many foods	Muscle catabolism
Phosphates, sulfates (acid forming)	Many foods, especially protein foods such as meats and cheese; soft drinks and other processed beverages	Metabolism of protein and/or fat
Calcium (base forming)	Many foods, especially milk	Mobilization of bone minerals
Organic acids, such as tartaric acid, citric acid, etc.	Many foods, especially fruits, vegetables, and fermented foods	Metabolism of carbohydrate, protein, and fat
Carbon dioxide	Many foods, especially fruits and vegetables	Metabolism of carbohydrate, protein, and fat

Table 12-11
Relationship Between Types of Foods and Urine Acidity-Alkalinity

TYPE OF FOOD	ACIDITY-ALKALINITY TENDENCY OF INGREDIENTS	ACIDITY-ALKALINITY OF URINE
Meats, fish, cheese, cereals (protein-rich foods)	Phosphates, sulfates, chlorides (acid residue)	Acidic urine
Most fruits and vegetables	Sodium, potassium, magnesium (alkaline residue)	Alkaline urine
Milk	Calcium effect surpasses protein effect (alkaline residue)	Alkaline urine
Plums, prunes, cranberries	Benzoic and quinic acids (not oxidized to carbon dioxide and water); converted in the liver to hippuric acid and tetrahydroxy hippuric acid; surpasses effect of sodium, potassium, and magnesium that are present	Acidic urine

Table 12-12
Classification of Foods According to Their Acid-Base Reactions in the Body

ALKALINE-ASH–FORMING OR ALKALINE-URINE–PRODUCING FOODS	ACID-ASH–FORMING OR ACID-URINE–PRODUCING FOODS	NEUTRAL FOODS
Milk and cream, all types	Meat, poultry, fish, shellfish, cheese, eggs	Butter, margarine, fats and oils (cooking), salad oil, lard
Fruits except plums, prunes, and cranberries	Plums, prunes, cranberries	Cornstarch, arrowroot, tapioca
Carbonated beverages	Corn, lentils	Sugar, honey, syrup
All vegetables except corn and lentils	Bread (especially whole-wheat bread not containing baking soda or powder)	Nonchocolate candy
Chestnuts, coconut, almonds	Cereals, crackers	Coffee, tea
Molasses	Rice, noodles, macaroni, spaghetti	
Baking soda and baking powder	Peanuts, walnuts, peanut butter	
	Pastries, cakes, and cookies not containing baking soda or powder	
	Fats, bacon	

kaline residue. Such foods can produce alkaline urine. The minerals responsible are sodium, potassium, calcium, and magnesium. Table 12-11 indicates the types of foods that can produce an alkaline or acidic urine. Table 12-12 categorizes foods according to whether they produce alkaline or acidic urine. Thus, the acidity of the urine can be regulated by eating more or less of the foods indicated in this table.

In clinical medicine, urine acidity has one important application. For example, an infection of the urinary tract may be due to some organisms that are sensitive to acidity. In this case, an acidic urine has the potential of eliminating the bacteria and thus the infection. Conversely, an alkaline urine may be as beneficial.

Because of the role that minerals play as essential nutrients, in this chapter you have seen that not only blood tests but also urine tests are used for diagnosis. You have also seen that hair analysis is used. Minerals are mined from the earth by plants, but they subsequently distribute throughout our bodies and must be considered high-grade ore in relation to our health and well-being.

STUDY QUESTIONS

1. Discuss the use of the terms *minerals, inorganic elements,* and *ash.*

2. In what six body processes are minerals important?

3. What distinguishes macroelements from microelements?

4. What can be said about the average person's sodium consumption?

5. What effect do calcium and potassium have on muscles?

6. How do oxalic and phytic acids influence the absorption of calcium and magnesium?

7. What three nutrients may be involved in rickets?

8. Discuss the relationships between calcium and phosphorus.

9. Under what conditions may borderline magnesium deficiency become serious?

10. Are iron deficiency and anemia inevitably linked?

11. Discuss some causes of iron toxicity.

12. Why is iodine deficiency especially damaging to children?

13. Discuss some reasons for a low intake of zinc. List at least four conditions for which zinc supplementation may be helpful.

14. What role is flouride thought to play in human health?

REFERENCES

Brewer, G. J., and A. S. Prasad, eds. *Zinc Metabolism: Current Aspects in Health and Disease.* New York: Alan R. Liss, 1977.

Crosby, W. H. "Lead-Contaminated Health Food Associated with Lead Poisoning and Leukemia." *J.A.M.A.* 237 (1977): 2627.

Hopkins, H. "Next to Mother's Milk, There's Infant Formula." *FDA Consumer* 14 (July/August 1980): 11.

Karcioglu, Z. A., and R. M. Sarper. *Zinc and Copper in Medicine.* Springfield, Ill.: Charles C Thomas, 1980.

Lecos, C. "Tips for the Salt-Conscious Consumer." *FDA Consumer* 15 (November 1981): 27.

Lecos, C. "Potassium: Keeping a Delicate Balance." *FDA Consumer* 17 (February 1983): 21.

Miller, R. "The Public Knows and Cares about Sodium." *FDA Consumer* 17 (April 1983): 10.

Smith, W. O., et al. "Vertical and Horizontal Nystagmus in Magnesium Deficiency." *South. Med. J.* 73 (1980): 269.

Taylor, F. "Iodine Going from Hypo to Hyper." *FDA Consumer* 15 (April 1981): 15.

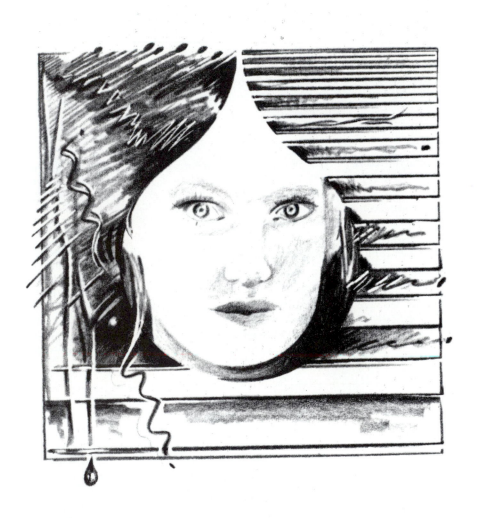

13

WATER:

MORE IMPORTANT THAN FOOD

Dehydration Maims an Infant

At the age of 6 weeks, Mary was placed in the care of her maternal grandmother. The grandmother felt that the child needed richer milk, as the child had recently recovered from bronchopneumonia. Accordingly, for the next five days, the grandmother fed the child undiluted evaporated milk. The child received this formula every three hours during the five-day period.

For the sixth and seventh days, the child received the milk diluted with an equal amount of water. She also received strained fruit. The child began regurgitating the "super-concentrated" formula, but no vomiting occurred. After two loose stools, the child ceased urinating. Her health deteriorated, and she was immediately taken to a hospital.

Upon admission it was determined that the infant had lost almost one pound during the preceding seven days. Her kidneys had ceased to function, and her feet and legs had turned blue. Her hands and eyelids twitched, and her body had tremors.

The hospital staff quickly realized that the infant was severely dehydrated and that both rehydration and kidney dialysis were necessary. She was given intravenous fluids. At this stage, Mary had high blood pressure and was losing consciousness. Her feet and legs continued to turn darker. On the third hospital day, the infant went into a deep coma. Sores developed on her upper legs and groin area, and her feet and lower legs turned a dark purple. Despite aggressive medical procedures, gangrene developed in her feet and in the lower portion of her legs. On the 19th day of hospitalization, a double amputation was performed (Abrams).

Mary was the victim of a loss of water balance. Figure 13-1 illustrates her condition. Specifically, the overconcentrated formula had low water content and a high solute (particles such as salt and protein) content. Because her fluid intake was deficient, there was not enough water to excrete the solutes. The infant's body was forced to draw upon its own water, causing dehydration, especially in the legs and feet. The solute load was too much for the child's immature kidneys. The combination of problems due to the overconcentrated formula directly resulted in the loss of the lower extremities and came very close to resulting in death.

Scientists consider water "the number one nutrient." In this chapter we'll discuss the rationale behind this claim (Hui; Lecos).

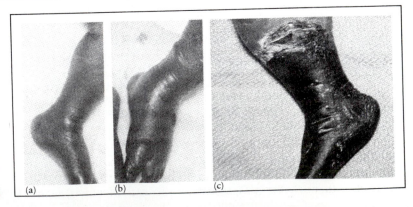

Figure 13-1: Severe dehydration. (a) Appearance of lower limb on patient's second hospital day. (b) Third hospital day. (c) Three weeks after hospitalization. Full demarcation and mummification occurred in both lower legs and feet. SOURCE: C. A. L. Abrams, et al. J.A.M.A. 232 (1975): 1136. Copyright 1975 American Medical Association. Reproduced with permission.

(a)   (b)   (c)

Water, Water, Everywhere . . .

Perhaps you do not immediately think of water when you think of nutrition, yet you probably know that for the most primitive tribes, water occupied an almost magical position. In many cultures, water has been viewed as a life force capable of curing illness, cleansing the spirit, and offering immortality.

Deny someone food and he or she can still live for days, even weeks. But death comes quickly—in a matter of a few days—if you deprive a person of water. Without air to breathe there is, of course, no life; but among all the nutrients that humans consume, water is, as one scientist described it, the "indispensable nutrient" on which all forms of life depend. Nothing survives without water, and virtually nothing takes place in the body without water playing a vital role.

From a scientific point of view, water accounts for 45 to 60 percent of the content of all living organisms. What is most important to realize about the water content of our bodies is that it does not consist of free-floating fluids but includes water contained in every cell. Scientists generally believe that it was water in which living cells first appeared, making water the initial environment of life as we know it, as well as the sustainer of life as we enjoy it.

The body uses water for virtually all its functions—for digestion, absorption, circulation, excretion, transporting nutrients, building tissue, and maintaining body temperature.

After Perspiring, We Feel Cool

Our bodies metabolize food to produce energy, some of which is released as heat. A portion of that heat maintains our body temperature, and the remainder is excess heat. We lose that heat through perspiration, and we actually perspire in two ways—by *insensible perspiration* and by *sensible perspiration*.

When smaller amounts of heat are dissipated, insensible perspiration occurs. It is "insensible" because we do not sense that it is occurring. Scientists have determined that about 600 kilocalories (kcal) are utilized in dispersing a liter of water from the body's surface. Although the rate of insensible perspiration is lower if body fat is high and more rapid for those with larger bodies, it is generally estimated that we use about 15 kcal per hour in disposing of 25 mL per hour via insensible perspiration.

Sweating—sensible perspiration—occurs when body heat becomes too high. Our sweating mechanism is a life-saving phenomenon; without it, we would suffer heat stroke that can cause cell damage and may even threaten life. Have you ever experienced a fever "break"? The profuse sweating that resulted was a perfect example of our body's heat regulation processes. As the perspiration evaporates from the skin, the resultant cooling effect lowers body temperature.

Moving Nutrients in Our Blood

Water also serves as a solvent in your body. In the utilization phase of nutrition, enzymes and hormones are dissolved in watery body fluids where they then act on such metabolites as carbohydrates, vitamins, minerals, and amino acids, which have also been dissolved. In the excretion phase of nutrition, wastes such as urea and carbon dioxide combine with watery body fluids for excretion. Water serves as a transport medium for nutrients traveling to cells and for wastes departing from cells.

Water is needed in each step of the process of converting food into energy and tissue. Digestive secretions are mostly water acting as a solvent for nutrients; in effect, water in the digestive secretions softens, dilutes, and liquefies the food to facilitate digestion. It also helps move food along the alimentary canal. Differences in the fluid concentration on either side of the intestinal wall facilitate the absorption process.

What Tears Are For

Beginning with the saliva in your mouth, water functions as a lubricant for digestion. It facilitates both chewing and swallowing in the form of saliva. We encounter it again in digestive fluids that continue the movement of food through the gastrointestinal tract. Shifting our view from digestion, we see water functioning as lubricant in our joints and for our eyeballs, and water additionally functions in tissues in the form of mucous secretions. Tears provide lubrication; that is why your eyes water when you walk into the wind. The tears offset the drying effect of the wind.

Some People Have More Body Water: Babies, Athletes, and Men

The quantity of water we contain varies with our size, age, and sex. As human embryo, we begin with over 95 percent water content. At birth, we are over 75 percent water. By adulthood our water content has about leveled off at 60 percent, but a gradual process of dehydration continues throughout life.

The distribution of water within our bodies varies according to tissue type. Our teeth are only 5 percent water, and our bones 10 percent, but our muscle tissue is almost three-quarters water. Body fat is approximately one-third water. As our fat content increases, the proportion of water in our body decreases, since fat tissue contains less water than muscle tissue. Thus, an obese adult might have over half of body weight as water, whereas a lean, muscular adult could have an additional 20 percent, making a total of almost 70 percent water content. Since women have more fatty tissue than men, on the average, women have a lower water content. Chapter 4 discusses this topic in more detail.

The Mystery of Osmosis

Basically, there are two categories of water in the body; the *intracellular* water that is found inside the cells and the *extracellular* water that is outside the cells. For example, a man weighing 155 pounds would have about 50 pounds of water in his cells and about 43 pounds outside the cells, including 14 pounds in the plasma. This water continually moves in and out of the cells. Yet we know the man actually contains about 93 pounds (60 percent of body weight) of water. The rest of his water is extracellular.

Minerals help maintain water balance. They ensure that different parts of the body contain a constant amount of water. The major minerals include sodium, potassium, chloride, and phosphorus, all of which are widely distributed in our diet. The chief minerals inside the cells are potassium and phosphorus, whereas the fluid outside the cells contains mostly sodium and chloride with smaller concentrations of other minerals. This characteristic—mostly sodium outside the cells and potassium inside—is found in virtually all living cells, plant and animal alike.

Water flows freely back and forth across the cell membranes that separate the inside from the outside of a cell. Yet the cells do not lose water, shrink, collapse, swell, or overfill. The water content is constant because of the minerals in the water.

Scientists explain that the movement of water across cell membranes is controlled by a force that is chemically known as osmotic pressure but is informally called *osmosis*.

Imagine this hypothetical situation: When two solutions of different concentrations are separated by a semi-permeable membrane or partition in a container, the dissolved molecules (solutes) should move from the solution of higher concentration to the other until both concentrations are equal.

As indicated above, body fluid is distributed between two areas—intracellular and extracellular. In a healthy individual, this distribution must be maintained in equilibrium at all times, either by (1) balancing the total concentrations of salt molecules within and without the cells, or (2) constantly shifting water between intracellular and extracellular compartments (such shifts are usually small and occur in both directions). Figure 13-2 shows how water moves from extracellular to intracellular compartments. Movement results from either a rise in the salt concentration in the intracellular fluid or a drop in the salt concentration in the extracellular compartment. The water moves because of osmotic pressure, which attempts to equalize the concentration of the particles (solutes) on the two sides of the semi-permeable cell membranes. In Figure 13-2, the extracellular fluid is hypotonic to the intracellular one; that is, the osmotic pressure of the intracellular fluid is higher than that of the extracellular fluid. The movement of water continues until equilibrium is reached.

As shown in Figure 13-3, water moves from the intracellular to the extracellular compartments when either the salt concentration in the extracellular compartment has increased or that of the intracellular compartment has decreased. In a normal person, equilibrium exists. In Figure 13-3, the osmotic pressure of the intracellular fluid is lower than that of the extracellular fluid, and water moves out of the cells to equalize osmotic pressure on the two sides of the membrane.

In sum, the dissolved sodium chloride outside the cell moves water toward itself (water follows salt) and potassium inside the cell draws water in from outside the cell. The delicate balance of sodium and potassium in the body is crucial to maintaining equilibrium of fluid distribution.

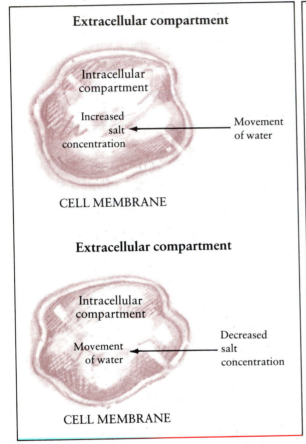

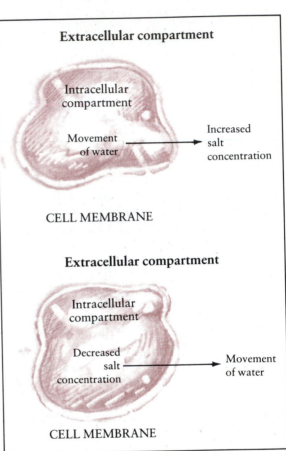

Figure 13-2 (Left): Movement of water from the extracellular to intracellular compartment.
Figure 13-3 (Right): Movement of water from the intracellular to extracellular compartment.

We Lose What We Drink

WATER NEED

While the average daily intake of water is about 2½ quarts, there is no formally established Recommended Dietary Allowance for water as there is for other nutrients. Need varies according to climate, age, size, level of activity, and health. The need for infants is approximately ½ quart to 1½ quarts by the age of 1. It is because of our level of need that practically all of us have heard that we should consume at least six to eight glasses of water daily. Table 13-1 shows daily water balance in a normal adult.

WATER GAIN

We obtain most of our water from foods and related dietary fluids. We average over 1 quart of water per day from drinking water, milk, coffee, tea, juices, soft drinks, and alcoholic beverages. Daily we obtain another

Table 13-1
Daily Water Balance in a Normal Adult

FACTORS AFFECTING WATER BALANCE	VOLUME OF WATER CHANGE (mL)
Sources of gain	
Food (meat, apples, etc.)	+500–1,000
Water, beverages, and liquid and semiliquid edible items (e.g., soups)	+1,100
Metabolic water (formed from chemical reaction, e.g., oxidation of food)*	+400
Total	+2,000–2,500
Sources of Loss	
Urine	−1,000–1,300
Stools	−90–100
Perspiration, respiration	−410–500
Insensible loss	−500–600
Total	−2,000–2,500

*The oxidation of 1 g of fat, carbohydrate, and protein produces 1.1, 0.6, and 0.4 g of water, respectively.

half quart from solid foods. Virtually all foods, except for fats, contain water, ranging from the 75 percent water content in fruits and vegetables to the 5 percent content of dry cereal.

In addition to dietary water sources, we obtain almost ¼ quart of water daily from our own bodies by means of such metabolic processes as nutrient oxidation. We also obtain water from our bodies through catabolism of fat, the breakdown of fat deposits.

WATER LOSS

Over a quart of blood passes through our kidneys each minute. Our kidneys filter waste products from the blood, producing urine; this is the primary mechanism by which we lose body water.

Urine production can average 1 quart per day, although the quantity depends on fluid intake. The function of our kidneys is vital not only for the removal of waste products but also for the maintenance of the body's acid-base balance, fluid balance, and mineral balance. That is, body acidity must be near neutral; the amount of water in different parts of the body must remain constant; and minerals inside and outside body cells must remain constant.

A small amount of water loss occurs through the feces, and a slightly larger amount is expelled through the lungs when we exhale. At high altitudes, such as in mountain climbing, or at times of strenuous exercise, respiratory water loss can increase to the point of dehydration (see later section).

Water loss through our skin accounts for the remainder of our daily water loss. As we saw earlier in this chapter, loss through the skin occurs through both insensible and sensible perspiration. Our perspiration loss, taken together with urine, feces, and respiration loss, totals between 2 and 2½ quarts per day, an amount relatively equal to our daily fluid intake, the ultimate measure of water balance.

Regulating Our Water Balance

Though no Recommended Dietary Allowance serves as an index of water need, that need is so critical to our health that our bodies contain systems for warning us when fluid levels are too low. For example, we sense thirst by dryness of the mouth and throat due to saliva decreasing as body fluids decrease. A section of our brain also reacts to decreased fluid levels by activating drinking behavior. This brain section can also be alerted by the heart's reaction to a low blood-sodium level. The various thirst reactions all advise our bodies that we need fluid intake.

The kidneys control most fluid output. By adjusting urine volume, the kidneys can slow or increase the amount of fluid leaving the body. Various hormones, including renin and aldosterone, regulate the "decision making" that goes on in our kidneys.

The Horror of Dehydration

Given our body's remarkable water controls, a logical question to ask is, "What could possibly disturb such a well-tuned machine?" This is an important question, because drastic changes in water balance can be fatal.

A major factor that can disturb our water balance is **dehydration**, a condition that can result either from decreased intake or excessive fluid loss. Excessive fluid loss typically results from vomiting, diarrhea, excessive bleeding, or profuse sweating.

When significant water loss occurs, the body also loses sodium. If sodium loss is accompanied by potassium excretion, the heart may fail.

Dehydrating conditions can be especially dangerous for both infants and the elderly. Infants contain little total water because they are small, so any significant water loss can cause death. In the case of the elderly, a low percentage of body water makes them similarly vulnerable. Thus, even in cases of mild diarrhea, fluid and electrolyte balance must be restored as quickly as possible. This can be accomplished by the consumption of tea, gelatin, water, fruit juice, soups, or soft drinks. If the direct dietary method proves unsuccessful, fluids must be given intravenously.

Profuse sweating not only results in water loss but also creates a danger of sodium and chloride dehydration. When salt depletion occurs, the subsequent intake of fluid to replace the water lost through profuse sweating can cause heat exhaustion related to the resulting water:salt imbalance. Heat exhaustion has the symptoms of muscle cramps, decreased blood pressure, and weakness. To avoid this condition, water replacement should be accompanied by salt replacement, with 2 g of salt per quart of water recommended if the replacement water is to exceed normal daily intake.

Especially for children, a rule of thumb has been developed: Loss of 5 to 10 percent of body weight in an infant due to fluid losses can cause skin to shrink and muscles to weaken. A loss of over 10 percent of body weight in a young child due to fluid losses can be fatal. The case history of Mary illustrates the danger of dehydration.

Other Things About Water You Should Know

WATER INTOXICATION

A condition similar to alcoholic inebriation is known as water intoxication. It can be fatal. If the kidneys cannot keep pace with the volume of fluid intake, all cells, including those in the brain, are affected. A water-intoxicated individual initially experiences confusion, dizziness, and lack of coordination. The condition advances to headache, nausea, vomiting, convulsions, and death. If salt is administered in the early phase of the condition and fluid intake is terminated, the condition can be controlled before it advances too far.

Though uncommon among the general public, water intoxication has been identified in some mental patients who drink water excessively.

DROWNING

If we think quickly of water as it relates to death, it is not water intoxication or dehydration that comes to mind, but drowning. Yet drowning can also be understood in many of the same terms as other water imbalance problems. For example, drowning in sea water places salt in the lungs that is four times the normal salt level of body fluids. This condition causes water from our own bodies to flow to the lungs to reduce the salt percentage. Death results from too much water in the lungs.

In the case of drowning by fresh water, the water pours from the lungs into the bloodstream, releasing massive amounts of potassium that damage the heart muscle and cause cardiac arrest.

WEIGHT LOSS

Although diuretics (see Chapters 20 and 24) are often used to promote weight loss, such loss consists of fluids, not fat. Also lost are both sodium and potassium. Weight loss resulting from the use of diuretics will, therefore, be regained. The minerals lost must be restored. For example, if a patient requires diuretics, mineral supplements may also prove necessary. Bananas and citrus fruits can help restore potassium.

MENSTRUATION

Water balance is also affected by female hormones. Water retention occurs at the start of menstrual periods and in the later stages of pregnancy. The female hormone estrogen causes water loss followed by sodium and fluid retention. A second female hormone, progesterone, interferes with the action of aldosterone. Although these hormonal effects are known, the effects vary among women and can vary at different times for an individual woman. Thus, the condition of premenstrual edema is not fully understood and may involve the effect of other hormones such as thyroid, and the interrelationships of hormones.

HANGOVERS

Related to the chemical effects of drugs and hormones, but in a class by itself, is the effect of ethanol, the alcohol in alcoholic beverages. Have you ever wondered what causes a "hangover"? Ethanol functions as a diuretic by inhibiting the secretion of certain hormones. The increase in urination following the consumption of alcohol is not solely from the fluid intake but also from such hormone inhibition. In this condition, fluids go directly to the urine. The headache-hangover effect is the body's signal that fluid loss requires replenishing.

ATHLETES AND DEHYDRATION

An area of study in need of further research concerns fluid loss experienced by athletes. On the average, a professional football player will lose 4 to 6 pounds during a practice session, which usually lasts longer than an actual game. Loss can be as great as 10 to 12 pounds in a training session. Most coaches try to schedule practice sessions during cooler parts of the day and while trainers and other experts are available. We do not know what long-term consequences may result from the significant and repeated water loss which will occur. Similarly, we do not know whether, for example, practice should stop for a player once 5 pounds is lost, or once a certain percent of body weight is lost. Such questions stand before researchers, and their answers could tell us all more about ourselves and about water nutrition.

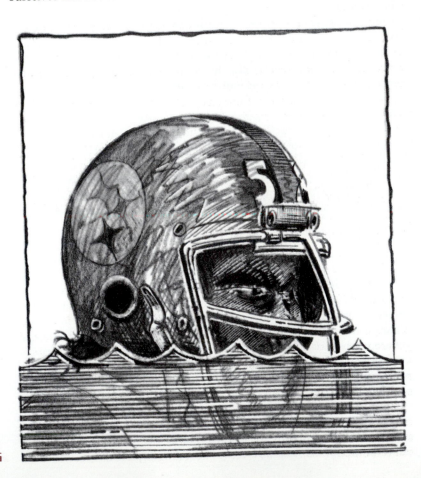

WHAT'S SO WONDERFUL ABOUT BOTTLED WATER?

The April 1983 issue of *Association of Food and Drug Officials Quarterly Bulletin* reproduces the speech given by W. F. Deal of the International Bottled Water Association during a 1982 meeting of the association. The title of the talk was "What You Should Know About Bottled Water." Part of the following has been adapted from this talk.

The bottled water industry in the United States began in the days of horse-drawn delivery wagons more than 100 years ago. The industry serves more than 10 million consumers who are concentrated in geographical areas where the esthetic quality of water is poor. This is changing somewhat, in that most areas of the country, regardless of the water quality, are using more bottled water. Nationwide, the use of bottled drinking water is increasing at a rate of about 10 percent annually.

One question frequently asked by those unfamiliar with the industry is why people buy bottled water. In the past, consumer demand for clean water and good taste were the prime motivators. Today, though the bottled water industry makes no health claims, customer inquiries and consumer interviews clearly show a growing public concern about health and especially about the safety of public water supplies. Bottled water is a safe alternative.

Most bottled water users are served by direct delivery of five-gallon bottles to homes and business establishments. This means that bottled drinking water tends to be purchased for all members of the family or work staff but may also be bought by individuals in supermarkets for general consumption or special dietary needs.

The industry distributes four generic types of bottled water, all of which must be derived from a protected source:

1. *Natural water* is water obtained from a protected spring or well.
2. *Mineral-free water* may be produced by distillation or by demineralization.
3. *Fluoridated water* may originate from a natural source or may contain added fluorides in an amount ranging from 0.8 to 1.7 mg per liter, depending on the annual average daily air temperature at the location where the bottled water is sold.
4. *Drinking water* is produced by demineralization, followed by the limited addition of minerals selected to achieve good taste.

Bottled water is one of the nation's most highly regulated and monitored drinking water supplies. All industry products must come from protected sources and must be bottled in facilities regulated as food plants, processed using manufacturing practices approved by the federal government, and delivered to consumers in bottles whose safety is assured by federal regulation. It must be labeled to provide public notification whenever the quality of any bottled water product is substandard.

Numerous bottled waters are available to the consumer, some domestic, some imported. In trying to choose among them, if price is excluded as a criterion, taste stands as the most reliable index. Conducting a taste test of bottled waters can be a most interesting experience (see box).

GIVING BOTTLED WATERS THE TASTE TEST

To be fair, you should test all the waters at the same temperature; for example, 45°F. Actually, you are not looking for a good taste so much as you are seeking to encounter no bad tastes. Whether the water is sparkling or still, it should be free of both sediment and color, and it should not have any unpleasant odors.

Just as with any other issue of taste, you want water to be refreshing, and that refreshing quality entails a clean taste that favorably stimulates your mouth to feel clean too. Generally there will be a barely discernible taste; it may be sweet, or perhaps slightly sour, or even bitter, but it will be a very slight taste, just enough to stimulate your mouth.

If the water is sparkling, the sparkle should give your mouth a tingling sensation. Water pays a taste price for being sparkling; that is, nonsparkling, still water will generally taste slightly better than most sparkling waters. This occurs because the carbon dioxide bubbles themselves have a very slight bitter taste.

In a taste test, one of the most popular sparkling waters, call it Brand A, was considered mildly bitter. In that same taste test, another leading sparkling water, Brand B, also tasted mildly bitter, to almost the same extent. Brand B had a slightly salty taste. Brand A also had that salty edge to it, but Brand A additionally had an aftertaste. When all was considered, Brand B rated the highest, and Brand A near the bottom, of all the sparkling waters.

Sparkling waters tended to have a salty taste caused by the presence of sodium, and a soapy taste due to high alkaline content. The alkaline content leaves a smooth, slick taste in the mouth. One water, Brand J, had both a salty taste and a soapy aftertaste, but its strongest taste was of plastic. The plastic taste is not uncommon to water sold in bulk, since water can "pick up" the slightest taint, even from its container. Selling water in bottles can avoid the problem, but at a higher cost. Brand J was rated the worst of all the waters, almost undrinkable.

Bottled water, especially that contained in plastic, will taste more plastic the longer it remains in the container. Temperature changes during bottling, distribution, and storage also affect taste. A taste test cannot control those factors. Chemical tests do, however, demonstrate that chemical differences of the waters do not seem to account for taste differences.

The overall results of the taste test showed that still waters rate higher than sparkling waters. Those with minerals added did not "outscore" the natural waters. The true test can not be based on anything other than the refreshing feeling measured on your taste buds.

THIRST QUENCHING

We begin to experience thirst when we lose 2 percent of our body water. Too great a loss leads to dehydration, the problem experienced by the infant Mary at the beginning of this chapter. The sensation of thirst is the first signal of a condition that can lead to fatigue, hallucination, loss of distance judgment, heat stroke, and high body temperature.

Most of us have favorite thirst quenchers. Some work better than others, and researchers have explored why they do. Temperature of the beverages is not an important consideration, but water content, taste, and sweetness are. For example, a sour-tasting drink quenches thirst better than a sweet-tasting one, even if both have identical water and sugar content.

Alcoholic beverages do not rate high on the thirst-quenching list because alcohol itself has a dehydrating effect. If an alcoholic beverage is preferred, though, beer proves the best choice since its water content is high—higher even than milk, lemonade, or nondiet colas.

Of all the beverages available, next to water the best choice is club soda. Club soda ranks high because it is all water, except for a less than 1 percent dissolved solid content. Using water content as the most important measure, favorite thirst quenchers would rank as follows:

Club soda	1
Iced tea and coffee	2
Diet cola and presweetened Kool-aid	3
Ginger ale and beer	4
Skim milk and buttermilk	5
Root beer and cola	6
Lemonade, sweetened Kool-aid, fruit sodas	7
Whole milk	8
Wine	9

National and International Issues

Chapter 23 addresses the subject of water in relation to oral health. Chapter 27 addresses the relationship between water and food production in the context of world hunger. Certainly the provision of potable water to a country's population is of high national importance.

Although we do not often think about it in those terms, water is a resource that does not grow. Rain is not new water; it is water "picked up" from the earth's surface. When you consider that our water has been recycled since the beginning of time, the subjects of water contamination and water pollution take on new meaning. If a portion of our water becomes permanently fouled each year by pesticides, chemical wastes, detergents, and other nondegradable products, we have lost a portion of the world's water supply. If the loss continues year after year, drinking supply becomes endangered.

Studies have been undertaken regarding various forms of water pollution. A recent problem, acid rain, comes to mind. Other studies have centered on carcinogens in water and the higher incidence of cancer in certain geographical areas.

A growing industry involves both bottled water and distilled water. Such sales occur because natural water supplies are considered untrustworthy or unsafe. Although the cost of such alternatives can be difficult to bear, if a community cannot adequately filter its water for contaminants, people have little choice but to resort to buying bottled or distilled water. The provision of clean water has thus become an increasing national and international priority, one upon which not only sanitation but also health and survival may depend.

WATER AND SANITATION-RELATED DISEASES: CLOSING THE LID ON PANDORA'S BOX

Cholera. Hookworm. Leprosy. Typhoid. Sleeping-sickness. These are but a few of the many water and sanitation related diseases that threaten the well-being of millions. About 100 million more people in the developing world were drinking dirty water in 1981 than in 1975; 400 million more did without sanitation than in 1975. In 1980, approximately 3 out of every 5 people did not have easy access to safe drinking water, and 3 out of every 4 had no sanitary facility—not even a simple pit latrine.

Control measures to reduce water and sanitation-related diseases can be relatively simple: improving water quality and sanitation practices; protecting water sources from contamination and avoiding contact with infecting organisms in the water; killing insect larvae and shielding water sources from insects that spread disease; and educating the public about the dangers of contaminating the soil with human waste and the merit of wearing shoes.

The U.N. International Drinking Water Supply and Sanitation Decade is 1981-1990. The goal is clean water and adequate sanitation for all by the year 1990.

AID (Agency for International Development) has been working on solving water supply and sanitation problems in developing countries since 1942 when the Institute of Inter-American Affairs was established. Since

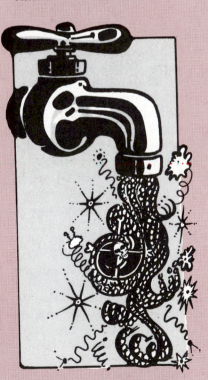

1973, AID has worked on 700 water supply and sanitation projects. Some of AID's current efforts include:

Provide a minimum of 20 to 40 liters of relatively safe water per capita per day

Improve water quality at reasonable cost

Introduce technologies that can be maintained and operated easily and that are acceptable within local cultures

Promote water conservation and reuse

Involve communities in designing and carrying out water projects

In 1980, AID's Office of Health created WASH—the Water and Sanitation for Health project. WASH provides AID managers with short-term, interdisciplinary technical assistance and information on water supply for rural and suburban settlements, sanitation, and environmental health. Over its first three years of operation, the WASH Project has worked on 170 projects for 54 countries.

SOURCE: G. Curlin. "Building for a Healthy Tomorrow." *Horizons* 3 (Spring 1984): 22.

STUDY QUESTIONS

1. List at least six major functions of water in the body.

2. Where is extracellular water found?

3. Define dehydration and edema.

4. What generally determines the passage of nutrients and wastes in and out of body cells?

5. Explain osmosis. What is osmotic equilibrium and how is it achieved?

6. Which body systems help to regulate body fluid and electrolyte balance? How?

7. Define the role of water in: water intoxication, drowning, weight loss, menstruation, and athletic training.

REFERENCES

Abrams, C. A. L., et al. "Hazards of Overconcentrated Milk Formula: Hyperosmalality, Disseminated Intravascular Coagulation, and Gangrene." *J.A.M.A.* 232 (1976): 1136.

Hui, Y. H. *Human Nutrition and Diet Therapy.* Monterey, Calif.: Wadsworth Health Sciences, 1983.

Lecos, C. "Water: The Number One Nutrient." *FDA Consumer* 17 (November 1983): 28.

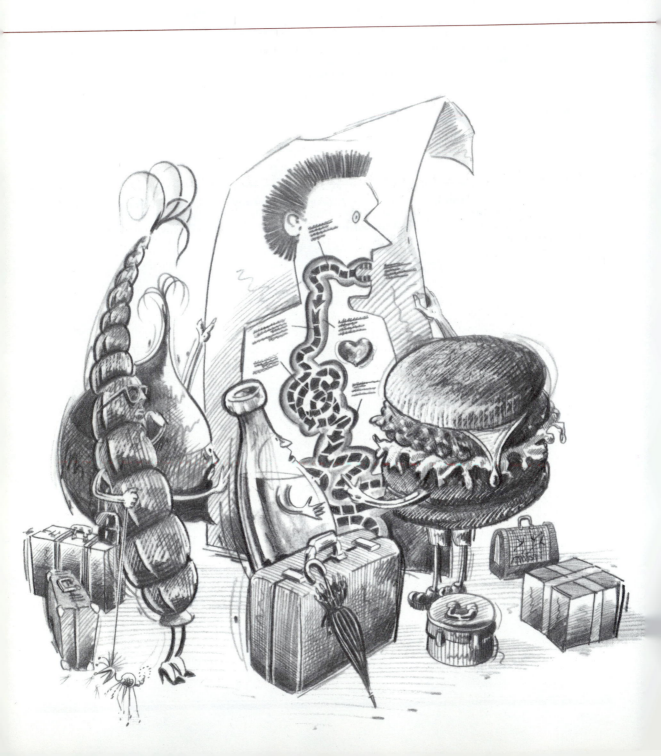

14

Metabolism:

THE INTERACTION OF ESSENTIAL NUTRIENTS

A BULLET OPENED A MEDICAL WINDOW

'Serendipity" is defined as the faculty of making fortunate and unexpected discoveries by accident. It was serendipity that made Dr. William Beaumont one of the most prominent physicians in American medical history. The accident occurred in 1822 when a French-Canadian trapper named Alexis St. Martin was shot in the left side. Dr. Beaumont examined St. Martin and predicted that his patient would not survive the wound, but St. Martin did far more than survive.

The accidental discharge that struck St. Martin came from a distance of just a few feet and sent birdshot tearing through his ribs and lower lungs. Part of a rib lacerated his stomach, and a portion of both lung and stomach protruded through the side wound.

Dr. Beaumont was unable to close the wound, but as St. Martin healed, a flap of tissue covered the opening in his side and into his stomach. This unusual opening in St. Martin's stomach made it possible for Dr. Beaumont to be the first person to view gastric digestion.

In a series of experiments, St. Martin was given different food substances to eat. Once a certain food was ingested and digestion had begun, Dr. Beaumont would remove the food through the opening. Beaumont was able to determine the time needed for digestion of various foodstuffs, and that gastric juices are formed from our stomach walls in response to food. He found that nonfood substances do not generate gastric juices. He also established that gastric juices are acid. Conventional wisdom had assumed that foods were digested in some order; for example, that all beef might be digested, then all vegetables, and finally all sweets. Beaumont's experiments were, of course, able to show that the theory was not true. His experiments served to advance the knowledge of digestion during a five-year period—which often saw St. Martin run away from Beaumont and have to be coaxed into returning.

Supported from Beaumont's salary as a military doctor, and ultimately put into a salaried position himself, St. Martin served as the subject for almost two hundred experiments.

While we remain indebted to the curiosity of researchers such as Dr. Beaumont, our indebtedness also extends to St. Martin. Due to the sacrifices of both, and those of others like them, we are able to share part of the discussion on digestive physiology in this chapter.

SOURCE: Adapted from *Nutrition Today,* September/October 1971, p. 28.

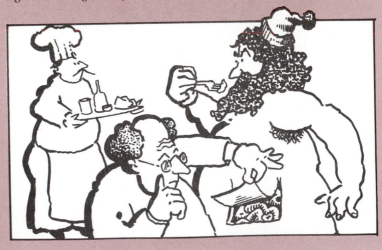

When Food Becomes Us

Most of us take the process of eating for granted, knowing that the body will take care of itself. But when we eat, hundreds of thousands of metabolic processes must take place before our cells can utilize dietary nutrients. In the process of **digestion**, food is broken down into particles of a size and chemical composition that the body can readily absorb. Figure 14-1 shows the digestive system through which food must pass from ingestion via the mouth to excretion of waste through the anus.

Absorption takes place mostly in the small intestine, where specialized cells transfer digested nutrients into the blood and the **lymphatic system**. In some cases, special changes are needed so that the nutrients can be *transported* to the cells where they are to be used or further

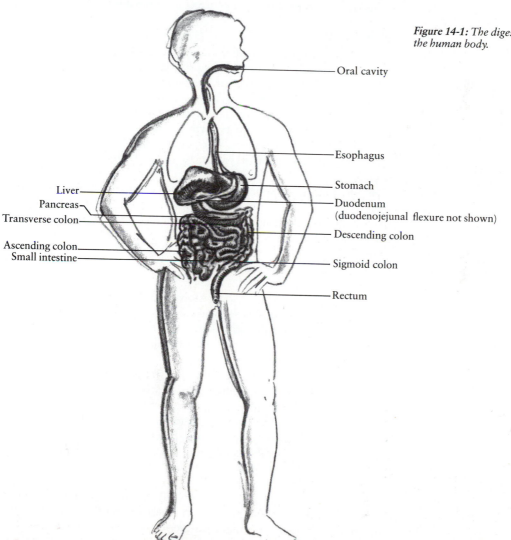

Figure 14-1: *The digestive system of the human body.*

Oral cavity

Esophagus

Stomach

Liver

Pancreas

Duodenum
(duodenojejunal flexure not shown)

Transverse colon

Descending colon

Ascending colon

Small intestine

Sigmoid colon

Rectum

processed. Within the cells, the nutrients may be stored, or they may undergo **metabolism**, the process by which they are broken down into simpler components for energy or excretion (*catabolism*), or used to synthesize new materials for cellular growth, maintenance, or repair (*anabolism*).

The complicated processes involved are different for each nutrient, although the paths that certain nutrients take do intersect at various points. This chapter provides a brief overview of what happens in our body to the foods we eat, with particular attention to the three major nutrients—carbohydrates, proteins, and fats (Hui). This chapter concludes with a look at some of the most common problems associated with a general understanding of body physiology and metabolism, those problems, such as heartburn, that affect a significant number of us.

The Food Path

The *alimentary tract*, or *digestive tract*, is the long tube whose parts include the mouth, the esophagus, the stomach, the small intestine (including the duodenum), the various sections of the colon, the rectum, and the anus. Some important accessory organs connected with the digestive tract are the salivary glands, the gallbladder, the pancreas, and the liver. Together, these organs form the **digestive system**. Along this tract, foods are broken down into small units, both physically and chemically, and then absorbed for use by the body. Figure 14-1 illustrates the digestive tract.

The food placed in your mouth is chewed, softened, and swallowed; in the stomach, it is churned, propelled into the small intestine and mixed with the bile from the gallbladder and with digestive enzymes from the intestinal walls. The nutrients released by digestion are partly or completely absorbed into either the portal vein (blood vessel leading to the liver) or the lacteal system (a special system of vessels that transport fat).

In the mouth, chewing (mastication) reduces large food lumps into smaller pieces and mixes them with saliva. This wetting and homogenizing facilitates later digestion. Individuals without teeth or with reduced saliva secretion have trouble eating dry foods and require a soft, moist diet.

Saliva facilitates swallowing and movements of the tongue and lips, keeps the mouth moist and clean, serves as an oral buffer, provides some antibiotic activity, and inhibits loss of calcium from the teeth by maintaining a neutral pH (not overly acidic or alkaline). Saliva contains a digestive enzyme (**ptyalin** or salivary *amylase*) and a special protein called **mucin**. Mucin lubricates food, and the enzyme digests carbohydrates to a small extent. Each day the "salivary glands" make about 5½ to 6 cups of saliva.

The bolus of food is propelled forward by rhythmic contractions of the entire intestinal system (peristalsis). These peristaltic waves move the food from the mouth, through the esophagus, and into the stomach. Certain individuals, especially nervous people, tend to swallow air when they eat. When part of the air is expelled through the mouth, belching

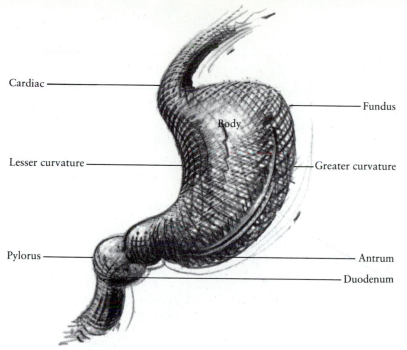

Cardiac

Fundus

Body

Lesser curvature

Greater curvature

Pylorus

Antrum

Duodenum

Figure 14-2: *General structure of the stomach.*

results; the remaining air is expelled as flatus (gas). Swallowing too much air leads to abdominal discomfort.

Food travels through different parts of the stomach (cardiac, body, greater curvature, the pylorus, and the duodenum; see Figure 14-2) and is well mixed there. The acid, mucus, and pepsin (another digestive enzyme) that these organs secrete cause partial digestion, and peristalsis mixes up the food. Food is then released gradually through the end of the stomach (pylorus) into the beginning of the small intestine (duodenum).

The digestive system breaks down complex carbohydrates, proteins, and fats into absorbable units, mainly in the small intestine. Vitamins, minerals, fluids, and most nonessential nutrients are also digested and absorbed to varying degrees. Foods are digested by enzymes secreted by different parts of the intestine. For reference purposes, Table 14-1 summarizes the major digestive enzymes and their actions. After the digestive process is complete, nutrients are ready for absorption, which occurs mainly in the small intestine. The absorption of each nutrient is discussed later.

After the nutrients have been absorbed, they enter the circulation in two ways. Most fat-soluble nutrients enter the **lacteal,** or **lymphatic system,** which eventually joins the body's entire blood circulation. Other nutrients enter the *hepatic portal vein* and are received by the liver, which eventually releases them to the bloodstream.

Enzymes, Coenzymes, and Energy Storage

After digestion and absorption, the nutrients exist as hexoses (mainly glucose and fructose; see Chapter 5), fatty acids and glycerols (see Chapter 6), and amino acids (see Chapter 7) and are then metabolized in various fashions. Many of the metabolic processes require the presence

Table 14-1
Characteristics of the Enzymatic System of Digestion

LOCATION	FOOD OR SUBSTRATE	PRODUCTS OF DIGESTION	ENZYME(S) INVOLVED FOR DIGESTION		
			NAME(S)	SOURCE(S)	ACTIVE IN ACID/BASE (pH)
Mouth	Starch	Maltose, dextrins, disaccharides, monosaccharides, branched oligo-saccharides	Ptyalin or salivary amylase	Salivary glands	Slightly acidic (6.7)
Stomach	Protein	Proteases, peptones, polypeptides, dipeptides, amino acids	Pepsin	Peptic or chief cells of stomach	Acidic (1.6–2.4)
	Milk casein	Milk coagulation	Rennin	Stomach mucosa	Acidic (4.0); requires calcium for activity
	Fat	Triglycerides; some mono- and diglycerides, glycerol, fatty acids	Gastric lipase	Stomach mucosa	Acidic
Small intestine (mainly duodenum and jejunum)*	Protein				
	Proteoses, peptones, etc.	Polypeptides, dipeptides, etc.	Trypsin (activated trypsinogen)	Exocrine gland of pancreas	Alkaline (7.9)
	Proteoses, peptones, etc.	Polypeptides, dipeptides, etc.	Chymotrypsin (activated chymotrypsinogen)	Exocrine gland of pancreas	Alkaline (8.0)
	Polypeptides with free carboxyl groups	Lower peptides, free amino acids	Carboxypeptidase	Exocrine gland of pancreas	
	Fibrous protein	Peptides, amino acids	Elastase	Exocrine gland of pancreas	
	Carbohydrate				
	Starch, dextrins	Maltose, isomaltose, monosaccharides, dextrins	α-amylase (amylopsin)	Exocrine gland of pancreas	Slightly alkaline (7.1)
	Fat				
	Triglycerides	Mono- and diglycerides, glycerol, fatty acids	Lipase (steapsin)	Exocrine gland of pancreas	Alkaline (8.0)
	Cholesterol	Cholesterol esters	Cholesterol esterase	Exocrine gland of pancreas	
	Nucleic acids	Nucleotides			
	Ribonucleic acid	Ribonucleotides	Ribonuclease	Exocrine gland of pancreas	
	Deoxyribonucleic acid	Deoxyribonucleotides	Deoxyribonuclease	Exocrine gland of pancreas	

Table 14-1 (*continued*)

LOCATION	FOOD OR SUBSTRATE	PRODUCTS OF DIGESTION	ENZYME(S) INVOLVED FOR DIGESTION		
			NAME(S)	SOURCE(S)	ACTIVE IN ACID/BASE (pH)
Small intestine (mainly jejunum and ileum)	Protein				
	Polypeptides	Amino acids	Carboxypeptidase, aminopeptidase, dipeptidase	Brush border of the small intestine	
	Carbohydrate				
	Sucrose	Glucose, fructose	Sucrase	Brush border of the small intestine	Acidic/alkaline (5.0–7.0)
	Dextrin (isomaltose)	Glucose	α-dextrinase (isomaltase)	Brush border of the small intestine	
	Maltose	Glucose	Maltase	Brush border of the small intestine	Acidic (5.8–6.2)
	Lactose	Glucose, galactose	Lactase	Brush border of the small intestine	Acidic (5.4–6.0)
	Fat				
	Monoglycerides	Glycerol, fatty acids	Lipase (enteric)	Brush border of the small intestine	
	Lecithin	Glycerol, fatty acids	Lecithinase	Brush border of the small intestine	
	Nucleotides	Nucleosides, phosphate	Nucleotidase	Brush border of the small intestine	
	Nucleosides	Purines, pyrimidines, pentose	Nucleosidase	Brush border of the small intestine	
	Organic phosphates	Free phosphates	Phosphatase	Brush border of the small intestine	Alkaline (8.6)

*The food is not grouped together, for example, all fat, all proteins, and so on. Instead the food is placed in an order that follows the sequence of digestion along the duodenum to jejunum. This attempts to present the digestive enzymes in their expected sequence of action.

of a *catalyst*, a substance that can facilitate a chemical reaction. Although participating in the process, the catalyst may or may not undergo physical, chemical, or other modification itself. Nonetheless, the catalyst usually returns to its original form after the reaction (Guyton).

In the body, most biological reactions require a special class of catalysts called **enzymes**. All enzymes are made of protein. Each enzyme catalyzes only one or a small number of reactions, so there are many enzymes, each with a specific responsibility. Without enzymes, most biological reactions would proceed at too slow a pace.

Coenzymes are accessory substances that facilitate the effect of an enzyme, mainly by acting as carriers for products of the reaction. In fact, most enzymes contain a coenzyme. Further, many coenzymes contain vitamins or their slightly modified forms as their major ingredient. A coenzyme can catalyze many types of reactions; for example, some coenzymes transfer hydrogens. Other coenzymes transfer groups other than hydrogens.

Everything your body does requires energy. Nature has provided us with a wide spectrum of methods that permit energy to be either released or stored and later released to satisfy energy need at that time.

When carbohydrate, fat, or protein is burned in the body, part of the energy is released as heat. One technique of storing the rest of the energy released from the oxidation of foodstuff is incorporating it into "ester bonds" between certain organic compounds and phosphoric acid groups. The resulting substances are called high-energy phosphate compounds, the most important of which is probably **adenosine triphosphate**, or ATP. This ubiquitous molecule is considered the energy powerhouse of the body. It releases its energy by combining with water. The energy released from this process can be used for such work as organ building, heartbeat, transportation across cell membranes, and muscle contraction. The role of ATP is illustrated in Figure 14-3.

What Happens to Sweet and Starchy Foods?

Of the carbohydrate we consume, over 95 percent (all but the fibers) is digested and absorbed. Later, when you see that some vital nutrients are only 50 percent digested and absorbed, you will realize how efficiently carbohydrates are utilized (Edholm and Weiner; Guyton).

During digestion, the carbohydrates are **hydrolyzed** (broken down by the addition of water) to their simplest units, monosaccharides. The breakdown begins in the mouth when food is mixed with the saliva enzyme amylase, continues in the stomach through the action of hydro-

Figure 14-3: The role of ATP in body energy metabolism.

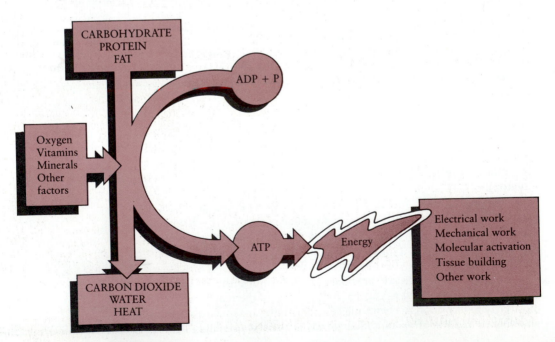

chloric acid, and concludes in the intestinal tract with amylase from the pancreas. This process is illustrated in Figure 14-4. (Table 14-1 may also be used as a guide.)

Carbohydrates are absorbed in the small intestine in the form of three monosaccharides—glucose, fructose, and galactose. From the point of absorption, the bloodstream carries the sugars to the liver, where fructose and galactose are converted to glucose and where some glucose is converted to **glycogen**. Glycogen is carbohydrate's storage form, whereas glucose is its active form, the form that can immediately be converted to energy. Among the various hormones that regulate the glucose level in our blood, **insulin**, secreted by the pancreas, is the most important. Insulin "tells" the liver when to store or release glucose.

When metabolism of glucose occurs, storage is referred to as anabolism; utilization or breakdown in the form of energy release is referred to as catabolism. Both activities are needed and occur in your body at the same time, and both are complex processes. The breaking down of glucose into its energy-releasing form of *pyruvic acid* and ATP (adenosine triphosphate) requires the aid of enzymes that bring about, or catalyze, the necessary chemical reactions. Such vitamins as thiamine, riboflavin, niacin, and pantothenic acid, and such minerals as iron, copper, and magnesium are necessary to the release of energy from glucose. Energy release from glucose relies on oxidation or burning of glucose, a process requiring oxygen. If oxygen supply is insufficient, as in the case of strenuous exercise, *lactic acid*, rather than pyruvic acid, results. The accumulation of lactic acid causes muscles to cramp.

Figure 14-4: Carbohydrate digestion.

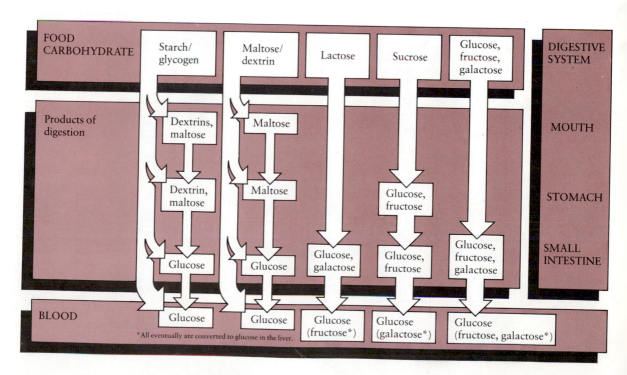

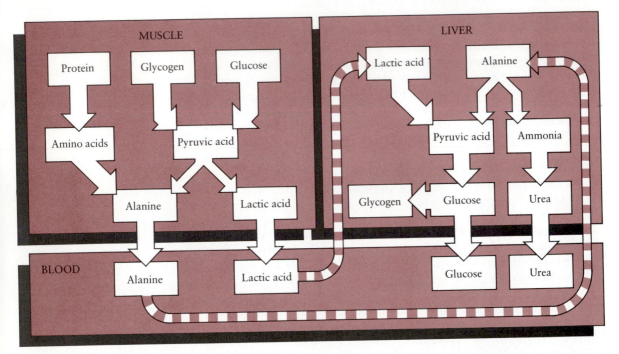

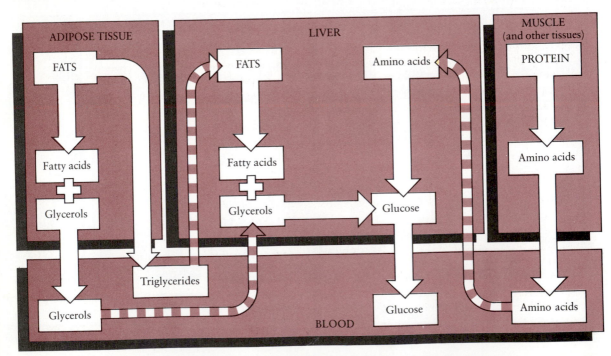

The metabolism of carbohydrates occurs concurrently with the metabolism of fats and proteins, and minerals and vitamins are necessary to the process, so all nutrients participate at the same time in fueling our bodies. Among the carbohydrates we consume are, however, a special group of carbohydrates—fibers, which function differently. Instead of functioning in the digestion process, they serve a cleansing function by scrubbing not only our teeth during chewing but also our intestines as the fibers move through the body to become waste. We do not fully understand the nutritional consequences of fibers, or roughage, beyond the cleansing function. Since the role of fiber has not been fully researched, proponents have suggested fibers can have a beneficial effect for every condition from heart disease to cancer, a claim discussed in detail in Chapter 5.

Figure 14-5 illustrates the role of liver and muscle in glucose formation, and Figure 14-6 provides an overview of glucose formation from fat and protein.

Figure 14-5(Opposite top): The role of liver and muscle in gluconeogenesis.

BLOOD SUGAR

In a normal person, blood glucose fluctuates within narrow limits—between 70 and 100 mg/100 mL of blood. This is achieved by a balance between the supply and removal of blood glucose (Hui). If blood glucose drops below the norm, **hypoglycemia** occurs. In a healthy individual, the blood sugar is restored to normal by the provision of glucose from three sources: (1) We may simply eat additional carbohydrates, thus increasing the absorption of monosaccharides, and the liver can then release more glucose. (2) The glycogen in the liver and muscle may be degraded to form more glucose. (3) Protein and fat may be degraded to provide glucose.

If a person's blood glucose rises above the norm, **hyperglycemia** occurs. If the person is in normal health, the body spontaneously lowers the blood glucose levels in one or more of the following ways: more insulin is released to drive glucose into cells for oxidation; more glycogen is formed in the liver and muscle; more glucose is changed to fat in more cells; and more glucose is excreted in the urine.

The **glucose tolerance test** is a simple test used to ascertain how well a patient tolerates an influx of glucose into the bloodstream. The rate with which glucose disappears from the blood is an indirect measure of how much circulating insulin is available to facilitate the entry of glucose into cells and tissues. The patient is asked to drink 100 g of glucose in a 25 percent chilled or flavored solution (usually water). Half an hour after the solution is given, a sample of venous blood is drawn, followed by additional blood samples at half-hour or hourly intervals for 3 to 5 hours. Most physicians prescribe a 3- to 4-hour test. The interpretation of the test results is complicated. The following example illustrates the extremes. If a patient shows a blood level of 200 mg glucose/100 mL of blood before the test and 250 mg 3 hours after glucose ingestion, then it is very likely that the patient is a diabetic. On the other hand, if the figures are 70 and 40 before and after the test, then the patient could have some form of hypoglycemia.

Figure 14-6 (Opposite bottom): An overview of glucose formation from fat and protein.

How the Body Utilizes Protein Foods

Protein digestion, absorption, and metabolism can be understood as even more complex processes than those for either carbohydrates or fats. The additional complexity results because numerous enzyme actions are necessary to reduce proteins to **amino acids**. The reductive, or digestive, processes occur in the stomach (where hydrochloric acid, pepsin, and protease, another enzyme, begin the digestion), in the duodenum (where the enzyme trypsin breaks proteins into dipeptides and tripeptides), and in the small intestine (where other enzymes ultimately break the peptides into amino acids) (Guyton). Table 14-1 clarifies this sequence of events. The amino acids then enter the bloodstream and travel to the liver. Figure 14-7 illustrates protein digestion. About 20 to 30 percent of ingested proteins are unabsorbed and are excreted in the stools.

Although normally only amino acids are absorbed, it is well known that in small infants some undigested proteins are also absorbed. The subsequent body reaction causes the child to develop an allergic reaction when ingesting the same protein foods later. This explains why so many infants are allergic to foods such as eggs and cereals. If adults show allergy to ingested protein foods, they probably remain capable of absorbing whole protein molecules. For the majority of the population, this ability disappears with age.

The liver holds amino acids until needed by cells in various parts of the body. When the cells require protein, amino acids re-form at the cell, with excess amino acids being returned to the liver. Amino acids not needed by the body can join either the carbohydrate or fat metabolic processes. If they enter carbohydrate metabolism, they are called *glucogenic amino acids* (that is, amino acids that can generate glucose). If they enter fat metabolism, they are called *ketogenic amino acids*

Figure 14-7: Protein digestion.

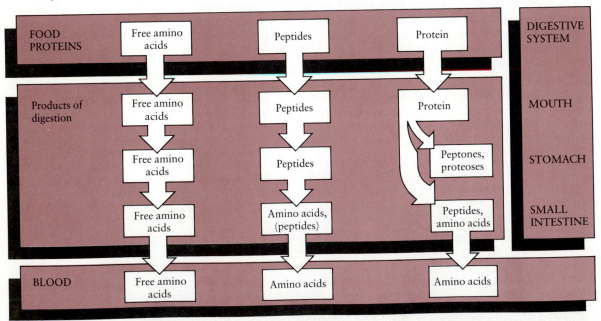

(that is, amino acids that can generate a special group of chemicals with a "keto" grouping attached). In the protein metabolic processes, hormones and enzymes play as large a role as they do in carbohydrate and fat metabolism.

For a protein to be synthesized, the appropriate type and number of amino acids must be available. There are eight to ten amino acids whose carbon skeletons cannot be synthesized or manufactured by the body. These essential amino acids, discussed in Chapter 7, must be supplied in the diet. In addition, there are ten to fifteen amino acids that the body can manufacture (including their carbon skeletons), which are the nonessential amino acids. If the appropriate carbon skeleton of an amino acid is present, the body can add, subtract, and transfer the "amino group" until the "right" amino acid is formed.

Of the three major nutrients—protein, carbohydrate, and fat—protein is the most important in the sense that it makes up our lean body mass (for example, muscle). Another factor that makes protein important is that body protein turnover is tremendous. For example, the formation of hair, skin, saliva, and sweat all involve large losses of protein that must be constantly replaced. How do we know whether we are eating enough protein? One acceptable technique is to measure the ingestion and excretion of nitrogen (nitrogen balance), because all protein has a relatively constant content of this element. Theoretically, if a young adult is in normal health and at a proper stage of development, the amount of nitrogen consumed should be equal to the amount excreted. This is **nitrogen equilibrium**. But depending on age, physiological condition, dietary intake, and other factors, some people are in **positive nitrogen balance** and others are in **negative nitrogen balance**.

Figures 14-8, 14-9, and 14-10 illustrate three sets of principles respectively: protein degradation, protein synthesis, and an overview of protein metabolism.

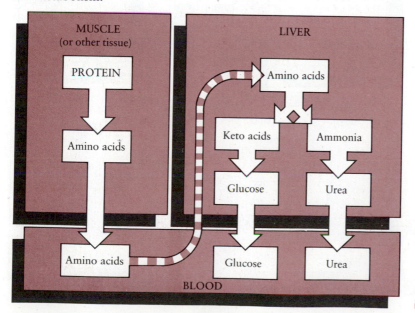

Figure 14-8: An overview of protein catabolism (degradation).

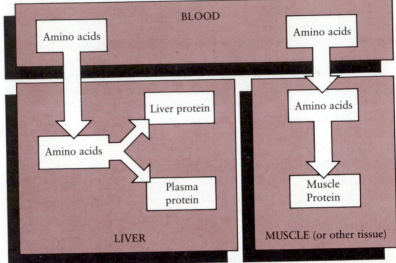

Figure 14-9: *An overview of protein anabolism (synthesis).*

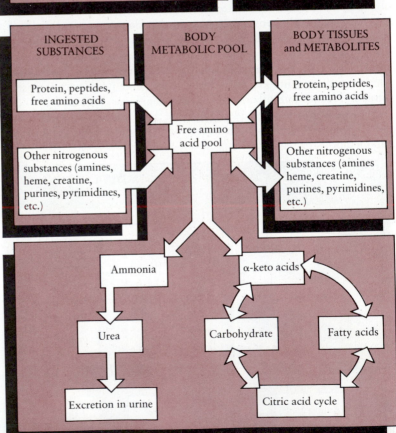

Figure 14-10: *An overview of protein metabolism, including nonprotein nitrogenous substances.*

The Metabolism of Fats

Of the fat we consume, over 95 percent is digested and absorbed, making it a nutrient as efficiently utilized as carbohydrate (Edholm and Weiner). Depending on the complexity of the fats (see Chapter 6), they may be attached to blood protein for transportation to the liver, or they may become very complex substances, called **chylomicrons**, before transportation.

Like carbohydrates, the fats are broken down by chewing and by the action of enzymes called *lipases*. Because fats are not soluble in water, they require combining with a water-soluble substance such as protein. Once the two combine, the resulting **lipoprotein** can be carried in the bloodstream to the liver. The liver then further refines the lipoproteins into phospholipids, triglycerides, and cholesterol. Figure 14-11 shows the digestion of fats, or triglycerides.

Triglycerides are the main storage form for fats, just as glycogen is the main storage form for carbohydrate. Cells in which the fat is stored are called *adipose tissue*. When required as energy, triglycerides undergo hydrolysis and are released to the blood protein for transportation to body cells. Both fats and carbohydrates are composed of hydrogen, carbon, and oxygen, so both produce water and carbon dioxide when fully utilized for energy (that is, upon oxidation). Fats are, however, the better energy source since they contain less oxygen and more hydrogen, a mix more easily oxidized, or burned.

Fat metabolism creates byproduct acids known as **ketone bodies**. Our kidneys draw body water to remove them, since their accumulation leads to a condition known as **ketosis**. Ketosis can cause kidney failure, dehydration, or coma. For this reason, it is important that we have

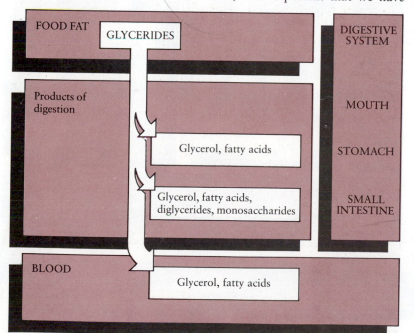

Figure 14-11: *Triglyceride (fat) digestion.*

sufficient carbohydrate intake along with fats, so our bodies do not depend too heavily on fats for energy.

About half of our dietary fats come from meats, eggs, and dairy products, with the rest coming from fats and oils added to other food products. Since much of our fat consumption is not recognizable as fat, we often consume far more fat than we think. Nutritionists have estimated that our average daily consumption may be as high as 150 grams (about 3 ounces), a level of concern because of the role of fats in such problems as heart disease (see Chapter 6).

Figure 14-12 provides an overview of fat metabolism.

Figure 14-12: An overview of fat metabolism.

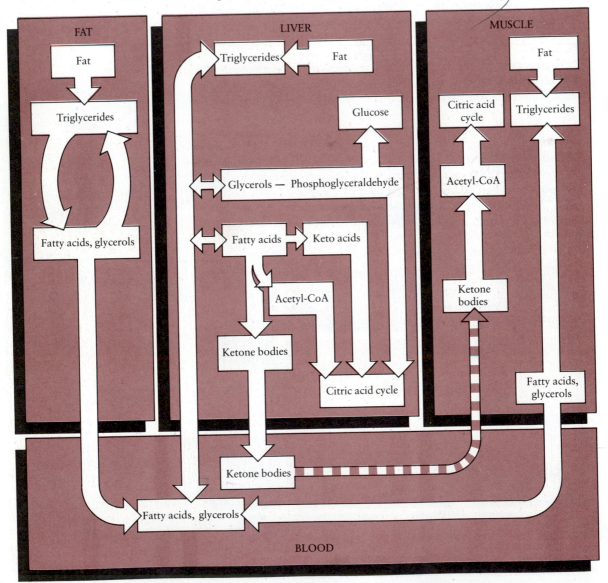

Metabolism of Nucleic Acids, Vitamins, and Minerals

NUCLEIC ACIDS

Practically everything we eat contains *nucleic acids*, which occur in cell chromosomes and are responsible for our heredity. During digestion, ingested nucleic acids are initially cleaved into smaller components called *nucleotides*. Next, nucleotides are broken up into smaller components, nucleosides and phosphoric acid. Nucleosides are further broken down to form sugars and two other smaller components, **purine** and pyrimidine, all of which are absorbed by the intestinal system. Figure 14-13 shows the digestion of nucleic acids.

Nucleic acids can also be synthesized by the body. In the body, purines, pyrimidines, and sugars are put together to form ribonucleic acid (RNA), deoxyribonucleic acid (DNA), and other related substances. Also, the liver can manufacture pyrimidine and purine.

Within a cell, although DNA is stable throughout life, RNA is in constant equilibrium with a metabolic pool (other free-flowing molecules of RNA in different parts of the body).

Figure 14-13: Digestion of nucleic acids.

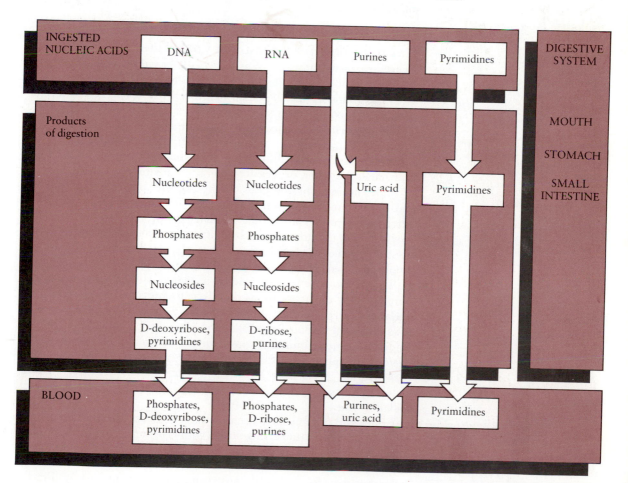

WATER, VITAMINS, AND MINERALS

From the stomach to the colon, water passes freely and reversibly between the intestinal space and the body organs or compartments, although less so in the stomach than elsewhere in the intestinal tract. Water moves in or out of the intestinal space to assure osmotic equilibrium between the interior and exterior of the intestine; otherwise the intestine would swell or collapse. After nutrients in the intestine have been absorbed, the excess water within it is passed out with fecal waste to maintain osmotic equilibrium.

All water-soluble vitamins are absorbed along the small intestine. Except for vitamin B_{12}, a healthy person can absorb these vitamins rapidly. All fat-soluble vitamins require the presence of pancreatic enzymes, bile salts, glycerides, and fatty acids for absorption, as does fat itself.

In a healthy person, all essential minerals are absorbed easily by the body, although the extent varies with individual minerals. What follows are some common gastrointestinal problems associated with body physiology and metabolism.

Heartburn: It's Been Around a Long Time

Heartburn, technically known as *gastroesophageal reflux*, has annoying symptoms that cause most sufferers to seek medical advice. That advice generally addresses diet, because heartburn has a characteristic relationship to food ingestion (Berk).

The problem of heartburn, or regurgitation, can be occasional or persistent. For example, it is common during the last three months of pregnancy but usually disappears after the birth of the child. Some individuals, however, experience regurgitation after every meal.

Under normal physiological conditions, the sphincter muscle at the end of the esophagus near the stomach (see Figures 14-1 and 14-2) exerts sufficient pressure on the esophagus to prevent food residue from moving out of the stomach and back into the esophagus. However, if the pressure in the stomach exceeds that against the lower end of the esophagus, then reflux, or regurgitation, can occur.

Various foods have been studied in regard to their effect on heartburn. Leading the list of foods that decrease pressure on the esophagus and thus open the door to heartburn are oils of plant extracts found in food seasonings, food flavorings, and after-dinner liqueurs. These include oils of peppermint, spearmint, onion, and garlic. Fat meals cause a decrease in sphincter pressure, protein meals cause an increase, and carbohydrate meals have little effect. Since fat content clearly has a causal effect on heartburn, whole milk can lead to heartburn while skim milk does not.

Coffee and caffeine have been the subjects of several heartburn studies since so many patients link coffee with heartburn symptoms. Studies have, however, shown that coffee increases rather than decreases esophageal pressure. This would indicate that coffee does not lead to reflux but may, for example, cause some similar symptoms by directly irritating the esophagus. Orange juice and tomato juice similarly irritate the esophagus without decreasing pressure.

Alcohol has also been studied in relation to reflux, and alcohol does negatively affect esophageal action, not only by decreasing pressure but also by slowing the clearance of acids from the esophagus.

Specific foods frequently cited by sufferers as causing reflux include fatty foods, fried foods, spicy foods, salad dressings, peppers, radishes, and tomatoes. As mentioned earlier, orange juice, coffee, and tomato juice do not decrease esophageal pressure, yet they too have been blamed by heartburn sufferers. Studies found, however, that all these cause irritation of the esophagus before they even reach the stomach, so the reaction to them is not a case of heartburn or reflux.

The practice of smoking a cigarette after a meal has been found to contribute to reflux. It is suspected that the loss in esophageal pressure results from either the effect of nicotine or the release of such natural body stimulants as epinephrine (adrenaline).

Because there are so many heartburn sufferers, antireflux diets are frequently prescribed. Small meals will decrease the likelihood of reflux, since they create less pressure in the stomach. Eating more frequently and losing weight are also beneficial.

High-protein/low-fat diets prove most beneficial. Meats should be baked or broiled. Skim milk and milk products provide the other protein need, and the balance of caloric need can be met by carbohydrate. Corn, potatoes, apples, and bananas rarely cause heartburn. Ice cream, baked cakes, soups, and candy also do not contribute to heartburn. Liquids can include water, skim milk, decaffeinated coffee, and apple juice. As with any food selection that is made to avoid specific problems, individual differences must be considered. For example, some sufferers may not be able to tolerate either decaffeinated or nondecaffeinated coffee.

What constitutes the best news for heartburn sufferers is that a healthy, balanced diet can be achieved while avoiding the foods that cause heartburn.

Talking About Ulcers

The term **peptic ulcer** is generally used to describe an ulceration found in the lower end of the esophagus (see Figure 14-2) or, more commonly, any part of the stomach or duodenum (Grossman). The affected area is thus exposed to the erosive effect of any acid or pepsin (a digestive enzyme) present.

The outstanding symptoms of a peptic ulcer are pain and discomfort (Hui). When located high in the abdomen, just below the front of the chest, the "midepigastric" pain is often described as steady, burning, and gnawing, like a severe hunger pain. The pain is periodic, occurring in attacks lasting a few days, weeks, or months, and is usually relieved by food. Frequently the patient is awakened at night with pain. In contrast, intestinal discomfort unrelated to ulcers, such as gas and indigestion, rarely awakens the patient.

A number of peptic ulcer patients lose weight. Other symptoms such as vomiting, nausea, and heartburn are less common, although they tend

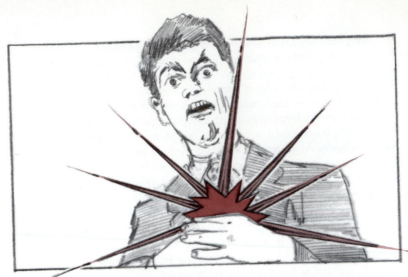

to accompany complicated (for example, bleeding) peptic ulcers. In these cases, the symptoms include pain radiating into the back and abdominal area. If the patient has a bleeding ulcer, other clinical manifestations include blood in the stools or vomitus.

At present, it is generally agreed that the ulceration may be the result of either too much hydrochloric acid, or an altered mucosal lining of the affected area showing lowered resistance to whatever amount of acid is present. Much research has attempted to determine what is responsible for the increased acid production and mucosal alteration.

Increased acid secretion can be caused by a simple defect in the body mechanism that produces the acid, or by rapid food movement, or frequent consumption of alcohol, caffeine, and similar stimulants. Heredity may be responsible for peptic ulcers in at least some patients. More men have ulcers than women. The incidence of ulcers in women apparently relates to the physiological phases of their life cycle. During active reproductive years, women seem to be protected from ulcers. For example, pregnant women rarely develop active ulcers, and the pre-pregnancy ulcer symptoms, if they exist, usually disappear shortly after conception, although they reappear shortly after delivery. Menopausal women are more susceptible to ulcer development, symptoms, and com-plications. Emotional instability may predispose a person toward ulcers. People who are chronically anxious or depressed are definitely more susceptible to ulcers than the population in general.

Certain professionals such as doctors, firefighters, and business ex-ecutives are more likely to have ulcers. The stress and hurry associated with these professions may exacerbate existing physiological tenden-cies. Bolting food and inadequate chewing are also possible factors for these people.

For a number of years, drugs and smoking have been implicated as one cause of peptic ulcers. Heavy smoking is associated with an increased incidence of peptic ulcers, and quitting smoking contrib-utes significantly to the healing of ulcers. But many nonsmokers also de-velop ulcers.

The goals of ulcer therapy are to relieve pain and discomfort, to hasten healing, to prevent complications, and to avoid recurrences. To achieve these goals, an ulcer patient is usually instructed to obtain mental and physical rest, revise the diet, avoid potentially aggravating agents, follow an appropriate antacid treatment, use certain medications, and, if conditions warrant, have surgery.

The relationship between peptic ulcers and irritating agents in the diet has been very controversial. In the past, the dietary treatment of an ulcer patient was very stringent. For example, the use of milk and bland foods and the avoidance of irritating agents were rigidly prescribed. However, such conservative diet therapy is now believed to pose a number of problems. Although milk can relieve pain, it has not been proved to heal ulcers. At present, no known clinical or dietary method can heal an ulcer permanently. But it is generally accepted that certain agents such as caffeine and alcohol can irritate the ulceration.

Milk has been used to relieve ulcer pain for more than 50 years. However, milk therapy has several drawbacks: The calcium in milk, when consumed in excess, can bring about calcium poisoning. Too much milk consumption can lead to weight gain, and increased levels of cholesterol and triglycerides in the blood. High cholesterol levels may predispose the person to heart disease.

Although some physicians still prescribe a bland diet for ulcer patients, its usefulness has been questioned.

The importance of antacid treatment cannot be overstated. Antacid can neutralize hydrochloric acid in the stomach and should reduce ulceration. Commercially available antacids vary in potency, effectiveness, and side effects. Antacids come in liquid (suspension) and tablet forms. Tablets are less useful because their neutralizing effect varies. They are also more expensive than liquid antacids, although they are convenient to use. If tablets are used, the patient should be instructed to chew them thoroughly. Most tablets containing aluminum hydroxide preparations are ineffective and should not be used. The usual prescription is an hourly ingestion of an appropriate number of tablets. Since one tablespoon of liquid antacid is equivalent in potency to three or four tablets, the liquid is preferred for patients with an active ulcer.

Depending on the type of antacid, the patient may suffer from diarrhea or constipation. Calcium carbonate may lead to constipation and calcium poisoning. Aluminum hydroxide gel may cause constipation and depletion of body phosphate. Mixtures of magnesium and aluminum compounds may cause diarrhea. Magnesium oxide preparations may also have laxative effects. One should read the label to identify the chemical contents. In general, noncalcium antacids, such as liquid magnesium hydroxide, magnesium trisilicate, and aluminum hydroxide, are preferred by many doctors.

An antacid has a very short-lasting buffering capacity when ingested on an empty stomach. The buffering effect is much longer when an antacid is taken 1 to 3 hours after a meal. Thus, during the acute phase of an ulcer, a patient is usually asked to take an antacid hourly after each meal, starting at breakfast and continuing until bedtime. However, many patients are awakened by pain at night (often at regular hours). Under these circumstances, the patient should wake up 1 hour before the expected pain and take some antacid. In most patients, this alleviates the pain.

How Common Is Constipation?

Constipation is a symptom of an underlying condition, not a disease in itself (Aman; Hui). A person suffering from constipation may have any of several symptoms. Bowel movements may be infrequent. Conversely, the patient may have frequent bowel movements in which small amounts of hard, dry stools are passed. There may be difficulty in passing stools, including general abdominal discomfort or even pain during a bowel movement.

What are the causes of constipation? Improper eating habits can easily lead to constipation. Conditions include a voluntary or imposed lack of food, insufficient dietary roughage, imposed dehydration, and insufficient water intake. Lack of water and a lack of dietary residue are the most common causes.

Constipation can also have a psychological origin. Stressful emotional states such as depression and anxiety can predispose a person to constipation. In these states, the patient may fail to respond to the need to defecate.

Of course, intestinal disease of various types also affects constipation. The use of drugs may be responsible. Finding and treating such causes of constipation is obviously important. Communication with the patient plays a very important role in that effort. The symptoms of constipation should be explained and clarified, and the adverse effects of commercially available laxatives emphasized. It is useful in this regard to suggest an easy home remedy for simple chronic constipation, as described below. Other appropriate clinical measures and obtaining a detailed medical history ensure good medical management of constipation.

COUNSELING THE PATIENT

Patients with constipation should know that good health does not depend on a daily bowel movement. However, if a problem exists, patients should be informed of common conditions that cause constipation. Among these are the omission of breakfast, irregular or strange dietary habits, very little activity or exercise, prolonged intake of certain drugs and laxatives, pregnancy, the use of contraceptive pills, and obesity. The connection between constipation and ignoring the urge to move the bowel should be explained. Various factors may be responsible for this inattention, such as a change in job or home environment, social activities, working routines, inconvenience, travel, increased age, convalescing from an illness, and emotional disturbances.

Older patients with constipation require special understanding. Their constipation problems may be directly related to age, to general weakness or to a dental handicap. The elderly patient may have little interest in food and its preparation. Older patients may dislike high-fiber foods such as raw fruits and vegetables or may be unable to afford foods with high roughage contents, which serve as laxatives.

The use of enemas and laxatives should be clearly explained to the patient. Long-term use of such substances weakens the muscles of the colon and the abdomen. The colon muscle must work normally and respond to regular stimuli for a bowel movement to be accomplished.

In the home remedy for simple constipation, the patient's habits must be changed first. Defecation should occur at about the same time each day. An after-breakfast routine is a good beginning. Drinking hot water and lemon juice after waking will help initiate intestinal motility. Walking and regular exercise of the abdominal musculature are also beneficial. Responding to the urge to defecate is important as well. The patient should avoid straining and should use a handrail or a footstool if necessary. The process should be completed in less than 15 minutes. The physician should try to find out whether the patient uses laxatives, and habitual use should be stopped.

Patients must also adjust their food and drink habits. They must consume adequate amounts of food and liquids; they should always include roughage in the diet and drink 5 to 8 glasses of water each day. If regular high-fiber foods are too expensive, they can use inexpensive unprocessed bran.

INCREASING ROUGHAGE

As indicated above, either regular high-fiber foods or unprocessed bran can be used to increase dietary roughage. If a patient chooses regular foods, an appropriate menu must be planned (see Chapter 15 for information). A high-fiber menu plan is shown in Table 14-2. Consult Chapter 5 for information on fiber content of foods.

Some high-fiber foods are whole grain cereals and bread, leafy vegetables, and raw and cooked fruits. Prunes, rhubarb, figs, dates, bananas, and applesauce are good laxatives as well as being high in fiber and residues. For individuals who cannot tolerate lactose and have developed constipation, milk and milk products may solve the problem at least at the beginning. Older people may be served food with soft residues, such as cooked vegetables and canned or stewed fruits.

Unfortunately, high-fiber diets can be expensive in some parts of the country. They may also be high in calories and may contain too many fruits and vegetables. In addition, these diets take some time to relieve constipation.

Eating unprocessed bran can also increase fiber intake. Bran is inexpensive and can be easily obtained. It serves as a laxative because it can not be digested and is able to absorb water, thus keeping the feces soft. It has been used successfully to treat constipation, irritable bowel syndrome, and diverticular diseases. Also see Chapter 5 for more information on bran.

A patient should take 2 teaspoons of unprocessed bran two or three times a day for 1 to 2 weeks. The bran can be taken in any way the patient prefers. It can be swallowed with water or juices, taken with cereals and milk, mixed with porridge, or added to flour in baking. The consistency of bran is like sawdust, and it is very difficult to swallow. If possible, the patient should eat it simultaneously with some other regu-

Table 14-2
A High-Fiber Menu Plan

BREAKFAST
Dried figs, stewed, 3
Oatmeal, 1 c
100% Bran*, 2 T
Toast, whole wheat, 1 sl
Margarine
Jam, 2 T
Coffee or tea

LUNCH
Fish, baked, 3 oz
Potato, baked, with skin, 1
String beans, ½ c
Lettuce and tomato salad: tomato, ½, lettuce leaves, 3
Bread, whole wheat, 1 sl
Margarine
Pudding, chocolate, ¾ c
Cookies, oatmeal and raisin, 2

DINNER
Beef stew, with vegetables, 1 c
Cole slaw, ½ c
Beets, buttered, ½ c
Muffins, bran, 2
Margarine
Ice cream, 1 c
Chocolate sauce, ½ c
Coffee or tea

SNACKS
Strawberries, ½ c
Ice cream, ½ c

Note: This menu contains approximately 12 to 13 g of undigestible fiber.

*A breakfast cereal marketed by Nabisco; it contains about 7.5% fiber.

lar foods that are high in roughage. The addition of bran may enable the patient to have one or two bowel movements of soft stools daily without straining.

After the initial trial, the patient should progress to 2½ or 3 teaspoons of bran until bowel movements with soft stools are regular. The treatment should be discontinued after the patient has established a good daily regimen. The patient should be told that initial consumption of bran may cause flatulence; this should not cause the patient to stop taking the bran. Some patients may also have abdominal pain, distention, and discomfort initially, all of which usually disappear with time. However, some constipated patients cannot tolerate unprocessed bran. Once the bowel has returned to normal, the patient should maintain a balanced diet with adequate daily roughage.

It should be emphasized that a high-fiber diet has a number of potential problems as discussed in Chapter 5.

Clinicians sometimes use other substances to promote defecation in a constipated patient. They may be administered orally or rectally. The common laxatives are divided into five types: lubricants, stool softeners, bulk producers, osmotically active chemicals, and irritants (stimulant purgatives). Physicians are usually careful about their usage and prescribe them only if necessary.

Passing Gas

A problem that plagues many people is the formation of wind, or gas, in the lower bowel. The presence of the gas, also called flatus, causes abdominal pain. There are various causes for gas in the bowel and various foods that contribute to its formation (Berk).

Flatus contains very little oxygen and is composed mostly of hydrogen, nitrogen, methane, and carbon dioxide. Gas occurs in the gastrointestinal system as a result of swallowing air and as a result of bacteria fermenting undigested food residue and producing the gas as a byproduct.

The unabsorbed foods that are metabolized by bacteria in the colon are generally carbohydrates; that is, sugars or starches. The foods have remained unabsorbed because some malfunction prevented their digestion and absorption. The malfunction can be a lack of sufficient enzymes to break down the foods or too rapid a transit time to enable their digestion.

Certain foods rate high as offenders in the production of bowel gas, with baked beans being the most notorious of the group. Milk is also a common offender because of its lactose content. Lactose is a double sugar that must be broken into two parts for absorption. For persons experiencing gas problems, elimination of milk and milk products from the diet will quickly demonstrate whether milk is the cause. If it is, another calcium source must be found.

No drugs have been found to be particularly effective in helping those with excessive flatus, so dietary control becomes most important. Since baked beans can increase flatus output to ten times its normal level, they should be avoided. Sugar tolerance testing can determine whether table sugar (sucrose) or milk sugar (lactose) is not being properly digested and absorbed. If they are the offenders, dietary change, especially withdrawal from milk sugar, can be effective.

Often prescribed is greater intake of fiber, especially bran and whole grain cereals in place of white bread and white flour products. These changes are especially beneficial for those suffering from spastic colon, a common cause of gas. This dietary change can diminish the gas resulting from spastic colon in about 3 weeks.

For those experiencing gas as a result of fat intake, the problem can be resulting from liver or gallbladder problems. If insufficient bile is present, fat digestion and absorption become impaired. If the gallbladder is diseased, it may have to be removed; however, that will not solve the gas problem. Reduced fat intake becomes the only practical solution.

Excessive bowel gas necessitates that the sufferer determine which foods cause the problem. Dietary change can then reduce the difficulty. Such dietary changes often require the assistance of a health professional to ensure that nutrient needs are met.

STUDY QUESTIONS

1. Define metabolism, catabolism, and anabolism.

2. Summarize the entire digestive system.

3. What is the role of enzymes? Of coenzymes?

4. To what form are all carbohydrates eventually reduced in the digestive process?

5. Discuss at least one way in which energy is released or stored in relation to carbohydrate metabolism.

6. How is blood sugar level usually maintained within a narrow range?

7. What is the end product of protein digestion? In what areas do protein digestion, absorption, catabolism, and synthesis take place?

8. Define nitrogen equilibrium.

9. What forms of fat can be absorbed and are therefore found in blood plasma? To what are they bound?

10. Define ketosis.

11. What happens to water, vitamins, and minerals that are ingested?

12. Discuss the clinical problems of heartburn.

13. Discuss the clinical problems of ulcer.

14. List some home remedies for constipation.

REFERENCES

Aman, R. A. "Treating the Patient, Not the Constipation." Am. J. Nurs. 80 (1980): 1634.

Berk, J. E., ed. Developments in Digestive Diseases. Philadelphia: Lea & Febiger, 1980.

Edholm, O. H., and J. S. Weiner. The Principles and Practice of Human Physiology. New York: Academic Press, 1981.

Grossman, M. I. Peptic Ulcer: A Guide for the Practicing Physician. Chicago: Year Book, 1981.

Guyton, A. G. Textbook for Medical Physiology. 6th ed. Philadelphia: W. B. Saunders, 1981.

Hui, Y. H. Human Nutrition and Diet Therapy. Monterey, Calif.: Wadsworth Health Sciences, 1983.

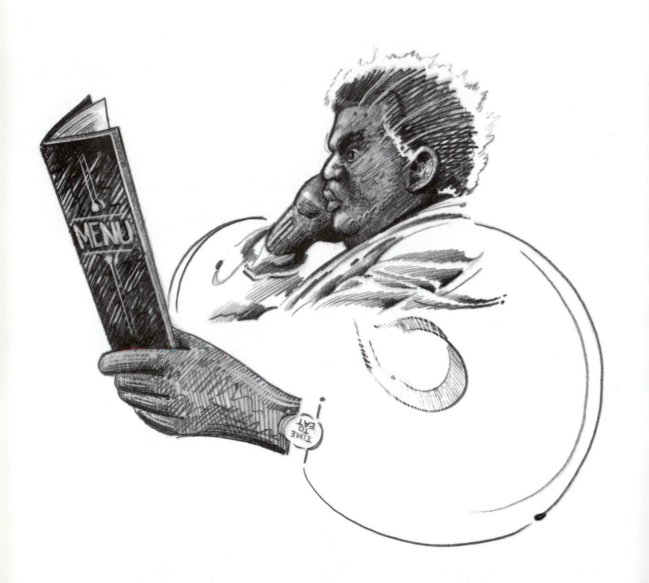

15

An Adequate
DIET
of an
ADULT

Cabbage, Cancer, and a Balanced Diet

Food supplementation can be legally complex as one California company learned (Ballentine). Drawing on a National Academy of Sciences report of an association between vegetable consumption and reduced incidence of cancer, the company began marketing pills composed of vegetables. The company's claims drew a reaction from federal and state authorities.

The Federal Trade Commission (FTC) began an investigation of the company's media campaign and finally charged the firm with false advertising. The FTC complained that the firm misrepresented the National Academy of Sciences' report and sought an injunction against the company's nationwide broadcast and print campaign. The Food and Drug Administration (FDA) also investigated the product and concluded that the company was making unsub-

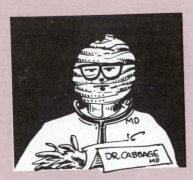

stantiated medical claims, a violation of federal law. The firm was advised by the FDA that the product was misbranded and was an unapproved new drug.

Although the company agreed to some labeling changes, it maintained its product was a food, not a drug, and that the disease-related claims were protected under the First Amendment's freedom of speech rights.

Finally, the Pennsylvania Department of Health brought misbranding charges against the

company, and the FTC obtained the federal court injunction barring the advertising of the product as a cancer preventive. This legal action ultimately resulted in permanently prohibiting the company from misrepresenting scientific findings, as well as from making health claims without "reliable and scientific evidence." Seizures of the product resulted, and the company filed for bankruptcy.

This case does not question that carotene-rich vegetables (dark green and deep yellow) and cruciferous vegetables (for example, cabbage, broccoli, cauliflower, and brussels sprouts) are healthful. Rather, it emphasizes that such items alone do not constitute an adequate diet. The consumption of these vegetables has been associated with a reduced cancer incidence, but a proper diet includes other foods too. What counts is a balanced diet.

Understanding the importance of various nutrients to our health is one matter; putting together daily diets with adequate quantities of all these nutrients is another. Nutritionists have devised a number of tools to meet this challenge. Food composition tables, Recommended Dietary Allowances (RDAs), nutrient labeling, and the four food groups are examples of such tools.

Chapter 2 also discusses food composition tables, RDA, and the four food groups, and you should review the information in that chapter before you proceed with materials in this chapter.

Daily food guides based on the four food groups offer a simple way for people to make certain that their diets are adequate.

In addition to examining these tools in this chapter, we will look at other factors that meal planners should consider (Hui). The frequency and timing of meals, the effects of cooking and processing on nutrient loss, and ways to keep food costs down without scrimping on essential nutrients are all important issues. These are followed by a discussion on nutrition labeling, organic foods, nutrient density, and adding nutrients to foods.

Daily Food Guides: The Four Food Groups

As discussed in Chapter 2, the four food groups are milk and milk products, meats, and equivalents, fruits and vegetables, and breads and cereals. Fats, sweets, and alcohol are considered as a fifth group by some individuals, and as supplementary foods by others, including the author of this book. For ease of reference, the four food groups listed in Chapter 2 are reproduced here, along with representative servings from each (Table 15-1).

MILK AND MILK PRODUCTS

We should consume at least a minimal amount of milk each day from among the following items:

Fluid milk: Whole, low-fat, skim, fat-free

Dry milk: Whole, low-fat, skim, fat-free

Other milk: Evaporated, condensed

Milk products: Yogurt, cheese, cottage cheese

Milk alternates: Soy milk, powdered soy milk, soy cheese

The recommendations range from 2 or more cups of fluid whole milk, for adults and children under age 9, to 4 or more cups for teenagers and nursing mothers.

The nutrient contents of cow's milk vary according to the characteristics of the cow, its lactation stage, and its diet. Milk bought at a grocery store contains a mixture of milk taken from many cows, further complicating analysis.

In general, however, milk's major contributions are calcium, protein, and vitamin B_2. Milk also contributes other nutrients, such as vitamins B_1, B_6, B_{12}, A, and D, niacin, and magnesium. Milk protein is cheap, easily digested, and of high quality; lactalbumin and casein make up about 80 percent of the protein in milk. The vitamin B_2 content of milk varies with the extent of light exposure. In a transparent container, the activity of the vitamin may be reduced by half. Paper cartons or opaque plastic containers help prevent this loss.

Milk is low in iron, manganese, copper, and vitamin C. A child under 6 months old will therefore receive an inadequate intake of iron if milk is the sole food source. Milk is low in vitamin C because of the heat applied during pasteurization. Sometimes, in the case of infant feeding, vita-

Table 15-1
Recommended Numbers of Servings from the Four Food Groups

FOOD GROUP	SERVING SIZE	NO. OF DAILY SERVINGS
Milk and milk products Fluid milk	1 c, 8 oz, ½ pt, ¼ qt	Children under 9: 2–3 Children 9–12: ≥3 Teenagers: ≥4 Adults: ≥2 Pregnant women: ≥3 Nursing mothers: ≥4
Calcium equivalent	1 c milk 2 c cottage cheese 1 c pudding 1¾ c ice cream 1½ oz cheddar cheese	
Meat and meat equivalents	2–3 oz cooked lean meat without bone 3–4 oz raw meat without bone 2 oz luncheon meat (e.g., bologna) ¾ c canned baked beans 1 c cooked dry beans, peas, lentils 2 eggs 2 oz cheddar cheese ½ c cottage cheese 4 T peanut butter	≥2
Fruits and vegetables	Varies by item: ½ c cooked spinach 1 potato 1 orange ½ grapefruit	≥4, including 1 of citrus fruit and another fruit or vegetable that is a good source of vitamin C and 2 of a fair source 1, at least every other day, of a dark green or deep yellow vegetable for vitamin C ≥2 or more of other vegetables and fruits, including potatoes
Bread and cereals	1 slice of bread, 1 oz ready-to-eat cereal ½ to ¾ c cooked cereal, corn-meal, grits, macaroni, noodles, rice, or spaghetti	≥4

min C is further reduced by repeated home sterilization. However, some manufacturers of infant formulas do add vitamin C to their products.

Fluid Whole Milk
The basic form of milk is fluid whole milk. It can be consumed as a beverage, used on cereals and desserts, and added to casseroles and soups.

To safeguard the quality of the fluid whole milk—and of milk products made from it—both federal and state standards have been established. Milk is *pasteurized*—usually by heating it to 161°F for fifteen seconds—to kill bacteria. Milk may also be *homogenized*—forced through small holes at high pressure to disperse the large fat globules and distribute them evenly.

Milk Products and Alternates

Products derived from fluid whole milk or products that imitate milk's flavor and nutrient content may be consumed in addition to or instead of fluid whole milk. Some people cannot digest fluid whole milk. It is now well established that some individuals are deficient in the intestinal enzyme lactase. They are therefore intolerant to lactose in milk. However, many of them can tolerate fermented products such as cheese, yogurt, or buttermilk, in which the lactose has been converted to lactic acid. Some of them can also drink a small amount of milk. Many children are actually allergic to milk, although some can become accustomed to the product if they drink gradually increasing amounts over a period of time.

When some dairy products are used in place of fluid whole milk, there are important nutritional considerations. If low-fat, skim, or nonfat milk is used, the intake of vitamins A and D and essential fatty acids may be low. If available, products fortified with these two vitamins are preferred. Also, chocolate milk has more calories than an equivalent amount of regular fluid milk.

Cheeses are popular substitutes for fluid milk. However, cheese is manufactured from the curds of skim or whole milk, after the whey is drained off—and whey contains some of the water-soluble vitamins. In the past, byproducts such as whey were discarded; much research is now being conducted to find a profitable use for these products. Cottage cheese prepared by acid coagulation should not be used as the sole substitute for fluid whole milk, since the content of calcium in this kind of cottage cheese is low and the drainage of whey reduces the water-soluble vitamin content. Cottage cheese is nevertheless a good source of protein.

Compared with fluid whole milk, cheeses tend to have higher fat and calorie contents and lower levels of protein, calcium, and vitamin B_{12}. Otherwise, the nutrient content of most cheeses resembles that of milk, although nutrient content varies with the method of processing.

Ice cream is made from milk, milk solids, cream, flavorings, and sweeteners. Nuts and fruits are sometimes added. Most commercial ice cream contains food additives to improve the texture, consistency, and appearance of these mixtures. Ice cream is higher in calories than milk.

Yogurt is made by fermenting milk (whole, skim, or low-fat milk or milk solids) with different strains of bacteria. Most commercial yogurts are low in fat and high (20%) in galactose. But more than half the weight of some commercial yogurts consists of added sugar and fruits.

Dairy or related products also include filled and imitation dairy products (for example, filled cheese). Most *filled* products contain milk solids and nonbutter fat; they come in many forms such as cheese and canned milk. An imitation dairy product is one that resembles real milk products, especially in flavor and cooking characteristics, but does not contain any milk solids. Instead, it contains nondairy ingredients.

How do we replace one milk product with another to derive equivalent amounts of nutrients? One cup (8 oz) of whole fluid milk is equivalent to: ¾ tablespoon butter plus 1 cup fluid buttermilk; ¾ tablespoon butter plus 1 cup fluid skim milk; ½ cup water plus ½ cup undiluted evaporated milk; ⅔ cup water plus ⅓ cup dry whole milk; or 1 cup whole milk yogurt. One cup (8 oz) fluid skim milk is equivalent to: ⅔ cup water plus ⅓ cup dry skim milk; 1 cup fluid buttermilk; or 1 cup skim milk yogurt. Table 15-2 shows the amounts of milk products that provide the same amount of protein or calcium as 1 cup of fluid whole milk.

In the last few years, the national consumption of dairy products has declined for various reasons. Technology has created a large number of nutritious beverages other than milk that cater to the taste and preference of some consumers. The threat of high blood cholesterol and obesity has also played a role; many consumers use dairy substitutes instead. In addition, many people are still ignorant about the value of milk.

MEATS AND EQUIVALENTS

According to the daily food guides (Table 15-1), we should eat two or more servings from the meat and meat equivalents group every day. In general, these two servings of meat provide approximately 50 percent of the protein, 25 to 50 percent of the iron, 25 to 30 percent of vitamins B_1 and B_2, and 35 percent of the niacin in the RDAs. Meat is not a good source of vitamins C and A or calcium. Common foods in the meat group are as follows:

Lean meat: Beef, veal, lamb, pork (fresh or cured), liver

Variety meat: Heart, brain, tongue, kidney

Wild meat: Squirrel, rabbit, bear, deer, buffalo

Fish: Shellfish, fresh and saltwater varieties (fresh, dried, frozen, canned)

Poultry: All fowl (for example, chicken, turkey, guinea hen, duck, goose) and their giblets

Table 15-2
Milk Products That Contribute as Much Protein and Calcium as 1 Cup of Fluid Whole Milk

| | AMOUNT OF PRODUCT CONTAINING GIVEN AMOUNT OF NUTRIENT | |
MILK PRODUCT	9 g PROTEIN	280 g CALCIUM
Nonfat milk	1 c	1 c
Cheddar cheese	1 ⅓ oz	1 ⅓ oz
Cottage cheese	1 ⅓ c	⅓ c
Ice cream	1 ½ c	1 ½ c
Cream cheese	30 T	9 T

Game birds: Pheasant, wild duck, grouse

Miscellaneous meats: "Turkey ham" (made from turkey meat but treated and smoked to look and taste like ham), "hot dogs" (made from a variety of meats including organ meats)

Dry legumes: Navy beans, lima beans, lentils, peanuts, others

Nuts: Nuts, nut butter

Peas: All split, dried peas, pinto beans, chick-peas, pigeon peas

Meat analogues: Textured vegetable proteins (TVPs), largely soy, which may be processed to simulate meat products such as sausage and bacon in shape and flavor

Meat equivalents: Eggs, cheese

The contents of iron and other minerals vary according to the type of meat. Muscle meats are high in iron, and organ meats are even higher. Pork liver is the richest and cheapest source of this nutrient. By contrast, chicken and fish have relatively low iron content. In addition to iron, muscle meats contribute zinc and phosphorus.

Although meats are a major source of protein, they have varying levels of the nutrient. For example, the content varies from about 12 percent in pork to 30 percent in some fish. The protein in fish is easily digestible and of good quality. Nonmeat alternates such as eggs, cheese, beans, peas, and peanut butter contain less protein, but they are cheap and provide good protein values when eaten with other protein foods. Dried beans and peas are 35 percent protein; nuts are 15 percent protein. Hard cheeses and cottage cheese may sometimes be considered part of the meat group because of their protein contents, but cream cheese does not qualify.

The fat content of the meat group may vary from 1 to 40 percent, according to animal feed, slaughter weight, the cut of meat, the extent of fat trimmed, and the method of preparation. Expensive cuts of meat have a high caloric content, since they have a significant amount of marbled fat. Prime beef is 25 percent fat; standard beef is 16 percent; and utility beef is less than 15 percent. By contrast, fish has only about 1 to 7 percent fat. Scientists are now attempting to modify the quality of fats in some animals. For example, some animals are being fed with varying amounts of fat and carbohydrate in experimental efforts to reduce the ratio of saturated:unsaturated fatty acids in their body fats.

Is Eating Meat Good for Us?

Those who observe dietary trends will find that many Americans continue to follow "meat-and-potatoes" food habits, while a growing number of people have sworn off meat in favor of vegetables, fruits, and nuts. Is meat healthful?

We know that nutrient need varies according to size and age, but assume that your need is for 56 g of protein per day. When you eat a steak dinner, you may ingest almost 50 g of protein, virtually your entire protein need. The excess amino acids are stored as body fat, posing the potential for obesity. A steak dinner also provides over 80 g of fat; close to 60 percent of the caloric content of the meal comes from fat. That is about twice the recommended level of caloric contribution from fat. Further, that fat is saturated, a type of fat with implications for heart disease. And the dinner probably lacked sufficient fiber, which aids in digestion.

In summary then, a meat-and-potatoes meal does not meet the essential definition of a balanced diet. Certainly the potential dangers can be offset by other meals in the same day, or by other meals during the week, but you should understand that those potential dangers are there.

Does that mean a vegetarian diet is healthier than a meat diet? To find out, refer to Chapter 7 for a detailed discussion of the advantages and disadvantages of a vegetarian diet. There you will find that vegetarian diets are not necessarily healthier.

FRUITS AND VEGETABLES

The daily food guides recommend four or more servings of fruits and vegetables each day, since this group makes many nutritional contributions to the American diet. Fruits and vegetables are responsible for the major intakes of iron and vitamins A and C; they are also good sources of calcium, magnesium, and folic acid. They contain small amounts of trace elements, depending on the type of soil in which they are grown, and some vegetables contribute protein. Fruits stimulate appetite, and their organic acid content helps in the absorption of iron and calcium, especially if a person does not produce enough stomach acid.

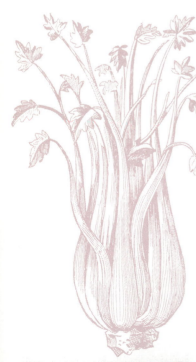

Most fruits and vegetables are nutrient dense, low in calories, low in fat, and high in cellulose. Because they provide roughage, cellulose, and bulk, the products in this group ensure a good intestinal environment. Some of them—such as celery, apples, and carrots—even help clean our teeth.

Although this group as a whole is a major source of vitamin A, very few vegetables and fruits contain good amounts of this vitamin. The major ones that are high in vitamin A are dark green vegetables, orange-colored vegetables, and orange-fleshed fruits, such as apricots, muskmelon, and mangoes (see Table 15-3).

Fruits and vegetables are our main sources of vitamin C. Citrus fruits are particularly high in vitamin C: a 4-oz serving of a citrus fruit juice provides 30 mg of the vitamin. Fruits such as cherries, strawberries, and cantaloupe also provide rich amounts of vitamin C. Vegetables such as spinach, cabbage, broccoli, and asparagus are good sources, especially when eaten raw.

The vitamin C level in many fruits and vegetables varies with the season, climate, variety of products, stage of maturity, storage period and temperature, and the plant parts utilized. Vitamin C loss after harvest, during oxidation, and in discarded parts is high. Since vitamin C is a very fragile compound that is subject to destruction by heat, air, and light, food should be prepared in ways that minimize its loss.

We derive about a quarter of our daily iron need from fruits and vegetables. In general, leaves contain more iron than stems, fruits, and

Table 15-3
Foods in the Fruit and Vegetable Group

VARIETIES RICH IN VITAMIN A AND CAROTENE
Dark green leafy vegetables: Beet greens, broccoli, chard, collards, watercress, kale, mustard greens, spinach, turnip tops, wild greens (dandelion and others)
Orange-colored vegetables: Carrots, pumpkins, sweet potatoes, winter squash, yams
Orange-fleshed fruits: Apricots, muskmelon, mangoes

VARIETIES RICH IN VITAMIN C
Citrus fruits: Grapefruit, oranges, lemons, tangerines; juices of these fruits
Other good and excellent sources: Muskmelon, strawberries, broccoli, several tropical fruits (including guavas), raw sweet green and red peppers
Significant sources: Tomatoes, tomato juice, white potatoes, dark green leafy vegetables, other raw vegetables and fruits

OTHER FRUITS AND VEGETABLES
Vegetables: Asparagus, lima beans, green beans, beets, cabbage, cauliflower, celery, corn, cucumber, eggplant, kohlrabi, lettuce, okra, onions, green peas, plantain, rutabagas, sauerkraut, summer squash, and turnips
Fruits: Apples, avocados, bananas, berries, cherries, dates, figs, grapes, nectarines, peaches, pears, pineapple, plums, prunes, raisins, rhubarb, watermelon; juices and nectars of many fruits

the parts grown in the soil. Because of the roughage and phytic acid in fruits and vegetables, the iron they contain is not well absorbed (about 5 percent absorption). However, the absorption is increased if meat is eaten at the same time.

Fruits and vegetables contribute a small amount of calcium. However, if the person's milk consumption is low or if a large amount of fruits and vegetables is eaten, the relative contribution of calcium from this food group is increased.

Legumes—vegetables such as soybeans, peas, and other beans—are good, acceptable sources of protein. Root tubers—such as potatoes—provide some protein too. Both groups are also high in carbohydrate calories. For example, root tubers contain 2 percent protein and 20 percent carbohydrate, whereas legumes contain 4 percent protein and 13 percent carbohydrate.

Although many fruits and vegetables are not high in calories by themselves, they are often consumed in combination with high-calorie foods, which increases the calorie intake. Broccoli, for instance, is often eaten with a high-calorie cream sauce or butter; canned peaches usually are packed in high-calorie sugar syrup.

CEREALS AND CEREAL PRODUCTS
In addition to recommending servings of milk, meat, and fruits and vegetables, the daily food guides recommend four or more servings of grain products each day. The major nutrients these foods contribute are calories, iron, niacin, and vitamins B_1 and B_2.

Cereals and cereal products include all grains served in whole grain, enriched, or fortified forms; for example, wheat, corn, oats, buckwheat, rice, and rye. Some common items in this group are as follows:

Breads: Yeast breads, rolls, quick breads, biscuits, buns, muffins, pancakes, waffles, crackers, others
Breakfast cereals: Ready-to-eat types, including flaked, rolled, and puffed forms; cooked types, including whole, grain, and rolled forms.
Other grain foods: Macaroni, spaghetti, noodles, flour, rice, cornmeal
Whole grain products: Whole wheat flour and its products, bulgur, dark rye flour, brown rice, whole ground cornmeal

The protein in grains is incomplete. Grains can be used to provide complete proteins, however, as discussed in Chapter 7. For example, if two or three different cereals are consumed at the same time, amino acids missing in one may be supplied by the others. We also tend to combine grains with protein-rich foods—macaroni and cheese, egg noodles, buns with hamburger, rice with chicken, and milk on cereals—and thus increase our amino acid intake. Finally, many baked goods contain liquid or dry milk, improving their protein quality.

Adding dry or liquid milk to commercial mixes for cereal products adds not only protein but also calcium and other nutrients. Many grain-related products are now enriched and fortified, an important health protection measure that is discussed later in this chapter.

Most nutritionists recommend eating some cereal products daily because they provide a fair amount of many nutrients at low cost. However, nutritional values of many breakfast cereals are being challenged by consumer groups. The main dispute concerns the practice of eating the cereals alone. A bowl of cereal with whole milk added is a nutritious food, but cereals by themselves contribute limited types and amounts of essential nutrients.

Refined, Enriched, or Whole Grain Bread: Which Is Better?

Since wheat is the primary cereal food and the most widespread crop in the world, significant attention has been paid to it. The approximately 50 kernels that cluster in the head of the plant at the top of the stem are milled to yield flour. Each kernel has four parts—germ, bran, endosperm, and husk. Only the husk, or chaff, has no nutritional use.

The germ is the part that can reproduce when planted. It is rich in niacin, thiamine, and vitamin E. The bran serves as a fiber source and is the coating or shell around the kernel. The soft, center portion of the kernel is the endosperm, which contains proteins and starch. From the endosperm, white flour is made from gluten, so white flour can be understood as using only a portion of the kernel.

As opposed to using only a portion of the kernel, whole grain wheat products utilize germ and bran as well as endosperm. Nutritionists have expressed concern about refining processes that remove the bulkier bran and germ, since those portions are richer in nutrients than is endosperm.

Nutrition surveys conducted in the United States as early as the mid-1930s discovered that many consumers had decreased their intake of thiamine, niacin, iron, and riboflavin. These were nutrients that had previously been obtained from unrefined bread, but the advent of refined bread resulted in a loss of these nutrients. In 1942, the Enrichment Act was passed. It required that nutrients be restored by enriching the refined flour with thiamine, niacin, iron, and riboflavin.

Although you can be confident that cereal products have the four basic wheat nutrients restored, nutritionists remain concerned by our use of highly processed foods. For example, fiber loss is not restored, nor are other nutrients such as chromium. Thus, many nutritionists continue to recommend whole grain products, which retain their chromium, zinc, folate, magnesium, and vitamins such as B_6—nutrients that are not restored by enrichment. In the case of chromium, some studies seem to indicate a correlation between diabetes incidence and chromium deficiency (also see Chapter 12).

The Foundation Diet and Supplementary Foods

A diet consisting only of the recommended numbers of servings from the four food groups is known as a **foundation diet**. An example of such a diet is shown in Table 15-4. A foundation diet provides more than 90 percent of most essential nutrients and over 75 percent of the calories in the RDAs, as shown in Table 15-5.

Table 15-4
A Sample Daily Foundation Diet for an Adult Using the Basic Foods

FOOD GROUP	NUMBER OF SERVINGS
Milk	2 c fluid milk
Meat	3½ oz broiled round steak
	1 medium egg
Fruits and vegetables	½ c cooked asparagus
	1 medium baked potato
	½ c cooked summer squash
	6 oz orange juice
	1 pear
Bread and cereals	3 slices enriched bread
	⅔ c corn flakes

Table 15-5
Nutrient Contribution by the Foundation Diet

NUTRIENT*	AMOUNT OF NUTRIENT CONTRIBUTED†	RDA FOR A 25-YEAR-OLD	
		MALE	FEMALE
Kilocalories	1,200–1,300	2,700	2,000
Protein	60–70 g	56	44
Vitamin A	1,100–1,400 µg RE	1,000	800
Vitamin E	1–5 mg	10	8
Vitamin C	125–135 mg	60	60
Thiamine	0.8–1.2 mg	1.4	1.0
Riboflavin	1.5–1.8 mg	1.6	1.2
Niacin	13.0–13.5 mg	18	13
Vitamin B_6	1 mg	2.2	2.0
Folacin	200–250 µg	400	400
Vitamin B_{12}	2–4 µg	3	3
Calcium	700–800 mg	800	800
Phosphorus	900–1,000 mg	800	800
Iron	10 mg	10	18
Zinc	5–8 mg	15	15

*Vitamin D and iodine are not included. All units used comply with the RDA system. Check the Appendix for more details.

†Because of the variation in the nutrient content of foods, only a range or an approximation is given.

WHICH FOODS ARE "SUPPLEMENTARY"?

We normally eat more than a foundation diet, however. We may eat extra servings of the foods in the four basic groups, and we may eat foods not included or listed in the four groups. These are called *supplementary foods*. They include spices, butter, margarine, and other fats. These are often ingredients in recipes or are added to other foods during preparation or at the table. Nutrient-light snacks and sweets, fabricated foods such as breakfast bars, and relatively nonnutritive beverages can also be included in this group.

Some common supplementary foods are:

Beverages: Coffee, tea, chocolate, soft drinks, alcoholic beverages

Fats: Butter, margarine, mayonnaise, cream, oils

Sweets: Sugar, jam, sweet desserts, candy, pastries, syrups

Snack items: Cookies, potato chips

Spices and seasonings: All spices, seasonings, flavorings, sauces

Although fats are now classified as supplementary foods, they are essential to health (see Chapter 6). Vegetable oil should be included among the fats used. Common sources of fats are butter, margarine, shortening, cooking and salad oils, cream, most cheeses, mayonnaise, salad dressings, nuts, and bacon and other fatty meats. Meats, whole milk, eggs, and chocolate contain some fat naturally. Many popular snacks, baked goods, pastries, and other desserts are made with fat or are cooked in fat.

Although supplementary foods may help round out meals and make them taste better, these foods tend to be low in nutrients. On the whole, each of the four food groups provides at least 25 percent of three or more nutrients to the diet. By contrast, nutrient contributions provided by the supplementary foods are relatively insignificant except for calories and fats. For example, supplementary foods contribute 20 percent of the total caloric intake, 30 to 35 percent of the total fat intake, and 10 percent of the vitamin A need. The approximate nutrient contributions of the different food groups to the average diet are shown in Table 15-6. The more calories one eats from the basic four food groups, the greater the likelihood of obtaining the RDAs. On a low-calorie diet, it is even more important that most of the foods come from the basic food groups rather than the supplementary foods.

The contributions of certain supplementary foods are controversial. One such group includes condiments, spices, and herbs. Usually of plant origin, these substances have been used by all known civilizations. During this century, numerous claims have been made about the therapeutic effects of herbs and related substances. Many therapeutic drugs are made from plant products, and some herbs and spices may contain pharmacological compounds. However, beneficial therapeutic effects from their regular use are not documented. On the other hand, there are reported cases of herbal tea poisoning as discussed in Chapter 25.

Table 15-6
Approximate Nutrient Contributions of the Different Food Groups

FOOD GROUP	MAJOR NUTRIENT CONTRIBUTED	PROPORTIONAL CONTRIBUTION TO THE AMERICAN DIET
Milk	Protein	1/3
	Calcium	2/3
	Riboflavin	1/2
Meat	Protein	1/2
	Thiamine	1/4
	Iron	>1/3
	Niacin	>1/3
Fruits and vegetables	Vitamin C	practically all
	Vitamin A and carotene	3/4
	Iron	1/4
Bread and cereals	Iron, thiamine, niacin, other B vitamins, fiber	>1/4
Supplementary foods		
Fats, oils	Calories, fat-soluble vitamins	varies
Sweet products	Fluids, calories, small amount of nutrients	varies
Spices and seasonings	Iodine	varies
Alcohol	Calories	insignificant to 1/3

Some individuals consume a large amount of substances such as sea salt and kelp, thinking them health giving. The safety of such practices has recently been debated. For example, arsenic contamination from seaweed and lead poisoning from bone meal have been reported. It is true that items such as seaweed, iodized salt, and chili powder can provide some minerals and vitamins. However, the importance of these contributions depends on the amount consumed.

Similarly, yeast can be a good source of vitamins, protein, and minerals if consumed in large quantities. However, most people do not eat much yeast, even when it is used in the leavening of bread.

COFFEE, TEA, AND COCOA

Among the supplementary foods that we consume in large amounts are beverages such as coffee, tea, and cocoa. All of these contribute some magnesium and potassium. In addition, tea provides a small amount of fluoride. But there has been much controversy recently regarding the effects of excess coffee and tea drinking on health. Although definitive findings are not available, some facts should be noted (Curatolo and Robertson).

Case reports of abdominal cramps and diarrhea from herb teas are discussed in Chapter 25. Tea also contains tannin, which has caused concern over the years, although not much evidence is available to substantiate claims about its adverse effects.

Caffeine is found in coffee and most cola beverages, theophylline in tea, and theobromine in cocoa. These chemical stimulants can keep us awake. Caffeine is also a diuretic and may increase urination, especially at night.

Caffeine has been one of the most studied individual foods. The first studies of caffeine showed that it countered fatigue. High doses produced increased motor activity, decreased reaction time, and increased attention. Such studies have also found that caffeine's effects vary depending on habitual use. For example, an individual who habitually uses small amounts of caffeine can have side effects such as headache, nervousness, insomnia, and irritability as a result of high intake. Yet in a habitual high user of caffeine, the same high intake can have positive effects.

Caffeine's effects have been studied among school-age children, because caffeine is found in many soft drinks. High caffeine users were found to be considered hyperactive by their teachers. Side effects and academic performance were not significantly different between high and low users. Among college age students, "high impulsive" personality types did better on tests after drinking caffeine in the morning, whereas "low impulsive" personality types did more poorly after morning caffeine. The pattern was reversed when evening consumption was tested.

ALCOHOLIC BEVERAGES

Cirrhosis, a condition of liver injury, is most often caused by chronic alcoholism. The liver cells are damaged by the alcohol and its negative effects on metabolism. The alcohol converts to *acetaldehyde* in the liver and yields an excessive production of hydrogen. The resulting fatty liver cannot be prevented by adequate diet, because the alcohol toxicity is doing the damage (Hui).

Fatty liver or cirrhosis usually progresses even more rapidly in the chronic alcoholic because the condition is compounded by malnutrition. Alcoholics tend to be malnourished because alcohol replaces food in the diet, providing calories but no nutrients. Twenty ounces of 80 proof liquor provides about 1500 kcal, one half to two thirds of daily need, but they are "empty" calories, calories devoid of nutrients such as protein, vitamins, or minerals.

Alcohol also interferes with absorption by causing inflammation of tissues in the digestive tract, retards the activation of vitamins that participate in digestion, and steals the B vitamins away from other functions to use them for its own digestion. Thus the chronic alcoholic often exhibits deficiency in protein, vitamins, and minerals.

Using the Food Guides in Meal Planning

Familiarity with the basic four food groups allows us to plan balanced and nutritious meals. Table 15-7 suggests a meal plan for an adult.

We all do not have to choose the same foods, however. Normal, healthy people can eat any food they like so long as they know how to combine it with other foods to provide a good diet. Lifestyles, national origin, religious beliefs, individual tastes, prices, and shopping and preparation times all influence the choices. We are fortunate in having a wonderfully abundant and varied food supply that gives us so many choices.

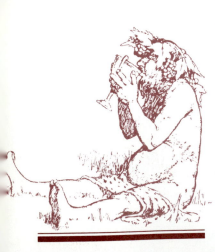

Table 15-7
Suggested Meal Plan for an Adult

BREAKFAST	LUNCH	DINNER
Fruit/juice, ½ c/1 serving	Soup, ½ c	Soup, ½ c
Cereal: hot/6 oz; dry/1 oz	Meat (regular/substitute), 2–3 oz	Meat (regular/substitute), 3–4 oz
Egg (regular or substitute), 1 serving	Vegetable (cooked/salad), ½ c	Fruit/juice, ½ c/1 serving
Meat: 2 strips bacon; 2 sausages;	Potato (regular/substitute), ½ c	Vegetable (cooked/salad), ½ c
1 oz regular meat	Salad dressing, 1 T	Potato (regular/substitute), ½ c
Bread, 1–2 slices	Bread/roll, 1–2 servings	Salad dressing, 1–2 t
Butter/margarine, 1–3 t	Butter/margarine, 1–3 t	Bread/roll, 1–2 servings
Jelly/jam/preserves, 1–3 t	Dessert, 1 serving	Butter/margarine, 1–3 t
Milk, 1 c	Milk, 1 c	Dessert, 1 serving
Hot beverage (coffee/tea), 1–2 c	Hot beverage (coffee/tea), 1–2 c	Milk, 1 c
Cream (regular/substitute), 1–3 t	Cream (regular/substitute), 1–3 t	Hot beverage (coffee/tea), 1–2 c
Sugar, 1–3 t	Sugar, 1–3 t	Cream (regular/substitute), 1–3 t
Salt, pepper	Salt, pepper	Sugar, 1–3 t
		Salt, pepper

In addition to considering nutrients and the form of foods that people will happily eat, meal planners should consider some other factors, including the frequency and timing of meals, nutrient loss in food processing and preparation, and ways of minimizing costs. Additional materials that are useful in planning an adequate diet are listed at the end of this chapter.

MEAL FREQUENCY AND TIMING

For a number of years, much effort has been spent on ascertaining what meal frequency and intervals are optimal for permitting the body to utilize ingested nutrients. So far it appears that the body can adjust to any pattern of eating, be it three equal meals; five or six small meals; or one small, one moderate, and one large meal. Some studies have confirmed that a number of small, frequent meals encourages the deposition of lean body mass, although the long-term effect of this regimen on the well-being of the body is unknown. On the other hand, other studies have shown that a nutritious breakfast raises blood glucose level and slightly increases the person's work efficiency throughout the day.

COOKING METHODS AND NUTRIENT LOSS

A second concern in meal planning is trying to minimize the nutrient losses caused by home cooking and commercial food processing. These occur even while food is being stored. For instance, oil becomes rancid if exposed to air for a long period. In the process, unsaturated fat and vitamins E and A may be oxidized. Refrigeration helps prevent oxidation. Cool temperatures and high humidity also help retain the nutrients in vegetables by delaying withering. But even in the freezer, the nutrients originally available in fresh foods may be slowly lost. Many frozen prepared foods continue to undergo oxidation at low temperatures.

Nutrient losses occur during precooking processing as well. A large piece of food has less surface area than the same food cut into smaller pieces, and thus fewer nutrients are lost. Most recipes, however, advise crushing, chopping, slicing, and shredding—practices that increase nutrient loss. Furthermore, trimming vegetables or removing the coarser outer leaves often results in a loss of vitamins A and C and calcium. Bruising vegetable tissues can have the same effect. Using sharp blades for trimming, cutting, or shredding fresh vegetables can avoid bruising.

High cooking temperatures may cause considerable nutrient loss. The high temperatures used in dry heat cooking—frying, roasting, baking, grilling, and broiling—may destroy any heat-sensitive nutrient. Vitamin C is unstable at dry heat cooking temperatures, and thiamine, folic acid, pyridoxine, and pantothenic acid are readily destroyed at these temperatures. Although beta-carotene (which becomes vitamin A in the body) is stable in most cooking operations, it suffers some loss during frying. The effect of dry heat on these unstable vitamins varies with the acidity of the food and the temperature and length of cooking. Dry heat denatures, or changes, the quality of proteins, especially if heating is prolonged. Polyunsaturated fatty acids are susceptible to heat and oxidation, and they become reduced in fatty foods cooked at temperatures typically used in dry heat cookery. Only mineral salts are not affected by the temperatures of dry heat cooking.

Oriental cooking methods, such as short-term frying at high temperature, reduce nutrient loss. Nutrient losses during frying, broiling, and roasting may also be reduced by using the juices in soup or gravy. If the fat contained in the juices is of concern, it can be removed.

Moist cooking methods, such as stewing or simmering in liquid, are less likely to destroy nutrients. Although protein is denatured during any type of heat treatment, moist heat cooking generally does not alter the protein's biological value (see Chapter 7). Mild heat like that used in moist cooking generally has no detrimental effect on the biological value of meat, fish, or poultry. However, if foods are cooked in a large amount of water, minerals and water-soluble vitamins are lost, especially if the fluid is discarded. If a small amount of fluid is used, nutrient loss is minimized. Alternatively, the fluid from cooking can be reused as a soup or base. In the American South, for instance, the "pot liquor" from cooking green vegetables is later used as a soup.

Not all changes in foods are undesirable. Heat treatment actually improves the digestibility and availability of certain nutrients in plant foods. Home or commercial fermentation of foods may result in the production of vitamins and other nutrients; some bacteria and molds (but not yeast) even make vitamin B_{12}.

FOOD BUDGETING
As the economy tightens, keeping food expenses low is of increasing concern to households and institutions. There are a number of ways to keep the food budget low without cutting nutritional values.

Planning Ahead

A shopper can save time, money, effort, and frustration if all needed items are listed ahead of time. It is especially helpful if foods located in the same parts of a store are listed together.

Sales, Specials, and Coupons

Grocery stores regularly run sales or specials on certain items. Sometimes newspapers, magazines, and other printed advertisements contain reduced-price coupons. Radio and television commercials are also used to promote sales. Of course, these opportunities are useful only if one needs the sale items and does not have to go to many different stores to purchase them.

"Generic" Brands

In the last few years, store brands and nonbrand items have become popular because they are cheaper than popular name-brand items. Savings of 5 to 10 percent are common.

Inexpensive-to-Moderate-Cost Items

People on fixed incomes or with low food budgets are accustomed to eating less expensive foods. But shoppers should be sure that such items are nutritious and contribute the same amounts of nutrients as costlier products.

Products in Season

Vegetables and fruits are abundant and therefore inexpensive when they are in season. Prices of such products will fluctuate. A wise shopper knows when to buy to save money. Some individuals save even more by freezing or canning seasonal products.

Wholesale or Quantity Purchases

If a freezer or storage space is available, purchasing a large quantity of nonperishable (or even perishable) items can save money. Of course, the wholesale store or warehouse should be within regular driving distance, and perishable items must be consumed before they spoil if money is to be saved.

Unit Pricing

The practice of displaying cost per unit (for example, per pound, ounce, or cup) instead of per package is gaining acceptance and is common in some stores. Not yet mandatory, unit pricing makes it easier to compare the cost of goods.

Cooperatives

Some parts of the country are witnessing an increase in the number of cooperative grocery stores, in which both members and nonmembers can purchase most staple items at wholesale prices. Because cooperatives are nonprofit, most of their products are somewhat cheaper than those in other stores. However, some consumers have complained about limited selections, occasional inferior quality, and high prices for some items.

BULK-FOOD MERCHANDISING CAN SAVE MONEY, BUT IS IT SAFE?

In an era of sprawling supermarkets and the glittering array of thousands of shelf-stacked food choices, a growing number of Americans are getting food from barrels and bins (Lecos). They help themselves to as much or as little as they want to buy.

This new food marketing concept—bulk-food merchandising—can save consumers money because packaging and (name-brand) promotion costs are less. Bulk-food displays usually include spices, flour, coffee, sugar, cake and other mixes, snack foods, pie fillings, dried beans, rice, and a variety of pasta.

Government health officials are concerned about bulk-food operations because these easily accessible foods may be open to human contact. Consequently, in April 1984, the Food and Drug Administration developed guidelines for such operations. Some of the guidelines are listed below.

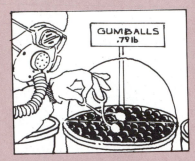

Foods should be in containers that are protected by close-fitting, self-closing covers. Operations should use self-closing lids that minimize consumer contact, product mishandling by children, and "environmental" problems (spills and insects).

Customer access to containers should be limited and controlled. Containers should not be so low that a customer who leans over might accidentally drop items from a shirt pocket into a container.

Customers should be provided with proper tools for removing foods, including mechanical dispensing devices (gravity dispensers, pumps, extruders, augers) and hand utensils such as scoops, tongs, ladles and spatulas.

Use of mechanical dispensers, where possible, is encouraged to eliminate customer contact with the food.

Tongs, scoops, ladles, spatulas and other utensils should be cleaned and sanitized at least once each day, more frequently if needed.

Containers and utensils should be made of safe materials that are corrosion resistant, nonabsorbent, smooth, durable and easily cleaned.

A supply of bags, cups, lids and other containers should be provided for customers to take food items home. Marking pens or labels should be handy so shoppers can identify their packages.

Less-Frequent Shopping
Some consumer studies have concluded that less money is spent when visits to grocery stores are reduced from once a week to once or twice a month. Obviously, this conclusion does not apply to purchasing fresh produce.

Fewer Fast and Convenience Foods
Fast and convenience foods are costly and should be avoided as much as possible. You can usually save money by preparing a dish yourself.

Despite the many aids to scientific meal planning, putting together nutritious meals that people actually like and eat is still a creative challenge. We all have our own preferences, and how a food looks, smells, tastes, and feels is usually as important to us as how nutritious it is.

In addition to individual preferences, those who plan meals for several people are typically confronted with a range of nutritional requirements and perhaps social problems. In later chapters, we will go beyond the general concept of an adequate diet to examine the special needs of the young, the elderly, and pregnant and nursing women. We will also look at diets that are either grossly inadequate or all too adequate—undernutrition and obesity. First, however, we will look at an additional concern in planning an adequate diet: nutrition labeling.

Nutrition Labeling

A rather new tool for planning an adequate diet is the nutrition information given on the labels of many packaged foods. In 1973, the Food and Drug Administration (FDA) completed a major rearrangement of regulations dealing with food labeling. Nutrition labeling, the most important of these regulations, involves a whole new practice—the listing of a food's nutrient contents on its label.

This practice is still largely voluntary. Nevertheless, both large and small food producers are providing nutrient analyses for many of their food products, greatly increasing the amount of nutrient information available to both consumers and nutritionists. The milk industry, for instance, has formed a task force to update information on the nutrient content of milk according to factors such as season, geographical location, and cow species.

Nutrition labeling is regulated by the federal government and is subject to constant changes as more scientific information becomes available. Therefore, a realistic approach to studying the discussion presented below is to supplement it with the latest scientific and legal developments. Such information may be easily obtained by writing or telephoning the nearest County Extension Agent. However, if experience and time permit, the *Federal Register* may be used to identify the current legal status of food and nutrition labeling. Also, a clear understanding of the discussion is possible only if the RDAs presented in Chapter 2 have been thoroughly studied.

U.S. RDAS

To establish nutrient intake standards of comparison, the FDA developed values based on the 1968 RDAs developed by the Food and Nutrition Board of the National Research Council of the National Academy of Sciences. The FDA used the 1968 RDAs to determine single values for the optimal intakes of different vitamins, minerals, and protein. These new values—called *U.S. RDAs*, or U.S. Recommended Daily Allowances—are used only for nutrition labeling. They give a *single* value for each nutrient rather than the range of values tailored to specific age and sex groups for the 1968 RDAs. In most cases, each single value is the highest value for each nutrient in the 1968 RDA for any age or sex group, excluding infants and pregnant and lactating mothers (different standards are applied to the labeling of foods for these groups). For some people, the U.S. RDA standards are therefore somewhat higher than their personal RDAs.

Exceptions to this procedure for determining the U.S. RDAs are calcium and phosphorus, each set at 1.0 g, and four nutrients not tabulated in the 1968 RDAs: biotin, pantothenic acid, copper, and zinc. The U.S. RDA for protein is 45 g if the protein efficiency ratio (PER; see Chapter 7) of the total protein in the food is equal to or greater than that of casein, and 65 g if it is less. Casein, the chief protein in milk, is used as the standard in measuring the growth-supporting quality of proteins.

One should bear in mind that unlike the RDAs, the U.S. RDAs are used only to provide consumers with information about the nutrient contents of foods. The nutrient composition of a labeled food is expressed as a percentage of the U.S. RDA, as shown in Figure 15-1, a frozen main dish label.

In the rules and regulations for nutrition labeling, the FDA states: "It is anticipated that U.S. RDA values will be amended periodically to concur with major changes that may be made in the National Academy of Sciences–National Research Council RDA values." At this time, however, the FDA has not yet updated its U.S. RDA values to reflect the 1980 edition of the RDA. The U.S. RDA values for labeled nutrients are listed in the Appendix and, within limits, can be compared with the 1980 RDAs in the same Appendix.

Figure 15-1: Frozen main dish label.

Nutrition Information
(per serving)

Serving Size = 8 oz

Servings Per Container = 1

Calories	560	Fat (percent of calories 53%)	33 g
Protein	23 g	*Polyunsaturated	2 g
Carbohydrate	43 g	Saturated	9 g
		*Cholesterol (20 mg/100 g)	45 mg
		Sodium (300 mg/100 g)	680 mg

Percentage of U.S. Recommended Daily Allowances (U.S. RDA)

Protein	35%	Riboflavin (Vitamin B_2)	15%
Vitamin A	35%	Niacin	25%
Vitamin C (Ascorbic Acid)	10%	Calcium	2%
Thiamine (Vitamin B_1)	15%	Iron	25%

*Information on fat and cholesterol content is provided for individuals who, on the advice of a physician, are modifying their total dietary intake of fat and cholesterol.

In 1973, the FDA completed a major revision of food labeling regulations. These regulations are now being revised again. Common foods, including most of those that contain added nutrients, can be labeled according to the "Nutrition Labeling" guidelines for the direct listing of nutrient contents of a food on the label. The "Special Dietary Foods" label is restricted to foods such as those used as the sole item in a diet (for example, a nutrition supplement consumed to the exclusion of all other foods) or those used under a physician's supervision.

Nutrition labeling is voluntary, with the exception of foods to which nutrients are added or about which nutrition claims are made. Enriched bread, breakfast cereals, and enriched milk products are among the foods to which nutrients have been added and for which nutrition labeling is mandatory.

As shown in Figure 15-1, nutrition labeling follows a standard format. The explicit statement "per serving" is required under (or following) the heading "Nutrition Information." To avoid confusion, all values on the table refer to the amount provided per serving. The size of a serving must be listed in common household units (such as cup) or as a recognizable portion (slice). The number of servings in a container must also be listed.

Caloric content is the next item in the format. Calories are listed in 2-cal increments below 20 cal, 5-cal increments up to 50 cal, and 10-cal increments above 50 cal.

Contents of protein, carbohydrate, and fat are then listed to the nearest gram. Information on fat composition or cholesterol content may also be provided, as discussed below. The protein content provides information to aid in comparative shopping for complex food products such as pot pies. Calorie and fat content information is probably of greatest use to those interested in losing weight or in fat-modified diets.

The amounts of eight nutrients—protein, vitamin A, vitamin C, thiamine, riboflavin, niacin, calcium, and iron—are shown as "Percentage of U.S. Recommended Daily Allowances (U.S. RDA)." These seven vitamins and minerals plus protein form the lower portion of the standard format and must always be listed. If quantities of any of these nutrients are minimal, they may be replaced by an asterisk, which refers to the footnote "Contains less than 2% of the U.S. RDA of these nutrients," or the missing nutrients may be listed as a footnote: "Contains less than 2% of the U.S. RDA of [list of missing nutrients]."

Sodium content may be listed without using nutrition labeling. But sodium content may also appear on a nutrition label as shown in the frozen main dish label in Figure 15-1. In both cases, it is listed in mg per 100 g, each declared to the nearest multiple of 5 mg.

FAT COMPOSITION

Final regulations have also been issued for the "Labeling of Foods in Relation to Fat, Fatty Acid, and Cholesterol."

If a manufacturer chooses to indicate on a label the composition of the fat and/or the amount of cholesterol in a product, it must also use

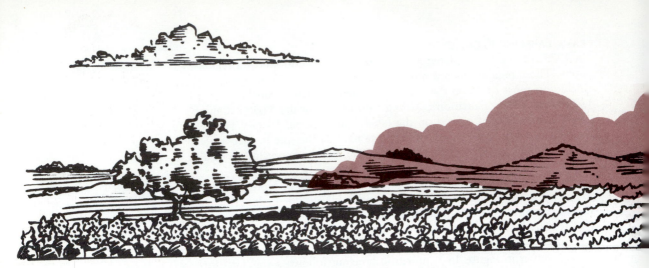

full nutrition labeling. This combination is shown in Figure 15-1. In addition to stating the total grams of fat, the percentage of calories provided by fat must also be stated. Below this, the grams of polyunsaturated fat and grams of saturated fat must be listed.

As indicated in Figure 15-1, the sum of saturated and polyunsaturated fats may not equal the total grams of fat. Certain unsaturated fats, short-chain fats, and some other forms of fat are not included in either "saturated" or "unsaturated." But the data on the label provide the ratio of polyunsaturated to saturated fats and also give the actual amount of polyunsaturated fat. These are the two figures that most dietitians and nutritionists want. In addition, a conditional statement must be made as follows: "Information on fat and cholesterol content is provided for individuals who, on the advice of a physician, are modifying their total dietary intake of fat and cholesterol."

CALORIE CLAIMS

Since the labeling regulations were established in 1973, new guidelines have been added concerning calories. These guidelines are as follows:

1. If the term *low calorie* or its equivalent appears on a label, it means that the food has a caloric density of 0.4 kcal or less per gram and provides 40 kcal or less per serving.
2. If the term *reduced calorie* appears on the label, it means that the food has a caloric reduction of at least one third of the regular item and is not nutritionally inferior to the higher-calorie counterpart.
3. Foods can be labeled "for calorie-restricted diets" if the basis for the claim is clearly stated on the label.
4. If a food is designed for a diabetic, the label must indicate this fact and state that the food may be useful in the diet "on the advice of a physician."
5. If a food is claimed to aid in weight control, an appropriate label statement is mandatory. Terms such as *dietetic, diet,* and *artificially sweetened* are reserved for low-calorie, reduced-calorie, or for calorie-restricted–diet foods. If the food contains a nonnutritive ingre-

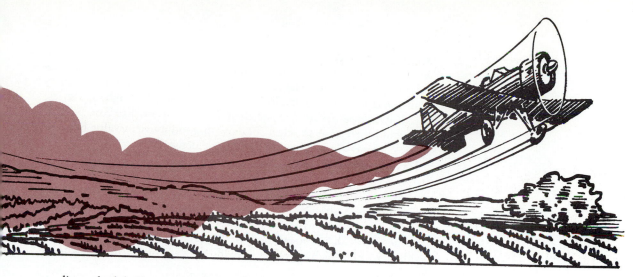

dient, the label must state the fact and indicate the percentage by weight the nonnutritive ingredient represents if it is not a sweetener.

Organic, Natural, and Health Foods

The industry that has developed around natural and health foods can be described as huge. Such foods are more expensive than traditional foods—often twice as costly. Given the potential expense, do the benefits justify the cost?

To answer that question, we address the claims made for organic, natural, and health foods. One such claim is for the curative or preventive powers of health foods. Studies have not shown that nutrients can work miracles. Nutrient intake beyond optimal requirements does not retard aging or promote virility. Further, many health foods, such as herbal teas, contain natural toxicants that can be dangerous.

The claim for organic food products is that they avoid dangerous pesticides and chemical fertilizers. Certainly we all agree that pesticides can be dangerous if misused. But studies question the logic of foods being pesticide free. For example, if pesticides can be found in fish swimming the ocean, how much more likely are they in plants grown on a farm located near other farms that use pesticides?

Concerning fertilizers, the issue is whether organic fertilizers prove more safe than chemical fertilizers. Studies of plants have shown that nutrition is equal regardless of fertilizer used. With both fertilizers, plants take up the same minerals such as nitrogen, phosphorus, and potassium.

The scientific conclusion is that organic foods do not offer a significant advantage over nonorganically grown foods.

In the case of natural foods, the claim for them is that they are safer and more nutritious since they avoid chemicals. The problem with this claim is that food itself is chemical. Although additives that may be used in processing must be watched, technology is not necessarily bad. Certainly natural foods do, however, avoid many additives. Safety of food additives is further explored in Chapter 25. Additional discussions on health foods and related subjects presented in Chapter 1.

Nutrient Density

On various occasions we have referred to "empty" calories, calories without nutrient value. The relationship between nutrients and calories is called *nutrient density*. If a food is low in nutrients but high in calories, we call it *calorie dense*. Assume then that you wanted to lose weight. You would then wish to select foods with good nutrient value but low caloric content—foods that are not calorie dense.

Foods can be analyzed according to their index of nutritional quality (INQ), a calculation that divides the percentage of nutrient standard, such as percentage of RDA, by the percentage of kilocaloric need. Calculation is a simple matter. For example, one cup of skim milk contains 25 percent of the daily calcium need and 100 kilocalories of a daily need of 3000 kilocalories, or 3 percent of daily caloric need. Dividing 25 percent by 3 percent yields an INQ of 8.3 for one cup of skim milk.

Consequently, each food has one INQ for each nutrient it contains. If we want to compare the nutrient densities of different foods, which

Bee POLLEN AS A HEALTH FOOD

It seems there's always someone willing to consider unlikely substances for curing an illness or promoting better health. In the case of bee pollen, the philosophy seems to be that what's good for bees will be better for humans. The idea of what's good for the bee is good for the beekeeper needs examination. Following are some claims made for pollen, along with scientific evidence and other facts associated with those claims (Larkin).

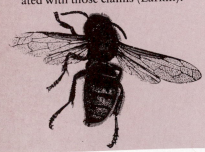

Claim
Pollen retards aging, as shown by the longevity of natives of the Russian Georgia mountains who owe it all to their pollen-rich diet.

According to a study of the eating habits of elderly persons in the Caucasus region of Soviet Georgia, "Sixty percent ate a mixed diet of milk, vegetables, meats, and fruits. Seventy percent of the calories were of vegetable origin and the remainder from meat and dairy products. Seventy to 90 grams of protein were included in the diets. Milk was a main source of protein." Although honey (which does contain some pollen) was sometimes included in the breakfast menu, along with cheese, bread and tea, the scientists conducting the study made no mention whatever of bee pollen, even though they were looking for some dietary clue that might explain why these people live so long.

Claim
Pollen is the richest source of protein known to science.

The major constituent of pollen is carbohydrate, not protein. And the protein quality of pollen varies, depending on the plant from which it comes. As pointed out by Dr. Hachiro Shimanuki, director of the Bee Laboratory at the U.S. Department of Agriculture Research Center in Beltsville, Md., the protein content nutrient's INQ will be the standard? The United States Department of Agriculture faced this problem when trying to ban the sale of certain foods at schools. A standard reached was that if the food product failed to provide 5 percent of the RDA for any nutrient per each 100 kilocalories, or per each serving, it was a food of limited nutritional value. In terms of INQ, if the INQ was not above 1.00 for any nutrient, the food product would not make the grade.

Adding Nutrients to Food

ENRICHMENT, FORTIFICATION, RESTORATION, AND NUTRIFICATION
The federal government permits the addition of nutrients to food to improve its nutritional value. In that case, the nutrients themselves are food additives, a topic to be discussed in detail in Chapter 25. To regulate the extent and safety of adding nutrients to food, the food industries must comply with guidelines and policies established by the FDA and the National Academy of Sciences. The four terms most commonly used in this practice are *enrichment*, *fortification*, *restora-*

varies, ranging from 5 to 28 percent. A study by the United Nations Food and Agriculture Organization shows that many foods contain more protein than even the bee pollen with the highest protein content. For example, soybean cake contains 46 percent protein; dry pumpkin seed, 29 percent; brewer's yeast, 39 percent. For comparison, round steak is about 20 percent protein.

Also, we do not really know what percentage of ingested bee pollen, if any, is actually capable of being absorbed by the human digestive system. It should be noted, however, that the amounts usually contained in a capsule of bee pollen provide an insignificant amount of protein.

It should also be pointed out that even if bee pollens were rich in biologically available protein, there are far less expensive protein sources, including filet mignon.

Claim
Scientific tests prove that bee pollen enhances athletic performance.

In a 1975 test sponsored by the National Association of Athletic Trainers, the Louisiana State University swimming team participated in a six-month experiment in which half the team took 10 pollen tablets a day, one-quarter received 10 placebo tablets (externally identical to the pollen tablet but devoid of pollen), and the other quarter received five pollen and five placebo tablets. There was no measurable difference in performance among the three groups.

The test later was repeated with 30 swimmers and 30 high school cross-country runners. As one of the researchers, Dr. John Wells of LSU, said, the bee pollen was absolutely not a significant aid in metabolism, workout training, or performance."

Claim
Bee pollen can alleviate a virtual encyclopedia of ailments, including sexual malfunction and tendencies toward suicide.

There is no valid scientific evidence for any therapeutic benefit from bee pollen. Under the law, since the pollen has not been shown to be harmful other than to those suffering from an allergy, bee pollen may be marketed as a food, provided no nutrition or therapeutic claims are made or implied regarding it.

If those selling bee pollen, or anything else, claim it can cure or alleviate any illness or produce some therapeutic benefit, the law says the product is a drug and must meet rigid scientific requirements for both safety and effectiveness.

tion, and *nutrification*. Each term has a separate meaning, but the first three are often used interchangeably. A knowledge of these terms will help us read labels accurately and plan an adequate diet (Vetter).

Enrichment refers to the addition of nutrients to food in compliance with legal regulations that specify: (1) the types of food that can receive additives; (2) the nutrients to be added; and (3) the amounts of the nutrients. For example, the nutrients vitamin B_1, vitamin B_2, niacin, and iron can be added to certain refined grain products, such as bread, flour, and cereals, which are then called "enriched."

Fortification is the addition of nutrients to foods for a variety of reasons. To improve nutritional intakes, margarine and milk (regular and skim) may be fortified with vitamins A and D, and table salt may be fortified with iodine. Fortification is voluntary in most states, though mandatory in some.

Restoration refers to the addition of nutrients that are lost because of processing. Adding vitamins to canned and dehydrated products is an example.

Nutrification is a process in which certain commercial meal equivalents and replacements, such as breakfast bars and canned mixed dishes (for example, beans and pork), are nutrified so that the manufacturer can indicate on the labels which nutrients are present and at what levels. For a product such as beans and pork, the label may compare the level of the nutrients added to that in the natural product.

PROS AND CONS

In the United States, the use of food additives to improve people's nutritional intakes started in the early 1920s. The practice successfully reduced the occurrence of such nutritional disorders as goiter, rickets, pellagra, and beriberi (see Chapters 9 and 12). Today, many additional foods are enriched or fortified with vitamin and mineral compounds. Some breakfast cereals, for example, are fortified with virtually all the vitamins and minerals for which the government has established U.S. RDAs (U.S. Recommended Daily Allowances; see previous discussion).

As discussed in Chapter 7, many plant proteins are incomplete; that is, they are either low or lacking in certain essential amino acids. Federal regulations require that the protein quality of certain commercially processed products meet minimal standards, thus forcing their fortification. A good example is formula milk derived from soy products, which is for infants having special needs. To assure the adequacy of the essential amino acids in the product, the formula is fortified with amino acids.

In the past, staple foods have been fortified for two reasons: to combat deficiency disease by providing nutrients lacking in the diet and to restore nutrients destroyed during processing and storage. But as eating patterns and food technology have changed, it has become necessary to ensure that alternate foods such as cheese substitutes and some meal equivalents (certain TV dinners), which constitute large portions of some people's diets, are also nutritionally balanced.

Some nutritionists now want to increase the use of nutrient addition to further improve public health. They point out that people in the

United States are now eating less, potentially shortchanging themselves on nutrients unless they eat a good variety of nutrient-dense foods. Proponents of increasing nutrient addition are skeptical about people's willingness to change their poor food habits, even after a quarter century of public nutrition education. According to their argument, why not try to make the foods people do eat—including "junk foods"—more nutrient dense?

Other nutritionists and scientists feel that extending enrichment and fortification programs would not be simple or altogether desirable. One objection stems from the variations among individuals and their eating patterns. How much we need of each nutrient depends on factors such as our age, sex, metabolic rate, body size, body composition, physical activity, personal body chemistry, health, and the drugs we may take. Individuals whose need for a certain nutrient is low or who are likely to ingest large amounts of a particular kind of food might ingest more of a nutrient than their bodies can safely handle. For instance, since our bodies store vitamins A and D, long-term high intakes of these vitamins could cause toxic accumulation. And our needs for trace minerals are so minuscule that even one dose of a trace mineral several times larger than the needed amount can be toxic.

Another major problem is insufficient information about eating patterns, the food supply, and nutrients themselves. Although great advances have been made in the science of nutrition, it is still a new and growing science. Certain issues—such as how much protein individuals actually need to lead a long and healthy life—are subject to varying opinions. If, as is currently thought, most Americans already consume enough protein every day, fortifying junk foods with protein would be pointless and might even have negative long-term results. Questions such as which foods should be fortified and with which nutrients involve value judgments that we may not yet be wise enough to make. And if foods are fortified with certain nutrients known to be essential to health but not with others, we run the risk of creating chemical imbalances in our bodies, since many nutrients must apparently interact at appropriate levels to create optimal health.

An additional set of problems involves the technology of enrichment and fortification. If nutrients are added to foods, they must be in a form that the body can use and that will not detract from the taste, appearance, or freshness of the food. And the food chosen must not contain elements that interfere with the body's use of the added nutrient. For instance, the oxalic acid in the bran of cereal can block the absorption of some mineral elements such as calcium. To choose whole grain bakery products as a carrier for calcium and certain other minerals would therefore be pointless. On the other hand, certain food ingredients actually aid the body's utilization of certain nutrients. Choosing good carriers for food additives will require detailed knowledge of such interrelationships.

To avoid random enrichment and fortification by food manufacturers that might lead to excessive or inadequate nutrient intakes or to the deception of consumers, government agencies have established some

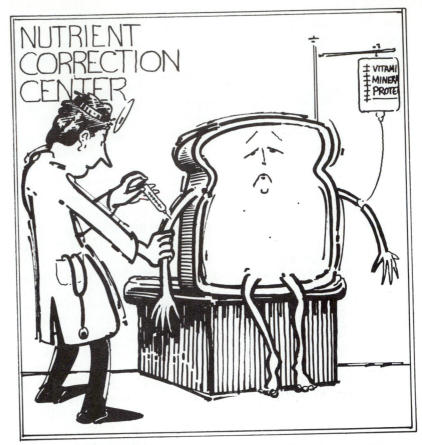

guidelines. The Food and Drug Administration (FDA) has established a fortification policy, guidelines for nutritional quality, and labeling regulations requiring that the nutritional contents of foods be listed to show which nutrients have been added. FDA policies also seek to prevent unnecessary fortification of foods. The Federal Trade Commission (FTC) oversees the "truth in advertising" regarding foods for which enrichment or fortification claims are made.

In general, the government encourages food manufacturers to: (1) correct nutritional deficiencies that scientists generally recognize; (2) restore foods to nutrient levels present before processing, storage, and handling; (3) balance the vitamin, mineral, and protein content of a food by adding these nutrients in proportion to the total caloric content of the food; and (4) make substitute foods nutritionally equivalent to the food for which they substitute. For example, infant formula replaces breast milk in many households. The manufacturers try to ensure that the nutritional contributions of infant formulas are at least equal to those of breast milk.

We see then that planning an adequate diet involves several considerations. Although the government has various programs in place to help us, we must do our part by being certain that we maintain a balanced diet, one from as wide a variety of foods as possible.

STUDY QUESTIONS

1. What is the purpose of food composition tables? What are their drawbacks?

2. What do the RDAs represent? Which agency or organization established them? How can the RDAs be used in conjunction with other criteria to determine a person's nutritional status?

3. What are the Four Food Groups? How many servings of each are recommended by the daily food guides? What are the major nutritional contributions of each group?

4. What is a foundation diet? Discuss the role of supplementary foods.

5. How does food processing or preparation cause a loss of nutrients? How can these losses be minimized?

6. List at least seven ways of keeping food costs down without scrimping on nutritional needs.

7. What are the U.S. RDAs? For what purpose are they used?

8. What type of information about fat composition may be given in nutrition labeling?

9. Using library resource materials, describe the legal status of "organic" food in each state in the country.

10. Define: enrichment, fortification, restoration, and nutrification.

REFERENCES

Ballentine, C. "On Cabbages and Cancer." *FDA Consumer* 18 (April 1984): 29

Curatolo, P.W., and D. Robertson. "The Health Consequences of Caffeine." *Ann. Inter. Med.* 98 (1983): 641.

Hui, Y. H. *Human Nutrition and Diet Therapy.* Monterey, Calif.: Wadsworth Health Sciences, 1983.

Larkin, T. "Bee Pollen as a Health Food." *FDA Consumer* 18 (April 1984): 21.

Lecos, C. "Making Bulk Foods Safe Foods." *FDA Consumer* 18 (April 1984): 17.

Vetter, J. L., ed. *Adding Nutrients to Foods.* St. Paul, Minn.: American Association of Cereal Chemists, 1982.

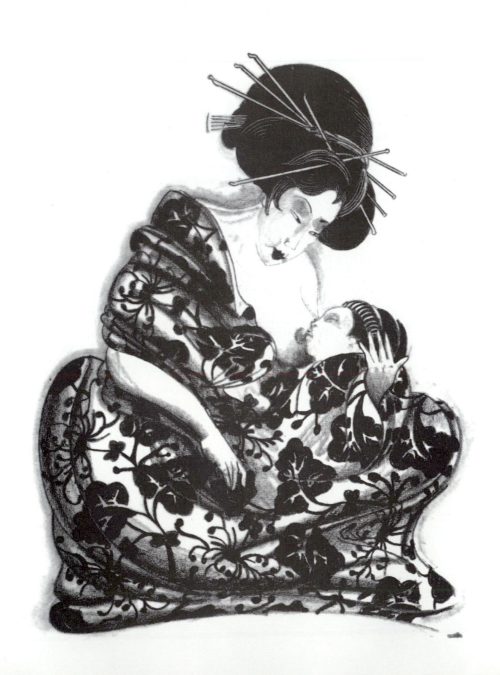

16

Nourishing the Pregnant or Nursing Mother

Rosalie is "Eating for Two"

Rosalie first visited the prenatal clinic in her eighth week of pregnancy. At 5′ 7″ and 115 pounds, she appeared to be a healthy 19-year-old, but she reported nausea and vomiting and occasional headaches, problems that she said had persisted for the last 4 weeks. She reported no history of diabetes, heart disorders, hypertension, or other major medical problems. Before her pregnancy she had taken birth control pills for 4 years.

Laboratory blood tests showed that Rosalie's hemoglobin (blood pigment) count was low but that all other values were within normal limits. After the clinic had ruled out any medical problems that might contribute to or cause her symptoms, Rosalie was referred to the clinic's dietitian.

The dietitian found that Rosalie's nausea and vomiting had caused her to resign from her job. She had eaten little since the inception of pregnancy and had lost 2 to 3 pounds in the 8 weeks. She regularly skipped breakfast, ate no fruit, drank little milk, and snacked on potato chips and soft drinks in the evening. She had not taken vitamins. Rosalie's weight was 20 pounds below ideal body weight for a nonpregnant female of her age.

The dietitian determined that the reduced food intake due to nausea and vomiting could precipitate nutritional anemia and recommended three meals per day with liquids or snacks between, and iron and folic acid supplements. Rosalie was shown how to incorporate milk, breads, and cereals into her diet, and was asked to bring a record of two-day food intake to her next appointment. She was especially encouraged to eat breakfast

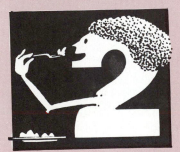

cereals with one or two soft-boiled eggs in the morning, and to drink more juices or milk between meals. The dietitian specifically advised Rosalie to avoid fried and greasy foods, especially if they tended to worsen her nausea and vomiting.

On a second visit some 2 months later, Rosalie said she was constipated. Her weight had increased by 4 pounds and her nausea and vomiting had sub-

sided, but her hemoglobin and hematocrit (red blood cell count) values had worsened. The dietitian suspected that Rosalie had been skipping her supplements, perhaps because of the constipating effect of ferrous sulfate (the iron supplement). She showed Rosalie how to increase roughage intake and suggested fresh fruits for snacks in place of cookies and soft drinks. Rosalie was given instructions on how to increase her consumption of calcium and protein by eating cheese, pudding, and ice cream. She was shown the importance of these nutritional matters to the developing fetus. The iron supplement prescription was changed to one more palatable and less likely to cause constipation. The dietitian also arranged for Rosalie to receive food stamp assistance, since she was unemployed. Another two-day food intake record was requested for the next appointment.

One month later, Rosalie showed a 5-pound weight gain, improved hemoglobin, and cessation of nausea, vomiting, and constipation. She felt better about herself and the health of the fetus. The dietitian provided her with recipe hints that would stretch her food budget while holding to principles of good nutrition.

Nutrition in Pregnancy

The common adage "eating for two" somewhat exaggerates the nutritional demands of pregnancy and nursing. Nevertheless, the expectant and nursing mother deserve special consideration. Another life besides her own depends on her nutrition.

PREGNANCY PROFILING

Numerous factors characterize the time span from conception to delivery, and these factors form the profile for any given pregnancy. Particularly influential to pregnancy profile is low income, which can cause both undernourishment and overweight conditions in women entering pregnancy. Deficiency in iron and folic acid, in vitamins A, B_{12}, and C, and in calcium and iodine are common. Although some of these deficiencies occur more frequently in adolescents than adults, all deficiencies are still found in the United States, especially among low-income women, ethnic women, and adolescent women.

Methods of contraception used prior to pregnancy can also affect pregnancy profile. For example, some contraceptive pills increase the amount of blood lost during menstruation. The use of an IUD may also cause blood loss. Any bleeding means loss of iron.

A well-nourished mother withstands the stresses of the gestation period, labor, and delivery. Her appetite continues, and her body changes in regard to digestion, absorption, and metabolism remain favorable. The well-nourished mother has minimal complications and delivers a healthy baby that experiences normal growth and development. The lactation period is also successful.

In contrast, the malnourished mother more commonly experiences pregnancy wastage: abortion during the first few weeks of pregnancy, intrauterine death, or stillbirth. Malnourished mothers may have an incompetent placenta—one smaller in size and having fewer cells than that of a healthy mother. Complications related to gestation, labor, and delivery increase among the malnourished. Infants born to such mothers are high risk, often suffering from such disorders as prematurity, low birth rate, reduced size, retardation, and birth defects, as well as high susceptibility to infection, kidney malfunction, and irregular body temperature. Such children do not develop normally during their first year or two.

Although exceptions to such generalizations can be found, *some* anthropological, epidemiological, clinical, and experimental studies have confirmed malnourished pregnancies as being higher in risks. Medical records from World Wars I and II confirm obstetrical problems among starved pregnant women. Clinical studies in the United States, Canada, India, and Guatemala have demonstrated that poor diet increases the incidence of stillbirths, premature births, and early infant deaths. When nutritional supplementation was used, healthier pregnancy profiles resulted.

Teenage pregnancy has long been associated with complications. Nearly one third of American teenage mothers are under 16 years of age, and half of all American women marry at 18 to 20 years of age. Teenage mothers give birth to about one fifth of the 3 million babies born each year. These teenage mothers have a dual nutritional need—their own development and the child's. Both suffer. Malnutrition occurs among young mothers for such reasons as poor diet and frequent attempts at weight loss, and offspring are typically high risk.

The importance of good diet has been demonstrated by studies that investigated diet before and during pregnancy in relation to health risk status of the infant. Results suggest that good diet before pregnancy even lessens the risk of poor diet during pregnancy. Because of the importance of diet to pregnancy profile, we will explore various diet-pregnancy relationships in detail in this chapter.

RISK FACTORS

Because malnutrition threatens both the expectant mother and the child, it is incumbent upon us to exercise special care at this time of life. Since the expectant mother's nutritional well-being is so important, obstetricians and gynecologists usually evaluate risk factors on the basis of her physical features: (1) overall physical appearance; (2) body development in relation to age; (3) body weight; (4) deficiency symptoms as seen in eyes, hair, skin, and nails; and (5) oral health. Physical findings are then correlated with the following nutritional risk factors (Hui; Ritchey and Taper; Rush et al.):

A. Reproductive history
   1. Unsatisfactory reproduction history/obstetrical complications.
   2. Long-term breast-feeding.
   3. First pregnancy when under 18 years of age.
   4. Repeated pregnancy with short intervals.
   5. Multiple births.
   6. Oral contraceptive use less than 6 months prior to pregnancy.
B. Current pregnancy profile
   1. Age under 17.
   2. Height under 5 feet.
   3. Over- or underweight.
   4. Clinical disorders.
   5. Therapeutic diet.
   6. Dietary faddism.
   7. Use of drugs (including cigarettes and alcohol).
   8. Other factors: low income; ethnic culture; emotional and psychological maladjustment.
C. Clinical progress of current pregnancy
   1. Restricted or excessive weight gain.
   2. Unsatisfactory fetal growth (example: over 42 weeks' gestation).
   3. Obstetrical complication (example: poor circulation, hemorrhage, abnormal presentation, toxemia).
   4. Severe dependent edema.

Comparison of the expectant mother's physical factors and the known risk factors yields a pregnancy profile that in turn can suggest nutritional modifications that will decrease the likelihood of a high-risk infant.

WEIGHT CHANGE

Obstetricians generally view normal weight gain during pregnancy as the key criterion of a healthy pregnancy. During early pregnancy, increase in breast size, uterus size, and blood volume all produce weight gain. Rosalie was a concern owing to her weight *loss*. During the fourth and fifth months, fat is stored as energy reserve, particularly for lactation. During the final two months of gestation, fetal size doubles, making that time period one of critical nutritional importance. Three factors influence weight gain: (1) the expectant mother's concepts; (2) her normal pattern of weight gain, and (3) instructions given to the expectant mother.

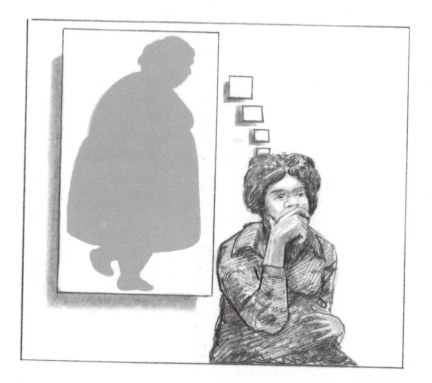

Expectant Mother's Concepts

Clinical experience indicates that most expectant mothers are concerned about excess weight. Those overweight at conception hope to lose weight so they will be slimmer after the birth. Some expectant mothers fear they will get stretch marks, be left with sagging and smaller breasts, and have poorly distributed and residual weight. Although social changes emphasizing a natural lifestyle and home birth have decreased many of the foregoing anxieties, they remain concerns that contribute considerably to poor health of both mother and child.

Mother's Pattern of Weight Gain

The acceptable pattern of weight gain during pregnancy constitutes the standard against which medical practitioners judge pregnancy profile. The standard has changed over the years. We present here the standard accepted by the National Academy of Sciences, the American College of Obstetrics and Gynecology, and numerous clinical nutritionists and physicians.

As you found in Chapter 3, ideal weight can be determined. A woman should be from 95 to 120 percent of ideal weight at pregnancy. In the case at the beginning of this chapter, Rosalie was too far below ideal weight. The average weight gain in the United States ranges from 27 to 29 pounds. The weight gain during pregnancy should be smooth and progressive, so it should be monitored not only at beginning and end but at intervals during gestation.

As shown in Figure 16-1, a slight gain in the first three months is followed by a steady rise. Most maternal storage occurs by midpregnancy. During the first 20 weeks, a 9-lb gain can be expected, at a rate of 2 lb per month. During the last 20 weeks, the gain averages 1 lb per week. Table 16-1 indicates the approximate distribution of pregnancy weight gain.

The fat reserve serves a significant need, since the fetus draws upon it if the mother's caloric intake is inadequate. Often the mother will also draw upon it during late pregnancy. The fat reserve thus reduces health risks to both mother and child while additionally providing cushioning

Figure 16-1: Weight gain during pregnancy.

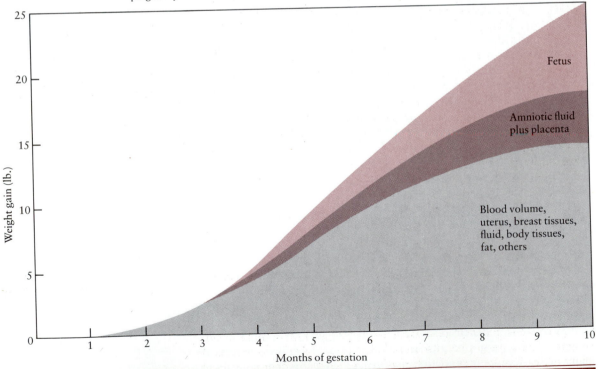

against physical injury. In most women, much of the fat reserve is deposited in breast tissues.

Instructions Given the Expectant Mother

Health care providers explain that weight gain varies because of individual differences. For example, the younger mother gains more than the older, the thinner more than the heavier, and a first-time mother more than repeat mothers. It is of paramount importance that fear of loss of waistline and similar concerns about appearance not interfere with healthy fetal development. Weight reduction efforts must be avoided.

Excessive gain can result in various clinical problems. The risk of **toxemia**—a pathological condition with symptoms including nausea, vomiting, liver enlargement, and convulsions—increases with excessive gain. The likelihood of a large baby that may have later life problems increases. Sudden and excessive weight gain, especially after 20 to 24 weeks of gestation, exposes both mother and child to higher health risks such as increased morbidity (sickness) and mortality (death). Excessive weight gain in successive pregnancies can lead to obesity.

If a woman's weight at conception exceeds her ideal weight by more than 20%, special problems can result. Statistically, she will have triple the medical and obstetrical complications of the woman whose weight at conception was ideal. Nutritional deficiency is common, since the pre-pregnancy excess weight typically consists of fat resulting from high-caloric but nutrient-light foods.

Weight gain evaluation during pregnancy is of significant importance. As we have seen, gain should be smooth and relatively predictable. Adequate nutrition does not lead to problems, but "adequate" should be defined in relation to dietary history, daily food intake, and blood and urine analyses. If gain is excessive, distinctions must be made between fat retention and water retention. Water accumulation is definitely more undesirable and dangerous than is fat storage.

Weight reduction prior to or after pregnancy is preferable to weight reduction during pregnancy. Contrary to popular belief, weight reduction during pregnancy does not make delivery easier and is, rather, dangerous for both mother and child. Starving or skipping meals can lead to **ketosis**, signaled by **acetonuria** (acetone in the urine). A starved person metabolizes body fat and protein. The process results in byproducts known as **ketone bodies.** Accumulated ketone bodies can cross the placenta and harm the fetus. A few studies have confirmed that these byproducts can result in mental retardation (Ritchey and Taper). The minimum recommended caloric intake during pregnancy is 1500 kcal per day—even when an obese expectant mother borders on toxemia—and vitamin/mineral supplements should be provided. The patient should be cautioned against the common practice of skipping meals prior to weigh-in at doctor appointments.

The converse problem of inadequate weight gain or existing underweight at conception presents risks similar to excessive weight gain. A slight increase in the risk of toxemia occurs, especially **preeclampsia** or **eclampsia** (convulsions and coma in a pregnant woman associated with

Table 16-1

Distribution of Weight Gain During Pregnancy

COMPONENT	APPROXIMATE WEIGHT (lb)
Fetus	7½ (5–10)
Placenta	1½
Amniotic fluid	2
Uterus	2
Mother's tissue fluid	3
Blood volume	4
Breasts*	½
Fat and other reserve†	3½
Total	24

*The increase is much bigger in some women and is considered as reserve.

†In some women, fat reserve may be as high as 8 lb.

TEENAGE MOTHERS
GET HELP AT ONE SPECIAL CLINIC

The medical center of the University of Alabama in Birmingham has a complications clinic for high risk pregnant women. Many of their clients are teenagers.

Peggy Davis, a nutrition consultant, described some of the nutrition-related problems she sees among the clinic's teenage patients.

"Many of the girls have low iron levels," she said. "Another problem I see is inadequate weight gain. Many girls are very figure-conscious. . . . They severely restrict their calorie intake so they won't gain weight . . . "

"When you're trying to talk to a teenager, it's very difficult for her to fully understand the importance of her diet," Davis said. "Many of these teenagers don't understand what's going on in their own bodies. They don't understand how they got pregnant. They don't understand where the baby is growing. I've had them talking about the baby growing in their stomach.

"And so I use a lot of pictures with them. I've got some picture books . . . that show the stages of pregnancy. . . and where the baby's growing in relation to the other parts of the body. You've really got to get down to basics with some of these kids."

A prenatal pamphlet she uses gives a breakdown of the weight expectant mothers should gain during pregnancy. "This is really important," Davis said. "The girls always think, 'If I gain 24 pounds, 7 of it's going to be the baby, and the rest is going to be me,'" "Once they understand where the weight really goes and how much the baby needs to be healthy," she said, "they are more likely to eat."

Timing Is Important

Davis said she might not give a girl a lot of nutrition information all at once, because many just aren't interested. "Many times it depends on their stage of pregnancy. If they're having a lot of nausea, that's not the time to talk to them about how they need to be eating. It's more important to talk to them about their specific problems and concerns," she said.

"I try to develop a rapport with them," she continued. If the girls don't follow her advice, she tries "not to be too judgmental."

"Usually when they get to the end of their second trimester or the beginning of their third, they're really coming around. Many of them are interested and want to take care of their babies.

"I think the most important thing in working with this age group is to show genuine concern," she said. "These kids are pretty sharp. They know when somebody's insincere. That's really the key to working with these girls—being compassionate."

Staff Offers Some Suggestions

Here are some suggestions the clinic staff made for those working with adolescent mothers:

Evaluate each teenager and see how mature her thinking process is. By age 15 or 16 teenagers may be beginning to think abstractly, but you have to be very specific and concrete with the younger girls.

Find out what they already know, and begin teaching from there. Don't make assumptions about what they know.

Use repetition and follow-up. Temper your remarks with understanding and concern.

Establish trust. . . .

Be authoritative without being authoritarian.

Teach them to reason for themselves and handle situations. Don't make them too dependent.

Foster peer relationships. . . .

Have a good balance of patients and staff, so there can be an informal group discussion rather than a lecture situation. But don't overwhelm them with staff.

Be aware of body language. Sit down and be eye level with the girls, rather than standing up.

*Adapted from L. Klein, *Food and Nutrition*, October 1980. pp. 9–13.

hypertension, edema, and other complications) if the weight gain is too small. Premature births and fragile infants are common. The risk of premature separation of the placenta increases. An overall increase in morbidity and mortality occurs for both mother and child.

The expectant mother builds her reserve at the expense of the fetus, and a woman underweight at conception and gaining insufficient weight during pregnancy experiences higher health risks. The proper weight gain for expectant mothers who have 95 percent or less of ideal weight at conception is calculated as the sum of normal weight gain during pregnancy, *plus* the mother's deficit at conception. In such underweight patients, the deficit generally occurred by choice, so aggressive nutritional counseling and behavioral modifications may prove necessary. The patient can be reassured that return to preconception weight can be hastened by breast-feeding. The general subject of *postpartum* weight loss generates significant debate among medical and nutritional experts. Table 16-2 presents the typical pattern as suggested by available data.

NUTRIENT NEEDS

Both pregnant and nursing women have heightened need for certain nutrients. You will find the RDAs for women at three physiological stages in Table 16-3. Of the various nutrients needed for pregnancy, seven deserve special attention (Hui; Ritchey and Taper; Rush et al.).

Table 16-2
Residual Weight Gain after Delivery

TIME POSTPARTUM	RESIDUAL WEIGHT GAIN (lb) OVER PREPREGNANT WEIGHT
Immediately after birth	8–9
6 weeks	4–5
6–8 months	0

Note: These data are statistical observations. The tendency to return to prepregnant weight varies with the particular individual.

Table 16-3
1980 RDAs for a 25-year-old Woman at Three Physiological Stages

NUTRIENT	DAILY AMOUNT NEEDED	ADDITIONAL DAILY AMOUNT NEEDED	
		PREGNANCY	LACTATION
Energy (kcal)	2,000	300	500
Protein (g)	44	30	20
Vitamin A (µg)	800	200	400
Vitamin D (IU)	200	200	200
Vitamin E (mg)	8	2	3
Vitamin C (mg)	60	20	40
Vitamin B_1 (mg)	1.0	0.4	0.5
Vitamin B_2 (mg)	1.2	0.3	0.5
Niacin (mg)	13	2	5
Vitamin B_6 (mg)	2.0	0.6	0.5
Folic acid (µg)	400	400	100
Vitamin B_{12} (µg)	3.0	1	1
Calcium (mg)	800	400	400
Phosphorus (mg)	800	400	400
Magnesium (mg)	300	150	150
Iron (mg)	18	>18*	>*
Zinc (mg)	15	5	10
Iodine (mg)	150	25	50

*The excess need cannot be supplied by a regular diet. Supplementation is needed.

Protein

Protein requirements increase by about 30 g daily during pregnancy. The expectant mother retains nitrogen at almost twice the rate of prepregnancy retention, and she deposits about 10 g of protein daily in placental and fetal tissues, and her own. During gestation, the protein gain will be 2.2 lb, half of which deposits in the fetus.

Satisfactory pregnancy profile correlates with adequacy of protein intake. Many studies have confirmed that infants of adequate to high protein intake during gestation are taller than those born to mothers with restricted protein intake. Similarly, clinical risks increase as protein consumption decreases. The smaller babies resulting from low protein intake have higher morbidity and mortality. Deficient protein intake has produced brain damage in animals that cannot be reversed through adequate feeding later in life, and some researchers suspect parallel effects in humans. Protein intake also influences the child's disease resistance; antibodies that are synthesized from protein in the mother's body in response to exposure to a particular antigen pass through the placenta, and the child receives passive immunity.

Calories

A pregnant woman needs an additional 300 kcal per day. If she consumes less than 1800 kcal per day, the nitrogen balance will be negative and will oblige the fetus to grow at the expense of maternal tissues. Low caloric intake results in low birth weight. Some studies show that supplementation can reverse the trend.

The total caloric need during gestation depends on energy expended by the mother. The entire gestation process requires approximately 80,000 kcal for growth of fetus, placenta, and the mother's organs, as well as for the mother's increased work and increased basal metabolic rate. Some pregnant women reduce their physical activity significantly, as much as 50,000 kcal during the nine-month period. Their additional kcal need would then be about 30,000. Conversely, a woman working full time until just prior to delivery might require more than 50,000 additional kcal.

Iron

The pregnant woman's need for iron increases 1 mg per day beyond the 18 mg RDA. The iron increase is necessary because of bleeding (spotting and delivery loss), transportation of greater nutrient load, and greater oxygen demands related to tissue increase. During the second to eighth month, the expectant mother's blood volume increases 20 to 30 percent.

The lack of menstruation somewhat offsets greater iron need, but absorption triples the prepregnancy level. During the second half of pregnancy, iron need becomes greater, since the placenta begins iron transfer to the fetus at that time.

Iron deficiency has numerous causes. Failure to replenish after repeated pregnancies and low-flesh diets are typical causes of iron deficiency existing prior to pregnancy. Anemia is common among women whose diet includes less than 10 percent of caloric intake from animal products. Since very few women have bone marrow storage of iron, the best recommendation is consuming an adequate amount of iron prior to pregnancy. Those eating 25 percent or more of their calories from animal sources realize low iron-deficiency risk.

High iron intake alone does not ensure freedom from iron deficiency, since absorption serves as the final measure of iron intake efficiency. Iron is less effectively absorbed from cereals than animal tissues. Additionally, oxalic acid or phytic acid in some cereals decreases iron absorption (see Chapter 12).

Unusual eating habits, especially the consumption of nonfood items, decreases iron absorption. *Pica*, the practice of eating nonfood items, is usually thought of in regard to children eating such items as dirt and paper. However, pica can result from iron deficiency, and pregnant women may crave ice, cornstarch, ashes, and clay. Moreover, low socioeconomic status women in the southern United States are known to practice pica as a regional habit. For those practicing pica out of iron deficiency craving, the materials eaten do not fulfill the nutrient need. Iron supplementation quickly and effectively reduces the practice of pica. However, at the present time, the exact cause of pica among most other patients has not been identified.

Both mother and newborn child may become anemic as a result of iron deficiency. Teenage mothers often have low blood hemoglobin, less than 10 g per 100 mL blood. If the mother is iron deficient, the baby will have little iron stored. Since milk is relatively low in iron, for the first three months after birth the child will actually be dependent on iron accumulated during gestation.

Iron deficiency anemia is the most common form of anemia during pregnancy and the period after birth, occurring in 15 to 20 percent of pregnant women. Anemia during pregnancy can be microcytic (from lack of iron) or macrocytic (from lack of folic acid). The two forms potentiate each other, so supplementing both is recommended. Unchecked, iron or folic acid deficiency can threaten life of mother and child alike.

Table 16-4 gives the level of iron supplementation recommended by some practitioners. Supplementation should begin not later than the second trimester and should continue until the end of lactation, or one month after delivery if the mother is not nursing. Supplementation commonly occurs through tablets (150 to 300 mg ferrous sulfate) but

Table 16-4
Some Guidelines for Iron Supplementation During Pregnancy

PERCENT OF DIETARY CALORIES FROM ANIMAL SOURCES	BODY IRON STATUS AT BEGINNING OF PREGNANCY	DAILY IRON SUPPLEMENT (mg)
30	Good	30
25	Below average	60
10	Deficiency prevalent, anemia	120–240

can be by injection if depletion is severe or if taking tablets is impractical for some reason.

Calcium

Adequate calcium levels during pregnancy can be maintained without supplementation. If adequate intake of vitamin D and calcium occurs, blood calcium will be at an appropriate level even during the last months of pregnancy when the absorption rate doubles and the excretion rate decreases. Low intake of vitamin D must be balanced by increased calcium intake. If emotional stress exists during pregnancy, as is common in teenage pregnancy, calcium absorption may decrease in spite of the increase resulting from pregnancy.

The deposition of calcium during pregnancy increases daily. Two thirds of the calcium in the infant's body is deposited in the last three months of gestation. Calcium deficiency at birth results in rickets and may permanently damage both deciduous and permanent teeth. During pregnancy the fetus draws on the mother's bones if her blood calcium is low.

Since jaws and teeth undergo formation during the last months of pregnancy and the first year of infancy, calcium and phosphorus are important to that time period. Malformed jaws and teeth, teeth more susceptible to decay, and crowded, unsymmetrical teeth all result from calcium shortage. These conditions frequently occur in underdeveloped countries.

Calcium deficiency may cause restlessness, twitching, insomnia, walking difficulty, thigh and back pain, and excess movement of the fetus. Leg cramps during pregnancy can result from low calcium intake or high phosphorus (eggs, milk, and meat) intake; calcium supplementation can be beneficial to leg cramps in such cases. If calcium supplementation is necessary for any reason, 0.5 to 1 g daily is recommended. Some clinicians suspect calcium deficiency predisposes the woman to uterine inertia during labor. They theorize that such difficult deliveries result from the weak uterus failing to mold the fetal head to the pelvic rim. No direct evidence supports this theory, although it has been established that if a woman has rickets as a child she is likely to have an unsatisfactory pelvis. Additional causes of unsatisfactory pelvis include combined gross calcium and vitamin D deficiency, and repeated pregnancy and long-term lactation with failure to replenish nutrients.

Sodium

Sodium intake during pregnancy has been a long-standing concern in relation to fluid retention. Many clinicians recommend decreased salt intake to avoid **edema**; however, recent animal studies have shown that reduced salt intake during gestation can adversely affect mother and child. Contemporary advice discourages indiscriminate restriction of salt intake.

Diuretics have been used to reduce body fluid, but some pose a hazard to both mother and child (see Chapter 24). Only a small number of diuretics are currently recommended for use during pregnancy, and then only when absolutely necessary. Diuretics used in combination with salt restriction must be carefully monitored.

Iodine

Partly owing to enhanced excretion, iodine need increases during pregnancy. Iodine deficiency in the mother, more common in teenage mothers, will result in infant iodine deficiency, as is the case with goiter in a mother. Salt restriction leads to reduced iodine consumption. High iodine intake during pregnancy can occur through excessive use of cough medicine, sea salt, and nutrient supplements and can cause the mother's thyroid to enlarge and pose a risk to the fetus as well.

Folic Acid

Although a detailed discussion of vitamin nutrition during pregnancy is not possible here, folic acid deserves special attention. (Chapters 9 and 10 should be consulted regarding vitamin nutriture during pregnancy.)

As we saw earlier in this chapter, folic acid and iron deficiencies lead to anemia. Folic acid deficiency results in **megaloblastic anemia** (also known as macrocytic anemia), characterized by lethargy, depression, nausea, and progressive appetite loss. Vomiting, diarrhea, **glossitis,** and gingivitis can be encountered too, as can pallor. Macrocytic anemia resulting from folic acid deficiency occurs in 2 to 3 percent of American pregnant women, is twice that common in England, and twenty times that in India.

Deficiency in folic acid is suspected as a cause of small placenta, premature labor, low birth weight, **abruptio placentae,** and hemorrhage. Less well documented is its role in fetal wastage or adsorption, miscarriage, and birth defects. The deficiency can occur in late pregnancy, the postpartum period, and lactation, and occurs most frequently in conjunction with iron deficiency. Also susceptible to folic acid deficiency anemia are women who have had several children (*multiparas*), women over 30, those with multiple and twin pregnancies, and those who fail to take recommended vitamin supplements. Women who do not eat animal products or adequate calories are at risk. There is speculation that women suffering megaloblastic anemia are anorexic, resulting in further decreased folic acid intake. Periodically consuming foods rich in folic acid should reverse the anorexia associated with the deficiency.

Many physicians who attend pregnant women routinely prescribe folic acid supplement. The supplementation starts during the second trimester and continues through lactation. Daily supplement is usually 5 to 10 mg. If the anemia fails to respond, parenteral (intravenous) vitamin administration may be needed. Simultaneous iron supplementation can enhance folic acid absorption. In cases of severe dietary limitation, protein supplementation can strengthen the effectiveness of folic acid supplement.

Megaloblastic anemia during pregnancy usually is not severe unless the expectant mother also has toxemia or systemic infection. If there is no improvement with folic acid treatment, blood transfusion may be necessary.

DIET

An expectant mother requires a well-balanced and nutritious diet that is best evaluated by comparing the recommended daily servings from the four food groups for prepregnancy, pregnancy, and lactation (see Table 16-5). Tables 16-6 and 16-7 present a sample meal plan and sample menu, respectively. Table 16-6 includes foods from the basic food guides. Table 16-7 includes both protective and supplemental foods.

The RDAs for a pregnant woman (see Table 16-3) show that caloric need and nutrient need increase over the prepregnant diet. Most women have difficulty fulfilling these nutritional demands over the period of gestation owing to the stresses of pregnancy. The use of nutrient supplements may prove necessary. The U.S. Food and Drug Administration has issued regulations governing such dietary products; for example, stated maximums for vitamins contained in commercial supplements. The intakes of five minerals and ten vitamins may be 50 to 150 percent higher than normal for pregnant women, owing to their increased nutrient need. Clinically, most frequently supplemented are iron, folic acid, and calcium. Vitamin B_{12} is also recommended for women who have been vegetarians. To reduce side effects, supplements should be taken in the food.

Nutrient supplementation should not be indiscriminate. Excessive intake of vitamins A and D can, for example, be harmful to both mother and child. Additionally, many commercial supplements may be high in the wrong nutrients and low in the ones most needed. The mother's excessive consumption of vitamin C can, for example, create an excessive vitamin need in the infant. For these reasons, supplementation should be under the direction of an expert.

CLINICAL PROBLEMS

Pregnant women may encounter several minor clinical problems in relation to food and nutrition. The examples addressed in the following section will provide you with an understanding of those most frequently experienced (Hui).

Table 16-5
Protective Foods for Women

PROTECTIVE FOOD*	RECOMMENDED NUMBER OF DAILY SERVINGS		
	NONPREGNANT, NONLACTATING	PREGNANT	LACTATING
Milk and milk products	3	4	5
Protein products	3	4	4
Grain products	3	3	3
Vegetables and fruits			
Rich in vitamin C	1	1	1
Green leafy vegetables	2	2	2
Others	1	1	1

*The grouping follows the basic four food groups (also see Chapter 15).

Table 16-6
Sample Meal Plan for Pregnant and Lactating Women

BREAKFAST	SNACK*	LUNCH	SNACK*	DINNER
Milk or milk products, 1 serving	Milk or milk products, ½ serving	Milk or milk products, 1 serving	Milk or milk products, ½ serving	Milk or milk products, 1 serving
Fruits or vegetables rich in vitamin C, 1 serving	Protein products 1 serving	Other fruits and vegetables, 1 serving		Green leafy vegetables, 2 servings
Grain products		Protein products, 1 serving		Protein products 2 servings
		Grain products, 2 servings		

*The snacks may be consumed at any time of the day.

Abnormal Appetite and Cravings

During the first three to four months of pregnancy, both appetite and thirst increase, though morning sickness may moderate this. Some pregnant women will consume large quantities of food during the early months of pregnancy. Experience has shown that frequent small meals are preferable in that they reduce nausea and vomiting and avoid the discomfort of stomach distention. Though the ravenous appetite must be satisfied with foods, extremes should be avoided, especially extremes in quantity at single sittings and extremes of any one food.

Cravings have not yet been understood, nor have the food dislikes that may occur during pregnancy. Although these preferences should be respected, pica, as we discussed earlier in this chapter, should be resisted.

Table 16-7
Sample Menu for Pregnant and Lactating Women Including Protective (Basic) and Supplemental Foods

BREAKFAST	SNACK	LUNCH	SNACK	DINNER
Orange juice, 4 oz	Salted peanuts, ½ c	Sandwich—whole wheat bread, 2 slices, tuna fish, ½ c, diced celery with onion, mayonnaise, lettuce	Oatmeal raisin cookies, 2	Roast beef, 6 oz
Oatmeal, ½ c	Milk, 4 oz		Milk, 4 oz	Egg noodles, ½ c with sauteed poppy seeds
Brown sugar, 1–2 t		Banana, 1 small		Cut asparagus, ¾ c
Milk, 8 oz		Milk, 8 oz		Salad—torn spinach, 1 c, sliced mushrooms, radishes, oil, vinegar
Coffee or tea		Coffee or tea		Milk, 8 oz
				Coffee or tea

Morning Sickness

The nausea and vomiting experienced by some pregnant women, especially after rising in the morning, may range from mild to severe. Severe symptoms usually accompany toxemia. These severe cases are known as pernicious vomiting of pregnancy, or *hyperemesis gravidarum*.

Morning sickness symptoms generally appear after the first missed menstrual period (week 5 or 6 of gestation) and terminate after the fourth or fifth month. Rarely will clinical effects of this condition be severe, despite the condition being common to 75 percent of pregnant women, most of them in second or later pregnancies.

The cause or causes of morning sickness remain unknown. Some clinicians and psychiatrists have postulated poor psychological adaptation to motherhood, emotional conflicts, resentment, or ambivalence. Certain clinical disorders such as hernia, ulcers, hepatitis, and gallbladder inflammation can cause nausea and vomiting during pregnancy. Vomiting is known to be more frequent in pregnancies with complications; for example, multiple births.

Experienced clinicians recommend various methods to reduce morning sickness symptoms. Initially, pregnant women should be assured that mild symptoms are common. Dry foods at frequent intervals are beneficial. Food aversions should be respected. Fats, odorous foods, and spice dishes should be restricted. Drinking distilled water and eating dry crackers in bed before rising have proved effective. Vitamin B_6 (50 mg per day) has been effective, as have sedatives and antiemetics. Use of drugs should be under prescription.

Persistent and severe vomiting during pregnancy—hyperemesis gravidarum—can be fatal if not controlled. Although the cause or causes of this clinical disorder remain unknown, it results in hospitalization in 2 of every 1000 pregnancies. The partial starvation resulting from the condition can lead to dehydration, **acidosis** or **ketosis**, weight loss, and nutrient deficiencies. Additional complications include toxic hepatitis (jaundice), eye damage, and hemorrhage.

Given the potential threat of hyperemesis gravidarum, medical treatment is stringent. Patients are hospitalized in private rooms, confined to their beds, and permitted no bathroom privileges. Visitors are not permitted until vomiting ceases. If the condition is not stabilized in two days, intravenous vitamin and protein supplementation begins, followed by tube feeding of a balanced diet via slow drip. Persistent symptoms can lead to therapeutic abortion.

Faintness

Especially during early pregnancy, temporary and sudden loss of consciousness may occur in response to an inadequate supply of blood to the brain. Causes for this vary. Postural hypotension, that is, low blood pressure related to sitting or standing can cut off oxygen to the brain. For example, if a woman sits or stands in a warm room for a long time, blood pools in the legs and pelvic area. Hypoglycemia before or between meals, common during pregnancy, can also cause faintness.

To reduce the risk of faintness, deep breathing should be practiced, and the pregnant woman should be more mobile than usual. Legs should be moved vigorously, but positions should be changed slowly. Small, frequent meals (five to seven per day) will reduce hypoglycemia, as will candy bars or oranges. Stimulants such as coffee, tea, and spirits of ammonia will reduce fainting due to hypotension.

Urinary Symptoms

Late pregnancy often produces frequent and urgent urination and so-called *stress incontinence* (release of urine when coughing or laughing, for example). These conditions result from fetal pressure on the bladder. Painful or bloody urination indicates urinary tract infection and should be clinically investigated. Bladder sedatives are available. If urinary urgency interferes with lifestyle, the expectant mother should avoid tea, coffee, spices, and alcoholic beverages.

Heartburn

Heartburn results from the regurgitation of stomach contents along the gastroesophageal tract. Stomach secretion and motility simultaneously decrease. Heartburn, also known as pyrosis or "acid indigestion," increases in late pregnancy. Upward protrusion of the uterine fundus can displace the stomach. A condition known as diaphragmatic hiatus hernia during late pregnancy causes 15 percent of expectant mothers to experience severe heartburn, leading to nausea and vomiting. The "tenting" of the diaphragm and "flaring" of the ribs return to normal after delivery.

Heartburn treatment can include drugs and acidifying agents. Drugs stimulate intestinal motility and secretion. An appropriate acidifying agent can neutralize whatever stomach contents that cause the heartburn. However, antacids should be avoided in early pregnancy, since the stomach acid level is already low at that time. Hydrochloric acid solutions should be avoided as they harm the teeth. Some pregnant women have found hard candy and hot tea beneficial, and positional adjustments can also relieve heartburn symptoms. During late pregnancy, aluminum hydroxide can reduce stomach irritation.

Muscle Cramps

Between the fourth and ninth months of gestation, women may experience cramping in buttocks, thighs, and calves. For some unknown reason, cramping decreases in the final month. Cramping generally occurs after lying down or sleeping and often accompanies toe pointing, which causes a sudden shortening of muscles.

High phosphorus or low calcium blood levels, or both, are suspected causes of cramping. Tiredness and slow blood circulation also contribute to cramping.

Relief of cramping can be achieved by standing barefoot on a cold floor, such as tile or linoleum, and rubbing the cramping area. Warm or hot compresses on the cramp area will also provide relief. During early pregnancy, calcium intake (drinking milk, for example) and phosphorus reduction (eating less meat, cheese, and potatoes) can minimize cramping. Medicines with excessive phosphorus should be avoided. Aluminum hydroxide can reduce blood phosphorus levels. Avoiding walking on the balls of the feet proves most helpful (in high heels, for instance), since that walking style points the toes forward, shortening muscles and precipitating cramping.

Milk and Egg Allergies

Milk and egg allergies present special nutritional challenges for the expectant mother, since the mother's allergies prohibit the consumption of foods that would otherwise benefit the unborn child. Such allergies can produce severe reactions, including abdominal pain and cramping, vomiting, diarrhea, and asthmalike symptoms.

Although carefully planned diet programs can often lead to desensitization, there may not be enough time to desensitize the mother. In these allergy cases, protein deficiency and attendant problems such as fatigue require especially careful meal planning and vitamin supplementation.

Mild Edema

About two out of three women in late pregnancy experience swelling of the lower extremities, such as the ankles. This mild edema results from sodium and water retention and is unrelated to toxemia. The retention can be brought about by one or more of the following: (1) venous congestion due to varicose veins, (2) steroid hormone increase in the blood (emanating from adrenal glands, ovaries, and placenta), (3) venous pressure increase in the legs, (4) sitting or standing too long, or (5) use of elastic garters or other too-tight clothing.

There is no sure treatment for edema. Common measures of prevention include sleeping with legs and feet elevated, avoiding tight clothing, and providing elastic support to varicose veins. Although salt restriction is a popular procedure, salt may be used with caution.

Constipation

Many expectant mothers are constantly plagued by constipation. Bowel sluggishness and resultant constipation during pregnancy come from reduced motility of intestinal smooth muscle, which in turn may result from excessive sex steroid hormones. The enlarging uterus also pressures and displaces parts of the intestine. Constipation may also cause hemorrhoids or worsen diverticular disorders.

General methods of treatment include a large intake of roughage and fluid and a consistent exercise program. Clinical therapy includes the use of laxatives. Strong laxatives must be used with caution, as they may induce labor. Medications such as mineral oil must be used sparingly because they can prevent the absorption of fat-soluble vitamins.

Abdominal Pain

Two categories of abdominal pain are experienced by expectant mothers. The first results from increased pressure. A sagging or dragging feeling and pelvic heaviness is experienced, resulting from the heavy uterus pressing on the abdominal wall. A heat compress, maternity girdle, and frequent rest periods of sitting or lying down will relieve the pain.

The second category of abdominal pain results from gas, bloating, or bowel cramping. As the swelling uterus compresses and displaces the bowel, the intestine loses tension and strength, resulting in the constipation previously discussed. Large meals, greasy foods, excess roughage, and cold beverages can also produce the reaction, so these should be avoided if discomfort occurs. Frequent small meals effectively reduce the abdominal pains, and changes in body position are also beneficial.

Tooth and Gum Problems

The incidence of dental decay is greater in pregnant than nonpregnant women. Reduced oral hygiene and increased sugar intake may be primary contributory factors. Gum infection may additionally be caused by hormonal imbalance. Some 50 to 70 percent of expectant mothers experience bleeding of the gums, and some develop swellings of the gums so severe that they are termed tumors.

The tendency for the gums to bleed at the slightest touch is due to the high vascularity of underlying connective tisue. All gingival changes are most marked in the second and third trimesters and return to normal within two months after delivery. Chapter 23 provides a thorough discussion of nutrition and oral health.

FETAL ALCOHOL SYNDROME

Fetal alcohol syndrome (FAS), a nutrition-related birth defect receiving increased attention, results if a mother consumes excessive alcohol during pregnancy (Hanson). Characteristic FAS defects include abnormal facial features, mental deficiency, malformed joints, low birth weight and shortened birth length, and reduced head size. All such defects are irreversible as the child matures.

Fetal alcohol syndrome remains a nutritional concern requiring further research, since the disorder was not recognized until the early 1970s. The precise relationship between quantity of alcohol consumed and extent of resulting birth defects has not yet been determined, but the correlation between alcohol and FAS has been confirmed. Animal studies have, for example, demonstrated that changes in alcohol dosage produce corresponding changes in defect severity. Scientific investigations have also shown that alcohol in the female's blood is critical to FAS but that alcohol in the male's blood is inconsequential.

Case histories have frequently involved mothers suffering from chronic alcoholism. In such cases the mother may consume an average of six beers and one bottle of wine per day during her pregnancy. Because of the alcohol dependency, one half of daily caloric intake may be from alcoholic beverages. In such cases, one third of the mothers produced children with readily identifiable FAS abnormalities.

Studies of FAS have further shown that mental impairment may not become obvious until the child's later life. Studies with rats and mice confirm the later-life effect of FAS. Based on such studies, estimates place the level of incidence in the United States at 12,000 births per year. If these estimates are accurate, FAS may be the largest single cause of birth defects.

The concern an expectant mother has for her unborn child leads to the question, "What is a safe level of alcohol consumption?" Although all aspects of nutrition vary according to individual metabolic differences, an unborn child is highly prone to alcohol injury. The safest level of alcohol consumption for the expectant mother is alcohol avoidance from conception to birth.

The case of Mary, a housewife, illustrates the risks of alcohol consumption to the unborn child. She and her husband waited until their early thirties to have their first child. Partly to celebrate the event and partly from lifestyle, she and her husband would have one or two mixed drinks before dinner, wine with dinner, and one or two after-dinner liqueurs, an average of four to five drinks each day.

Their child was born undersized, with head circumference even smaller than would be normal for the reduced size. The child's eyes were set quite close together and had folds in their inner corners characteristic of the mongoloid race. The nose had virtually no bridge at the juncture with the forehead, and the lips were misshapen. As the child grew, mental impairment became increasingly obvious, and the child remained too thin despite attempts to increase body weight. Mary's child was a certain victim of fetal alcohol syndrome.

Figure 16-2 provides a clinical example of FAS.

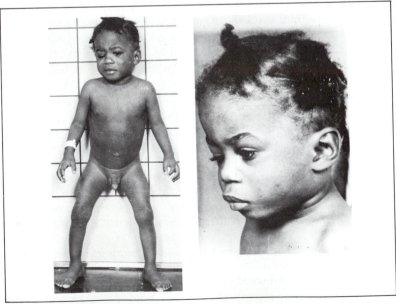

Figure 16-2: Fetal alcohol syndrome. This child is 23 months old and weighs 18 pounds. His forehead is flat and bald, and he has a drooping right eyelid and a high-pitched cry. His mother had been an alcoholic for 10 years.
SOURCE: J. J. Mulvihill, et al. "Fetal Alcohol Syndrome: Seven New Cases." Am. J. Obs. Gyn. 125 (1976): 937.

Nutrition in Lactation

BREAST-FEEDING

Observers of nutritional trends in the United States have noted that breast-feeding is on the increase. Expectant mothers face a decision about breast-feeding versus using formulas. Chapter 17 addresses infant nutrition, and this section provides you with information for those who choose to breast-feed and with information on the nutrient needs inherent in that decision.

The decision to breast-feed is best made at midpregnancy to allow sufficient time for nutritional choices that will benefit the decision. Numerous factors influence the production and secretion of breast milk. Primary among those factors is a nutritious and balanced diet, one high in caloric intake, coupled with adequate fluid intake. Additionally, the mother needs: (1) a strong desire to breast-feed, (2) support and encouragement from family and friends, (3) a satisfactory nutritional status, and (4) some knowledge of the breast-feeding process, including "letdown" and suckling.

A woman may make more milk if her breasts are large. If she has little breast tissue, often a result of severe malnutrition as a child, she may produce very little milk. A healthy mother will produce more milk if nursing is frequent. Interspersal of formula supplements will decrease milk production because suckling occurs less often when formula is used. More milk results when breast skin temperature is high. Contrary to popular belief, no evidence supports the influence of substances such as beer or garlic on milk production.

NUTRIENT NEEDS

The optimal nutrient need for a nursing mother remains elusive. We do not know the rate and volume of milk production and their variation in nutritional composition of milk formed at different times in the lactation period (**colostrum**, transitional, and mature milk). Some nutrient levels remain consistent in breast milk; others fluctuate in relation to the woman's physiological condition, the time of day, and the length of time since delivery. We do know that all essential nutrients are required for proper storage, repair, and maintenance of the woman's body and for the production of milk that is nutritionally sound.

Underdeveloped countries have been the subject of studies confirming that good-quality milk can be produced for periods of three to four years if nursing is permitted to continue. Such milk must be assumed to be produced at the expense of the mother's nutrient reserve, since these women have inadequate diets. Milk nutrients such as vitamins, protein, calories, and minerals can be obtained from the mother's storage.

As was indicated in Table 16-3, RDA values enable determination of a nursing mother's nutrient needs. Although similar to those of a pregnant woman, nutrient needs are somewhat higher because the child's demand increases daily with growth. The mother needs protein, vitamins, minerals, and especially calories to ensure nutritionally sound breast milk and to rebuild her own storage. The mother's needs are influenced by variables including her nutritional status; her body size; the rate, volume, and efficiency of milk production; and infant demand.

For the first two weeks following delivery, the mother is recovering and tires easily yet must provide for the nursing child through frequent feedings. Under this stress, nutrient storage preceding and during pregnancy is called upon for the proper production of milk. In the remainder of this chapter we will discuss the nursing mother's needs for calories, fat, iron, calcium and phosphorus, and vitamins.

Calories

An infant needs about 850 mL of milk per day, and the mother expends about 90 to 100 kcal for each 100 mL of milk produced. The mother's energy expenditure goes into the milk, the nursing process, and milk secretion. The mother's daily calorie cost will be 760 to 850 kcal, with 600 to 700 kcal actually contained in the milk. The mother's fat reserve following childbirth can provide 200 to 400 kcal, leaving a daily intake need of about 500 kcal to fuel the nursing process.

Approximately two to three months following childbirth, the nursing mother returns to her prepregnancy weight, though she can eat 500 to 1000 kcal more in foods. Experience has convinced many women that nursing helps them lose weight, regain their appetite, and retain a trim figure, even after several pregnancies.

Fat

The RDAs established in 1980 do not specify the fat intake needed during nursing. Though the fat level of the milk does not reflect the mother's intake, the nature of the fat does. For example, a large intake of polyunsaturated fats will result in a higher proportion of these fats in the breast milk. About 6 to 9 percent of the caloric contribution of breast milk is from linoleic acid. Breast-milk fatty acids are primarily of medium-chain length, though small amounts of 10-carbon ones can occur (see Chapter 6).

Iron

Iron need undergoes changes during nursing. During the first three to four months of nursing, iron supplementation plus an adequate diet enables replenishment of the mother's depleted storage. After these first months and until menstruation returns, a nursing woman's diet should provide sufficient iron nutrition without the need for supplementation.

As discussed in Chapter 12, a menstruating woman can experience difficulty in receiving sufficient iron, even with a satisfactory diet. Physiologically, a nursing mother is not expected to menstruate; however, some nursing mothers do have menstrual periods.

Within limits, the iron content of breast milk is not affected by the woman's intake. For the first three months following birth from a healthy mother, the infant's iron storage is sufficient in combination with breast milk to provide adequate iron.

Calcium and Phosphorus

Calcium need increases for the nursing mother, partly for milk production and partly for body storage. Although calcium level in breast milk is not directly related to the woman's calcium intake, the secretion of calcium in the milk continuously draws upon the woman's calcium reserve. Negative calcium balance will occur if the drain is not compensated for by increased intake or supplementation. For months after the cessation of breast-feeding, continuous reduction of calcium absorption occurs, further boosting the calcium need. An imbalanced phosphorus intake also occurs. Dietary intake of calcium and phosphorus must be carefully evaluated to prevent a negative body balance of both elements.

Vitamins

The RDAs for vitamins (see Table 16-3) show the nursing woman's needs are 150 percent greater than the nonpregnant woman's. Within limits, the breast-milk levels of vitamins C, B_1, B_2, B_6, and B_{12} reflect the mother's dietary intake. The folic acid nutriture requires careful monitoring. Chapter 17 provides composition of breast milk and cow's milk.

DIET

What should a nursing mother eat? We have seen that an adequate diet must be balanced and that supplementation is necessary in certain situations and for certain time periods. Table 16-5 presents recommended amounts of protective foods for the lactating woman. Table 16-6 gives a sample meal plan, and Table 16-7, a sample menu. If a new mother follows these dietary regimens, she and her nursing child will receive adequate nutrients.

STUDY QUESTIONS

1. What nutritional deficiencies are common among women entering pregnancy? What health risks are greater among malnourished pregnant women than among well-nourished pregnant women?

2. Describe the currently recommended pattern and extent of weight gain during pregnancy. Why is a fat reserve important?

3. When is weight loss in an overweight woman preferable: before, during, or after pregnancy? Why?

4. What are the risks of being underweight when entering pregnancy? What advice should such women be given?

5. What nutrient needs are increased during pregnancy? What can be said about the intakes of calcium, sodium, iodine, and vitamins A, D, C, and K during pregnancy?

6. What general dietary advice should be given to a pregnant woman? Plan 1 week's menu for a 25-year-old pregnant woman.

7. Name at least six minor health problems in a pregnant woman that may be related to nutrition. What dietary or related advice may be helpful in each case?

8. How does the recommended diet for a nursing mother differ from that for a pregnant woman?

REFERENCES

Hanson, J. W. "Alcohol Use in Pregnancy: Implications for Fetal Welfare." In *Alternative Dietary Practices and Nutritional Abuses in Pregnancy.* Proceedings of a workshop. Washington, D.C.: National Academy Press, 1982.

Hui, Y. H. *Human Nutrition and Diet Therapy.* Monterey, Calif.: Wadsworth Health Sciences, 1983.

Ritchey, S., and L. J. Taper. *Maternal and Child Nutrition.* New York: Harper & Row, 1982.

Rush, D., et al. *Diet in Pregnancy.* New York: Alan R. Liss, 1980.

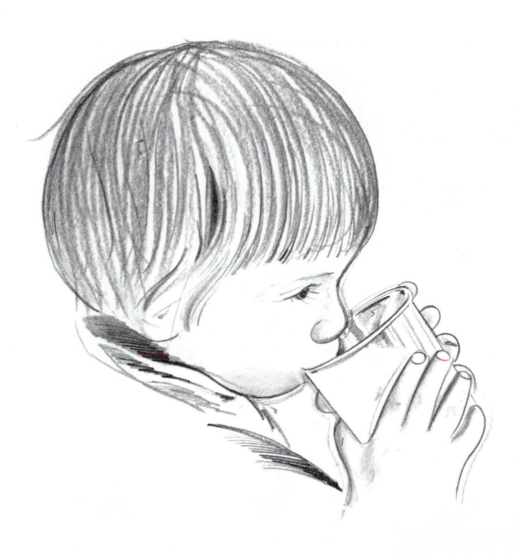

17

NUTRITION FOR INFANTS, CHILDREN, AND ADOLESCENTS

Raw goat's milk for an infant?

Seven-month-old Jerry was admitted to the hospital as a result of fever, vomiting, and sore mouth and tongue. The child was irritable, dehydrated, and had an elevated temperature. He had been consuming 30 to 35 ounces per day of raw goat's milk for the last five months.

Laboratory tests showed severe folic acid deficiency, but the fever persisted even after vitamin administration, and a body rash developed. Further tests were conducted, and *toxoplasmosis* was found. Toxoplasmosis is the disorder resulting from infection by the organism *Toxoplasma gondii*, a protozoan.

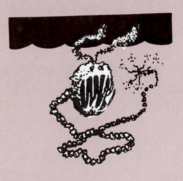

An examination of milk from the various goats composing the source of milk for the infant showed that the organism was present. Other potential sources of the infection (cats, flies, cockroaches, blood transfusion, congenital infection) did not prove likely, so it was concluded that the unpasteurized goat's milk was the source of the infection.

Despite the growing trend to rely on "natural foods," the use of unpasteurized milk represents a clear danger. The use of pasteurized milk diminishes the chance of contracting such diseases as toxoplasmosis.

This case history illustrates two basic principles (Riemann et al.). Certain forms of milk are nutritionally inadequate for a newborn infant; milk for infants must be sterilized in some way to prevent food poisoning.

Parents and health professionals are understandably concerned about the diets of infants, children, and adolescents. The need for nutrients is high during the growing years, and deficiencies at that time can create health problems that persist in later life. In infancy, questions of breast- versus bottle-feeding and the introduction of solid foods are important concerns. During childhood, feeding problems, snacking, obesity, food allergies, and nutrient deficiencies are the major issues. Similar problems, aggravated by emotional stress and peer pressure, continue through the adolescent years. Throughout this period, sound nutritional education is crucial for both parents and children to help them make wise food choices.

Nutrition and Infants

All newborns need an adequate amount of essential nutrients for the proper development of body organs, cells, and tissues. One major index of health for a newborn infant is its growth rate. Table 17-1 shows the weight gain from birth to age 1. Standard growth charts for infants at different ages are given in the Appendix.

Of particular concern to health workers, nutritionists, and parents is the normal development of the child's brain in structure, size, and function. Animal experiments have confirmed that a newborn's brain development can be adversely affected by undernourishment. However, in humans, whether the effect of malnutrition during infancy on mental development and learning potential is permanent has not yet been established.

As discussed in Chapter 16, the nutritional status of a newborn is partly determined by the health of the mother and her nutrition during pregnancy. But it has been shown that if a child is born with nutritional problems because the mother is malnourished, there is a good chance of complete recovery if the child receives adequate nutritional care thereafter. This assumes, of course, that the nutritional lack experienced by the infant has not been extreme. High-risk newborns can have a multitude of nutritional problems that may or may not be correctable. For information on this last clinical topic, use the references at the end of this chapter.

PROS AND CONS OF BREAST-FEEDING

Ever since World War II, the debate over the pros and cons of the two major types of infant feeding, breast and bottle, has preoccupied the public and scientists. It is still one of the most emotional and controversial issues in nutrition. The following sections discuss the advantages, disadvantages, and techniques of breast-feeding.

Nutritional Benefits

A number of nutritional benefits are associated with breast-feeding. First, the higher level of lactose in breast milk creates a better intestinal environment, and the mild fermentation allows a better bowel movement. The child becomes hungry and eats more frequently. Sometimes lactose can complex with calcium and permit more of the mineral to be absorbed. This improves bone development in the child and serves as a major benefit of breast milk for many years. Recently, synthetic lactose can be added to commercial formulas due to technological advances. Furthermore, lactose can increase the absorption of amino acids and magnesium, and it is the major contributor of galactose for the formation of myelin, a substance that coats certain nerve fibers.

Second, breast milk contains a protein-splitting enzyme that is relatively intact, whereas the enzyme in formula milk has been destroyed by pasteurization. This enzyme permits better protein digestion in a breast-fed infant. Third, the high level of polyunsaturated fatty acids in breast milk encourages easy digestion and utilization of fat by the infant. Fourth, breast milk tends to contain more vitamin C and B_1, since they are partially destroyed in cow's milk by pasteurization (however, most currently available commercial brands of formula milk are fortified with these nutrients). Finally, observations in many developing countries have confirmed that even a malnourished woman secretes milk of acceptable quality and quantity.

Table 17-1
Weight Gain from Birth to 1 Year Old

AGE (mo)	AVERAGE WEIGHT VALUES	
	WEIGHT (lb)	WEIGHT GAIN RATE (lb/mo)
0	7½	1
4–6	15	2
10–12	22–23	3

NOTE: Consult the Appendix for the standard growth grid.

Allergy Is Less of a Problem
Breast-fed infants tend to develop fewer allergies. Since the intestinal system of an infant just a few weeks old permits the absorption of large protein molecules, absorption of "foreign protein" from cow's milk may directly result in allergic reactions or may predispose the child to lifelong allergies such as milk-induced colitis.

Breast Milk Protects Against Infection
It has been well documented that breast-fed infants are less likely to develop intestinal infection due to **Escherichia coli** (a bacterium that can cause diarrhea). Because this benefit of breast milk has not been duplicated by any other milk, bottle-fed infants are more likely to develop diarrhea. Clinical observations indicate that diarrhea in a bottle-fed child can be stopped by switching to breast milk from a breast-milk bank or from another lactating mother. In the United States and many other countries, higher morbidity and mortality rates from diarrhea among bottle-fed as compared with breast-fed infants have been documented for many years. Breast-fed babies also have fewer constipation problems than bottle-fed ones. It is suspected that the higher content of lactose in breast milk may be responsible for this difference.

What are the antiinfective factors in breast milk? No satisfactory answer is available, although there are many theories. More research is being conducted. Human milk itself is probably not sterile when it reaches the newborn. The sources of bacteria are most likely the nipples and fingers. Nevertheless, breast milk somehow protects infants from infection. The following briefly analyzes several other popular theories.

Colostrum, the yellowish fluid that comes before the white milk, is suspected of providing the child's intestinal system with passive immunity. One possibility is that certain colostrum corpuscles or particles that escape destruction by gastric juice and intestinal enzymes are able to reduce the number of intestinal bacteria. Another theory suggests that macrophages in colostrum may produce lactoferrin, which may inhibit bacterial growth.

Like colostrum, milk may contain lactoferrin that can inhibit the growth of bacteria. Breast milk contains the antibody immunoglobulin A (IgA), which is active against *E. coli*. Milk may contain lysozymes that have an antiinfective property. The presence of a specific factor in breast milk permits the growth of *Lactobacillus bifidus* (a bacterium), which can directly stop the multiplication of undesirable organisms or indirectly crowd out pathogenic bacteria such as *E. coli* or viruses.

Other reports indicate that breast milk can also protect some infants against nonintestinal infection. For instance, breast-fed babies have a lower incidence of respiratory infections. It is suspected that breast milk contains an antistaphylococcus factor.

Breast-feeding Creates a Bond
The psychological benefits of breast-feeding are often cited. For example, many women feel that human milk is designed for human infants and is therefore the best food for them. Women who breast-feed often

feel that they have established an important bond with the child. It appears that a woman's desire to breast-feed increases if she is permitted a direct and immediate contact with the child in the delivery room. Such women have a better chance of successful breast-feeding.

Oral Structures Get a Workout

The process of sucking milk from the breast is different from that of sucking milk from a bottle. An infant has to work harder to suck milk from the breast. Some suggest that this effort improves the utilization and coordination of the oral muscles, jaws, teeth, and tongue. The consequence may be the absence of overcrowded teeth and the development of stronger oral tissues.

Some studies have claimed that breast-feeding has a beneficial effect on the speech development of the child. For example, the natural act of sucking can accelerate the development of the neuromuscular system involved in speech. Also, since the holes in an artificial nipple are slightly larger than those in the breast, the child is forced to use tongue thrusts to arrest the rapid flow of milk. Some professionals claim that this increased tongue thrusting may adversely affect the child's later speech development.

The Uterus Returns to Normal

Clinical reports have confirmed that breast-feeding brings about a vigorous contraction of the uterus, which returns to its normal size in a shorter time than in a woman who chooses not to breast-feed. Also, bleeding of the uterus is reduced.

Additional Benefits

Other benefits from breast-feeding include contraception, weight reduction, and the reduced risk of breast engorgement and trauma. Years of observation have shown that unimpaired breast-feeding is an effective contraceptive method during the first few weeks after delivery. In most mothers with successful lactation, ovulation is postponed until at least the tenth week after childbirth. The period is longer if mothers maintain full breast-feeding without any formula supplement. The logic is that early weaning leads to early ovulation and accelerates the possibility of another pregnancy.

Some women do not have confidence in this contraceptive explanation, since they experience menstruation two or three months after delivery. However, a possible explanation is their frequent use of supplemental feeding, which interrupts the sucking and flow of milk and thus disrupts the hormonal prevention of ovulation. Some women actually do become pregnant while breast-feeding and are understandably dissatisfied with this method of contraception. On the other hand, the hormones in some oral contraceptive pills can suppress lactation and be passed on to the infant, posing a risk. For reasons not yet clear, mechanical devices such as the IUD can increase lactation.

Many women find that breast-feeding is effective in reducing weight, although this beneficial effect fails to occur in some nursing mothers.

Breast-feeding is also a natural prevention for the engorgement of the breast tissues from milk. Women who choose to bottle-feed their infants find their breasts initially painful and tender from engorgement. Some suggest that this may increase their susceptibility to breast trauma and cancer. The milk supply gradually dries up if there is no sucking, but some physicians prescribe medications to arrest milk production.

Finally, as discussed later, formula feeding has a number of disadvantages, most of which can be avoided if the child is breast-fed.

Drawbacks

Contrary to the claims of many enthusiasts, breast-feeding can have some problems. One is the mother's failure to produce enough milk for breast-feeding to be successful. A woman who wants to nurse but is unable to make enough milk often becomes disappointed and anxious. It is important that the woman drink sufficient fluid, eat enough calories, sustain a strong desire to nurse, and provide a peaceful period for breast-feeding. Some failures are due to a negative attitude and confusion over the difference between colostrum and mature milk. Often a woman's milk production relates directly to her emotional state and degree of fatigue. Any fluctuation in the quantity of milk secreted affects the child's satiety and weight gain and may prompt excessive use of supplemental bottle-feeding. This further reduces the amount of milk formed because of a lack of stimulation of the breasts.

A second disadvantage for some women is the fear that breast-feeding may distort their physical appearance. Although most are able to lose residual pregnancy weight when breast-feeding, some are afraid that their breasts will remain enlarged for a long time, making it difficult to return to their prepregnancy weight. On the other hand, some women's breasts shrink after repeated breast-feeding.

Some women oppose breast-feeding because it restricts their freedom of movement. Obviously, nursing is difficult if a mother holds a full-time job that does not permit regular intervals for nursing.

If a woman uses drugs frequently (whether prescription, over-the-counter, or illicit), including cigarettes and alcohol, the chemicals may appear in the milk. The risk to the infant varies with the type of drug (see Chapter 24). Any accidental ingestion or inhalation of minute amounts of pesticide and industrial chemicals can be transferred to the milk, although the clinical hazard posed by this has not been documented.

A newborn infant may have sucking difficulty for the first two to three days (or sometimes longer) if the mother was sedated because of difficult delivery and long labor. After this period, sucking improves, and the difficulty rarely recurs.

Finally, some women are afraid that nursing may increase the risk of breast infection. Also, as discussed later, breast milk is lower than cow's milk in a number of nutrients.

THE TECHNIQUE OF BREAST-FEEDING

During pregnancy the breasts are prepared for lactation. Influenced by body hormones, they enlarge from the deposition of fat and a moderate collection of fluid. Hormones also prepare the secretory cells for milk production. During the last weeks of pregnancy, an amber fluid (usually thin) called colostrum is often secreted from the nipples. This fluid also appears during the first days of breast-feeding. Colostrum is high in protein and minerals and, as mentioned earlier, may contain antibodies capable of providing the child with passive immunity. The mature milk, higher in carbohydrate and fat, is formed about the third day after birth. However, the newborn should be put to the breast within the first 24 hours of birth because its sucking will stimulate milk production. Normal white milk production is established at the end of the first week in the amount of about 500 mL daily.

In general, the breast-feeding woman should assume a position that is comfortable for both her and the infant. The child should be held close to the breast, whether the mother is reclining in bed or seated in a chair. A chair with low arms will give more support to the mother, although many mothers prefer a rocking chair. To initiate sucking, the nipple should be held toward the child's mouth, and brushing the baby's cheek next to the breast will cause it to turn its head in that direction as a reflex action.

The nipple should be held by the mother so that both nipple and areola are in the baby's mouth; this procedure maximizes the flow of milk. If the infant is permitted to suck only the end of the nipple, milk flow is reduced, and the nipple may become very tender and sore. Both breasts should be used alternately at each feeding.

Nursing time may vary from 5 minutes (for a tiny infant) at each breast to 20 minutes. When the baby is satisfied, it will stop nursing and often go to sleep. After and perhaps during the feeding, the infant should be held to the shoulder and patted on the back to help expel any swallowed air. Experienced mothers are familiar with other ways to "burp" the baby. The intervals between feeding are shorter for the newborn and gradually extend to 3 or 4 hours.

To produce an adequate amount of milk, the mother should eat nutritious meals, drink an adequate amount of fluid, and be relaxed. Normal care of the breasts during nursing includes washing them with plain water and the adequate support of a properly fitted brassiere. Clean white cotton fabric (or nursing pads) may be placed in the brassiere cup to absorb any milk leakage. Plastic-lined brassieres are not advised because they prevent air circulation and drying of the nipple areas.

PROS AND CONS OF FORMULA FEEDING

If a woman wants to breast-feed she should do so, since breast milk is nature's food for a human infant. But in the last 50 years clinical observations have confirmed that a child grows equally well when bottle-fed, as shown in Table 17-2. If the mother and doctor have decided that the child is to be bottle-fed, the ideal is to modify cow's milk so that it approximates breast milk's nutrients in quality and quantity. As Tables 17-3 and 17-4 illustrate, whole cow's milk is higher in certain nutrients and lower in others than breast milk. Cow's milk can be modified in

Table 17-2
Growth Rates and Body Size of Infants by Method of Feeding

TYPE OF FEEDING	GROWTH RATE (MO)		BODY SIZE AT 2 YEARS
	0–5	5–24	
Breast	Faster	Slower	Same
Bottle	Slower	Faster	Same

various ways to make it similar to breast milk, as indicated below.

The protein and some minerals in cow's milk must be reduced in quantity. This is accomplished by heat, acid, alkali, enzyme, bacterial action, or dilution with water. The last technique is the most common and can effectively reduce protein and calcium levels, although it also decreases the caloric density. This loss is usually compensated for by adding a carbohydrate such as sucrose, dextromaltose, or lactose to either commercial or home-prepared formulas. Because of the high content of sodium in cow's milk, the mineral is usually partially removed by dialysis to approach the concentration in breast milk, although this

Table 17-3
Approximate Nutritional Content of Colostrum, Breast Milk, and Whole Cow's Milk*

NUTRIENT PER 100 mL	COLOSTRUM	BREAST MILK	COW'S MILK
Water (mL)	87	87	87
Kcal	59	75	68
Protein (g)	2.8	1.2	3.5
Lactose (g)	5.5	6.9	4.9
Fat (g)	2.8	4.4	3.7
Calcium (mg)	30	34	120
Phosphorus (mg)	15	14	94
Sodium (mg)	45	160	505
Potassium (mg)	75	407	1,360
Iron (mg)	0.1	0.13	0.1
Vitamin A (IU)	200	210	150
Vitamin D (IU)	No information	0.5	2.0
Vitamin E (mg)	1.0	0.6	0.06
Vitamin K (μg)	No information	1.4	5.8
Vitamin C (mg)	5.0	4.3	1.8
Vitamin B_1 (mg)	13	16	41
Vitamin B_2 (μg)	25	40	160
Vitamin B_6 (μg)	No information	10	50
Vitamin B_{12} (μg)	No information	0.03	0.4
Folic acid (μg)	0.05	5	5
Pantothenic acid (μg)	180	190	340
Niacin (μg)	70	170	90

*Information obtained from a number of investigators' reports. All values are averages.

Table 17-4
Comparison of Vitamins and Minerals in Breast and Cow's Milk

NUTRIENT	BREAST MILK	COW'S MILK
Vitamin B_1	More	Less because of destruction due to pasteurization
Vitamin C	More	Less because of destruction due to pasteurization
Overall minerals	Fewer if distilled water is used in supplemental feeding	Varies with the type of feed and drinking water
Strontium	Amount varies	About six times more
Calcium:phosphorus	≈1.9:1.0	≈1:1

method again involves a loss of other minerals. When whole milk is diluted, the curd formation is reduced with a *flocculent*, an additive that gives the milk a soft texture for easier digestion. Table 17-5 compares the

Table 17-5
Comparison of Protein in Breast and Cow's Milk

PROTEIN QUALITY AND QUANTITY	BREAST MILK	COW'S MILK
Quantity	Standard amount	Twice as much
Type	Mainly lactalbumin	Mainly casein
Amino acid profile	Pattern resembling human protein	Pattern slightly different from human protein
	More essential amino acids	Less essential amino acids
Digestion	Soft and flocculent curd, rapid and easy digestion and absorption	Hard curd, more difficult digestion and absorption
Cysteine and methionine content	Higher, making more efficient use of methionine	Lower, making less efficient use of methionine
Proteases (enzymes)	Higher level, facilitating degradation by splitting protein to less complex forms	Mostly destroyed by pasteurization, thus making protein digestion a little more difficult

protein in breast and cow's milk before the latter is modified for formula feeding.

Because of the high ratio of saturated to unsaturated fat in cow's milk, part of its butterfat is replaced by a vegetable oil such as corn oil, which has a high level of long-chain, polyunsaturated fatty acids, especially linoleic acid. To prevent oxidation, an antioxidant such as vitamin E may be added. Table 17-6 compares the quantity and quality of fat in breast and cow's milk before it is modified for bottle-feeding of infants.

Table 17-6
Comparison of Fat in Breast and Cow's Milk

FAT QUANTITY AND QUALITY	BREAST MILK	COW'S MILK
Amount (g/100 mL)	4.4	3.7
Percent of total calories	53–55	47–49
Linoleic acid (g/100 g fat)	10–11	2–2.5
Percent of total calories	6–9	1–2
Cholesterol (mg/100 mL)	19–21	13–15
Fatty acids		
Saturation	Fewer	More
Carbon chain	Mainly 10–14	Mainly less than 10
Digestion	More effective (95%)	Less effective (60%)
Free palmitic acids	Releases very little free palmitic acid in the intestine, thus reducing interference with calcium absorption	Releases more free palmitic acid in the intestine, thus increasing interference with calcium absorption
Ratio of polyunsaturated fatty acids to saturated fatty acids	Is increasing because of general increase in unsaturated fats consumption in this country	Constant if animal feeding practices remain unchanged
Fat variation with each feeding	At the end of each feeding, level of fat in the milk increases, making the infant satisfied and thus spontaneously regulating total milk intake	Remains constant

Disadvantages

Although bottle-fed formulas can be made nutritionally similar to breast milk, formula feeding has a number of drawbacks. One is the possible lack of sanitation in preparing the formula, which can result in infection. This problem is especially common in families of low socioeconomic status and in underdeveloped countries.

Underdilution of a formula may cause dehydration and pose the major hazard of solution overload. This may happen when the mother does not pay adequate attention to the preparation instructions. Even when properly diluted, the high levels of protein and sodium in cow's milk are of major concern. Refer to the case history in Chapter 13.

Formula-fed babies have a higher incidence of allergy and constipation, diarrhea, and infection of the gastrointestinal and respiratory tracts than breast-fed babies. The tendency for a formula-fed infant to overfeed is also high, probably because of the easy access to the food.

The preparation of some formula milk calls for the addition of syrup or sugar. There are documented cases of mothers using salt instead of sugar by accident, with disastrous consequences. Containers for salt and sugar must be clearly labeled.

Because of the high fat content of some formula milk, it is possible that an infant fed such milk accumulates lipids in its blood. High blood cholesterol and triglycerides may pose a risk later in life.

An infant may be conditioned to prefer sweet things because of exposure to sugar, honey, or syrup added to a bottle containing milk, juice, vitamin C supplement, or plain water. A higher incidence of cavities may also result as the child grows. Obviously, the effect is exaggerated if the child sucks the bottle for a prolonged period. Dentists and physicians have recently identified a "nursing bottle syndrome" or "dummy reservoir syndrome," in which the teeth and gums of youngsters show excess rotting because as infants they were permitted to fall asleep with a bottle of sugary liquid in the mouth. The sugar solution soaks the mouth for hours and causes the decay. Refer to Chapter 23.

Another potential disadvantage of bottle-feeding is the option of changing formulas. Frequent changing of infant formulas (from ready-to-serve to evaporated milk, for example) is not advised, since it varies the child's caloric intake and tampers with its hunger-satiety rhythm.

Advantages

On the other hand, bottle-feeding has many advantages. First, the mother enjoys freedom of movement, especially valuable for the many women who are joining the work force. Second, breast milk is not necessarily cheaper than formula; the price comparison varies with the formula used and the diet of the mother. Third, breast-feeding is not recommended for women who drink and smoke excessively, use contraceptive pills and illicit drugs, receive medications, or are exposed to chemical compounds in their occupations. Fourth, some babies fed breast milk do not gain weight satisfactorily or may develop an occasional allergy. For these infants, bottle-feeding is preferred.

There is a variety of milk that can be used to feed an infant. But the use of skim, nonfat, or low-fat milk has a number of problems. Nutritionally, the product is not appropriate as the only food for infants of any age. The child may suffer linoleic acid deficiency. The minimal requirement of an infant for this nutrient is 1 to 3 percent of total caloric intake. For breast milk, skim milk, and commercial formulas, the figures are about 6 to 9 percent, 0 to 1 percent, and 10 to 20 percent, respectively.

Some infants are susceptible to diarrhea because of low intestinal fat if fed skim milk. Because of the partial or total removal of fat, the supplies of vitamin A and D are low, and cases of their deficiency have been documented. Fortification with these nutrients does not guarantee an adequate intake, since the lack of fat decreases their absorption. Some infants fail to gain weight and store very little body fat. The decreased intake of cholesterol may interfere with proper myelin formation.

The high nitrogen and sodium content of skim milk may pose hazards, and a child who drinks skim milk should be provided with enough fluid to excrete the waste in the urine. The low level of iron and copper in skim milk may pose a risk. This explains why using boiled skim milk to treat diarrhea in infants is ill advised, since the dehydration caused by the diarrhea will be intensified by the large load of solute in the milk.

Feeding low-fat milk to decrease cholesterol intake and avoid obesity is a preventive measure in health care, but its actual benefits have not been substantiated. The use of condensed milk to feed an infant is not advisable, since it contains too much sugar, which may cause the baby to become overweight.

BASICS OF BOTTLE-FEEDING

For infants under the care of a pediatrician, the formula to be used will be prescribed or recommended. Normally, the base of the formula is cow's milk, which is diluted with water to reduce its protein and mineral contents and supplemented with sugar, syrup, and/or lactose to raise the carbohydrate content. The form of milk used is determined by convenience, cost, and special needs. Commercial powdered or liquid formulas can be used, although some prefer fresh, evaporated, or dried milk. Nutrient supplements may or may not be needed.

Enough formula for 24 hours' feeding may be prepared at one time. With the increasing use of commercial formulas and availability of disposable utensils, most nursing mothers do not have to practice *all* the details of terminal or aseptic sterilization. Also, pediatric and public health clinics provide free brochures with easy-to-follow instructions if any form of sterilization of tap water and feeding equipment is needed or practiced by a nursing mother.

IS A MILK DIET NUTRITIONALLY ADEQUATE?

How adequate is an all-milk diet for an infant? The answer varies with the baby's age, milk intake, and the type of milk.

The amount of milk consumed by a baby varies from about 3 oz per pound body weight during the first 5 to 10 days of life to 1½ to 2 oz per pound during the second and third months. For example, an average infant may consume about 1 qt of milk daily during the first 2 to 4 weeks. The exact volume of milk consumed depends on body size, growth rate, appetite, and supplemental liquids. Also, we must consider the varying feeding schedule. Early feeding may be five to ten times daily, decreasing to four to six times at about 3 months.

Assume that an infant under 3 months needs and normally consumes about 800 to 900 mL of milk. For the most part this amount, especially if breast milk, satisfies the child's RDAs during the first three months. However, between 3 and 5 months of age, iron intake may not be adequate if the child is on a milk diet only. The remedy is using infant iron supplement or commercial formulas that have been fortified with iron. A fluoride supplement may also be needed, depending on water fluoridation, formula content, and so on.

Some formula-fed infants may need vitamin C supplementation. Liquid commercial ready-to-serve formulas with added vitamin C are acceptable. However, if the formula preparation involves commercial pasteurization or home sterilization, vitamin C supplement may be needed, since vitamin C is destroyed by heat. Such formulas include regular whole milk, evaporated milk, and other formulas requiring home sterilization. The RDA for the vitamin may be met by a liquid supplement or 1 teaspoon of orange juice per day. At the beginning, the juice is diluted with another teaspoon of water. Gradually the amount is increased to 2 teaspoons of juice a day, with proper dilution for tolerance. Some infants are allergic to the oil extract in the juice; if so, a liquid nutrient supplement may be used. Some evidence suggests that if the mother consumes an abnormally high amount of vitamin C during pregnancy, the newborn baby may be conditioned to an excessively high requirement of the vitamin.

The need for vitamin D supplementation varies under different circumstances. Because regular and evaporated milk and most commercial formulas are fortified with vitamin D, the intake should be adequate. However, breast-fed infants over 3 months old should be provided with an additional source of vitamin D. If the child's exposure to sunlight is sufficient (30 to 60 minutes daily for a clothed infant), no other measure is needed. Otherwise, the child should be provided with a supplement. The availability of water-miscible vitamin D has reduced the use of cod liver oil, which poses the risk of being aspirated into the lungs. Premature or high-risk infants tend to be deficient in vitamin D, which frequently must be administered. Nevertheless, the possibility of vitamin D toxicity cannot be underestimated, especially for very young infants.

Cow's milk contains less vitamin E than breast milk. Because of the difficult passage of the vitamin through the placenta, a premature infant tends to be deficient in vitamin E because of its shorter gestation period. Most commercial formulas now have vitamin E added.

Some infants have a tendency toward hemorrhage that can be managed by an injection of vitamin K. This applies especially to the breast-fed newborn and infants consuming relatively small amounts of formula milk during the first few days of life.

Two final points should be mentioned. First, goat's milk does not have enough folic acid to sustain a growing child. The case history illustrates this. Second, infants of strictly vegetarian mothers may be deficient in vitamin B_{12}, especially if a supplement is not used by the mother or given to the child.

INTRODUCING SOLID FOODS

People have argued for nearly a century over when to wean a young infant from milk and introduce solid foods. Table 17-7 shows some

Table 17-7
Practices in Introducing Solid Foods to Infants

YEAR	PEDIATRICIAN-RECOMMENDED TIME TO START SOLID FOODS
1900	>12 months old: meat and cereal supplementing milk
1920	8–12 months old: meat broth supplementing milk
	>12 months old: solid foods supplementing milk
1960	2–6 weeks old: cereal supplementing milk
	4–5 months old: meat, eggs, vegetables, fruits, cereal
1980*	0–4 months old: milk, nutrient supplements
	4–6 months old: solid foods supplementing milk

*In 1980, 90 percent of U.S. infants were fed solid foods before 3 months of age.

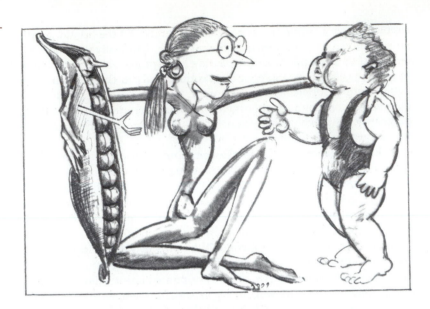

trends in the practice of introducing solid foods. Factors to be considered when introducing solid foods to an infant are: (1) The nutritional requirements of the infant; (2) the appropriate physical and physiological development, especially of the child's digestive system; (3) relative advantages and disadvantages of introducing solid foods early; and (4) the importance of establishing eating habits that will lead to good nutritional intake throughout life. Some aspects of these considerations are discussed below.

When Can a Baby Eat Solid Foods?

One important consideration is the oral development of the child. An infant under 2 months old can perform three basic oral functions: rooting (searching for the nipple), sucking, and thrusting (extruding the tongue). Exactly when the child starts to swallow is unknown, although it is generally agreed that this ability develops at about 3 months. At about 2½ to 3 months, the child can manipulate its tongue to convey liquid food particles to its throat. If solid food is fed at this young age, then the caretaker must place the food at the back of the child's mouth. The use of force here will encounter resistance, frustration, and a generally unhappy feeding atmosphere. The child may eventually develop uncooperative eating habits because of this unpleasant experience.

Another important consideration is the physiological development of the child. The child's digestive system should be mature enough to handle solid foods. When a child is under 1 month old, its enzyme system is appropriate only for digesting milk protein. Salivary amylase for digesting starches is not present until age 2 or 3 months, but lactose and sucrose in milk do not require salivary enzymes for hydrolysis. Only at 4 or 6 months of age do most infants acquire the appropriate enzyme system to digest nonmilk protein. Thus, introducing solid foods too early may result in an excess protein intake that cannot be digested properly by the child. Since the child's kidney functions are not fully developed, an excess solute load from sodium and protein may then pose a problem.

In areas with a hot climate, calorie-dense foods can cause dehydration. Because of the high concentration of nitrate and nitrite in such vegetables as celery, spinach, carrots, and lettuce, homemade baby food with these ingredients should not be fed to babies under 6 months old to prevent the clinical disorder known as *methemoglobinemia* (also see Chapter 25).

Pros and Cons of Early Solid-Food Feeding

In addition to questions of whether the child is physiologically capable of swallowing and digesting solid foods at an early age, the practice of introducing solid foods early has been criticized as nutritionally unwise. For one thing, if the child can eat only a small amount of solid foods, then nutrient intake will be limited. Solid-food feeding may not be worth the work, time, cost, and risk of contamination. Second, many solid foods have a higher caloric density than breast or formula milk. If the child eats solid foods and drinks large quantities of milk, it may overeat and become obese. A third possible problem is that forced feeding of semisolid foods before 9 to 12 weeks of age will increase the feeding problems and food dislikes of the infant. If the child is not yet ready, it will fight back and become resentful.

Infants introduced to a variety of foods at an early age may have an increased incidence of food allergy. This is an especially important consideration if the child has a family history of allergy. For such children, feeding sensitive foods such as fruits, vegetables, and even rice cereal should be delayed. If the child is fed such foods, the exposure should be kept brief by switching to other foods.

Some claim that tongue extrusion or thrusting is a natural process. Prolonged spoon feeding resulting from the early introduction of solid foods may thwart this natural instinct and cause frustration in self-feeding, delay in manipulating finger foods, and even maladjustment in the childhood eating pattern.

On the other hand, some people feel that if a child eats solid foods early, this is a superior achievement. Another unconfirmed claim suggests that introducing solid foods at an early age will keep the infant sleeping through the night. Most professionals accept the decision of the mother to feed the child solid foods early because most infants appear to tolerate the foods well. In addition, the practice is so common that nothing much can be done about it. Probably the best advice is to avoid telling the mothers to start solid foods at precisely 4 or 6 months. Rather, they should be asked to postpone the introduction of solid foods as long as possible, preferably after 4 to 6 months. Recently, nutritionists and pediatricians have been adopting the term *beikost* (introduced by

Dr. S. J. Fomon of the University of Iowa) for infant foods other than milk, although its use is not widespread.

Guidelines for Solid-Food Feeding

Professionals have suggested certain guidelines in introducing new foods to an infant, since the order in which solid foods are usually introduced is only semiscientific and strongly traditional. These guidelines are given in Table 17-8. It is important that the infant be made familiar with new

Table 17-8
Nutritional Aspects of Introducing Solid Foods to Infants

FOOD*	SOME OBSERVATIONS
Single-grain cereals	Popularly started first; good iron content, cheap, least allergenic, easily prepared and stored
Strained vegetables and fruits	Avoid those that can cause gas and irritation to the intestine
Egg yolk	Usually introduced early; provides protein, iron, vitamins A and B_{12}†
Meat	Provides the RDAs of several nutrients

* Items arranged in chronological order of introduction (meat last). With each item, start with small quantities and progress to larger ones.
† A small amount should be given first to ascertain whether the child is sensitive to the substance.

foods one at a time. A new food should not be introduced until the child is accustomed to the last one. Mixtures of foods should be avoided, especially if they contain a new food.

Each new food is tried for a few days to detect tolerance. The caretaker should not feed any food the child finds objectionable. Like adults, infants have food preferences. Any food preferred by the child for the first few days and then genuinely disliked and rejected should not be given. As the child grows, it may come to like a food it once rejected.

Most infants are given a very small amount of a new food at first and then slightly larger portions. The texture of the food must be appropriate. The smaller the child, the less viscid the food. Initially, solid foods are mashed, pureed, strained, or blended. All these processes increase the softness of a food and minimize the residue. A soft food is followed by chopped solid food or bits of solid food. The transition depends on the child's ability to chew. The initial inability to move food back with the tongue for swallowing is indicated by the frequency with which the child spits it out, although this outward tongue thrusting may also indicate a dislike for the food or some other individual factor. The child should be permitted to eat as much and as slowly as it wants unless there is a reason to suspect that the child is not eating adequately. In any case, the child should not be forced to eat more than it wants.

The use of sugar, salt, and other seasoning is generally avoided, although certain cultural groups may prefer to use special spices or herbs. As the child becomes increasingly accustomed to solid foods, its preferences can be broadened by providing a large selection of items, serving a combination of foods (such as egg and formula or vegetables and milk), and not allowing the child to see an adult show any sign of dislike for food (especially nutritious ones).

The Technique of Solid-Food Feeding

Solid foods are given when the child is ready; for example, when it develops the ability to move food from the front to the back of its mouth with the tongue, which usually occurs at about 4 or 5 months. Otherwise, the food is placed at the back of the mouth to avoid spitting. During the feeding process, the child sits on the lap of or in front of the caretaker. Sitting upright, the child is fed with a spoon and should be able to see the entire feeding process. The child progresses to holding its own bottle or drinking from a special cup. At 5 to 7 months of age, the child may be given family table food.

The feeding sequence of liquids, soft (pureed) foods, chopped foods, and solid foods of biting size is recommended to assure that the child learns how to coordinate the different oral structures (teeth, jaws, tongue, palate, and so forth). When the child shows preference for crackers and cookies, it can bite them. A child 8 to 9 months old can swallow mashed and cut-up vegetables and chopped-up moist meat. Feeding techniques for a child between 1 and 3 years are given in the references for this chapter. Table 17-9 shows a list of suitable supplemental foods for infants during the first year.

Table 17-9
Suitable Supplemental Foods for Infants During the First Year

FOOD	USUAL AGE WHEN SUPPLEMENTED
Orange juice, tomato juice (source of vitamin C)*	10 days
Well-cooked cereals	2–4 months
Strained, pureed vegetables and fruits	3–5 months
Pureed, strained meats	4–7 months
Mashed home-cooked vegetables, potatoes, carrots	6–9 months
Mashed egg yolk	6–7 months
Crackers, zwieback, dried bread	7–9 months
Regular cooked cereals, meats, eggs	10–12 months

* If vitamin C supplementation is necessary and the child cannot tolerate juices, administer liquid ascorbic acid supplement.

Care and Preparation of Baby Foods

An important aspect in infant feeding is the proper care of baby foods. All leftover foods must be handled with care to prevent spoilage. Unused portions should be placed in an appropriate storage container and stored in a refrigerator for the next feeding. Leftover food that has been handled or placed on the infant's plate should be discarded to avoid contamination and spoilage. Once a jar of baby food has been opened, the contents should be used within 2 or 3 days, even if it is refrigerated.

Homemade baby foods are becoming increasingly popular, although they may or may not be economical. Spicy and strong foods (sausage, some salad dressings, and the like) should be avoided. Plain family food is preferred. A strainer, blender, or grinder can be used to make baby food that is frozen and used later. For example, cooked potatoes or bananas are easily mashed and then frozen for later use.

FORMULA FEEDING IN THE THIRD WORLD: A CONTROVERSY
Commercial infant formulas became popular following World War II. As the number of infants in the American and European populations began to decrease, companies started to sell to developing nations. That practice has caused some concerns related to lack of sanitary facilities, contaminated water, and illiterate parents. Who is responsible for determining that products are properly used?

Concern that marketing techniques for infant formula had contributed to infant malnutrition in developing countries ultimately resulted in international conferences under the sponsorship of United Nations agencies. Qualified scientists and medical practitioners have appeared on behalf of both sides of the controversy.

Arguments Pro and Con
Poverty is at the heart of the controversy, but so is the belief that breast milk is preferable. Spending scarce resources on bottles, formula, and attendant materials can worsen the poverty condition. Parents may try to stretch formula by diluting it beyond recommended levels, thereby depriving infants of protein and calories. Breast milk contains antibodies to help fight diseases, whereas formula does not. Breast-feeding proponents also note that breast-feeding provides a natural method of birth control since maternal hormones inhibit ovulation. Those opposed to use of formula thus argue that bottle-feeding can worsen overpopulation. Breast-feeding proponents also point out that the closeness between mother and child is vital.

Defenders of bottle-feeding contend that widespread malnutrition in developing nations translates into improved health for infants if formula is used, since the lactating mothers often have breast milk that is deficient in nutrient supply. Bottle-feeding defenders maintain that any close contact between mother and infant will create a bond, that the extra nutrients needed in a lactating woman's food intake are just as expensive as formula, and that breast-milk supplementation is often necessary anyway since the mother may be ill, may have insufficient volume, or may have breast infection.

Two further arguments against bottle-feeding focus on contaminated water and inadequate sanitary facilities and on high-pressure sales techniques. Supporters of bottle-feeding argue that a 1976 study by the U.S. Agency for International Development found in an eleven-country survey that local water supplies are mixed with other foods for feeding infants from the third month on. Such supplemental feedings are less nutritious than formula, so formula would be an improvement on existing conditions, even if facilities are not ideally sanitary. Defenders of bottle-feeding also cite studies showing that the desire for bottle-feeding often precedes advertising, so they claim that it is not advertising that has caused the industry's growth in developing nations.

Critics of bottle-feeding have accused its proponents of using doctors and hospitals to promote their products, citing such practices as free samples to doctors and hospitals. Formula companies sponsor seminars on nutrition at hospitals. Walls are decorated with formula posters and similar advertising devices.

Bottle-feeding defenders explain that their practices promote the health of infant and family.

International Responses

In October 1979, the World Health Organization (WHO) and UNICEF hosted a meeting to review infant and child feeding. They developed a code of conduct for industry marketing. The three principal tenets of the code are: (1) There should be no sales promotion of breast milk alternatives; (2) there should be no free samples to health care providers; and (3) industry employees should not be allowed to work in the health care system.

In May 1981, these recommendations came up for a vote at the World Health Assembly. The United States cast the only negative vote.

Nestlé Boycott Lifted in 1984

The front page of the January 27, 1984 issue of the *San Francisco Chronicle* carried the news that a six-year boycott against Nestlé Company had been lifted.

The boycott had been organized by the Infant Formula Action Coalition in protest of Nestlé's promotion, marketing, and sales of infant formula in developing nations. Boycott organizers had argued that formula, due to unsanitary conditions and nutritional deficiencies in the developing nations, was a dangerous substitute for breast-feeding.

What ended the boycott was Nestlé Company's agreement that it would follow the recommendations of the World Health Organization and UNICEF regarding the marketing of infant formula to the Third World.

Controversy Continues

Debate continues on whether bottle-feeding causes malnutrition and death in developing countries. There is evidence for both sides of the argument. Debate also continues on the promotional tactics of the bottle-feeding industry in developing countries. Clouding both debates are the issues of poverty and social trends.

Breast-feeding is the most healthful method for nourishing an infant, if the mother's milk is adequate and nutrient filled. If it is not, supplementation proves necessary. If supplementation occurs, then sanitary conditions, adequate education, safe water, and sufficient income to obtain an adequate supply of supplementary products all become factors in the continuing debate.

Nutrition and Children

The nutritional and dietary need of children has been much debated. Some major concerns are children's nutritional status, feeding problems, questions about milk's reputation as a near perfect food, snacking, obesity, anemia, cavities, and food allergies. School lunches and sound meal plans are useful ways to improve nutrition during the childhood years.

NUTRITIONAL STATUS

The nutritional status of children under 6 years of age has been reported in several national surveys, including the Preschool Nutritional Survey (1968–1970) (G. Owen, *Pediatrics* 1974; 53:11 [supplement]), the Ten-State Nutrition Survey (1968–1970) (Department of Health, Education and Welfare publication No. [HSM] 72-8132), and the Health and Nutrition Examination Survey (1971–1974) (Department of Health, Education and Welfare publication No. [HRA] 74-1219-1).

From these surveys, it appears that the nutritional status of most children in the United States is satisfactory, although family income has an undeniable influence. For example, children from poor families have slightly arrested body growth, whereas those from well-to-do families tend to consume more essential nutrients.

Iron deficiency was the most prevalent nutritional disorder among American children. Anemia was reported in 7 to 12 percent of all children studied, especially youngsters from poor families. On the other hand, about 5 to 10 percent of children were overweight, many of them from families with moderate to high incomes. Protein intake was in general higher than the RDA. One quarter to nearly one half of the children were being given vitamin supplements. However, some black and Hispanic children were receiving a substandard amount of vitamin A, and about 10 to 15 percent of children had a low intake of vitamin C. About 10 to 30 percent of children, especially blacks, did not eat an adequate amount of calcium.

COPING WITH FEEDING PROBLEMS

Feeding children sometimes becomes a problem. Nutritionists recommend a number of pointers for avoiding or managing eating problems.

One is to take the child's food preferences into account. Like adults, children have likes and dislikes about foods. Table 17-10 summarizes some general attitudes of children toward foods. The caretaker should be familiar with these criteria and should tailor meals to the child's preferences. Quite often, the child's eating preferences reflect those of the parents; for instance, both parents and children may dislike vegetables. Since in many families foods are prepared according to the preferences of the father, the child's attitude toward certain foods may reflect the father's behavior. If the child is known to prefer moist foods, his or her fluid intake should be studied, for he may not be producing adequate saliva. If children prefer mildly flavored foods, they should initially be allowed to eat what they like. Flavors can gradually be made more intense by adding cream, juice, sauce, and other dressings to the diet until the child accepts normal food flavors. Sometimes children may not like a food at first but may develop a taste for it after repeated exposures.

Guardians should note that a child eats better in a happy and attractive environment. Foods requiring manipulation should be slowly introduced as the child's motor development and manual dexterity allow. The care giver can help the child relax before mealtime. Many children have a difficult time settling down to eat. The adult can read the child a story or have the child sit and talk for a few minutes before mealtime. The child should be discouraged from eating any food for at least an hour before a meal. If children do not eat at mealtime, they should not be allowed to fill up on snack foods later.

Refusing to eat is one way of attracting a parent's attention. Hovering over the child and fretting about her or his refusal to eat may actually reinforce this behavior. Is the child getting enough attention at other times of the day? If not, he or she may be trying to make up for it at mealtime.

It is not unusual for children suddenly to have a favorite food that they want to eat every day. Such food obsessions rarely last more than a week or two, because the child tires of having the same thing over and over. There is no need to go to great lengths to indulge the child, but it will not hurt if the child does have a favorite food every day.

Some families have a hard and fast rule that a child must eat everything on the plate before leaving the table. Nutritionists are beginning to wonder whether this practice accounts for the fact that there are so many overweight people in our society. Perhaps adult overeating can be traced to this "clean-plate policy" of early childhood years. Adults

Table 17-10
Criteria for the Acceptance of Foods by Children

FOOD CHARACTERISTICS	PREFERRED BY CHILDREN	DISLIKED BY CHILDREN
Texture	Soft, e.g., thin soup or puddings, tender beef, moist ground meat, soft mashed potatoes, soft bread	Thick, tough, stringy, dry, e.g., stringy beans, dry toast, coarse bread, thick soup, dry fish
Temperature of foods	Lukewarm; e.g., milk that is out of the refrigerator for a while; slightly melted ice cream	Very cold or hot; e.g., hot soup, cold rice, and meat
Flavor	Normal, unspoiled flavor	Any off flavors; e.g., slightly colored (e.g., very light yellow) or scorched milk, strong cabbage or onion flavor unless they are creamed to modify the flavor
Color	Colorful meal setting including the food, plate, table, and room decoration	Strange color such as blue or purple foods
Serving portion	Small portions and small utensils	Large portions and large utensils
Food shapes	Forms that they can manipulate with their hands rather than with utensils; e.g., strips of vegetables or meats	Shapes and forms that they cannot manipulate with their utensils and hands

TOMMY WON'T LISTEN

Tommy pays almost no attention to his teacher's directions, so his schoolwork suffers. He constantly gets out of his seat and disrupts other students. He almost seems incapable of sitting still. On the playground he exhibits a violent temper and cannot get along with his peers. His mother reports frequent episodes of crying and foot-stamping if Tommy doesn't get his own way. Despite an early bedtime, he usually fails to fall asleep until after 11 o'clock, yet he regularly rises by 7 o'clock.

Tommy's mother will welcome any "magic formula" that will change her son's behavioral problems.

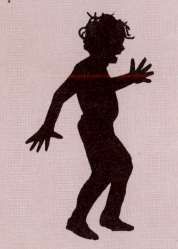

should let children eat until they are just satisfied, rather than using adult appetites as a guide.

If a child has a real eating problem, professional help is needed. Behavioral modification together with an aggressive program in nutrition education can improve the eating habits of many children.

FOOD ADDITIVES AND HYPERACTIVITY

Increasing medical attention has been directed toward a problem, experienced by children, that is known as *hyperactive syndrome*. The condition generally results in learning and behavior problems due to distractibility and ease of attention disruption; however, there are many symptoms. No known cure exists for hyperactive syndrome.

Many factors have been related to the condition, including exposure to toxic substances, allergies, nutritional deficiency, social factors, and environmental factors (Denny; Kolata). Attention recently focused on an allergist's hypothesis that food additives constitute toxic substances that can cause the syndrome. To combat the possibility that food additives can be a causative factor, the allergist recommended the restriction of certain foods, a practice that has come to be called the Feingold diet after Dr. Ben Feingold, its originator.

The Feingold Diet

To many parents, Dr. Feingold's diet offers an alternative to drug therapy. The diet recommends elimination of artificially flavored foods such as candy, soft drinks, chewing gum, preserves, ice cream, and baked goods. It recommends elimination of foods using the artificial colors known as Blue #1, Blue #2, Green #3, Red #3, Red #40, Yellow #5, and Yellow #6. Additionally, Orange B can be taken only in hot dogs, and Citrus Red #2 only in orange skin. The diet eliminates foods using either the preservative butylated hydroxytoluene (BHT) or butylated hydroxyanisole (BHA). Finally, the diet eliminates foods containing natural salicylates (the active chemical ingredient in aspirin): almonds, apples, apricots, cherries, cloves, coffee, cucumbers, currants, grapes, green peppers, nectarines, oranges, peaches, pickles, plums, prunes, raisins, tangerines, tea, and tomatoes.

Some experts have questioned the diet, pointing, for example, to the similarity in chemical composition between artificial flavorings and natural flavorings (Mailman and Lewis). Despite those questions, parents with hyperactive children who have successfully followed the diet suggest that the diet is viable. They claim that some items, especially those containing salicylate, can often be restored if they cause no resumption of symptoms.

What One Survey Shows

One researcher (Springer) conducted an informal survey of Feingold diet followers. The survey showed improved family relationships due to improved behavior of the hyperactive child. The survey also determined that the worst food for hyperactive children was flavored and colored beverages, followed by candy. Apples were the worst fruit, followed by tomato dishes such as pizza. Next came colored and flavored breakfast cereals, followed by luncheon meats, baked goods, chocolate, and table sugar. Symptoms could follow ingestion immediately or within the first 24 hours, with liquids bringing a more rapid reaction than solids. Adverse reaction can last up to five days after ingestion.

The survey of those who responded positively to the diet found that the diet's average calorie count per day slightly exceeded 2000. Carbohydrate contributed almost half the calories, followed by fat. Protein contributed about 15 percent of the total calories. It was found that dietary supplementation was necessary for some of the children, especially in regard to calcium.

Anecdotes Can Be Misleading
Does the above survey mean that we can cure our children's hyperactive tendency by complying with Dr. Feingold's diet? Even though parents and teachers report anecdotes of improvement, no controlled research studies have confirmed such observations. Studies do suggest that further research is needed in regard to absorption differences and food additive interactions. If, however, parents choose to try the diet, despite the absence of research findings, professional assistance is recommended to ensure that the child is getting the appropriate RDAs.

IS MILK A "PERFECT FOOD" FOR CHILDREN?
Although milk is advocated by all professionals as a good food for children, it is by no means a perfect food. It has a short shelf life and deteriorates rapidly. Pasteurization and refrigeration are needed. Milk is low in iron and copper and some vitamins, and whole milk is high in fat and cholesterol. Some individuals have lactose intolerance or milk allergy. In some, milk causes constipation or intestinal bleeding. Milk can also be a cause of obesity if too much is consumed. Finally, the waste byproducts of commercial milk production are environmental pollutants.

SNACKING
Snacking among children has been one of the most controversial issues in nutrition. It is well confirmed that excess snacking, especially when it occurs close to mealtime, will decrease appetite. However, since children have small stomachs, they cannot eat a large amount of food during regular meals even if they have not been snacking. Even if children consume large meals, they may still not get enough food, especially during periods of rapid growth. In this case, snacks solve part of the problem. There is no doubt that some snacks are nutritious and others are not. Aggressive nutrition education of children and parents can mold their snacking pattern in healthy ways.

Snacks are bad if a child gobbles up foods that are loaded with sugar, salt, and fat but low in protein, vitamins, and minerals. But if children use snacking to supply their bodies with nutritious foods that are lacking in their regular meals, then snacking is a great idea. A slice of cheese, a wheat cracker, or a banana eaten at midmorning or midafternoon can help supply the energy needed to keep children from tiring.

WEST VIRGINIA
TRIES A "JUNK" FOOD BAN

West Virginia has not experienced success with a state law that banned the sale of non-nutritious food in vending machines at schools (Medical World News). Many people looked to that state for guidance after the USDA proposed a law that would prohibit sales at schools, until after the lunch period, of foods containing less than 5 percent of the recommended daily needs for eight nutrients per 100-calorie portion.

A. Ellis, assistant director of education for West Virginia's child-nutrition program, advised that such a law would simply cause youth to wait until after lunch to "hit the vending machines." West Virginia law totally banned the sale of candy containing more than 40 percent sugar, all ice bars, and soft drinks with less than 20 percent juice. Sales fell dramatically when soup, granola bars, fruit juices, raisins, nuts, and yogurt were substituted.

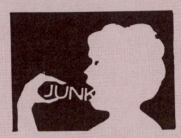

At the high school in Glenville, the principal, W. J. Percy, reported that sales were one-third those of "junk" food, despite the selection having increased from 5 items to 34. At Parkersburg High School near Wheeling, R. L. Kincaid, the principal, reported that sales were cut in half. Since the vending machine sales often help fund school activities, the effect was devastating. To raise funds for the school's debate team, students went into the community selling candy.

As reported, the effect of a "junk" food ban in West Virginia schools was simply one of causing students to bring "junk" food from home. No increase in cafeteria sales resulted, and no decrease in the daily consumption of "junk" food by students resulted.

Despite the findings in West Virginia, some nutritionists and parents believe the ban should ultimately be beneficial. Since the ban is not legally mandated, it is uncertain whether other states will adopt similar policies.

OBESITY

Pediatricians find that obesity is a big problem in infancy and childhood. The major cause is too much food. To determine the extent of childhood obesity, one should ask whether the child is obese or overweight (see Chapter 3) and whether the extra weight consists of fat, bone, or muscle. The child's weight:height ratio is a more accurate indication of obesity than weight alone.

Many factors must be considered in identifying the child at risk of becoming an obese adult. Since obesity may run in a family, if one or both parents are obese, the child is more likely to become obese. The child's weight pattern between 4 and 7 years of age, the weight pattern during the first 6 months of life, and the birth weight may show an emerging pattern of obesity. For example, babies that are overweight from excess fat have a higher tendency to become obese adults. The family's eating habits should also be taken into account.

To manage an obese child, care givers must first find the reasons for the obesity. They should then help the child establish a good eating habit. Balanced diets with a variety of foods should be fed. The inclusion of foods such as gravies, pastries, pork, greasy beef, and fried foods should be reduced in the family diet. The child should reduce snacking and eat nutrient-dense items when he or she does snack. Foods should not be used as a reward or reprimand to regulate the child's conduct at home or school. Overfeeding should be avoided, and the child should be encouraged to become aware of when he or she is full. Care givers should make certain that the child does not depend on food for emotional or social comforts. For example, a child may overeat because he or she is not loved or is not accepted by other children. As the child grows, he or she should be educated in nutrition and increasingly allowed to choose his or her own foods. The child should be taught to follow a good exercise program. Children often exercise little, watch too much television, and overconsume soft drinks, and fat babies and children are not as active as their thin counterparts.

The goal of such measures is for the child to achieve an appropriate weight:height ratio. In many cases, the child need not actually lose weight but should rather maintain a constant weight while gaining height. Depending on the child's age, caloric intake should be kept about 1200 to 1400 kcal per day.

Parents can practice some preventive measures to avoid obesity in infants and children. If possible, a child should be breast-fed with minimal but adequate supplemental feeding. A fat baby should not be fed solid foods before 3 or 4 months of age, preferably at 5 or 6 months.

Among children, the *Prader-Willi* syndrome is one of the better-known pathological conditions of obesity. Apart from obesity, a child with the Prader-Willi syndrome shows other clinical characteristics. Its cause is unknown, although some cases could be due to damage (for example, drug accident) received during pregnancy. The newborn child is usually of low weight and fails to thrive after birth. As the child grows, bone development and height are arrested, and obesity becomes evident. Mental retardation may be evident in addition to undeveloped muscle tone and a lack of motor coordination. Some children have undeveloped genitals, especially males. Other outstanding physical abnormalities include small feet and hands, triangular upper lips, and Oriental-like eyes. These children also have difficult personality traits (violent reactions, hurting other children, disobedience, and so on), delayed language development, and feeding difficulties when young. A tendency to develop diabetes during adolescence is also common.

Children with Prader-Willi syndrome have some common nutrition and feeding problems. Abnormal mouth development may affect sucking ability to the extent that feeding by *gavage*, or dropper, is necessary. Affected children start to gain weight after 1 year of age and tend to become obese between the ages of 1 and 3. Their appetite is difficult to satisfy, and they eat constantly. Body fat is concentrated on the feet, hands, and lower part of the body. These children also tend to have many cavities. In view of the diabetic tendency, the care taker may have to face the task of feeding a diabetic child.

Before a long-term dietary management program is developed for a child with this syndrome, feeding difficulties must be identified and corrected. If an afflicted child is not obese, an aggressive program should be implemented to prevent the child from gaining weight in the future. On the other hand, a child who is already obese must lose weight. If cavities are rampant, the child may have to learn new eating habits and avoid sugar foods. As in other instances of chronic health problems in children, the dietitian, nutritionist, nurse, parents, and child must work together as a team.

Caloric and other nutrient needs must be determined for each child with the Prader-Willi syndrome. Early feeding training must include the conditioning of muscles involved in eating, such as those of the jaws, gums, cheek, and tongue. Daily food records should be maintained, and the child's nutritional status should be evaluated regularly. Information such as weight and height gains and problems with food intake should also be recorded.

Children with this syndrome should be conditioned to the diet and environment. For example, if their food intake must be restricted for a prolonged period, they must learn to adjust. It is definitely inadvisable for such children to eat indiscriminately. Thus, they may have to explain to friends and relatives why they must refuse certain foods.

Figure 17-1 shows a child with the Prader-Willi syndrome.

Figure 17-1: The Prader-Willi syndrome in a 14-year-old patient. (a) 206 lb (93.5 kg) before therapy. (b) 148 lb (67.54 kg) after 18 months of intensive diet therapy with an occasional dose of Fenfluramine. SOURCE: Widhalm, K., Deutsch, J. "Behandlung der exzessiven Adipositas am Beispiel des Prader-Willi-Labhart-Syndroms." Pädiatrie und Pädologie 11, 297–304. Wien–New York: Springer, 1976.

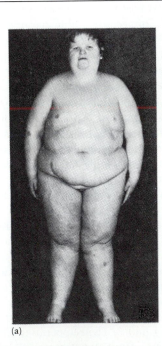
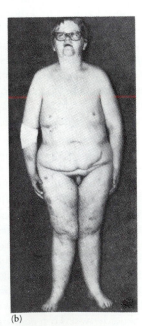

(a)   (b)

ANEMIA

A number of surveys indicate that many youngsters suffer iron deficiency anemia. The blood hemoglobin of these children is less than 10 g per 100 mL. Many of them come from poor families, and their poor diets may be the cause of their low iron intake. Some experts suggest that the children's parents do not feed them the right foods because of ignorance or cultural traditions rather than poverty. Some suggest that the children may be harboring intestinal parasites or that some may have *occult* (nonapparent) bleeding from excess milk drinking.

CAVITIES (DENTAL CARIES)

Dental cavities among children mainly result from consuming too much fermentable carbohydrate. Children must also have a good diet to have strong teeth and oral tissues. At present, nutritionists propose the following preventive measures.

1. Avoid foods that tend to cause cavities, mainly carbohydrates (sugar, pastries, and so on).
2. Replace sweet snacks with tasty fruits and vegetables, cheese, nuts, and so on.
3. Reduce the consumption of sweetened carbonated beverages.
4. Avoid all forms of sticky candy and sweet gums.
5. Eat a well-balanced and nutritious diet.
6. Make sure that there is a source of fluoride and calcium.
7. Practice good oral hygiene.

More information is provided in Chapter 23.

FOOD ALLERGIES

The term **allergy** refers to an excessive sensitivity to substances or conditions such as food; hair; cloth; biological, chemical, or mechanical agents; emotional excitement; extremes of temperature; and so on. The hypersensitivity and abnormal reactions associated with allergies produce various symptoms in affected people. The substance that triggers an allergic reaction is called an **allergen** or *antigen*, and it may enter the body through ingestion, injection, respiration, or physical contact (Hui).

Although food allergy is not age specific, it is more prevalent during childhood. Because a reaction to food may impose stress and may interfere with nutrient ingestion, absorption, and digestion, the growth and development of children with food allergies can be delayed. Half the adult patients with food allergy claim that they had a childhood allergy as well. Apparently, a childhood food allergy rarely disappears completely in an adult. If a newborn baby develops hypersensitivity in the first 5 to 8 days of life, the pregnant mother was probably eating a large quantity of potentially offending foods, such as milk, eggs, chocolate, or wheat. The child becomes sensitized in the womb, and the allergic tendency may either continue into adult life or gradually decrease.

Children may also develop a food allergy called the delayed allergic reaction or hyperactivity. The classic sign of this is the tension-fatigue syndrome. Children with this syndrome have a dull face, pallor, circles under the eyes, and nasal stuffiness. A delayed food allergy symptom is more difficult to diagnose than an immediate one.

The first step in dealing with food allergy is to eliminate the offending food from the diet. This task can be relatively easy if the food can be isolated; however, the task becomes more complex if it is a food that occurs as an ingredient in other foods. For example, milk and eggs can be individually eliminated, but they also are used in numerous other foods. Parents must read labels to identify hidden allergens.

Childhood allergy to cow's milk is probably the most common food allergy in the United States, affecting 2 to 4 percent of all infants and children. It can occur in a child of any age. Milk allergy runs in the family, and pediatricians can sometimes predict likely victims. Milk allergy is frequently, though not always, associated with allergic reactions to egg white or citrus fruit. The symptoms of milk allergy are diarrhea, skin reactions (eczema), respiratory difficulties, asthma, headache, irritability, and tiredness. Symptoms can be quite severe, as seen in Figure 17-2. One must distinguish some children's intolerance for milk (due mainly to a lack of intestinal lactose) from actual milk allergy. Sometimes heating milk before serving can denature the offending protein, although the heat destroys some of the nutrients.

Substitutes may also be found. For example, an allergy to cow's milk

Figure 17-2: (a) Severe atopic dermatitis in an infant allergic to milk. (b) Same infant after changing to a milk-free formula diet. SOURCE: A. Holzel. Postgrad. Med. J. 51 (1975), Supl. 3: 71.

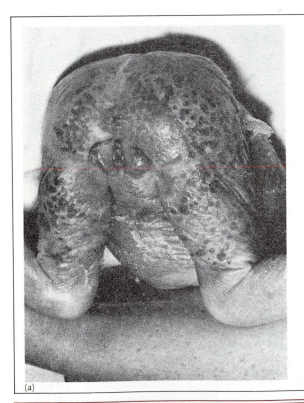

(a)

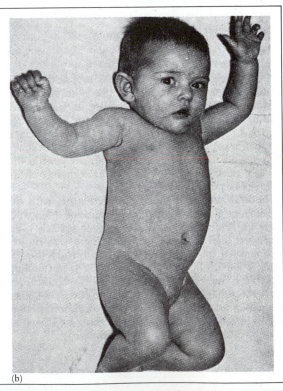

(b)

may necessitate the use of soy milk or formula. An allergy to wheat may call for the substitution of rice, soy, rye, or potato flour. An egg allergy will eliminate not only eggs but also noodles, most baked products, and some ice creams. It thus becomes necessary to obtain, for example, ice cream and bread that do not contain egg.

Obviously, children with food allergies can be nutritionally at risk. If allergic reactions are severe, the child may develop an aversion to eating. If the child has multiple allergies, the nutritional risk is simply that much greater. Energy intake can be too low. Milk allergies can cause calcium and vitamin D deficiency, and cereal allergy can cause a deficiency of B vitamins. As long as the allergy persists, supplements may prove necessary.

Children and infants are also frequently allergic to such foods as cola drinks, chocolate, peas, corn, tomatoes, citrus fruits, cinnamon, and food colors (for example, tartarzine). Since allergy tends to run in a family, doctors in general request parents to pay particular attention to such foods. Foods such as nuts, eggs, and seafood (especially fish) can produce an immediate allergic reaction, whereas others such as chocolate, corn, milk, and wheat may produce a delayed reaction. (See also Chapter 25.)

SCHOOL LUNCHES AND BREAKFASTS

Since school-age children may eat five meals a week at school, school lunches have been seen as a way to improve their nutrition. The U.S. Department of Agriculture (USDA) administers many child nutrition programs.

The USDA administers the school lunch program at the federal level (USDA). In most states, the state education agency operates the program through agreements with local schools or school districts. The program offers federal financial assistance for each lunch served, technical guidance, USDA-donated foods or cash, and additional financial assistance for each lunch served free or at a reduced price to eligible children.

Any public or nonprofit private primary or secondary school is eligible to enroll in the program. Also eligible are public and licensed nonprofit, private residential child care institutions such as orphanages, homes for retarded children, and temporary shelters for runaway children. To reach as many needy children as possible, participating schools and institutions send information to parents and the news media each year to explain how families can apply for free and reduced-price lunches.

For participating schools to be reimbursed for meals served through the program, lunches must meet USDA requirements, which are shown in Table 17-11. The pattern is designed to provide about one third of the RDAs for key nutrients established by the National Research Council of the National Academy of Sciences (see Chapter 15). This pattern also encourages serving a wide variety of conventional foods, including whole grain breads and fresh fruits and vegetables.

Meals must be not only nutritionally adequate but also prepared and

Table 17-11
School Lunch Pattern—Approximate per Lunch Minimums

COMPONENTS	MINIMUM QUANTITIES				RECOMMENDED QUANTITIES
	GROUP I, AGE 1–2 (PRESCHOOL)	GROUP II, AGE 3–4 (PRESCHOOL)	GROUP III, AGE 5–8 (K–3)	GROUP IV, AGE 9 AND OLDER (4–12)	GROUP V, 12 YEARS AND OLDER (7–12[2])
Milk: Unflavored, fluid low-fat, skim, or buttermilk must be offered[1]	¾ cup (6 fl oz)	¾ cup (6 fl oz)	½ pint (8 fl oz)	½ pint (8 fl oz)	½ pint (8 fl oz)
Meat or meat alternate (quantity of the edible portion as served):					
Lean meat, poultry, or fish	1 oz	1½ oz	1½ oz	2 oz	3 oz
Cheese	1 oz	1½ oz	1½ oz	2 oz	3 oz
Large egg	1	1½	1½	2	3
Cooked dry beans or peas	½ cup	¾ cup	¾ cup	1 cup	1½ cup
Peanut butter or an equivalent quantity of any combination of any of above	2 tbsp	3 tbsp	3 tbsp	4 tbsp	6 tbsp
Vegetable or *fruit*: 2 or more servings of vegetable or fruit or both	½ cup	½ cup	½ cup	¾ cup	¾ cup
Bread or bread alternate (servings per week): Must be enriched or whole grain—at least 1½ serving[3] for group I or one serving[3] for groups II–V must be served daily	5	8	8	8	10

[1]If a school serves another form of milk (whole or flavored), it must offer its children unflavored fluid low-fat milk, skim milk, or buttermilk as a beverage choice.
[2]The minimum portion sizes for these children are the portion sizes for group IV.
[3]Serving 1 slice of bread or ½ cup of cooked rice, macaroni, noodles, other pasta products, other cereal product such as bulgur and corn grits, or as stated in the Food Buying Guide for biscuits, rolls, muffins, and similar products.
SOURCE: *Code of Federal Regulations*, Title 7, Section 210.10, 1981.

served attractively. The USDA periodically reviews and revises program meal requirements to take into account new information about eating patterns, food preferences, and the nutritional needs of children.

One point must be emphasized. Fundings for programs such as school lunches must be allocated by Congress annually and will vary with the political climate.

One of the fields of nutrition study that has received increased attention is the relationship between nutrition and school performance. The public's belief that a definite relationship existed caused the National School Lunch Program to be expanded to include breakfast. Subsequent studies regarding the breakfast-learning connection showed the relationship to be statistically significant. Students skipping breakfast do more poorly on arithmetic tasks and continuous performance

Table 17-12

Suggested Meal Plan and Sample Menu for 3- Through 6-year-olds*

MEAL PLAN	SAMPLE MENU
Breakfast	*Breakfast*
Juice or fruit	Apple
Cereal (hot or dry)	Bran flakes with milk
Egg, meat, or toast	Egg (soft-boiled) with whole wheat
Milk	toast
	Milk
Snack	
Dry fruits or nutritious cookies	*Snack*
	Dates
Lunch	
Meat, egg, or alternate	*Lunch*
Potato, bread, or alternate	Peanut butter and jelly sandwich
Vegetable	Vegetable soup with rice
Butter or margarine	Margarine
Milk	Milk
Dessert	Custard pudding
Snack	*Snack*
Milk or juice	Orange juice
Crackers, pudding, or dried fruits	Apple wedges with peanut butter
Dinner	*Dinner*
Meat, cheese, poultry, or alternate	Fish sticks
Vegetable or salad	Sweet corn
Potato, bread, roll, or alternate	Baked potato
Butter or margarine	Butter
Dessert	Fruit pudding
Milk	Milk

*Serving size varies with the child. Other nutritious items not shown may be used; e.g., jams, oatmeal, cookies, peanut butter. Their inclusion must be integrated into the child's overall daily intake of calories and nutrients.

tasks than do those eating breakfast. Although studies focusing on general diet or individual meals (e.g. breakfast) can provide some insights, studies that focus on one food are preferred.

MEAL PLANS

What is a nutritious meal for a child? Table 17-12 provides meal plan and sample menu for children 3 to 6 years old. The meal plan in this table is based on four basic food groups discussed in Chapter 15. When it is used to feed a child, serving sizes must be adjusted to the age, development, activity, and appetite of the child.

Nutrition and Adolescents

You are already familiar with the growth spurt that signals the beginning of puberty for both boys and girls. You are also aware that girls typically experience the onset of puberty between the ages of 10 and 13, whereas boys experience comparable changes about two years later. You also know that once boys begin their growth spurt, they generally become both taller and heavier than girls during adolescence and adulthood. An integrated discussion is provided in Chapter 4.

If nutrition has been inadequate during childhood years, puberty can be delayed by as much as two years; but, with adequate nutrition during puberty, a previously underfed person can enter adolescence with good nutriture. Puberty thus provides an opportunity for catching up with nutriture.

NUTRITIONAL STATUS

Nutritional need differs between boys and girls during puberty and adolescence relative to energy. Boys gain lean tissue rather than fat tissue, their skeleton becomes heavier, and their red blood cells increase. Girls gain more fat tissue than lean tissue, also experience skeletal change, but have less blood cell development. These differences result in boys' requiring more energy during adolescence than girls require; that is, boys need more of the nutrients that go into building lean body mass. This difference translates into a daily kcal need of 2400 for girls and 2800 for boys. During late adolescence, the energy need for girls can be 2100 kcal, whereas boys may have a need of 3000 kcal.

Other than the difference in energy need, other recommended dietary allowances are similar for boys and girls during adolescence. For example, both have increased need for calcium, phosphorus, and iron. Vitamin need increases, and, as would be expected owing to the earlier onset of puberty in girls, the increased vitamin need by girls precedes that for boys.

Adolescence is, however, a very trying time, one that can lead to poor nutriture. As adolescents assert their individuality, they may reject familiar dietary practices. Increased social activities can also interfere with established dietary patterns. Figure consciousness and related peer pressure may result in poor nutriture.

United States dietary studies show that adolescents often have deficient intakes of calcium, iron, vitamin C, vitamin A, and the B vitamins. Both Australia and Canada have conducted surveys of adolescents that showed deficiency of the same nutrients.

EATING HABITS

Teenagers are influenced by their family background, the combined effects of physical, physiological, and emotional development, and their changes in lifestyle, characterized by increased mobility and independence. Teenagers are usually lacking in nutrition education. They like to eat outside the home and share meals with their peers, but when they do, their nutritional intake is frequently poor.

If a teenager's eating habits are tied significantly to social acceptance by peers, dietary habits are more likely to be unsatisfactory. On the other hand, if health and family relationships are important, the teenager may develop wise food choices.

The season also affects the eating habits of teenagers. Young adults tend to have a more regular eating pattern in winter than in summer, and so they generally eat a wider variety of food during the winter.

Adolescents have a number of bad food habits, such as the omission of meals, especially breakfast; not taking time for regular meals; dislike for nutritious foods such as milk; frequent consumption of unbalanced meals outside the home; and concern for body weight. Hair and skin problems, especially acne, can also affect eating habits.

Currently, there is much concern regarding the dietary habits of teenagers, especially as they affect physical, physiological, and emotional development. It is claimed, but not totally substantiated, that dietary inadequacies are common among adolescents. The occurrence of tuberculosis among young adults may be the result of nutrient deficiency. Nutrient deficiencies among teenage girls are especially critical.

Teenage girls who become pregnant impose a heavy demand on their nutritional storage. A young mother's nutritional status has a profound effect on the outcome of the pregnancy and the health of the newborn (see Chapter 16).

Many young adults skip breakfast. Reasons commonly cited are being in a hurry, lacking time, having no appetite, preferring to spend more time on personal appearance, trying to maintain weight, and having no company to eat with. Boys eat breakfast more frequently and in greater quantity than girls. Because many homemakers also omit breakfast, it has been suggested that young girls copy their mothers. Young adults in small towns do not skip breakfast as frequently as those in cities or rural areas. Although people who skip breakfast may still eat adequately, they may not be able to satisfy their nutritional need by two meals and snacks. Because such practices as skipping breakfast are so common among teenagers, the need for good nutrition education is clear.

With the wide selection of fresh, processed, and convenience foods, a nutritious breakfast can be easily put together. Traditional breakfast foods such as eggs, fruits, milk, juice, bacon, toast, and hot cereals are readily available, as are processed items such as beverages, dry cereals, and snack bars. A breakfast should contribute approximately 500 kcal and is especially important for contributing calcium and vitamins C and B complex, maintaining a normal to high level of blood glucose, and reducing the appetite for snacks.

In recent years, snacking by teenagers and concern over this habit have been on the rise. According to a current estimate, daily snacks may make up one fourth to one third of adolescents' RDA of calories. Although girls snack more frequently than boys, they do not necessarily have more nutritional problems. Whether snacking is good or bad for a person depends on his or her dietary intake.

Some snacks contribute a significant amount of nutrients without reducing the appetite for regular meals. There is no doubt that excessive snacking on nutrient-light foods is undesirable, especially if they are eaten just before bedtime. However, if the habit of snacking persists, should several small meals a day be encouraged that include nutritious snacks?

Some nutritionists propose that nutritious foods be made available at such strategic places as home refrigerators, school lunchrooms, vending machines, and grocery stores near schools. There is, however, a strong feeling that banning nutrient-light snacks is not a key to good dietary intake. Nutrition education is still the most important step.

Fortifying popular snack foods with nutrients that are likely to be lacking in teenage diets is another suggestion, since one survey has shown that some teenagers who snack have inadequate intakes of nutrients such as calcium and iron.

OBESITY

Obesity frequently occurs as a problem among adolescents and proves difficult to control. For this reason, significant efforts have been made to identify children who may be at risk for obesity in later years. Efforts have also been made to correct familial lifestyles and associated factors that place such children at risk.

Are Many Adolescents Obese?

Studies have shown that over 80 percent of youth who are obese by ages 10 to 13 will be so 20 years later. Studies of obese adults have shown that about one third of them were obese juveniles. Given that obesity generally causes low self-esteem; predisposes the person to hypertension, heart disease, and diabetes; and often leads to discrimination in school, career, and society in general, the problem is a significant one.

Although obesity can result from environmental factors, statistical studies suggest it can also be hereditary. Although less than 10 percent of average-weight parents have obese children, over 60 percent of obese adolescents have one or more obese parents. Inherited body type may well contribute to obesity.

An environmental factor affecting childhood obesity is parent lifestyle. Parents who are relatively inactive and sedentary can have children who become obese while ingesting no greater quantity of calories than peers who do not become obese. Infant feeding patterns can also contribute to obesity. For example, an early introduction to semisolid foods can lead to overfeeding. Some studies have found that children who have feeding problems during infancy tend to be obese. Obesity can also result from parental insecurity or parental guilt. In such cases, the parent overfeeds the child to relieve guilt or to express care and affection.

Prevention and Treatment

Although obesity can have various causes, it results when energy intake exceeds the energy utilized for body maintenance, growth, and activities (also see Chapter 20). Since parents control the food available to younger children, nutrition education is primarily directed to the parents for controlling or preventing obesity in the younger years. Adolescents, however, control their own food intake. For all ages, individual willpower must be developed as soon as possible. Weight control requires as much assistance as possible to be successful.

Adolescent obesity is estimated to involve about 10 million adolescents in the United States. Rigid diet and parental control do not prove effective in curing the problem. Since growth spurt and attendant weight gain are natural during adolescence, the problem of controlling obesity is complex. Treatment must consider the extent and duration of obesity, maturation, motivation, mental state, eating patterns, and socialization.

If the adolescent is immature, depressed, socially withdrawn, dependent on parents, and has low self-esteem, counseling must precede weight control efforts. If adolescents exhibit maturity and motivation, dietary guidance, exercise, and counseling can be beneficial.

Since studies have shown that teenage obesity proves a difficult problem to solve, realistic goals, patience, counseling, and positive reinforcement are vital. Some success has been achieved by involving adolescents in such activities as caloric calculations, nutrition planning, examination of food labels, and maintaining food records. Such activities give adolescents a sense of responsibility and a sense of accomplishment.

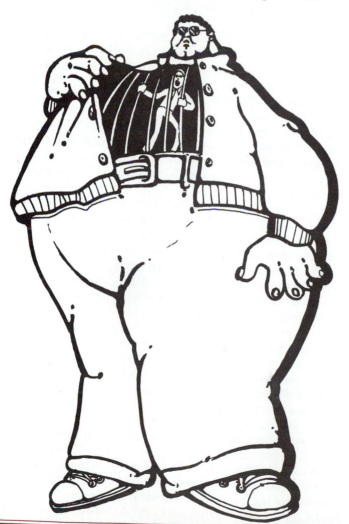

American teenagers desperately need nutrition education, and implementing this knowledge is as important as acquiring it. Good eating habits will develop if the person is motivated. A young adult pays much attention to personal appearance, emotional fluctuations, and peer opinions, but health usually does not play an important part in eating choices. Thus, in addition to learning about good dietary intake, teenagers should be introduced to behavioral modification (discussed in Chapter 20) to change old eating habits to positive new eating behaviors.

Fast Foods: Are They "Junk"?

A favorite topic of the news media is fast foods. The general public appears to have the idea that fast foods such as hamburgers, french fries, fish and chips, and thick shakes or milkshakes are bad for us (Appledorf). We will see.

Americans, especially children and adolescents, consume a significant quantity of fast foods. Estimates place one fifth of the meals we eat as being consumed away from our homes, but only one in four of those meals is eaten at a fast-food restaurant. Despite the fact that the level of fast-food consumption proves lower than many had thought, fast foods continue to be open to criticism.

Those who criticize fast foods typically cite two reasons. First, they favor natural or organic foods and thus are opposed to processed, preserved, or manufactured foods. Second, they favor protein, vitamins, and minerals and thus oppose fast foods as typically being carbohydrate, fat, and sugar.

Those criticisms can be seen as overly harsh if you consider that "fast" really does not refer to the food but to the service. When we realize that such foods as fried chicken and Mexican-American foods are typically included among the fast foods being criticized, we begin to realize that the foods may be unfairly indicted.

Rather extensive nutrient analysis of the foods typically served in fast-serve restaurants has occurred. A typical fried chicken dinner with roll, milk, potatoes, and cole slaw utilizes foods from the four basic food groups. A cheeseburger with vegetables on it, plus fries and a milkshake, also meets the four-food-group goal, as does pizza.

Using a different standard of measurement, the foods from fast-serve restaurants also fare well. U.S. Dietary Goals encourage that total caloric intake be 60 percent from carbohydrate, 30 percent from fat, and 10 percent from protein. Limits are also recommended on sugar, salt, and cholesterol intake. Pizza and hamburger meals meet those goals, too. Fried chicken dinners prove somewhat high in the caloric contribution from fats.

The verdict for foods served in fast-service settings is that they are acceptable to adequate diet planning. As with any other food, food selections should be balanced to prevent excessive intake of any particular food.

STUDY QUESTIONS

1. Discuss some nutritional benefits of breast milk. What are some other advantages of breast-feeding? What are the potential disadvantages?

2. What are some differences between the modified milk in most common infant formulas and regular cow's milk?

3. Discuss some advantages and disadvantages of bottle-feeding.

4. Discuss the nutritional adequacy of milk for the first 3 months and for the next 3 months. What supplements may be needed and under what circumstances?

5. What are some reasons why feeding solid foods to an infant during the first few months of life is not recommended?

6. What are some nutrition problems revealed by national surveys of American children?

7. What is the current thinking among nutritionists about the "clean-your-plate" rule often laid down by parents?

8. Does snacking have any potential benefits?

9. Using an appropriate reference source, compile a list of foods to which children are commonly allergic.

10. Using library resource materials, research and discuss the current research status of the relationship between diet and hyperactivity.

11. What is the *latest* meal pattern requirement for school lunches? (You may have to check into your nearest school lunch program.)

12. Why is it important that teenagers learn not to skip breakfast?

REFERENCES

Appledorf, H. "How Good Are 'Fast foods'?" *Professional Nutritionist* 14 (Winter 1982): 1.

Denny, F. W., chairman. "National Institutes of Health Consensus Development Conference: Statement on Defined Diets and Childhood Hyperactivity. *Am. J. Clin. Nutr.* 37 (1983): 161.

Hui, Y. H. *Human Nutrition and Diet Therapy.* Monterey, Calif.: Wadsworth Health Sciences, 1983.

Kolata, G. "Consensus on Diets and Hyperactivity." *Science* 215 (1982): 958.

Mailman, R. B., and M. H. Lewis. "Food Additives and Childhood Hyperactivity." *Contemporary Nutrition* 8 (June 1983): 1.

Medical World News. "'Junk Food' Ban in Schools Unlikely to Improve Nutrition." *Medical World News* 20 (1979): 41.

Riemann, H. P., et al. "Toxoplasmosis in an Infant Fed Unpasteurized Goat Milk." *J. Pediatrics* 87 (1975): 573.

Springer, N. S. *Nutrition Case Book on Developmental Disabilities.* Syracuse: Syracuse University Press, 1982.

USDA. *The National School Lunch Program and Diets of Participants.* Washington, D.C.: USDA, Human Nutrition Information Service, 1982.

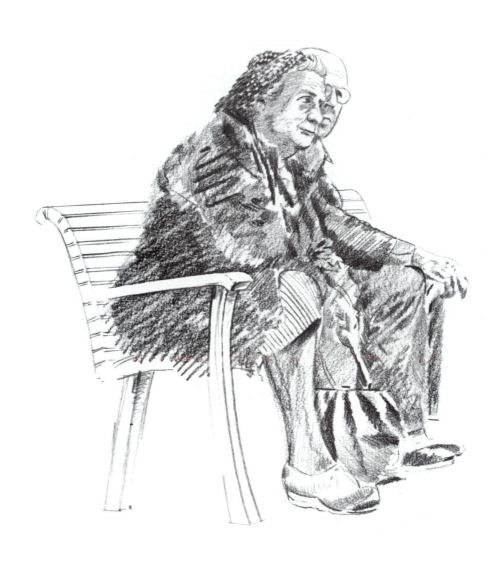

18

Nutrition AND Health OF THE Elderly

THE INCREDIBLY OLD— THE INCREDIBLY REMOTE

For years we have heard about phenomenally long-lived people who live in remote villages high in the mountains. In the early seventies, such leading publications as *National Geographic*, *Nutrition Today*, and *Scientific American* carried articles on three such isolated villages: Vilcabamba located in the Andes of Ecuador, Abkhazia located in the Caucasus Mountains of Russia, and Hunza located in the Himalayas of Pakistan. All three had villagers claiming ages well beyond 100, and nutritional secrets were rumored.

The public wanted very much to believe that these populations, living simple, isolated lives in remote mountain regions, might have found a secret to prolonged life. Some people's hopes suggested that there might be a special water, a secret herb, or a unique combination of foods that might slow the otherwise inevitable processes of aging. Rumors circulated that a fermented dairy product like yogurt with apricot kernels might be the secret.

Preliminary reports suggested that villagers in these three remote regions seemed to live extraordinary long lives characterized by especially good health. Witnesses testified that some centurians could swim long distances and climb tall mountains with little effort.

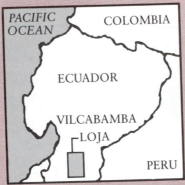

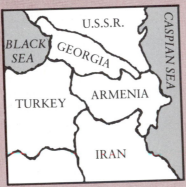

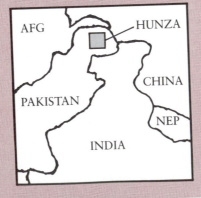

These initial findings logically called for the gathering of scientific evidence.

Dr. Alexander Leaf of Harvard Medical School, who had conducted investigations of the elderly population of Vilcabamba through interviews and site observations, returned to Ecuador to research the villagers' claims. He subsequently discovered that age exaggeration is a cultural characteristic. Other researchers had similar findings when examining village records of events such as marriage, baptisms, and births. The records revealed that age exaggeration ranged from 20 to 40 years. These follow-up studies demonstrated that the Vilcabambians are not a population of exceptional age. For example, the oldest villager was found to be 96, despite claims of some local residents being 150.

The studies showed that there is no fountain of youth in the Andes. While similar follow-up studies have not been conducted in Russia or Pakistan, the same results would be expected. Our knowledge of nutrition tells us that long-term, good dietary practices will result in quality old age, in living a little longer while enjoying good health. Miracle foods and miracle waters are not part of the world's bounty.

Adapted from: "A Staff Report: Paradise Lost." *Nutrition Today* 13 (May/June 1978): 6.

The life span of an individual has increased during the twentieth century. In the first decade of this century, life expectancy was only about 50 years; in the 1970s, the average life span was 65 to 70 years for males and 70 to 75 years for females. This older population now constitutes the fastest-growing minority group in the United States. In the early 1900s, only about 3 million people were older than 65; in 1976, there were more than 25 million. Because of the larger number of older people, many of their problems, such as housing, income, diet, and health, are now given more recognition. This recognition and subsequent study of the problems could eventually lead to further changes in the formulation and implementation of solutions. We will first consider the health status of the elderly.

Health Problems of Senior Citizens

About 60 to 70 percent of people over 65 have at least one chronic illness, and 30 to 50 percent are chronically disabled. Seniors of low socioeconomic status have more health problems, and many of the elderly have low and fixed incomes. The health status of the elderly is also affected by their degree of independence, which is best illustrated by comparing the health of those who are institutionalized with those who are not.

Many known physical factors can affect the health of an older person (Rivlin). These include heredity or genetic condition, the quality of the air and water, deleterious substances such as pesticides and harmful bacteria, tobacco in any form, alcoholic beverages, drugs, and short- and long-term nutritional intakes.

Since illness frequently accompanies old age, an older person obviously has more health concerns than a younger person. And although many of the health problems of the elderly are real, others are imaginary. Further, some can be managed, others cannot. Preoccupation with health is common in this age group, especially the functioning of the gastrointestinal tract.

The health problems of old people can be complicated by a lack of health knowledge and a surplus of misinformation. Because older people want to be healthy, possess youthful vigor, and live longer, they become very susceptible to quick cures or the unsubstantiated benefits of "patent medicines." They may be more vulnerable to quacks than are younger, healthier people.

CONSIDERATIONS IN NUTRITIONAL AND DIETARY CARE

With the understanding that health problems of the elderly are only partially related to nutrition, we look now at factors affecting older people's food intake and nutrient utilization: body changes with aging, personal factors, and specific nutrient needs (Roe).

HOW THE BODY CHANGES WITH AGING

The mechanism of human aging is still unknown, although the types of physiological and anatomical changes associated with the aging process are well documented. Various organs show progressive changes or deterioration, which are reflected in altered physiological functions. Some of these alterations have a direct impact on the nutritional and dietary status of the person, whereas others, though of clinical significance, do not. It is suspected that many changes that affect nutritional status are responsible for some of the degenerative diseases associated with aging. The major biological changes of old age are described below.

Changes in the Heart and Lungs

As a person ages, the capacity of the lungs decreases, thus decreasing the oxygen supply to various organs. This has a direct effect on the basal metabolic rate of the body.

The pumping action of the heart, blood flow, and heart muscle sensitivity to oxygen all decrease in old age. Such changes can slow blood flow and allow fatty chemicals to deposit on the walls of blood vessels. Blood clotting problems and heart disease become more likely. The smooth muscle of blood vessels is replaced by hyaline and fibrous tissue, thus reducing vascular elasticity. This causes an increase in the systolic blood pressure and pulse pressure.

Changes in Muscles, Kidneys, and Blood

As people age, muscular strength, endurance, and agility decrease. The loss of the elasticity of muscles in the abdomen and pelvis contribute to problems in defecation and urination. Also, the nitrogen content in the urine increases because the lean body mass atrophies. As indicated in Chapter 7, atrophy is a wasting condition.

The kidney eliminates waste products less efficiently. Urinary tract changes are marked by an excessive need for nighttime urination. The filtration rate of the kidney and the rate of renal blood flow are also reduced. Renal stones are more frequent, possibly because of a reduction in their solubility and a change in urinary acidity and alkalinity.

An older person may suffer forms of anemia from a variety of causes including malnutrition, malabsorption, and chronic diseases such as infections, arthritis, and cancer. Other disturbances of the intestinal system, such as bleeding from hemorrhoids, may also contribute to anemia.

Hormonal Changes: Why Grandpa Sets the Thermostat Up

Aging also involves hormonal changes. One example is that cells become less sensitive to the action of insulin in some elderly diabetics. This may increase the blood glucose level. Other hormonal changes may affect body nutrient metabolism. The atrophy of muscle or lean body mass may be partially explained by the disturbed hormonal balance.

Temperature maintenance seems to be less reliable in the aged. This fact accounts for many of the tragic deaths of older persons who succumb to extreme heat or cold.

Eating and Digestion Change, Too

In an older person, changes in the alimentary tract affect nutrient intake, digestion, and absorption. Changes occur along the entire canal—the oral cavity and the gastrointestinal system.

Elderly patients have numerous problems with the mouth: dryness, pain, a burning sensation, tongue fissures, cracking of the lips and corners of the mouth, loss of taste sensation, and difficulty in chewing and swallowing. In the oral cavity, taste, odor, and saliva all undergo changes. Taste-bud and olfactory sensitivity are altered, resulting in a loss of taste sensation and loss of the desire for food. Food becomes less appealing. Further, among many patients with upper dentures, taste sensitivity for bitter and sour decreases, though remaining normal for salty and sweet. However, many elderly people with full dentures become conditioned to this loss of taste acuity for bitter and sour.

The loss of taste sensation, especially for salt, in an older person may result from a specific nutrient deficiency (such as inadequate folic acid), degeneration of nerves supplying the oral cavity, and/or *epithelial keratinization* (structural changes of the surface layer of cells) of the tongue.

The tongue undergoes an aging process itself; in *edentulous* people (those with no teeth) it loses some of its papillae and also becomes larger (*hypertrophies*). The latter may occur because the tongue now does most of the mastication and thus increases in size. However, specific nutrient deficiencies are occasionally responsible.

The aging process definitely affects the salivary glands, causing them to make less saliva. Food becomes less palatable, and the person has difficulty in masticating, which normally involves mixing with saliva and swallowing. Saliva content also changes. There is less ptyalin (or amylase, and enzyme) and more mucus, and the saliva is ropier and more viscous. The partial digestion of starch in the mouth is reduced because of insufficient ptyalin. As a result of these saliva changes, more dental plaque forms. This, together with increased sucrose intake, permits bacteria to grow that cause tooth decay. Some elderly people are reported to have a large number of cavities. Others develop a dry mouth. The oral mucosa is often translucent and pale, although it is inflamed and atrophic in some older people. In some patients, sore spots develop under the dentures because of a lack of saliva to lubricate the area. In addition, the dentures do not stay in place well because of the reduced saliva flow. This partially explains why the elderly prefer liquid and soft diets.

There are also major changes in the gastrointestinal system. The stomach has a lower acidity because of a decrease in hydrochloric acid formation. Fewer digestive enzymes are formed and released, interfering with digestion. The intestinal mucosa becomes physically altered, which impairs digestion and absorption. Because of the decreased formation and release of bile, an older person has more difficulty in digesting fat. Reduced intestinal blood flow usually accompanies a decrease in motility of the stomach and intestines. Because of a decline in a number of intestinal absorptive cells, nutrient transport systems are modified. Loss of peristaltic tone increases the likelihood of constipation. Calculus (stone) formation in, or calcification of, the liver or gallbladder increases with advancing age. Finally, both prescription and over-the-counter drugs, which are commonly consumed by the elderly, have a profound effect on the gastrointestinal system (as discussed in the next section and in Chapter 24).

LIFESTYLE AFFECTS NUTRITION

In addition to debilitating body changes, elderly individuals may be subject to a number of personal factors that limit the adequacy of their diets. These include food habits, financial problems, limited resources, physical handicaps, psychological problems, clinical conditions, and drug use.

Lack of Money and Related Problems

Very few people do not like foods; both young and old enjoy eating. However, the past eating habits of an older person may be bad. But even though an unwholesome eating pattern should be modified as age advances, this frequently proves to be very difficult. All the unavoidable changes in later years, such as limited income, solitude, and physical handicaps, affect the traditional dietary pattern, even if an elderly person has been following a wholesome diet throughout life. The elderly also face some difficulties in adjusting to a new nutritional pattern.

Food prices keep rising, but the income of a senior citizen is usually fixed. As a result, food selection is limited, and even occasional eating out may prove impossible. The belief in the miraculous benefits of special foods such as supplements, yeast, and seaweed has drained some of the financial resources of the elderly, since most of these items are relatively expensive.

The lack of cooking utensils, refrigerators, adequate housing, storage, and kitchen facilities can affect the eating pattern of an older person. Purchasing food is sometimes difficult or impossible because of a lack of transportation. Other problems include the decreasing number of neighborhood grocery stores, unsafe neighborhoods, and the confusingly wide selection of foods in a modern supermarket. Also, for a person who cannot cook, walking to a distant restaurant can be tiring.

Loneliness and Lack of Interest

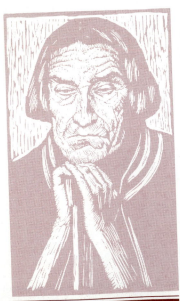

Some elderly people are very fragile, which poses numerous problems in food shopping, cooking, and eating. Many have poor teeth or none. Some elderly suffer from "old age" conditions of the esophagus such as achalasia, hiatus hernia, spasm, and diverticula, all of which can affect eating and drinking. Some may be unable to feed themselves because of the paralysis resulting from a stroke. Other physical handicaps of the aging and aged may hinder their eating and drinking ability.

The emotional and psychological makeup of older people has a tremendous influence on their nutritional and dietary intakes. Some psychological factors that can affect this population group include death of a spouse or a dear friend, lack of meaningful work or interactions because of retirement or the departure of children, loss of youthful vitality and deterioration of health, maladjustment to changes in self-image and self-regard, uneasiness after relocating, lack of social activities and companionships resulting in slow alienation, and constant fear of death.

These psychological problems can make an older person susceptible to depression, which may lead to either disinterest in food or overeating. Some individuals suffer a loss in interest and desire to shop and cook because it is troublesome to prepare meals for one person. Boredom, inconvenience, and lassitude can therefore lead to undesirable eating habits and patterns. Sometimes people may express their anger, resentment, and dejection by rejecting food or overeating.

Clinical Conditions

As a person ages, two types of clinical entities occur, those of old age, or those of *diseases* of old age. Either can lead to disability or death. It is generally agreed that good nutrition throughout life helps prevent or delay the diseases of old age, although its specific impact on delaying the aging process is still unknown. Many older persons are fit and independent without any sign of old age diseases if they follow good eating and exercise patterns. On the other hand, some older people suffer from nutritionally related clinical problems. The major ones are listed below.

Anemia. Old people are very susceptible to nutritional anemias because of deficiencies in dietary iron, folic acid, and vitamin B_{12}.

Diabetic tendency. For unknown reasons, as one ages, glucose tolerance is impaired. In some patients this results in clinical diabetes, although most patients never proceed to this stage.

Cardiovascular diseases. Heart disease is recognized as a serious problem among older men. This is further complicated by the frequently high lipid blood profiles among the elderly. High blood pressure is also common in this population group. Circulatory complications from high blood pressure may be related to a high salt intake.

Muscle atrophy. As discussed in Chapter 4, a decline in lean body mass, or muscle atrophy, becomes more evident as one ages. The resulting negative nitrogen balance is one of the fundamental signs of deteriorating nutritional status. The loss of body fat will exaggerate any protein malnutrition that may exist.

Weight imbalance. Probably the two most obvious clinical signs of nutrient imbalance are underweight and overweight. Some older people are highly susceptible to either deficient or excessive caloric consumption. More details on this topic are presented later in this chapter.

Nutrient deficiencies. Deficiencies of dietary nutrients among older Americans occur in all segments of the population, although the extent varies. However, those elderly who are alcoholic or indigent make up a sizable portion of those with nutrient deficiencies. More information on nutrient deficiency is presented later in this chapter.

Bone Diseases

Many older people, especially women, have **osteoporosis**, a disease that accounts for much bone trouble such as fractures and back pain. Chapter 12 provides some background information. Because of the importance of this disease, the following provides additional details.

Osteoporosis is a debilitating bone disorder common among American women over 60 years old. Although it also occurs in men, osteoporosis is definitely more prevalent among postmenopausal women. Experts suspect that hormonal change is one cause of the disease.

Osteoporosis literally means porous bones (bones with holes). The deteriorating condition of the bones can affect teeth and is definitely related to dental problems such as periodontal diseases and cavities. Deafness can also occur as a direct result of osteoporosis of the ear cochlea. Figure 18-1 shows the characteristic signs of osteoporosis. Although osteoporosis often is not diagnosed until its advanced stages, when serious bone fractures begin to occur, simple test procedures are available. Bone density measurement can be done by a radiologist. The test involves low radiation levels and is recommended for women who are thin, petite, sedentary, and postmenopausal.

The exact cause of osteoporosis is unknown, but inadequate dietary intake of vitamin D, calcium, and fluoride may play a role. Among these three nutrients, the biggest culprit is calcium.

Though the RDA for calcium for adult women is 800 mg, recent research indicates that typical consumption is 450 mg daily. Bone experts advise that the average consumption level creates a negative calcium balance that can result in a 1.5 percent bone loss per year.

In the first decade following menopause, a woman could lose 15 percent of her bone structure. To offset that risk, 1,000 mg have been recommended by some experts for premenopausal adult women, and 1200 to 1500 mg following menopause.

Such foods as milk, yogurt, hard cheese, sardines, turnip greens, broccoli, and mustard greens also constitute good calcium sources. Calcium carbonate serves as a fine supplement source and should be taken through the day, rather than all at once, for better absorption.

Figure 18-1: The "dowager's hump" in a patient with osteoporosis. Some patients with the appearance are asymptomatic.
SOURCE: J. Ingham. Drugs, 8(1974):290

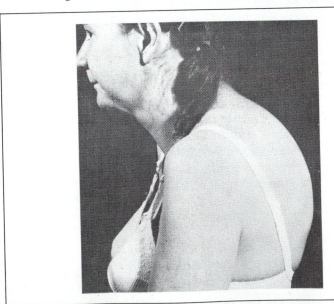

Calcium supplements may slow or stop bone loss, but by themselves they cannot increase bone mass. Presently, physicians prescribe sodium fluoride for osteoporosis victims in addition to calcium supplement. Some patients have benefited from such double treatment. However, the use of fluoride should be monitored by a physician in view of its toxicity.

Exercise proves the most effective natural way of increasing bone mass. Stress on bones strengthens them, so walking, jogging, bicycling, and dancing are activities that can help prevent osteoporosis. Exercise must, however, be balanced. Inactivity results in bone loss, but excessive exercise can, especially for women, result in ultrathinness.

Drugs

Because debilitating conditions are common among some elderly people, drugs are frequently prescribed. The drugs most frequently used are aimed at correcting problems of the mind, the heart and circulation, blood pressure and chemistry, pain, infection, the alimentary tract, and nutritional deficiencies. Complete information on the relationship between drugs and nutrients in the body is presented in Chapter 24, but we will give a brief overview of the effects of drugs commonly prescribed for older people here (Hui).

Drugs prescribed for the mind include those that treat mental disorders, are antidepressant, or produce sedation. Chlorpromazine (Thorazine) is used to treat mental disorders, especially in the elderly. Because it stimulates food intake, overconsumption and overweight can become problems. Monoamine oxidase inhibitors (for example, isocarboxazid) are antidepressants; they can interact with tyramine in such foods as cheese to produce hypertensive crisis. Frequently, high blood pressure is already a problem in an older person. Other antidepressants may cause constipation and paralytic ileus (intestinal obstruction).

Sedatives are employed by elderly people to combat anxiety, insomnia, or nocturnal restlessness. Popular prescriptions include barbiturates and benzodiazepines (Librium, Valium, and Dalmane). These chemical compounds affect the nutritional status of individuals in many ways. Barbiturates may induce vitamin deficiencies by interfering with absorption and secretion. In some cases, because of the strong effects of these sedatives and hypnotics, an elderly person may become confused and take an overdose. As a result of such drug-induced confusion and forgetfulness, he or she may also neglect food and liquid intake, which may, in extreme form, result in dehydration and starvation.

Drugs for the heart and circulation are prescribed for a large number of elderly people. Common ones such as digitalis glycosides and quinidine can confuse the patient and precipitate nausea and vomiting. Because of this reaction, the older patient may eat less, although the nausea and vomiting may help an obese patient lose weight. Nevertheless, using these drugs to control weight is obviously unacceptable.

Control of high blood pressure in the elderly is a major task in geriatric medicine. However, antihypertensive chemical compounds such as hydralazine may induce vitamin deficiency, and the use of diuretics to control blood pressure can create numerous problems. For example, the use of furosemide (Lasix) may increase potassium excretion and result in hypokalemia in the patient. Often the symptoms of low blood potassium, such as lethargy and muscular weakness, are passed off as signs of old age, but hypokalemia can complicate other existing clinical conditions in the patient and may be fatal.

Many older patients are treated for other problems related to the blood, including such common illnesses as anemia, blood clots, and varicose veins. Some of the therapeutic chemicals used to treat these illnesses have an adverse effect on nutritional status. On the other hand, anticoagulants such as coumarin may be counteracted (negated) by the vitamin K included in some vitamin supplements when the patient uses these supplements at the same time. Long-term use of large doses of iron may produce constipation or diarrhea, although the use of hematologic agents does not necessarily produce such problems.

The need to relieve pain in some older patients necessitates the use of analgesics and antiinflammatory agents (for arthritis) such as aspirin (salicylates) and corticosteroids. The former may cause intestinal bleeding; the latter may cause ulcers. The use of antibiotics in older people, though not a common practice, can have a profound effect on body nutrients. As an example, neomycin interferes with the absorption of essential nutrients (Chapter 24).

Probably the drugs most "abused" by older people are those that regulate intestinal functions. Older people frequently use antacids to treat indigestion and heartburn. One complication of the long-term use of certain antacids is the excessive consumption of sodium. Laxative usage by American senior citizens has become legend, so much so that a large percentage of prime-time TV commercials are devoted to the sale of these products. Some common side effects from frequent use of laxatives are prolonged constipation, dehydration, and electrolyte (mineral) imbalance. Psychological and physiological dependence on laxatives occurs in many patients. Also see Chapter 14 regarding these common intestinal problems.

In the United States the pursuit of health has made many elderly people believe in the miracle of vitamin and mineral supplements. Sometimes they are prescribed by physicians to correct genuine nutrient deficiencies. However, indiscriminate use of these supplements can cause poisoning. The adverse effects of high doses of niacin, ascorbic acid, and vitamins A and D are discussed in Chapters 8, 9, and 10.

NUTRITIONAL NEEDS

Like people of all ages, an elderly person must have an adequate intake of nutrients and food. It is generally agreed that the consumption, digestion, absorption, utilization, storage, and excretion of nutrients are all affected by nutrition and the physiological, psychological, social, economic, and cultural changes associated with old age. However, there have been very few controlled studies to ascertain the appropriate nutrient intakes of the elderly. One thing is certain: There is no single "special" or "right" food for someone who is growing old.

Although there is very little documented information to indicate the exact nutrient requirements of the elderly, experts in the field generally assume that, with the exception of calories, the RDAs of an older person are about the same as those of a 25-year-old. A brief analysis is provided below (Roe).

Calories

According to the current RDAs, the daily caloric requirement for people over 50 decreases. Some reasons for this decline include a decrease in the basal metabolic rate, atrophy of the lean body mass, and decreased activity. Retirement, a relaxed attitude, disability, or chronic illness can decrease daily activities. Many older women expend less energy because their children have left home.

Experts agree that a man between 60 and 70 uses about 75 to 90 percent of the calories of a 25-year-old. There is no fixed daily caloric recommendation for ages above 50, although caloric intake should correlate with the person's age, physical activity, and body function. Being underweight or obese should be avoided.

Protein

We can study the protein need of an elderly person from a number of perspectives. According to the latest RDA, an adult needs about 0.8 g of protein per kg of body weight. It is estimated that the senior population in this country consumes about 40 to 50 g of protein a day, less than is recommended for most of them. One study concluded that many women under 40 years of age consumed nearly twice as much meat, poultry, and fish as women over 70. However, given the many factors involved in the nutritional and dietary care of an older individual, it is difficult to conclude exactly what the most appropriate amount of protein for an older person is.

It must be emphasized that the protein consumption of an older person should not be excessive, since kidney problems increase as age advances. A large amount of ammonia and urea must be excreted if too much protein is eaten. On the other hand, many clinical problems of the elderly may be related to insufficient protein intake, including such complaints as fatigue, backache, and hair loss. Low protein consumption usually means that the intake of many essential nutrients occurring in protein-rich foods is also inadequate.

There are many possible reasons why the protein intake of an older person may be less than what is recommended. Since most protein foods are expensive, many senior citizens have few opportunities to get good and tasty protein-rich products such as meat, fish, and poultry. Another good source of protein is milk. A decline in consumption of dairy products may be due to high cost or adverse intestinal reactions such as lactose intolerance or constipation.

Another major reason for the decreased intake of good protein food among senior citizens is dental problems. Loss of teeth and poor-fitting dentures make it difficult to chew meat. Because of the decline in the total intake of food or calories among the elderly, much of the protein they consume is actually used as energy sources. The overall result is a decrease in both protein intake and utilization efficiency.

Because many elderly people have chronic illnesses, protein absorption and utilization and nitrogen retention may all be affected. Older people characteristically have an unusually high nitrogen content in their urine. Their ability to retain nitrogen may be decreased or may become less efficient with a concomitant slow atrophy of the lean body mass. One additional cause may be common psychiatric problems such as depression. Emotional instability has been related to decreased nitrogen retention. There is also some nitrogen loss because of reduced physical activity.

Carbohydrate

Carbohydrate should provide 50 to 55 percent of an older person's total daily caloric intake. Carbohydrate and protein intakes should be co-ordinated so that there is sufficient carbohydrate to "spare" protein but not so much that protein intake is limited.

About 40 to 45 percent of carbohydrate consumption should be starch and other complex forms, with sugar intake limited to about 5 to 10 percent. An older person should be careful not to eat too many sugary products, because they may increase dental problems, are notoriously "empty-caloried," and can inhibit the intake of essential nutrients. Persons over 40 are susceptible to the development of diabetes. Pancreatic malfunctioning, decreased cellular sensitivity to insulin, or glucose mal-utilization may impair glucose tolerance.

Lactose in milk products poses a difficult problem; intolerance to this disaccharide is being recognized more frequently in older people, although the reason is unknown. One should always ascertain whether an elderly person can drink milk and eat dairy products without intestinal discomfort.

Fat

There is much controversy surrounding the quantity and quality of fat needed or eaten by older people. The major question is the effect of dietary fat on the cause and outcome of heart disease. It is also noted that an aging digestive system provides less pancreatic lipase for fat digestion and absorbs fat less efficiently. Currently, it is recommended that the fat intake of people over 50 should make up about 30 percent or less of their total caloric intake.

Vitamins and Minerals

Vitamin and mineral deficiencies in elderly people are common. Vitamin deficiency in the elderly progresses in five stages: (1) body storage depletion; (2) an abnormal biochemical profile; (3) physiological maladjustments such as general tiredness and anorexia; (4) general clinical manifestations such as anemia, hair loss, and weight loss; and (5) identifiable clinical symptoms with organs manifesting pathological conditions.

The elderly have the same stated requirement for vitamins as 25-year-olds, although old people are suspected of having a higher need. A brief analysis of the vitamin needs of senior citizens follows.

Vitamin C is the vitamin most likely to be low in the diet and blood of older people, especially those who are chronically ill or living alone. The body's ability to retain the vitamin appears to decline, and there is definitely a reduced level of vitamin C in the tissues, blood, and cerebrospinal fluid of older people. The low intake of this vitamin in some senior citizens is probably related to their lifelong eating habits; others limit their intake of fresh fruits and vegetables because these foods are expensive and contain undigestible cellulose. The need for vitamin C may be especially high during old age, possibly because of decreased efficiency in utilization, although the relationship between vitamin C metabolism and old age is very complex. As discussed earlier, drug use can decrease the absorption and increase the excretion of vitamins, including vitamin C.

Thiamine (vitamin B_1) deficiency in old age can be brought about in several ways. First, old age itself may increase the need and decrease the efficiency of utilization of thiamine. Second, certain drugs can decrease absorption, increase excretion, and distort proper metabolism of the vitamin. For example, diuretics can increase excretion. Third, excessive alcohol consumption can result in the well-known Wernicke's disease, although this syndrome is actually associated with multiple nutrient deficiencies. Fourth, because of the decreased secretion of hydrochloric acid in the stomach, thiamine can be inactivated there. Fifth, clinical circumstances such as fever, cancer, or the intravenous administration of dextrose may precipitate thiamine deficiency. Finally, a low-cost, starchy diet can precipitate deficiency, since the metabolism of carbohydrate requires a large amount of thiamine.

For vitamin B_2 (riboflavin), an increased need because of old age is suspected. The clinical use of testosterone therapy and tissue repair from trauma such as bedsores may increase the requirement. The types and quantity of intestinal flora may adversely affect the utilization, synthesis, and secretion of riboflavin.

The need for pyridoxine, or vitamin B_6, is governed by a number of factors. Generally increased need during old age; the use of drugs such as isoniazid or penicillamine, which induce deficiency; adverse effects of the intestinal flora on the absorption and synthesis of the vitamin; and decreased intestinal mucus secretion of vitamin B_6 all can occur. Finally, urinary tract infections may be associated with vitamin B_6 deficiency.

Folic acid deficiency is common in old people. Reasons for the deficiency are an increased body need, the effects of drugs, an insufficient intake, destruction during cooking, a decreased absorption and utilization, reduced intestinal synthesis, and decreased intestinal mucus secretion.

As discussed in Chapter 9, there is a very important clinical relationship between folic acid and vitamin B_{12}, since vitamin B_{12} deficiency can be masked by a large dose of folic acid. The deficiency of vitamin B_{12} in older people may reflect decreased absorption, gastric atrophy with a decrease in intrinsic factor (see Chapter 9), or abnormal bacterial growth in the small intestine. Although serious vitamin B_{12} deficiency can result in neurodegeneration, the relationship between psychiatric problems in the elderly and vitamin B_{12} deficiency is not clear. However, some studies have shown that when older patients are given B_{12} injections or even oral doses, the symptoms of fatigue disappear and the person's sense of disorientation and confusion can be alleviated. Other studies have reported negative results.

Vitamin B_{12} and folic acid can be affected by iron intake; a decreased iron intake will decrease their absorption. Iron, B_{12}, and folic acid are responsible for the well-known nutritional anemia in some older Americans.

The absorption of all fat-soluble vitamins is affected by a low fat intake, insufficient secretion of bile, pancreatic failure, and extensive dependence on antibiotics and laxatives. The conversion of provitamin A to the vitamin may be affected by old age. Deficiencies of vitamin D (and thus calcium) are partially responsible for osteoporosis. For example, low milk consumption and little exposure to sunlight are major factors in vitamin D deficiency. Excessive consumption of vitamins A and D in supplements is always hazardous, but especially so for older people. For those older individuals for whom a diet high in polyunsaturated fat is prescribed, the requirement for vitamin E may be increased to preclude oxidation of the fat. Some clinicians therefore prescribe vitamin E supplement for these individuals.

Vitamin K may be deficient in some older people, but not from insufficient dietary intake. A number of clinical conditions predispose older people to this vitamin deficiency, including liver and gallbladder disease, excessive use of antibiotics, excessive use of aspirin or related chemicals (salicylates), decreased intestinal synthesis of the vitamin for various reasons, and the excessive use of mineral oil. Ecchymosis (bruising) is a sign of possible vitamin K deficiency.

According to the 1980 RDAs, an older person requires the same essential minerals as a 25-year-old, including calcium, phosphorus, iodine, iron, magnesium, and zinc. Older people may, however, have a special need for fluoride, although this has not yet been confirmed. Iron, calcium, and fluoride intakes require special attention because of the incidence of nutritional anemia and osteoporosis in the older population. Since calcium absorption is related to the dietary intake of phosphorus, the latter is of obvious importance.

Calcium deficiency plays an important role in the development of osteoporosis (see Chapter 12). Low calcium intake may be due to consuming too few dairy products. However, osteoporosis has multiple etiologies. For example, many patients show clinical improvement when given sodium fluoride.

Iron deficiency among the elderly is common and may result from many causes, including a low intake. Elderly women living alone who consume only doughnuts, coffee, and a limited number of other food items are commonly affected by iron deficiency anemia. Fortunately, anemia can be easily identified in an older person. In general, iron deficiency is less common among elderly men.

The water and fiber requirements of an older person are especially important. As indicated earlier, aging is accompanied by decreased intestinal muscle tone and reduced peristalsis. This condition usually results in constipation. To manage constipation, a person should drink 6 to 8 glasses of water daily and eat abundant whole grains, fresh fruits, and vegetables that will contribute fiber or cellulose. If desired, the liquid may be hot bouillon (not recommended if salt is not advised), coffee, tea, fruit juice, or vegetable juice to add variety. Consult Chapter 5 for more information on the importance of fiber in the diet. Also see Chapter 14 for more details on constipation. Nutrition education may be needed if the person does not like some of the suggested foods.

Assessment of Nutritional Status in Older People

The assessment of the nutritional status of a given population group proves a formidable task, one with many options. For example, as discussed in Chapter 22, nutritional status can be determined on the basis of food intake, on the basis of physical and biochemical tests, on the basis of frequency of health complaints or the incidence of clinical conditions, or on any combination of these methods.

The elderly constitute a population group whose nutritional status has been the subject of surveys. Three such national surveys can be reviewed for the insights they provide concerning the nutriture of our elderly. Details about these surveys, especially their limitations, are presented in Chapter 22. The following summarizes the results of the three surveys (Kart and Metress).

HOUSEHOLD FOOD CONSUMPTION SURVEY, 1965–1966

In general, this survey showed that older men fulfilled recommended daily allowances for more nutrients than did older women. The aged tended to be most low in vitamin B_6 and magnesium, though iron, calcium, vitamin A, thiamine, and riboflavin were often low as well. An important finding of the study was that inadequate diet correlated with low income. Two thirds of those with less than $3,000 in after-tax income had less than adequate diets.

In regard to the use of vitamin and mineral supplements, the elderly were high users. One third of those over 75 used such supplements. The use of supplements was found to increase in relation to income.

TEN-STATE NUTRITION SURVEY, 1968–1970

Among the aged, those 60 and over consumed far less than needed for good nutriture. The elderly had lower calorie intake than young individuals. The elderly, however, obtained their calories from better nutrient sources. For example, elderly females had good protein, vitamin A and C, and iron intake. Blacks showed a high vitamin A intake, whereas Mexican-Americans were low in that vitamin.

Generally the survey found that those residing in the lower-income southern states had lower intakes of protein, niacin, and iron.

The physical assessments made showed periodontal (gum) disease occurred in over 90 percent of those aged 65 to 75. The gum disease appeared to be associated with lack of dental care rather than with malnutrition. In terms of obesity, 45 percent of black women were found obese in the 55 to 65 age group. One third of the white women in that same age group were obese. Higher income was associated with obesity in both black and white males.

HEALTH AND NUTRITION EXAMINATION SURVEY, 1971–1972
Low caloric intake was significant among those 60 or over. For those who were low income, 27 percent of the white and 36 percent of the black aged had daily caloric intake below 1000 calories. Protein intake was closely related to total caloric intake.

Iron and vitamin A intakes were below standards for over half of those 60 and over. For blacks below the poverty level, 55 percent had less than adequate vitamin C intake. Whites below the poverty level were more likely to have substandard iron intake than whites above the poverty level.

Obesity patterns were similar to those of the Ten-State Survey. A moderate risk of niacin deficiency was found for all the aged in this survey. With the exception of blacks, the aged showed little risk of vitamin C deficiency.

Practically all nutritional surveys done in this country show that our elderly are nutritionally vulnerable. This vulnerability appears to be not so much a consequence of age as it is a consequence of poverty.

Planning a Good Diet

In providing dietary care for the older population, providers of care should remember that each person has unique problems and must be evaluated individually. The multiple considerations discussed in this chapter should be reviewed. The elderly as a population group can be aided nutritionally only when those who work with them can perceive the entire environment in which a particular individual lives. The nutritional and dietary care of senior citizens must be supplemented by a complete understanding and consideration of the social, economic, psychological, environmental, and clinical factors involved (Hui).

Care givers should take into account the person's present nutritional status and eating patterns, age, lifelong eating habits, income, social standing, education, activity, illnesses, physical handicaps, psychological problems, and living arrangements (independent living versus institutionalization). Nutrition education may be needed, for although it is never too early or late to establish good eating habits, the eating habits of an older person may be more ingrained than those of a younger person. All abnormal physical and other conditions that may result in poor nutritional status should be corrected as much as possible. Some elderly people may need advice on how to spend money wisely on food.

In diet planning, the total calories of an older person should be reduced, but all other essential nutrients must be provided in adequate quantities. Chapter 15 should be consulted for some basic information about planning a balanced diet. Using the basic four food groups is a good start. The foundation diet for an older person should contain about 1100 to 1200 kcal a day (see Table 18-1).

Table 18-1
Suggested Foundation Diet for an Elderly Person

FOOD GROUPS*	SAMPLE SERVING
Milk and equivalent; e.g., yogurt, ice cream	2 to 8 oz milk
Meat and equivalents; e.g., eggs, legumes, peas, peanut butter	2 to 4 oz cooked lean meat
Vegetable and fruit	½ c yellow or deep green vegetables ½ c other vegetable 1 medium cooked (baked) potato 6 oz tomato, orange, or grapefruit juice (citrus juices) 1 serving other fruit or juice, such as apple, banana
Cereal and equivalents; e.g., bread, macaroni	3 sl bread ⅔ c cereal

* For complete information on different food items in the food groups, consult Chapter 15

The diet shown in Table 18-1 meets the RDAs for older people in all nutrients except calories. When one uses this foundation diet in meal planning, the foods mentioned may be combined in the cooking process and need not be consumed in the forms listed. The food items listed may not be very flavorful by themselves, since they lack the fat and sugar normally found in pastries, honey, cream, butter, and gravies. All these appetizing additions may be used, although overindulging in any of these items should be avoided.

In using the foundation for older people, good protein foods include meat, poultry, fish, and cheese, especially if they are cooked until tender. Many elderly individuals do not include such items in their diet for reasons such as low income, ignorance of protein value, and poor dental condition. Many elderly people have problems with milk. It is costly, it may cause diarrhea or constipation, some older people simply do not like it, and it may not be advisable for some people because of its high saturated-fat and cholesterol content. All these parameters must be taken into consideration when planning menus with milk as a major source of calcium, vitamin B_2, and possibly protein. For some older people, low-fat or skim milk can be used as a beverage or in cooking. If fluid milk must be totally excluded, more tender meat, canned fish, cheese, and similar protein-rich foods (such as yogurt) may be used; however, the calcium intake must be monitored if milk is excluded from the diet.

In determining how many calories should be added to the foundation diet to meet a particular older person's needs, body weight is the major index.

It can be assumed that a person 60 years old should weigh the same as when he or she was 25. If the person is not underweight or overweight and is doing a fair amount of activity such as walking or light gardening, a daily intake of 1,600 to 1,900 kcal for a male and about 1,500 to 1,700 kcal for a female is sufficient. If the person is underweight or overweight, the caloric intake should be adjusted so that he or she will achieve the optimal weight and then maintain it.

In planning menus for older people, the foods should be those that they like, with as few restrictions as possible. This will ensure that similar foods can be found in restaurants or friends' homes. A reasonable arrangement is to use a combination of the foundation foods and a fair amount of those other items that the person likes. Foods with low-fat sauces will help those with a reduced saliva flow. The family, patient, or nursing home operator must be carefully taught how to provide the diet, with special attention to food preparation and the size of serving portions. Table 18-2 gives sample menus for 7 days for an elderly person.

Under- vs. Overnutrition

An older person with an intestinal problem may have many nutritional and dietary complications. However, for healthy elderly individuals, inadequate dietary intakes and overeating are probably the most widespread problems.

Inadequate dietary nutrient intakes may result from many factors, including a decreased intake of food or a selective eating habit (that is, eating the same one or two foods daily). Those who do not eat enough food may be suffering from dental problems, lack of money, loneliness, or other factors discussed earlier. Many are underweight and exhibit old-age symptoms such as backache, tiredness, weakness, loss of alertness, and nutrient deficiencies or a borderline nutritional status. Some may have other pathological conditions, such as chronic illness.

GERTRUDE—
A CHALLENGE FOR A NURSING HOME

After several falls at home, Gertrude was placed in a nursing home by her only daughter. Gertrude was overweight at admission as she had been for most of her 81 years.

The nursing home staff noted that Gertrude had several health conditions that affected her nutritional status. She suffered from constipation, poorly fitted dentures, and confusion. She also had difficulty holding utensils, and chewing and swallowing, so she rarely finished a meal because it cooled and lost its palatability.

The staff considered what dietary regimen would be most appropriate for Gertrude. Of her various conditions, the weight problem was the most obvious, but the staff knew there were several considerations. For example, if Gertrude were placed on a diet, she *might* follow it if she could be convinced of the importance the doctor placed on it. Her reaction to the diet, however, might be adverse. Rebelling against it could lead to anger and frustration that would elevate her blood pressure. Or, she might violate the diet by getting

food from her daughter, other patients, or vending machines.

Assuming that Gertrude would conclude her life in the nursing home (unless she were transferred to an acute care facility), what courses of nutritional and dietary care would *you* recommend for her? Is there a dietary approach that will recognize Gertrude as a complete human being? Using library resources, find information that supports your recommendation.

Table 18-2
A Week's Sample Menus for an Older Person

Snacks: Some suggested items are fresh fruit; soft, dried prunes; whole wheat crackers with cheese; cheese sticks; peanut butter on toast; and yogurt. Snacks may be served in mid-morning, mid-afternoon, and/or before bedtime.

BREAKFAST	LUNCH	DINNER
Monday		
½ c orange juice	1 c creamed tuna on noodles	1 c chicken, rice, and pea casserole
Poached eggs	Celery or carrot sticks	½ c buttered spinach
Whole wheat toast	1 c skim milk	Fresh fruit; banana, melon
2 slices bacon	1 orange	Decaffeinated coffee
Tuesday		
½ c grapefruit juice	Cottage cheese with pineapple salad	3 oz broiled fish
½ c cooked oatmeal, sugar, and milk	Banana	½ c mashed potato
1 fruit or 2 sausages	Toasted raisin bread with butter	½ c creamed peas
	Tea or decaffeinated coffee	Celery sticks
		Gingerbread, 1 square
		Decaffeinated coffee
Wednesday		
Sliced banana and milk	1 c split pea soup	1 c beef and vegetable stew
2 bran muffins	Tomato and shredded lettuce salad	½ c cabbage coleslaw
1 baked egg with cheese	Crackers and cheese	½ c rice pudding
1 orange	Skim milk	Decaffeinated coffee
	1 pear	
Thursday		
3 stewed prunes	1 c minestrone soup	3 oz hamburger steak
2 French toast slices with butter and syrup	Cottage cheese and peach salad	½ c mashed potatoes
8 oz skim milk	2 crackers	½ c buttered broccoli
	Skim milk	1 sliced tomato with dressing
	Decaffeinated coffee	2 oatmeal cookies
		½ c gelatin
Friday		
Sliced orange	Tomato and rice soup	1 c tuna noodle casserole
1 c puffed rice with milk and sugar	⅔ c potato salad	½ c mixed vegetables
Sliced cheese	Celery or green pepper sticks	½ c lettuce salad
Hot tea	½ c strawberries	1 slice angel food cake
	Skim milk	Decaffeinated coffee
Saturday		
Melon or fresh fruit	1 c creamed chicken and mushrooms on toast	1 c spaghetti and meatballs in tomato sauce
3 hotcakes	½ c carrot and raisin salad	½ c string beans
2 sausages	Fresh fruit	½ c fruit gelatin
8 oz skim milk	Skim milk	Decaffeinated coffee
Sunday		
3 stewed figs	2-egg cheese omelet	1 baked pork chop with applesauce
½ c hot cream of wheat	½ c steamed rice	½ c buttered peas
Milk	½ c asparagus	1 baked potato
2 slices crisp bacon	Celery or carrot sticks	Lettuce wedge
8 oz hot chocolate made with skim milk	8 oz skim milk	½ c custard
		Decaffeinated coffee

NOTE: Each day's caloric contribution is about 1,800 kcal. The amount can be increased or decreased by adjusting the serving sizes. Thus, the serving sizes of some items are not provided. If there is concern about the cholesterol in eggs, replace some egg servings with lean meat (e.g., turkey), fish, and so on.

Those whose diets provide plenty of calories but are lacking in nutrients will not be underweight, but they may have the other symptoms of old age, such as backache. Their main problem is eating foods that are high in calories and low in essential nutrients. This inclination may be related to physical or physiological handicaps. For example, dry mouth and ill-fitting dentures predispose them to eating processed foods such as frozen dinners, sugary pastries, and canned spaghetti. Many of these prepackaged foods are soft, require minimal cooking, and are tasty. But they are high in cost and low in good proteins and essential vitamins and minerals.

Why are some older Americans overweight? Some health professionals believe that many of them eat too many calories and drink too many alcoholic beverages. Foods such as fatty beef, potato chips, and pastries are all fattening. Individuals who eat these foods may or may not have essential nutrient deficiencies. Inactivity is also a major cause of obesity in this population group; the elderly often lead sedentary lives with little exercise and too much sleep (8 to 12 hours versus 6 to 10 hours for young adults). Some elderly people eat excessively because of psychological problems, and others have carried obesity from childhood into old age.

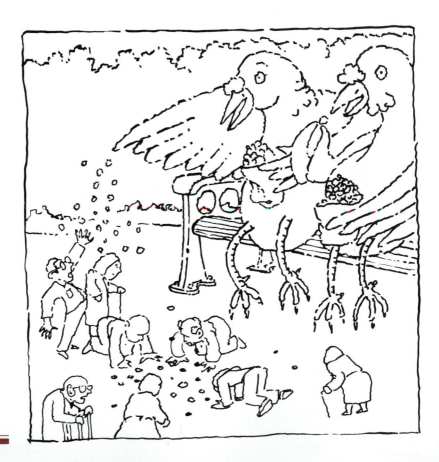

Programs Benefiting the Elderly

THE FOOD STAMP PROGRAM

For background information on the Food Stamp Program, consult Chapter 22. In 1976 a Department of Agriculture survey found one or more elderly persons in 17 percent of the food stamp households. This statistic projects to over 1 million elderly participants, about half of whom were living alone. The majority of the single-person households were women. The Food Stamp Program has been viewed by various observers as being the single most important program for providing assistance to all needy families, especially the elderly. It is one directly focused on nutrition.

TITLE III OF THE OLDER AMERICANS ACT

Title III of the Older Americans Act was established in 1978 to combine various services, including nutrition, for older Americans (Hui). An important forerunner to this legislation was Title VII (Public Law 92-128), the National Nutrition Program for the Elderly, which was passed in 1973. (At the time of this writing a proposed federal budget cut would have eliminated this program partly or completely.)

This legislation is currently administered by the Administration on Aging, Office of Human Development, Department of Health and Human Services. Its major responsibility is to grant money to each state for specific nutrition projects that are designed for individuals over 60. Some basic aims of this legislation are to provide the elderly with (1) nutritious and hot meals at a low cost, (2) food and nutrition education, (3) an opportunity for socialization and recreation, (4) information on other health and social assistance programs, and (5) low-cost and convenient transportation. Aggressive outreach programs and personal approaches to the elderly provide senior citizens with the incentive to use these services.

Although the federal government provides the money, private or public nonprofit organizations such as churches and women's clubs usually run the food programs. Any such organization should have an advisory board consisting of local citizens and professionals. Each organization is required to have a dietitian or nutritionist on its staff to provide professional advice about the foods and nutritional needs of older citizens.

At present, two special programs are common: home-delivery programs ("Meals-on-Wheels") and congregate meals programs. In the first program, meals are served to individuals at their homes for various reasons. They may be living in isolated spots far away from large meal centers, or chronic illnesses or disability may make it inconvenient or impractical to transport them to a meal center. The second program appears to be more common, although accurate statistics are lacking. Older citizens come to a central kitchen where they are served hot, nutritious meals and at the same time engage in social interaction.

The policy on the cost of the meals is simple. Older citizens who prefer to pay may do so; otherwise, the meals are free. Meals served at home may be paid for with food stamps, but congregate meals may not.

The meals served should contain:

1. Milk or other source of calcium (one serving; e.g., 8 oz of milk).
2. Meat, fish, or poultry (one serving; e.g., 3 oz).
3. Bread or equivalent (e.g., 1 or 2 slices).
4. Vegetables and fruits (2 servings of green/yellow vegetables and other fruits.
5. Desserts such as pastries, pie, or cake (one serving).

Although the number of meals served each day has declined from 1978 levels, the program continues and has a significant nutritional focus. As with all meal planning for older people, these special feeding programs must take into consideration the person's situation and his or her environment.

THE SOCIAL SECURITY ACT

Since its inception in 1935, the Social Security Act has been amended to add various benefits. Originally it was a pension program and a federal-state unemployment insurance system. In 1948, just 13 percent of those 65 and older were receiving social security benefits. With the 1983 amendments, almost all workers are covered by the program.

Social security eligibility is based on work rather than need. The average monthly benefit for a retired worker in 1980 was $330, a level below the maximum because many retired workers either retired early and forfeited the maximum benefit or else did not have sufficient covered employment during their work years to qualify for maximum benefits.

The social security program has significantly reduced poverty among the aged. Accordingly, since we know that nutrition and income are linked, the program has significantly improved the nutrition of the elderly.

Supplemental Security Income (SSI) is a section of the Social Security Act that provides assistance for the needy, the blind, and the disabled. Over 4 million people are aided by this special section of the legislation. It provides monthly payments, with a maximum that is below the average worker benefit; however, these supplemental payments are not based on work earnings but on need as evidenced by an assets test.

MEDICARE

Although Medicare is also an amendment to the Social Security Act, it deserves special recognition as being our nation's system of individual health services for the elderly. The program has further been amended since its inception in 1966 to provide assistance to the disabled and to those with chronic kidney disease.

Almost 100 percent of the United States elderly are enrolled in the portion of Medicare that provides a hospital insurance plan. The other portion of Medicare coverage, that for supplemental medical insurance, involves over 95 percent of the elderly. Both portions of Medicare pay part of the patient's expenses.

In 1981, Medicare payments were almost $1,300 per aged person, an

NUTRITION EDUCATION FOR THE ELDERLY: ONE WORKABLE PROGRAM

The North West Division of Talman Home Federal Savings and Loan Association in Chicago and a local consulting dietitian demonstrated (Bonnett and Carlson) just what nutritionists and dietitians can accomplish when they are alert to new opportunities to provide nutrition education. The association's manager of financial planning services realized that a significant segment of their customers were senior citizens concerned about scarce financial resources, health, and fitness. With the help of a registered dietitian, a program was designed.

Titled "You're in Command: Finances for Food and Fitness," the program was developed to enable senior citizens to improve their financial management skills and to understand the basics of a nutritious diet. The senior citizens were shown how the Consumer Price Index works and how it can be used to make and adjust financial plans according to price trends. The seniors were also shown how a management plan for food costs is composed of: (1) serving nutritious meals within a dollar limit, (2) preparing definite written plans such as menus and shopping lists, (3) fulfilling the plans, and (4) evaluating the accomplishments.

To enable the senior savers to better understand nutritional

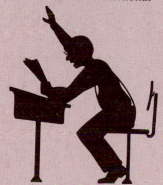

planning, a dietitian reviewed with them such issues as aging's effects on dietary habits. Especially addressed were dental and periodontal changes, decreased motility, lowered caloric need, osteoporosis, and new research findings.

Participants were asked to identify themselves as belonging to one of three groups, based on dietary habits: (1) whose who snack all day long, (2) those who eat three or four meals daily but meals built around tea and toast, or (3) those who strive to eat from the four basic food groups. Recipes were given to participants.

The program's theme of being in command emphasized the participants' choices. They could choose to cut food costs, to have more nutritious meals, to have fewer health problems, and to look and feel healthy.

The use of such audiovisual aids as transparencies and filmstrips enhanced the program. Posters also added to the atmosphere of the training session. Some forty publications were given to participants.

The collaboration of a consumer educator and a nutrition educator brought about an effective program design for reaching a specific group, the elderly. The approach offers a challenge to others who wish to accomplish creative nutritional education.

annual expenditure of over $32 billion! A companion program, Medicaid, covers many costs that Medicare does not, such as nursing home care. Another $9 billion was paid to nursing homes in 1981. The Medicaid program is jointly funded by federal and state government.

PUBLIC HOUSING

The Housing Act of 1937 initiated federal involvement in housing and was considered in 1956 to specifically address housing for the elderly.

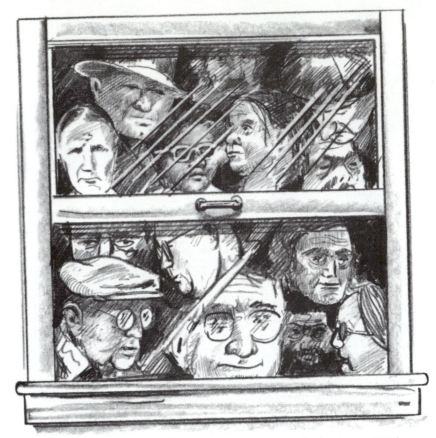

The program is administered by the Department of Housing and Urban Development. Over three-quarters of a million people have benefitted, and 80 percent of those live in housing for the elderly.

Most public housing for the elderly consists of high-rise apartments. Tenants pay rent on a sliding scale based on their ability to pay. A special section of the Housing Act, Section 202, provides for independent living for the elderly, as well as for handicapped persons. Section 202 enables nonprofit organizations to obtain loans to develop and operate multi-family units. By 1979 some 45,000 units had been constructed at over 300 project sites. The sites are generally in residential neighborhoods, and most occupants are middle-income whites.

Section 8 provides house rent subsidies for the elderly. Low-income families pay no more than 25 percent of their income for rent. If the fair rental value of the housing is higher than that, the government pays the difference. About one-quarter of a million rent subsidies are paid each year, and about 25 percent of those are received by the elderly.

Although such programs as public housing do not address nutrition, they do indirectly improve the nutrition and health of our elderly in two ways. They provide a secure, warm environment that permits the person to conserve body heat. They also provide some relief from costs that would otherwise leave little money for food.

STUDY QUESTIONS

1. Describe the health status of older people in this country according to the latest statistics.

2. Explain the effects of aging on at least five of the following body systems: respiratory, urinary, musculoskeletal, blood, hormonal, thermoregulatory, cardiovascular, and digestive.

3. What are some physical, psychological, and financial conditions that may contribute to malnutrition in elderly people?

4. What clinical problems are common among older people?

5. Name some drugs commonly used by older people, and explain their potential effects on nutritional status.

6. How do the RDAs for an elderly person generally compare with those for a 25-year-old? Discuss the effects of a deficient or excessive protein intake on the elderly.

7. What vitamins are most likely lacking in the diets of older people? Why? Inadequacies of what nutrients may be responsible for nutritional anemia?

8. Why is a high intake of both water and fiber recommended for older people?

9. Why is milk sometimes omitted from diets planned for older people? How can its nutritional contribution be compensated for in these diets?

10. Describe the aims of the National Nutritional Program for the Elderly. What kinds of programs are currently used to meet these goals?

REFERENCES

Bonnett, J. L., and M. J. Carlson. "Teaming Up to Teach Fitness Programs for Senior Years." *Food Nutr. News 54* (September/October 1982): 5.

Hui, Y. H. *Human Nutrition and Diet Therapy.* Monterey, Calif.: Wadsworth Health Sciences, 1983.

Kart, C. S., and S. P. Metress. *Nutrition, the Aged, and Society.* Englewood Cliffs, N.J.: Prentice-Hall, 1984.

Rivlin, R. S. "Nutrition and the Health of the Elderly: A Growing Concern for All Ages." *Arch. Intern. Med.* 143 (1983): 1200.

Roe, D. *Geriatric Nutrition.* Englewood Cliffs, N.J.: Prentice-Hall, 1983.

Nutritional Consideration for Special Individuals

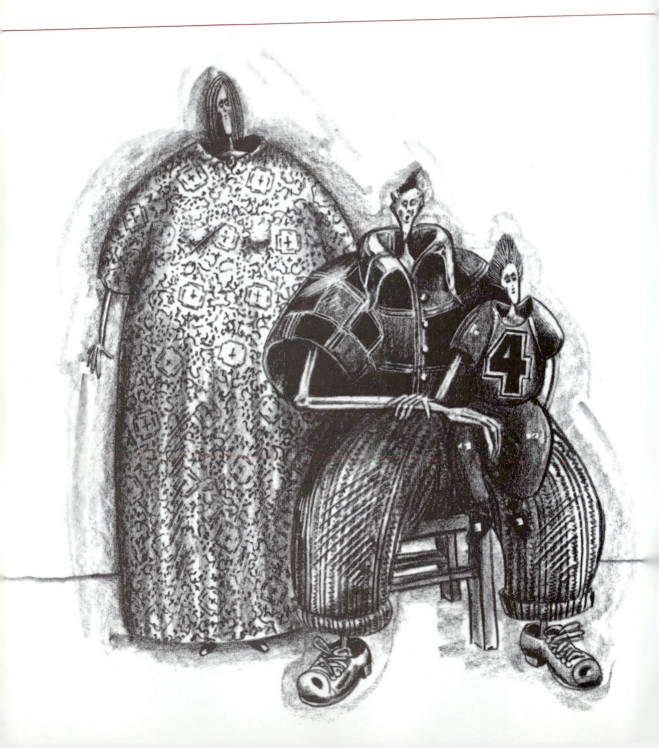

19

UNDERNOURISHED PEOPLE

Malnutrition from Ignorance

Larry weighed only 3½ lb at birth and was the fourth living child resulting from his mother's ten pregnancies. The mother's other pregnancies had been unsuccessful because of chronic hypertension.

When Larry was 6 weeks old, his mother became concerned about mucus in his throat, and she decided, without benefit of medical advice, that milk caused Larry's mucus problems. She placed Larry on a diet consisting of fruit juices, cereal, rice, and baby fruit—a diet that excluded all milk and milk products.

At 10 weeks of age, Larry contracted pneumonia. He was hospitalized, and his mother instructed the hospital that he should not have milk. The hospital gave him a protein formula during the treatment of pneumonia. He had no adverse reactions to the formula, but his mother

placed him on the original diet after his release from the hospital.

Eight weeks later Larry was readmitted to the hospital. His symptoms included generalized swelling, cracked skin and lips, and fussy behavior. In addition to a low body temperature, Larry's blood chemistry was abnormal. He was undersized,

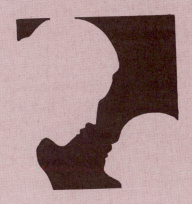

would not smile, and had a weak cry. He would not reach or turn over. His hair was sparse and straight, and it fractured easily.

The hospital immediately began feeding Larry a protein formula, baby cereals, fruits, vegetables, and eggs. He began to gain weight. Upon his discharge from the hospital at 7 months of age, he weighed 11 lb, had normal blood levels, and was smiling and active.

Larry had developed an illness resulting from malnutrition, an illness known as **kwashiorkor**. Although Larry's case represents one of the few cases that occur in the United States (Lozoff and Fanaroff), the illness is common in underdeveloped countries. As an illness of malnutrition, it can be corrected, as it was in Larry's case, by feeding sufficient amounts of protein, vitamins, calories, and minerals.

What We Mean by Undernutrition

In comparison with the recommendations presented in Chapter 13, many people's diets are grossly inadequate. A number of different terms are used for degrees and types of inadequacy. The terms *hunger, semi-starvation, total starvation, general inanition, underfeeding,* and **undernutrition** all refer to the lack of essential nutrients in the human body caused by insufficient food intake. The term **malnutrition** is frequently used interchangeably with undernutrition. However, it actually means "bad" (*mal-*) nutrition, which may or may not be caused by inadequate food intake.

Undernutrition exists in the United States among some population groups, such as Mexican-Americans and American Indians, but the extent and severity of this undernutrition are not comparable to its occurrence in India, the Philippines, West Africa, Ethiopia, Ghana, Guatemala, Brazil, and other underdeveloped countries. On the other hand, malnutrition from a number of causes is quite widespread in the United States.

Alcoholism has caused malnutrition in many American men and women. Deficiencies of minerals and vitamins (especially thiamine), liver malfunction, neurodegeneration, and anemia are all complications of excessive alcohol consumption. Overconsumption of sugary foods causes cavities and gum diseases. Obesity predisposes people to diabetes and high blood pressure. Hospital malnutrition has recently been documented. Suspected causes include a patient's inability to adopt new eating habits, the attending physician's ignorance or underestimation of the ramifications of nutritional inadequacy, and among other factors, a lack of communication within the medical team.

Most of these topics are explored in other chapters in this book. This chapter will focus on undernutrition: its occurrence in the United States and in underdeveloped countries, undernutrition syndromes that are all too common in these countries, ways of treating undernutrition, and current attempts to provide high-protein foods to alleviate the great suffering and ill health caused by hunger.

Undernutrition in the United States

The majority of documented cases of undernutrition in the United States involve newborn infants, children, adolescents, college students, and the elderly. Each year, about 5 to 10 percent of newborns in this country are of low birth weight. Although underweight in newborns can have many causes, a major one is the mother's improper nourishment before and during pregnancy (see Chapter 16). The population groups most affected are the indigent. The pregnant mother cannot afford to purchase good protein foods and is deprived of the opportunity for good prenatal care. There is no doubt that uterine malnutrition can cause growth retardation in the fetus, although whether this has a permanent effect on mental development is still being debated.

In the United States, children of many ethnic origins (Native Americans, blacks, Mexican-Americans, and Puerto Ricans) and impoverished white population groups are substandard in weight:height ratio. The causes of clinical undernourishment are many: lack of food, unsanitary living conditions, poor housing, unsafe and inadequate drinking-water supplies, unemployment, lack of parental education, and other social, geographical, and cultural factors.

In addition to infants and children, high school and college students and the elderly occasionally show evidence of undernutrition. They come from different socioeconomic levels and ethnic backgrounds, and the causes of their inadequate diets vary. A teenage girl may try to lose weight to keep up with social trends, and her deliberate avoidance of food results in underfeeding. Such tendencies can lead to serious clinical conditions. One of these, anorexia nervosa, will be addressed later in this chapter. A high school student on the wrestling team may undergo semistarvation to obtain a lower weight classification; undernourishment from this practice has been documented. A college student who adheres to an ill-planned vegetarian diet may lose too much weight. Documented cases of undernutrition among senior citizens have been traced to a variety of causes including poverty, ill-fitting dentures, physical handicaps, and disinterest in cooking for themselves.

Clinical rehabilitation of undernourished individuals with various medical problems such as diabetes and surgery requires special attention and is outside the scope of this book. However, if an adult or a child is simply underweight without other clinical problems, the best way to gain weight is by following a high-calorie, high-protein diet. Refer to Chapter 13 for methods of meal planning.

Undernutrition in Underdeveloped and Developing Countries

Gross or class undernutrition, which is widespread in many impoverished countries, is characterized by a number of general symptoms. They are most often seen among children of countries with minimal resources. After reviewing these general symptoms, we will examine two of the most common syndromes of gross undernutrition: marasmus and kwashiorkor (Hui).

GENERAL SYMPTOMS

When a person is deprived of food for any reason, the body adapts to the stress, at least initially. As the lack of food continues, other more profound and overt changes take place. The functioning and physiological turnover of organ tissues slows down, and the organs' demand for nutrients declines; the individual unconsciously (or consciously) reduces physical activity in order to expend less energy. If inanition continues, a child's growth will be retarded, with the risk of permanent brain damage. As starvation progresses, victims manifest general wasting and emaciation, especially after body fat (in the buttocks, abdomen, and breasts) and part of the muscle mass have disappeared. The victims become quiet and separate themselves from activities and people. This withdrawal, together with a general apathy, is part of the body's efforts to conserve energy. Other specific changes that may take place include:

Hair—The hair becomes dry and falls out with the slightest teasing, and keratin (a special skin protein) occasionally accumulates near the hair roots.

Skin—Skin shows "color" changes because of the appearance of pigments over the different parts of the body surface, especially the face. White skin may become gray or red, although the discoloration usually appears as brown spots or patches. In cold weather the skin becomes cyanotic (blue from insufficient oxygenation); in warm weather it is pale, dry, and easily lifted, and it does not spring back when pinched because it has lost its fat and elasticity.

Body Weight—Wasting and emaciation are characterized by a gradual loss of body weight, which sometimes dwindles to 50 to 60 percent of the original weight. Water, fat, muscle, skin, and organs such as the liver and intestine all suffer losses, as the body obtains energy by "burning" these important tissues.

Edema—The accumulation of water during inanition is observed in some but not all individuals. If present, edema is clinically identifiable. Although a depressed level of plasma protein has been suggested as one of its causes, the actual reasons are still being debated. The affected person urinates frequently as the body attempts to get rid of excess fluid, although there may be nothing wrong with the kidneys.

Cardiovascular system—Most normal functions relating to the cardiovascular, or heart-circulation, system are depressed. For example, blood pressure decreases, the output and beat of the heart slow down, and the heart shrinks in size.

Respiratory system—The rate, depth, and efficiency of the respiratory system decreases.

Basal metabolic rate—Body metabolism slows down. The body's loss of ability to adjust to cold temperatures increases the person's vulnerability to death by hypothermia (lowering body temperature).

Hormonal modifications—Hormonal changes vary. For example, growth hormone decreases, but adrenal and thyroid secretions remain within the normal range. In many females, ovaries and associated organs atrophy slightly, menstruation ceases, and sexual desire and drive (libido) are reduced. Loss of libido can also be identified in some male victims.

The nervous system—If important vitamins are deficient, the person may still reason and think well, but overall behavior changes. For example, apathy, irritability, and failure to concentrate are evident.

Gastrointestinal system—The victim may suffer malabsorption and diarrhea. The stomach may not make enough hydrochloric acid, and the small intestine secretes fewer and less-active enzymes.

Anemia—Anemia develops in some patients.

Activities—In addition, the adult victim is unable to work or move around easily because of the lack of energy and muscle, a reduced capacity of the cardiovascular system, and anemia.

The overt signs described above are easily identified in a malnourished individual. Health professionals working in the public health and community nutrition area can estimate to some extent the nutritional status of an individual by a detailed clinical examination. Chapter 22 provides some guidelines on identifying symptoms and signs of malnutrition.

SPECIFIC FORMS OF UNDERNUTRITION

The clinical manifestations of gross undernutrition described above are especially common among children of countries with minimal resources. These children are deficient in energy and in protein, vitamins, minerals, and other essential nutrients, although some are less severely deficient than others. For many years such classic undernutrition has received much attention and has been given many names. One description is *protein-calorie malnutrition*, or PCM (in this case, the term "malnutrition" refers to a lack of food). Despite its name, the condition of PCM inevitably includes a deficiency of vitamins and minerals, since high-calorie and protein foods that are lacking in the diet contain the essential vitamins and minerals.

The term "PCM" covers a wide range of nutritional deficiency diseases. At one end of the spectrum is nutritional **marasmus**, which is characterized by a deficiency of calories and nearly all other essential substances, as in simple starvation. At the other end is kwashiorkor, characterized by a severe lack in quantity and quality of dietary protein (deficiency in one or more of the essential amino acids), an adequate or even excessive intake of calories, and a mild to moderate lack of other essential nutrients. However, in a clinical situation, the two diseases are not always easily distinguishable. Between the two extremes are some manifestations of both conditions and varying degrees of combined energy and protein deficiencies, usually accompanied by infections and vitamin and mineral deficiencies. These are simply referred to as PCM or as marasmic kwashiorkor.

In general, the symptoms of an adult suffering from protein-calorie malnutrition are less defined than those of infants and children. Figure

Figure 19-1: Undernutrition in an adult in Bangladesh. SOURCE: Agency for International Development.

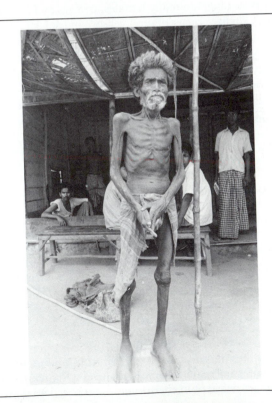

Table 19-1
Comparison of Marasmus and Kwashiorkor Symptoms in Children

CRITERION	MARASMUS	KWASHIORKOR
Clinical symptom		
Subcutaneous fat	Little	Some
Lean body mass	Wasted	Wasted
Edema	No	Yes
Potbelly	No	Yes
Hair	Changes common	Changes very common and severe
Skin	Occasional minor changes	Characteristic dermatosis
Liver	Frequently enlarged	Very frequently enlarged
Anemia	Usually mild	Varies from mild to severe
Symptoms from vitamin deficiencies	Yes	No
Mental status	Usually normal	Apathetic
Age of occurrence	Under 1 year old	After 1 year old
Prognosis	Fair	Good
Permanent damage		
Liver	No	No
Neurological	Yes	No
Body organs and tissues	Major	Somewhat
Some chemical and biochemical analyses		
Body potassium depletion	Mild	Severe
Fatty liver	No	Yes

19-1 shows an adult suffering from PCM. Malnutrition is a serious problem in many parts of the world, and marasmus and kwashiorkor in infants and children are devastating. Table 19-1 compares some characteristics of children suffering from these two conditions. Figure 19-2(a) shows drawings comparing a marasmic child with a child suffering from kwashiorkor. The following sections describe in greater detail marasmus, kwashiorkor, and the infections that frequently complicate these conditions.

Marasmus

Marasmus is derived from a Greek word meaning "to waste," and the term has been used for centuries. *Nutritional marasmus* refers to wasting because of a lack of food. An affected child is usually under 1 year old. The victim loses weight, fails to thrive, and is irritable. For unclear reasons the child has no appetite, although he or she may be hungry. A marasmic infant is usually bright eyed and alert, although the face is shrunken, like that of a wizened monkey or a little old man (see Figure 19-2). Growth is retarded, and there is a loss of fat and muscle. The child is skinny and bony and may lose up to 50 or 60 percent of body weight, although skeletal development is usually unaffected in the beginning.

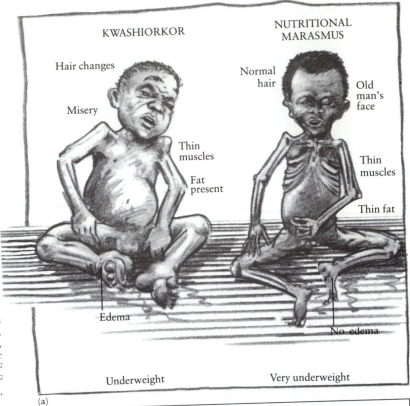

KWASHIORKOR

NUTRITIONAL MARASMUS

Hair changes

Misery

Normal hair

Old man's face

Thin muscles

Fat present

Thin muscles

Thin fat

Edema

No edema

Underweight

Very underweight

(a)

Figure 19-2: Children with marasmus and kwashiorkor. (a) Comparison of marasmus and kwashiorkor. (b) A child in Chad with kwashiorkor. (c) A marasmic child in Uganda.
SOURCE: *(a) Adapted from D. B. Jelliffe.* Clinical Nutrition in Developing Countries. *Washington, D.C.: U. S. Department of Health, Education, and Welfare, Public Health Service, 1968. (b) UNICEF photo by Diabate. (c) UNICEF photo by Arild Vollan.*

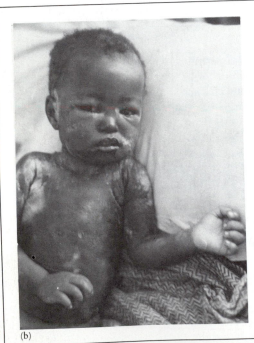

(b)

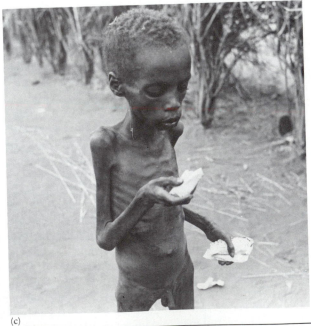

(c)

The patient shows no edema. Changes in the skin, hair, mouth, mucous membranes, and liver are less noticeable than in kwashiorkor but may appear. Watery diarrhea with acid stool is common and may lead to dehydration. Because of the thinness or shrunkenness of the abdomen,

CAMBODIA, A PORTRAIT OF MASS STARVATION

Cambodia is a devastated nation, one that suffered the ravages of the Vietnam war. Cambodia was a target of repeated bombings because of its occupation by hostile troops. The country's government has declined aid out of fear that the food supplies will fall into the hands of their enemies.

Estimates place the number of Cambodians who might starve to be a staggering 2.25 million. Thousands of Cambodian refugees have managed to make their way to such neighboring countries as Thailand. The refugees are sick and starving. The quantity of food supplies that can be delivered by boat or plane to Cambodians and Cambodian refugees, far less than what could be delivered by truck if permitted, must be contained in small packages because they are destined for a people too weak to carry anything heavy.

As they flee from certain starvation, refugees eat grass and tree bark. Neither contain sufficient nutrients. Yet many consider the refugees to be the lucky ones, in comparison with those too weak to escape their certain death. The refugees have described heartrending scenes of children thrown beside the road, their limbs no larger around than the bones within them, eyes sunken and unresponsive.

Death by starvation is a slow, painful process. Without food, the body burns its own reserves. It breaks down the protein of muscle mass, draining strength from the body. Even the heart is robbed of protein in the process. The body automatically reduces its energy consumption to conserve. Pulse rate and blood pressure drop. The body's temperature lowers. Women cease menstruating and men become impotent. Children stop growing.

With just a small amount of food and water, the body can fight death for several months, but the damage is being done. As the body literally eats itself, illness begins to take its toll.

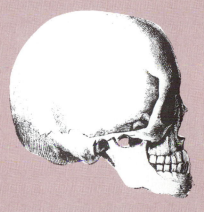

Diarrhea usually becomes constant. The heart can stop as a result of water and mineral loss. Infection thrives on the weakened state. Deficiency diseases such as rickets, pellagra, beriberi, and scurvy become common. Often, the sufferer simply loses the will to live.

Perhaps the greatest irony of prolonged starvation occurs for the seemingly fortunate few who receive a large meal. The resultant shock can be fatal because the heart and digestive system have been weakened. For the infants and children who survive prolonged starvation, the mental damage resulting from the terminated brain growth can be irreversible.

Cambodia gives us a stark look at the face of starvation, one of the most pathetic of human conditions. In the case of Cambodia, starvation involves such large numbers of people that those observing the nation find the people's condition overwhelming. Cambodia presents what may be the most poignant example of a more widespread nutritional issue, world hunger, but undernutrition and malnutrition are even more widespread. Malnutrition lacks the drama of starvation. It is more clearly understood as a crippler.

SOURCE: Adapted from *Time*, Nov. 12, 1979, p. 42.

one can see the movement of peristalsis, although occasionally a patient's abdomen may be distended with gas.

It is very rare that the patient suffers only caloric insufficiency. This nutritional marasmus may occur together with respiratory and intestinal infections, tuberculosis, and parasitic infection. Vitamin deficiencies can be very severe in some victims, and classic symptoms of these deficiencies are identifiable.

Kwashiorkor

The word *kwashiorkor* comes from the language of Ghana, an African country. It was introduced in 1933 by Dr. Cicely Williams, who obtained it from the natives of the Ga tribe living near Accra, the capital of Ghana. The term is commonly used in two ways. Dr. Williams defined it as the "sickness the older child gets when the next baby is born." One interpretation is that the mother is unable to breast-feed two babies at once and so has to give up nourishing the first child. Many health workers who have cared for these children equate the term "kwashiorkor" to "red boy," referring to the patches of red and brown pigment that appear on the affected child's skin.

A kwashiorkor child is usually over 1 year old. The child loses weight, but this loss is less extreme than in marasmus. Apathy, irritability, diarrhea, and anorexia are all present. The child is miserable and withdrawn and sometimes has a whimpering cry that is monotonous and weak. There is muscle wasting, but some body fat remains. Edema is present, and the water and fat around the jaws gives the child a moon face (see Figure 19-2). Skeletal measurements remain unaffected, at least in the beginning. More details on specific symptoms are given below.

Edema. Edema is a characteristic diagnostic symptom of kwashiorkor. Its extent varies from slight to great and is directly related to the degree of protein deficiency and the amount of salt and water in the diet. Serum albumin level is frequently used to monitor the extent of edema; the higher the level, the more severe the disease. The edema is concentrated in the lower parts of the body, although it affects almost every part. Figure 19-3 shows the edemic condition of a kwashiorkor child; note the characteristic potbelly. Also see the swollen face of a kwashiorkor child in Figure 19-2(b).

Hair. The hair has a fine texture, is easily plucked, and is thin, sparse, and soft. The curly hair of Africans becomes straight. The length of the hair may become pigmented, with streaks or patches of gray, blonde, or red. The color change is more common in black children than in those of other races. Among Caucasian children with straight hair, depigmentation appears as "flag" signs—alternating bands of white, black, and/or another color along the length of the hair. This unique pattern of discoloration is frequently interpreted to mean that the child has been exposed to good and bad nutrition alternately. Because it takes time for hair to grow, the hair color presumably reflects what the child has been eating for 1 to 3 months before the change takes place. Figure 19-4 shows the unique hair changes in a kwashiorkor child.

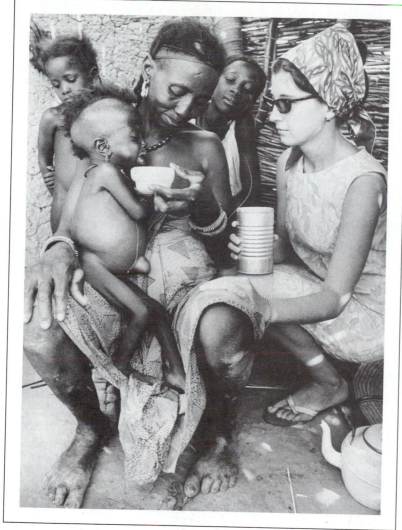

Figure 19-4: *The flag sign in the hair
of a child with kwashiorkor.*
SOURCE: *N. S. Scrimshaw and M.
Behar. Science 133 (June 30, 1961):
2039–2047. Copyright 1961 by the
American Association for the
Advancement of Science.*

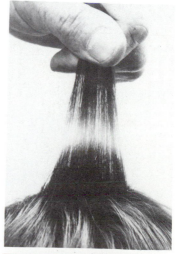

Liver. The child shows a fatty liver that is frequently enlarged.

Skin. Skin changes in a kwashiorkor child are also unique. The skin discoloration (pigmentation or depigmentation) affects every part of the body, especially the lower parts, groin, and buttocks. The changes are more frequent and severe in dark-skinned children and are characterized by patches of pigments. Because the skin also desquamates (scales), it sloughs off like a bad sunburn and has been described as looking like "flaky paint." In nonblack children, skin pigmentation affects the forehead, with desquamation and dark spots on the skin frequently described as "mosaic" or "crackled." Skin discoloration is not influenced by sunlight. Some of the affected areas may develop sores or ulcers with cracks, or bleeding and lesions in the skin folds resembling burn damage. If accompanied by infection, the skin flaking

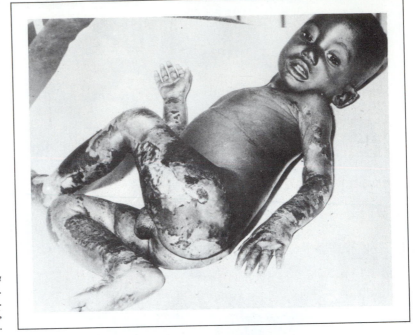

Figure 19-5: Skin lesions in a kwashiorkor child.
SOURCE: *A. J. Radford and A. J. H. Stephens.* Lancet *(December 7, 1974): 1391.*

and lesion can be debilitating and even fatal (see Figures 19-2(b) and 19-5).

Anemia. The victim may develop anemia, although the degree of severity varies. The causes of anemia may be deficiencies of iron, folic acid, protein, and/or other essential nutrients. It is difficult to generalize about the type of anemia, since practically any form can be identified in different kwashiorkor children.

Mucous membranes. Many kwashiorkor children develop oral inflammation, lesions and cracking at the corners of the mouth, tongue atrophy, and ulcers around the anal membranes.

INFECTION IN MALNOURISHED CHILDREN

Cases of malnutrition such as marasmus and kwashiorkor are frequently associated with either intestinal infection caused by parasites or systemic infection brought on by agents such as viruses and bacteria. Infection can deal a severe blow to the child who is suffering from malnutrition. It can intensify the negative nitrogen balance already existing, whereby less nitrogen is being absorbed and more excreted. As a result of the additional atrophy of lean body mass, more vitamins and minerals are excreted. Malnutrition and infection work together to arrest body growth and produce a subnormal weight:height ratio. The infection can also severely reduce appetite, resulting in the patient's refusal to eat solid food and further compounding the undernutrition problem. In addition, any treatment for systemic or intestinal infections can have adverse side effects. For example, antibiotics can further lower the victim's im-

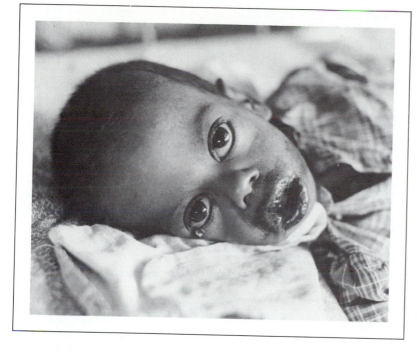

Figure 19-6: Oral infection in a
malnourished child.
SOURCE: Agency for International
Development.

mune defense mechanism and simultaneously interfere with nutrient
absorption.

It has been suggested that half the world's malnourished children,
especially the younger ones, may also be suffering from infection. Malnutrition and infection are often linked because the lack of dietary
calories and protein impairs the body's four major immune systems.
Figure 19-6 shows oral and facial lesions of a malnourished child with an
oral infection.

MANAGEMENT OF PROTEIN-CALORIE MALNUTRITION
The rehabilitation of a severely undernourished adult follows the same
standard clinical procedures for treating a patient under such stress as
surgery or burns. Such topics are not within the scope of this book.
However, the nutritional and dietary care of a child suffering PCM
requires special considerations and is conducted in two stages: immediate treatment and long-term rehabilitation.

Immediate Treatment
When a child is admitted to a hospital because of severe malnutrition or
infection, the immediate treatment includes restoring fluid and electrolyte (mineral) balance, antibiotic therapy, and blood transfusion. But
the measures adopted depend on the condition of the child. The next
therapy is diet therapy.

Most children suffering from malnutrition or infection require vitamin and mineral supplements in addition to possible electrolyte compensation. Any specific vitamin deficiency can usually be corrected,

although large doses of all vitamins can be given with careful consideration to those likely to elicit toxic reactions. When antibiotics are considered for treating an infection, their potential interference with nutrient digestion, absorption, utilization, and metabolism is weighed against the risks of the infection itself (see Chapter 24).

Calorie and protein needs are usually supplied in the form of milk, although milk may be inadequate for an older or a very malnourished child. In any case, too much milk should not be given in the beginning. Modern commercial nutrient supplements are an excellent source of calories and protein (see some examples in Chapter 27). If these are unavailable, the child should be fed progressively, first with a small amount of milk, then a larger quantity, and finally a concoction of milk, potato, mash, plantain, and banana or any other combination of locally available nutrient-dense foods that are acceptable to the child. Hand feeding, holding, and touching the child gives a feeling of comfort, security, and emotional and physical support. Tender care and a good diet are the best medicine.

Since hypothermia (lowering of body temperature) may be fatal, the child should be provided with a comfortably warm environment. The child's improved well-being, good appetite, subsiding edema, and normal reactions to environmental stimuli indicate recovery from the emergency stage. There may actually be weight reduction in some children because of water loss, but others will gain weight steadily. Satisfactory recovery may be apparent at the end of one month, with severe cases taking three to four months. Figure 19-7 shows mothers feeding

Figure 19-7: Emergency feeding of malnourished children.
SOURCE: UNICEF photo by H. Dalrymple.

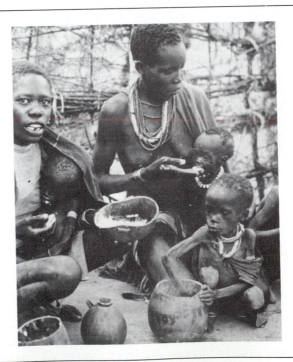

their emaciated children at the Kaabong emergency center in drought-stricken Karamoja Province.

Long-Term Rehabilitation

After emergency or lifesaving measures have been successful, the question of the child's long-term rehabilitation remains. This is especially important in most poverty-stricken countries, where food may not be

My DAUGHTER AN ANOREXIC?

Diana was a 15-year-old white girl from an upper-middle-class family. When she was 7, her mother died from a diabetic coma caused by excessive alcohol consumption. Her father remarried when she was 9. Her stepmother had a 10-year-old daughter and a 5-year-old son from her previous marriage. Diana's father worked nights two to three days a week. When Diana was 14 years old, the family doctor felt that this girl was immature, lacking in self-confidence, and verbally and socially inhibited. The parents sought medical help. After 10 months of psychotherapy, she showed some improvement.

When she was 15 years old, she started dieting. Although her weight was normal, she felt that her hips and thighs were fat. Within 5 months, her weight decreased from 110 lb to about 85 lb at a height of 5'5". She had practically abstained from eating, and her parents were very worried about her deteriorating condition. The family physician placed her in the hospital for observation and treatment.

The girl had a repulsive appearance resembling the emaciated state of a concentration camp victim. The doctor conducted a complete endocrinologic (hormonal) workup and was unable to find any defects. Results of skull and upper gastrointestinal x-ray studies were also normal. The attending physicians were unable to find any cause for her weight loss. At this time Diana's weight was 73 lb. She frequently experienced indistinct auditory hallucinations. For example, she said that her stepmother cried repeatedly to her "Eat, eat!" and that voices from the air-conditioning came from a crowd of people. She was depressed, had very little self-confidence and motivation, and was socially withdrawn. The doctors concluded that she was most likely suffering from anorexia nervosa, and a specialist in this area was consulted.

After a careful study, the health team developed several approaches to her treatment. The doctors began giving her 200 mg/day of the drug Elavil to control her emotional instability. She was placed on an aggressive behavior modification program

that required her to gain weight in exchange for rewards such as cosmetics, mirrors, or permission to watch her favorite television programs. Apparently, this program and the drug were effective, since her depression gradually disappeared and she gained 14 lb during the first 5 weeks in the hospital. But during this period she complained frequently about everything and was manipulative, dependent, and hostile. There were many episodes of self-induced vomiting that were witnessed by the hospital staff, although she denied them when questioned. Her parents confirmed that she had frequent self-induced vomitings at home.

Because of Diana's manipulative behavior, the therapeutic and administrative functions in caring for her were assigned to different groups. Among many strategies implemented by the health team, one important approach was to involve Diana in every step of the treatment plan. She was encouraged to express how she felt and to value herself as a human being (Hui).

abundant. The complicated and tragic subject of world hunger will be explored in Chapter 28.

Anorexia Nervosa in the Western World

Anorexia nervosa refers to the clinical condition in which a person voluntarily eats very little food. As a result, there is a large weight loss with all its concomitant symptoms. The disorder is more common among females, especially teenage girls, although it has been identified in men and older women. Typically the teenage female patient comes from a middle- to upper-middle-class family. Before the problem occurs, the patient is usually healthy and cooperative and has made good progress in school. All indications point to a "model" student and child. Then, at some identifiable time, the child develops psychological problems leading to resentment of her obesity (which may be real or imagined), and she embarks on a self-prescribed starvation diet. She continues to abstain from food even when she has achieved an ideal weight. After that, her health deteriorates.

CLINICAL MANIFESTATIONS

The anorexic patient presents several clinical manifestations. No desire is present for food or drink. The patient refuses to eat, although occasionally the patient has an uncontrollable urge to gorge, which is followed by self-induced vomiting. Because of this, anorexic patients may lose 25 to 35 percent of their body weight and become emaciated and wasted. (The appearance of an anorexic patient is shown in Figure 19-8.)

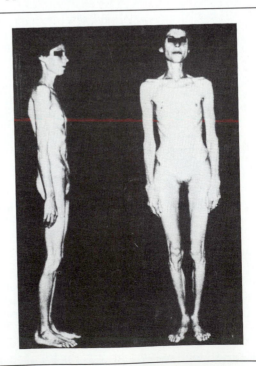

Figure 19-8: An 18-year-old anorexic girl, height 165 cm, weight 31 kg.
SOURCE: H. Bruch. "Anorexia Nervosa." Nutrition Today, September/October 1978. Courtesy of Dr. H. Bruch and reproduced with permission of Nutrition Today *magazine*, P. O. Box 1829, Annapolis, MD 21404. Copyright September/October 1978.

Electrolyte (mineral) imbalances occur, and female anorexic patients develop hair over various parts of their bodies and cease to menstruate. Body metabolism is decreased, hands and feet are cold, blood pressure is lowered, and sensitivity to insulin is reduced. Anorexic patients exhibit abnormal behavior such as frequent self-induced vomiting, excessive use of cathartics (laxatives), and overexercise (hyperactivity). In some patients, such actions may lead to death. Recently, medical authorities define the specific practice of "gorging and vomiting" as *bulimia*. No such distinction is made here.

The causes of anorexia nervosa are unknown. Two proposed causes are a brain disorder and psychological maladjustment. Because the hypothalamus (part of the brain) is related to eating, there is speculation that a defective function of this part of the brain may be responsible for the decreased food intake and lowered basal metabolic rate. However, some health professionals believe that a decreased food intake lowers the body metabolism, which in turn triggers the hypothalamus to produce a distorted body hormonal profile, which then produces all other clinical manifestations.

There are many psychological theories about a patient's refusal to eat. One is that a normal, healthy adolescent desires to be slender and that this desire becomes obsessive. Another is that the patient wants to do what he or she wants without interference. A female adolescent's fear of transition from girlhood to womanhood may lead to a perverse attempt to maintain a little girl's appearance.

A number of events can spark the beginning of a voluntary, continuous reduction of food intake. A worsening mother-daughter relationship may set it off. Or a sudden, highly emotional conflict between the patient and someone else may do so. Other possible causes are an abrupt failure in schoolwork and the emotional turmoil over beginning or continuing a sexual relationship.

In-depth studies by psychologists and psychiatrists of anorexic patients have indicated a common psychological profile. These patients show a lack of feeling for hunger, satiety, tiredness, and sometimes even physical pain. They generally have a distorted image of their physical size. Some anorexic patients think that they are 40 to 50 percent larger than they in fact are. Consequently, they become obsessed with dieting. In addition, these patients commonly feel inadequate in identity (role in life), competence (work or school performance), and effectiveness (in communication, controlling events, and so forth). This loss of faith in personal ability leads to an attempt to control the environment by controlling body weight. Food binges, guilt about eating, and a reluctance to admit abnormal food habits are the typical attitudes of anorexic patients.

The treatment for a patient with anorexia nervosa consists of psychotherapy, behavior modification, drug therapy, and hospital feedings.

PSYCHOTHERAPY, BEHAVIOR MODIFICATION, AND DRUG THERAPY
Anorexic patients must undergo intense psychological treatment to overcome negative perceptions of self and to normalize their food intake.

Clinicians must identify the causes or initiating events of each patient's illness. All correctable family conflicts that are relevant must be resolved. But psychotherapy is best started after a patient has gained a little body weight and should be maintained even after the patient has attained normal weight. Clinical experience shows that a patient may revert to abnormal eating behaviors if underlying problems have not been resolved.

Some clinicians use behavior modification in treating anorexic patients. This therapy consists of using rewards and reprimands to make the patient eat. For example, an agreement is reached between the patient and the practitioner that if there is any weight gain (such as 1 lb), the patient can do or receive certain things that she or he likes. If the patient fails to gain weight, activity will be restricted. Some clinicians claim reasonable success with this method, with some patients gaining 2 to 6 lb per week. Other clinicians warn against this practice, believing that a patient may feel cheated, frustrated, or despondent because of being forced into doing things he or she does not like. The insecure feelings that may ensue can thus aggravate feelings of inadequacy, which may be the source of the patient's problem.

Some clinicians use drugs such as amitriptyline and other antidepressants as treatment. This usage is based on the possibility of a brain defect. However, antidepressants have not been consistently effective in treating anorexic patients.

Because anorexia nervosa represents a growing problem in the United States, and because many patients could help themselves avoid this serious and potentially fatal condition, we need to understand the ultimate consequences of treatment.

HOSPITAL FEEDINGS

Patients with anorexia nervosa are best hospitalized, because the eating environment can be controlled and family involvement is minimized. Some patients eat better in a hospital because they do not have to make any decisions about what and when to eat. In general, the dietary care requires careful planning, an experienced staff, and a tremendous amount of concern and understanding. Because of the difficulties involved, a detailed management procedure is necessary (Crisp).

Upon admission to the hospital, the patient should undergo a thorough physical examination and psychiatric evaluation. A complete medical history should be obtained. The results of these evaluations can confirm a diagnosis of anorexia nervosa. Confirmation is crucial, since other clinical conditions may cause the patient's symptoms.

Once anorexia nervosa has been diagnosed, the first major responsibility of the health team is to develop a dietary and nutrition program. Any deviation from the established treatment procedure must be approved by the doctor or the assigned coordinator. There should be complete understanding and communication among the health team members to avoid inconsistency or friction precipitated by the patient. This is important, since the patient may try to manipulate the health personnel and parents to avoid food intake and secure an opportunity to exercise. Most anorexic patients want to maintain a starved appearance.

The nurse can coordinate all activities to ensure that the program is implemented and that all parties involved are providing full support and sympathy for the patient. If the patient stubbornly refuses food, visits by the dietitian may be necessary to assess the situation. The patient may be asked to help formulate a new basic strategy to encourage eating.

Full communication should be maintained between the patient and health personnel. The doctor should describe the treatment procedures to the patient, preferably in the presence of the primary nurse and the dietitian or nutritionist. The parents should also be fully informed of the treatment procedures, but preferably not in the presence of the patient. As the patient improves, restrictions may be removed progressively.

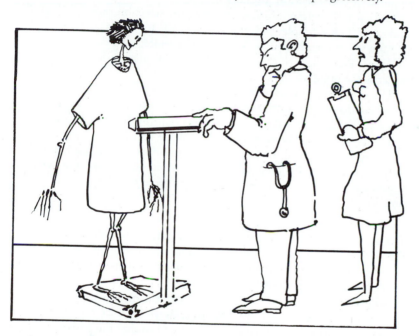

Body Weight Determination

Obviously, the patient's weight should be closely attended. The patient should be weighed before breakfast twice a week with the same scale. The patient should be clothed only in a hospital gown that does not have a pocket, since some patients may hide food they don't want to eat. No food and only a minimal amount of fluid should be consumed before weighing. The weight record should not be accessible to the patient or the parents to avoid any friction over weight changes. The record is best kept at the nursing station or similar location. Talking about the patient's weight in the presence of patient and parents is definitely not advisable. It should be made certain that weight gain is not due to an excessive fluid intake. No overtly edematous spots should be visible on the patient, or the specific gravity of the urine can be analyzed to ascertain whether the urine is dilute.

The benefits of any proposed reinforcement system to encourage weight gain must be weighed against its risks. For example, a promise of special privileges if there is weight gain and penalty if there is none may increase the patient's despair. Similarly, it is not advisable to promise patients that they can go home if, for example, they gain 50 lb.

Anorexic patients have a mixed reaction to any weight gain. On the one hand, they feel relieved and assume that they will be discharged earlier. On the other hand, the weight gain is contrary to their heartfelt desire to lose weight. They thus feel sad and outraged that they have not lost weight instead.

Diet Therapy

The diet prescription for anorexia nervosa is not very complicated but requires special attention. Initially the dietitian interviews the patient to obtain a list of preferred foods, although the selection must be carefully evaluated. For example, the patient may ask for fruits and vegetables that are not common or in season or for so much food that it cannot be provided. Regardless of the requests, the meal plan should contain the prescribed number of calories.

The attending physician will prescribe a diet after studying the patient's condition. Most practitioners start with a diet containing 1,000 to 3,000 kcal and progressively increase the intake by 200 to 400 kcal every 3 or 4 days. The intake is continued until the patient eats normally. To avoid any misunderstandings, all changes in caloric intake must be made by the doctor or an assigned coordinator in the form of a written request. A cooperative patient can be fed three main meals and occasionally a snack.

Feeding Routines

The nurse should be fully informed of the patient's condition, including the treatment protocol. Most important, the attending nurse should monitor the patient's eating behaviors and pay full attention to some of the following feeding routines:

1. Check that the foods served comply with the meal plan.
2. Pay attention to the patient's hands constantly.
3. Assume a friendly and supportive attitude so that the patient will not feel spied on.
4. Leave the room only in an emergency, since the patient may try to get rid of some foods.
5. Prevent food disposal by keeping all containers (such as facial tissue boxes, wastebaskets, or flower pots) away from patient during the meal and checking the meal tray after the patient has finished eating. The patient may hide food under napkins or smear butter under the bed and on the window sill.
6. Permit a maximum of one hour for eating a meal.
7. If feasible, arrange for the patient to eat alone (separate from other patients) and be monitored by the same nurse.
8. If possible, the patient should be wearing a pocketless hospital gown while eating.
9. Insist that the patient rest for ½ to 1 hour after a meal and insure that she does not leave the bed, since she may induce vomiting.

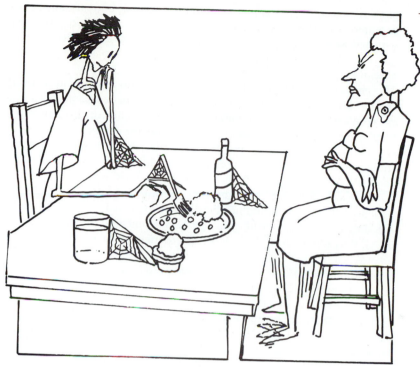

During mealtime, anorexic patients tend to exhibit certain behaviors. For instance, they may indicate that they are not hungry or do not feel like eating because they do not feel well. Patients may purposefully prolong eating time to encourage the nurse to end the meal or leave the room, in which case food may be hidden or thrown away. Some patients show a sudden eating binge and gulp down large portions of food. One patient may be sincerely eating, whereas another will induce self-vomiting after the nurse has gone.

Patients may try to get rid of food by any available means including discarding food and beverages in the toilet, exchanging empty trays, cups, and glasses with roommates and seeking help from relatives and friends.

After each meal, the dietitian should use the record obtained from the nurse and the serving tray to calculate whether the patient has eaten the required calories. Any missing amount is then made up by providing a high-calorie beverage. The routine of supplemental feeding should already have been clearly explained to the patient. The patient should know that supplemental beverages must be drunk within 15 to 30 minutes of being served. To ensure this, straws or cans that can prolong drinking time should not be used. The patient should also be aware that any part of the beverage not drunk voluntarily will be tube-fed.

Forced Feeding
Forced feeding is done only if all attempts to get the anorexic patient to eat voluntarily have failed. Obviously, if the patient resists this measure,

physical restraints may be necessary. Tube feeding is tried first, before parenteral nutrition is administered. Both success and failure have been reported with the forced feeding of patients with anorexia nervosa.

Special Considerations

The patient must be provided with emotional understanding to overcome a difficult time of life. For this reason, an experienced nurse should be assigned to an anorexic patient. A student nurse or any nurse not familiar with the patient's condition may delay the patient's recovery. An experienced nurse will know, for example, that the patient's room should not have any weighing equipment and that the room should be constantly checked to ensure that no food has been stored or hidden.

All health personnel must be very sensitive when dealing with the patient. The patient should not be slighted, ridiculed, or treated condescendingly even if she or he cheats, is temperamental, throws tantrums, or exhibits other unruly behavior. The patient must not feel alone or abandoned even if any acutely ill patient in the same room receives a great deal of attention. If circumstances permit, a private nurse may be needed to provide constant care.

Many activities or practices are definitely not advisable for anorexic patients. For example, any exercise, including walking, should not be permitted, since it will lead to caloric loss. Further, patients should not be permitted to participate in any form of work that is tiring. The staff should attempt to ensure that: (1) Parents and relatives are not allowed to visit at mealtime; (2) the patient is not permitted to interact with or help other patients during mealtime; (3) the patient does not have access to records or to the nursing station; and (4) the patient is not alone for any period of time.

Treatment Outcome and Recovery

The management of anorexic patients can be very complex and difficult, because the patients are accustomed to use foods as a manipulative weapon. Some patients pose special problems when they deliberately expend a large amount of calories. Recovery is a long and difficult process that may last from 6 months to 1 year or more. About 60 to 70 percent of all patients may recover after several years of treatment; the remaining patients may die. Genuine recovery is extremely important, since most of these patients are so mentally unstable. The following guidelines should be used to determine whether recovery has taken place:

1. The patient attains and maintains a normal body weight.
2. The patient shows no abnormal food behavior, such as sudden food binges or self-induced vomiting.
3. The patient resumes regular menstruation and establishes a normal relationship with peers, friends, and relatives.

Anorexia nervosa has been considered an undernutrition extreme in that it has been characterized as "intentional," at least in comparison with the "forced" or "involuntary" undernutrition that occurs due to poverty or food shortage. We know, of course, that a physical condition that may result from psychological problems cannot be considered intentional. Anorexia nervosa is, then, a specific condition within the undernutrition spectrum, one that provides significant challenge to health practitioners.

STUDY QUESTIONS

1. Write a paragraph describing the difference between the terms *undernutrition* and *malnutrition*.

2. In the United States, which age groups are most likely to be undernourished? Why?

3. Describe the general symptoms of gross undernutrition.

4. What is protein-calorie malnutrition? In what way is this term misleading?

5. What is the theoretical difference between kwashiorkor and marasmus? Describe some characteristic symptoms of each condition.

6. Research and develop a protocol of behavioral modifications for a teenage *boy* with anorexia nervosa.

7. Talk to your friends and relate some of their (or your) experience with anorexics.

REFERENCES

Crisp, A. H. *Anorexia Nervosa: Let Me Be*. London: Academic Press, 1980.

Hui, Y. H. *Human Nutrition and Diet Therapy*. Monterey, Calif.: Wadsworth Health Sciences, 1983.

Lozoff, B., and A. A. Fanaroff. "Case Reports: Kwashiorkor in Cleveland." *Am. J. Dis. Child* 129 (1975): 710.

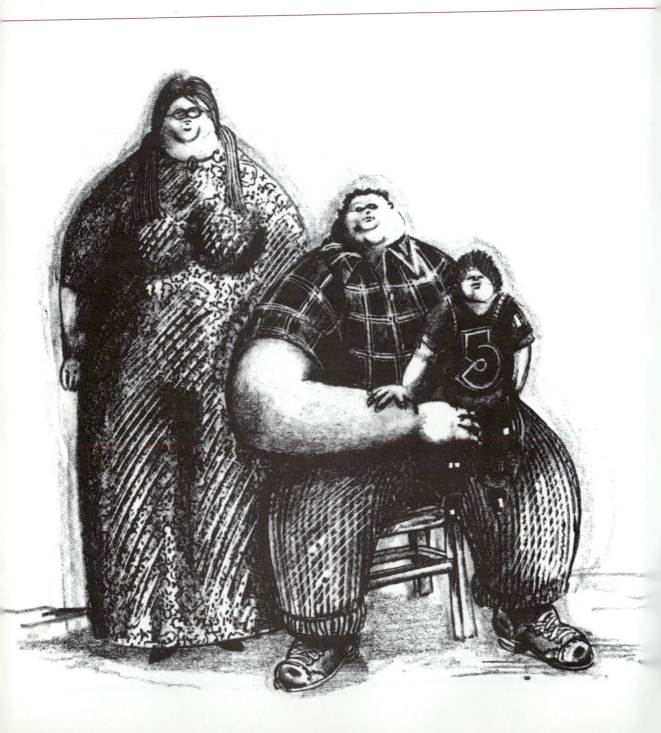

20

OVERWEIGHT & OBESE
PEOPLE

"WHOOSH! THAT'S TOTAL BODY CARE?"

It is hard to describe the boots I was wearing. Long, plastic hip-high boots that alternately blew up like a balloon and then suddenly deflated with a whoosh. I saw the needle on the air compressor, which was attached to the boots by hoses, going up and up, past 30, 40, 50, and finally stopping at 60 milligrams per square centimeter pressure. My legs inside the boots started feeling the squeeze, and I wondered if the things would ever stop inflating. The boots got bigger. The squeezing got tighter, then suddenly, whoosh! The air rushed out. This happened first to one leg and then the other for 15 minutes as I sat with just a towel around me. The timer on the air compressor finally buzzed; the attendant unhooked me; and the boots came off. I could leave. My cellulite treatment was over.

This was my experience in a New York salon that specialized in cellulite treatment claiming "the most up-to-date approach to total body care ever conceived." . . .

Inside the salon the carpet was deep and plush, and on the wall were huge photos of a very slim young model going through the various treatments the salon had to offer. Why were there no "before and after" pictures? "Oh, but they wouldn't show you anything. You would have to know when they were taken,

how long the treatment had been. You wouldn't learn anything just looking at pictures," was the answer. What did the treatments cost, then? There was no uncertainty about this: One appointment was $45, and there was a special rate of 12 treatment sessions for $475.

A fortyish woman with a French accent, attractive, but not especially trim herself, showed me to a private room and looked at my legs and buttocks. "Oh, yes, the cellulite is starting here and here and here," she said pointing. Apparently it was creeping down my legs to my knees, and for some reason my left thigh was worse than the right. She said I perhaps needed to lose some weight, too. At 5'3" and 112 pounds I was rather startled to hear that, although I had to acknowledge that the women in my family seem to have chubby thighs no matter what we weigh.

Another attendant came in and the treatment started with a "subaquatic massage"—a whirlpool bath—in a brightly colored tub with lots of dials and hoses at one end. As soon as I stepped into the tub, jets of water started spurting from the sides, and the attendant tried to guide me so the jets would hit my thighs. We then went into a curtain-lined cubicle, where she started in on my cellulite with a vengeance. A green, gel-like material was massaged into my

skin by hand, and then she used an electric massager that had three different heads. The third head had rotating spiky points and looked like a torture instrument. Although it felt bumpy rolling up and down my leg, it was not painful.

The pièce de résistance came next—those inflatable hip boots. While I was immobilized inside them, the woman with the French accent returned with instruction on a diet to follow and exercises to do at home. Most of the exercises amount to bouncing on the floor on my buttocks and occasionally beating my knees together. The diet suggested I eat lots of fresh fruits and vegetables, drink eight glasses of water a day, and cut down on sodium to reduce water retention.

Along with this came a warning that I could fail to get rid of all the cellulite if I didn't keep exercising at home and coming back for monthly follow-up treatments.

"Cellulite has to be attacked on all fronts—diet, exercise, massage," she said as she unhooked me from the hip boots. "It takes discipline and persistence. You have to do your part. That's very important."

What she was actually saying was that even for $475, there were no guarantees.

SOURCE: Adapted from L. Fenner. "Cellulite—Hard to Budge Pudge." *FDA Consumer*, May 1980, p. 4.

Not Just Fat

Later in this chapter we will specifically address cellulite, but first we need to understand excess body weight. The medical problem of being overweight or obese—the accumulation of excess body weight—can affect anyone regardless of age or sex. Although there is no known cure for obesity, it can be controlled.

A technical distinction can be made between the terms **overweight** and **obesity,** but the actual definitions of these terms may vary among clinicians. For the purposes of this book, when you weigh more than your ideal body weight (see Chapter 3), you are overweight. This excess can be fat, but it can also be cell solids or muscle mass. And, when you are obese, the excess is fat, rather than water, muscle, or bone, and the ideal body weight is exceeded by 15 to 25 percent. The term *grossly obese* is used to apply to those cases in which ideal body weight is exceeded by over 25 percent. In our discussion, we use obesity and overweight interchangeably, but with the understanding that the excess weight is fat.

Obesity results from the constant accumulation, over a long period, of calories from overeating. To prevent such an accumulation, calories consumed must equal energy expended. Calories *do* count: this applies to all healthy individuals. One pound of *pure* fat contains 4,086 kcal. One pound of *body* fat contains approximately 3,500 kcal, since body fat is 85 percent fat and 15 percent water and cell components. We can say that one gram of body fat contains 7.7 kcal.

What this translates to for you is that if you eat 3,500 more kcal than you require for your energy level, you will gain one pound of body weight. As an example of how easy it is to gain weight, suppose that a young woman suddenly decides that she likes to consume an extra ¾ cup of celery soup and one slice of toast as an afternoon snack, and that she does this three times a week. If her other daily meals and activities remain unchanged, this woman will gain 8 to 9 lb of body fat within one year.

Studies of Americans have shown that about one fourth of those over 30 years of age are 10 to 25 percent above ideal body weight. Women start to gain weight after age 20, and men between 25 and 40. Adult males can lose weight slightly more easily than females. What is important for you to understand, however, is the effects of excess weight.

An Obese Person Has Numerous Problems

An obese person definitely has more problems than a person of normal weight (Hui). Medical complications may include: (1) shorter lifespan; (2) becoming sick frequently; (3) respiratory difficulties; (4) multiple problems with the heart and circulation such as blood clots, hypertension, heart attack, and stroke; (5) diabetes; (6) gallbladder trouble; (7) hernia; (8) arthritis; (9) complicated pregnancy; and (10) chronic illness.

In addition to such medical complications, psychological problems can occur. "Distorted body image" can cause an obese person to blame his or her weight for everything that goes wrong. Obese people in such a condition can become preoccupied with weight, heaping blame on themselves, feeling inferior, and becoming withdrawn and passive.

For the obese child or adolescent, parental and peer pressure and ridicule can generate significant unhappiness. Schoolchildren who cannot participate in sports may be targets of ridicule that creates a long-lasting stigma. Obese individuals have reported discrimination in college admissions and in job placement. Because of social rejection, obese individuals often turn to eating for the sense of comfort it gives, further adding to their obesity. Using food for comfort can be especially common for those who are rejected by the opposite sex.

Obese people have a higher cost of living, since clothes, food, and even furniture and transportation can be more expensive for them. Moreover, obese people often suffer inconvenience and discomfort. The burden of extra weight may lead to back problems and aching feet. Such difficulties may combine to frustrate the obese person and make him or her unhappy with life.

What Makes a Person Fat?

Given the numerous disadvantages of obesity, you surely must ask what causes a person to overeat to such an extent. Theories abound in regard to that question. Except for those cases resulting from clinical disorders, there is no single, satisfactory answer. Table 20-1 presents the currently accepted possible causes of obesity.

The Weight Wars

As Dr. A. J. Stunkard of Stanford University stated in 1958: "Most obese persons will not stay in treatment for obesity. Of those who stay in treatment, most will not lose weight and of those who do lose weight, most will regain it." Although this statement remains basically true, it is encouraging to note that the number of obese persons who are successfully losing their excess weight and maintaining their ideal weight is on the increase.

Perhaps you have already experienced the process of losing weight by choice. If you have, you know it is not an easy task. One major difficulty is that all of us like to eat. The other major difficulty is that life's problems tend to interfere with our weight loss resolve.

Table 20-1
Some Proposed Causes of Obesity

FACTOR	ANALYSIS
Genetics	
Body build by birth	All types: round, plump, thin, fragile, heavily muscular. For example, a person born thin, fragile, and linear may grow up to be a small person and underweight.
Familial traits	If parents are obese, their children have a higher chance of being obese.
Defective hunger and satiety center	Hypothalamus does not respond normally. Usually, it responds to hunger and informs the person to stop eating when full. Its failure to do so results in obesity.
Defective body metabolism	Defects in an obese person: inability to release energy efficiently (from ATP, for example), reduced lipase (enzyme) activity to mobilize fat, and overactive fat storage enzyme system.

Table 20-1 (*continued*)

FACTOR	ANALYSIS
Genetics	
Body fat cell type	An obese person may be born with a large number of fat cells or a special type of fat cell that can hypertrophy easily.
Anthropological factors	
Cultural acceptance	Obesity is considered good fortune or a beautiful attribute in many countries.
Food and hospitality	The expression of hospitality through food and drink makes food more available. In an affluent society like the United States, this increases food consumption.
Eating habits	
Overeating	Obese people like to eat. They eat more calories than they expend.
Meal pattern	Eating three meals a day may predispose some individuals to deposit more fat. Nibbling the same quantity of food throughout the day may enable the body enzyme system to use the calories more efficiently, and less fat is deposited.
Childhood conditioning	
Infancy eating maladjustment	Solid foods given too early, excess high caloric-density milk, and excess food consumption all may result in large weight gain. A big baby (from too much fat) is not necessarily a healthy baby.
Overeating	A fat child can grow into an obese adult.
Psychological factors	
Eating as an emotional outlet	If the person wants to stay away from food, he or she must be convinced to use another means of emotional support.
Eating to allay anxiety, tension, frustration, and insecurity	The greater the level of anxiety, tension, frustration, or insecurity, the more food a person eats and the more likely he or she is to gain weight.
Eating as a substitute or demonstration of love and affection	The relationship between family members is expressed with food. To show love and affection, one person serves more food to another. Or to replace loss of love and affection, a person eats more or is served more food.
Eating as a substitute for whatever is missing (e.g., no job)	In this context, food is similar to excess alcohol drinking and heavy smoking.
Physiological factors	
Hormones	Hypothyroidism or decreased metabolism may result in weight gain and therefore obesity.
Basal metabolic rate	BMR decreases with age, while the caloric consumption is undiminished and there is a decrease (or no increase) in daily activity.
No exercise or activity	Eating a lot of foods without a good exercise program results in obesity.
Environmental factors	
Trauma and emotion	Certain individuals are susceptible to traumatic and emotional experiences and will eat more food.
Family eating habits	One develops an overeating habit if parents and other members in the family eat too much.
Sedentary job	A job requires constant sitting, with minimal movement.
Abundance of foods	Obesity is more common in affluent societies.
Advertisements	A person is conditioned to the type of foods advertised on television and in magazines, most of which are high in calories.
Living comfort	Comfortable ambient temperature, light clothing, minimal shivering, and lack of heavy work all contribute to reduced expenditure of calories.
Convenience of food preparation	Minimal preparation time and labor. Less activity, more food consumed.
Smoking or alcohol	When a person tries to stop smoking or drinking, he or she may eat more and gain weight.

Not only do we like to eat, but we also have eating patterns. There are certain quantities you have become accustomed to, and there are certain foods you prefer. Given your set of eating habits, sticking to a low-calorie diet and avoiding what may be favored foods requires a significant modification of behavior. Assuming you have sufficient will-power to change behavior, the next task becomes that of staying with your resolve until your goal is attained.

When we try to lose weight we want quick results. Yet losing 5 to 10 pounds of excess weight can easily require two to three months. For example, during the first two to three weeks of a moderately low-calorie diet, there may be no weight loss because empty fat cells may temporarily be filled with water. It takes two to three months to produce a real loss. If a 50- to 100-pound weight loss is desired, and 1 to 2 pounds of excess weight is lost each week, it can take one to two years to achieve the goal. It takes significant perseverance to stay with a weight loss program through all the various adversities of life that can arise in a two-year period.

A third problem involves seeking professional help. When an overweight patient goes to a doctor to seek help, the slightly protruding abdomen of an overweight, middle-aged physician may shatter the patient's confidence at the first interview. Even if the doctor is in good shape, clinical experience indicates that every obese person seeking medical assistance expects dramatic results. Often the relationship between patient and doctor results in a waste of time and money with very little weight loss. The patient blames the doctor and the other weight reduction schemes he or she has followed previously, and the doctor feels that the patient has failed to follow instructions to reduce eating and increase exercise.

Nevertheless, experience has shown that if overweight people are given *free* advice regarding a low-calorie diet, perhaps by an acquaintance who is a nutritionist or dietitian or by a professor in nutrition, they are likely not to follow the instructions. However, if they go to a clinic and are charged for the office visit, they are likely to comply with the low-calorie diet with some enthusiasm, even if the information is nearly the same. In any event, the earlier an overweight person seeks medical advice, the easier it is to lose weight.

Following the desired weight loss, the second half of the battle involves maintaining ideal weight. The best possible program for maintenance of ideal weight includes a balanced diet, an adequate exercise program, and good eating habits. If developed in childhood, such an ideal weight lifestyle is more easily maintained in adulthood.

ENCOURAGEMENT CAN BE PIVOTAL

Weight loss should follow certain patterns. First, the best and safest method involves a 1- to 2-pound loss per week. Second, exercise is necessary to a successful effort. Fifteen to 20 minutes of meaningful exercise or activity makes one feel better, helps spend calories, and conditions muscular tone. Third, during the process of weight reduction, nearly every obese person reaches a "plateau"—a stage of stabilization when the body seems to refuse to shed any more poundage, at least for some time. Fourth, weight loss must be followed by weight maintenance.

A fifth consideration applies to those who seek to help a person lose weight: All overweight or obese individuals need encouragement and support. Any negative and condescending attitudes should be avoided. Concerned health personnel (doctors, nurses, dietitians, and nutritionists) should become familiar with some pertinent psychological supports for the patient.

When an obese patient undergoes medical treatment to lose weight, all communication between health personnel and that patient should be sensitive and supportive—not tainted with value judgments such as "An obese person eats like a horse" or "All fat people have no willpower." If patients fail to reduce eating and lose weight, they should not be made to feel bad, embarrassed, or discouraged. Rather, they should be told that even just maintaining the current weight is a bonus and encouraged to never stop trying. Although obesity increases the risks of a number of health problems, there is no need to frighten patients. Explain clinical implications that apply to the particular patient, and emphasize that not every obese person experiences the same health problems. The patient's willingness to come to a clinic should be considered a praiseworthy preventive action.

The success of any weight reduction process is greatly enhanced if the patient fully understands the details of the regimen, including the treatment method, the ease or difficulty of any step, and the expected success rate. When the patient specifically expresses disapproval or unwillingness to go through a certain procedure, an alternative should be seriously considered.

A patient's maladjustment to social interaction such as dating, clothes, or housing should be viewed with sympathy and understanding. For example, a fat patient may feel that he is unable to rent a good apartment because he will be discriminated against. Perhaps he can be convinced that such pressure is not so important or that it may not even exist. There is no reason why a patient should suffer from other people's lack of consideration.

Losing Weight the Scientific Way

You will find in Table 20-2 a listing of the various scientific methods utilized for weight reduction, and you will find a brief analysis of each. Though no one method is successful for everyone, each has its place and is worthy of discussion here.

CALORIES DO COUNT

Eating less stands as the most obvious weight reduction technique. Any successful weight reduction diet should have certain characteristics. The diet should be nutritionally adequate in all aspects but low in calories. The RDA for the particular individual is used as a guideline to plan the diet. The daily dietary allowances are best divided into three or four meals a day with some carbohydrate, protein, and fat in each meal. A minimal distribution provides at least 250 to 350 kcal per meal. The

Table 20-2
Some Scientific Methods of Reducing Weight

TREATMENT METHOD	ANALYSIS
Reduced caloric intake	If done without medical supervision, caloric intake should not be less than 1,200 kcal per day. May be accomplished with the help of a doctor, nurse, dietitian, nutritionist, or other allied health personnel.
Increased exercise	May be accomplished by oneself or with the supervision of a doctor, exercise physiologist, or other similarly trained personnel.
Behavioral modification	May be accomplished by oneself or with one-to-one or group counseling with a trained therapist, clinical psychologist, or psychiatrist.
Group program	May be accomplished by organizing one's own group weight reduction program, joining national groups, and participating in commercially supervised (nonclinical) weight reduction enterprises.
Hypnosis	May be achieved under the care of a clinical hypnotist or by learning self-hypnosis.
Jaw wiring or lock-jaw	Some success when conducted by experienced medical personnel.
Forced exercise	Some success when performed under the direct supervision of a physician.
Drug therapy	Overall effectiveness is not sure. Physician's prescription required.
Surgery	Some success, although some techniques are accompanied by severe side effects: high morbidity and mortality.
Starvation or fasting	1. Semistarvation. Reduction of dietary intake to 500–1,200 kcal per day requires the direct supervision of a physician. 2. Protein-sparing modified fast. Requires the direct supervision of a physician. 3. Total starvation. Requires the direct supervision of a physician.
Comprehensive medical weight reduction program	Some success. Must be conducted under direct medical supervison.

consumption of fat and carbohydrate should be small to moderate, whereas protein (meat, cheese, eggs, fish, poultry, and skim milk) should be served liberally. Staple and satisfying items such as potatoes, noodles, rice, and bread should not be completely eliminated, because they provide satiety value. Whenever feasible, foods with maximal satiety and minimal caloric values should be provided.

Special attention and control should be exercised over the following foods: starches, pastries, alcoholic beverages, thick gravies, cream, mayonnaise, table sugar, and fats. Any foods eaten between meals must be accounted for, whether they are fruits or cocktails, doughnuts, cookies, peanuts, sodas, or ice cream. The habit of nibbling and snacking during meal preparation and cleanup must be avoided. Since practically all foods provide some calories, avoiding any quantity—a bite, a mouthful, a piece, a wedge, or a cup—contributes to weight loss.

A successful diet is also appetizing, tasty, and acceptable to the patient and does not require special preparation. This ensures that the meal plans can be integrated into the entire family's eating routine and will not bore the patient, since he or she may have to stay with it for a long period.

When one is on a weight reduction program, a number of tips are important in preparing foods. Skim milk can be used when whole milk is called for. Visible fats should be removed from meat and meat products. Natural meat juices should be used rather than thick gravies. Fruits or plain desserts can be offered rather than high-calorie sweets. Artificial sweetener may be used if available. Green, yellow, and red vegetables are generally low in calories. Lemon juice, low-calorie dressings, or vinegar can be used on fruit and vegetable salads in place of high-calorie dressings. Meats should be baked, broiled, boiled, or roasted rather than fried. When meat is roasted, a rack should be used to keep it from remaining saturated with fat. In recipes that call for frying, foods can be steamed or simmered instead, and nonsticking cooking utensils can be used to avoid the use of cooking fats.

Fats from juices, soups, stews, and casseroles can be skimmed off after cooking and refrigeration. Butter or margarine consumption can be reduced by using whipped products and very small servings. No fat should be used on vegetables after cooking. To improve flavor, bouillon cubes can be used instead. The cook should become familiar with new or gourmet cooking methods that minimize the use of fat and gravy. The attractiveness of foods can be improved by using herbs, spices, artificial sweeteners, or diet dressings.

Some planning and learning processes are required on the part of the person who is trying to lose weight. People on a weight reduction regimen should learn about basic nutrition and new eating habits. They should make meal plans early and know what is to be consumed in the next meal. For example, they can plan at least one day ahead of time or even a few days. One way to do so is to cook a large amount of some specific dishes, divide them into portions, and freeze the portions in separate plastic bags. Each portion will thus provide the correct meal contribution. Once a diet plan is fixed, dieters should not skip meals. Dieters should also learn to recognize their own tendencies to binges and compulsive eating. These occurrences can be anticipated by setting aside a specific number of calories for them, but meals should not be skipped nor basic nutritional needs sacrificed.

People on a weight reduction regimen should make special plans for meals eaten away from home, such as restaurant dining, bag lunches, picnics, banquets, holidays, and festivals. Written instructions for such occasions should include what foods to eat, their caloric contribution, and preparation methods. Many reputable books provide easy, convenient, low-calorie diets for such occasions. They include guidelines, tips, and specific instructions that apply to eating out and at home.

Those seeking to reduce their caloric intake can make other preparations as well. They can compile a list of nutritious, tasty, and low-calorie snacks and regular foods; the list can be carried everywhere; and another copy can be posted in the kitchen. A list of commercial dietetic products that are low in calories can also be compiled; for example, water-packed fruits and tuna, chewing gum, soft drinks, margarine, pies, and canned goods.

Overweight people can carry out these preparations on their own, but many sources of help are available. Free classes are often given by adult schools, colleges, and church organizations, and there are many good publications on food preparation, dieting, menus, calories, and nutrition. If the cost of a publication is prohibitive, specific pages can be photocopied or books borrowed from local libraries. University instructors, hospital dietitians, and public health nutritionists are all willing to provide advice as well.

Although calories do count, dieters should not overdo calorie counting. To do so will be frustrating to themselves and irritating to friends and relatives. Instead, every effort should be made to reduce dependency on foods. For example, dieters can make new friends and find activities and pleasurable tasks that will help reduce their loneliness and opportunities to eat.

THE ART AND SCIENCE OF CALORIE COUNTING

Before starting a low-calorie diet, one must know how low it should be. After one has ascertained his or her ideal body weight, the daily caloric need according to routine activity level can be obtained by one of the methods described in Chapter 3. Assume that the caloric need of a hypothetical patient is 2,100 kcal per day. For this particular person, the safest starter is a diet of 1,500 to 1,600 kcal per day. This will permit a loss of 3,000 to 4,000 kcal, or 1 pound of body fat, per week. Eating less than 1,000 to 1,200 kcal per day should be under medical supervision. There are four ways to plan a 1,500-kcal-per-day diet without unnecessary inconvenience (Hui). (Additional considerations may occur as new products of dietetic or reduced caloric content are introduced.)

A Daily Eating Guide

A daily eating guide tells the dieter the approximate number of servings of each category of food he or she can eat daily. Table 20-3 describes a guide that provides 1,000 to 1,500 kcal per day, depending on the number of servings of each food type consumed. Table 20-4 provides a few examples of food servings that give an approximately equivalent amount of calories within the food type. The Appendix provides many examples of each food type to use in developing a good daily menu plan.

Table 20-3
A Core or Daily Eating Plan Providing 1,000 to 1,500 kcal Per Day

FOOD TYPE	SERVING	APPROXIMATE CALORIC CONTRIBUTION	REMARKS
Milk	2–2½ c	Skim milk: 170–255 kcal Whole milk: 330–495 kcal	If interested in cheeses, ice cream, cream, and other dairy products, make calculations and replace.
Meat	4–6 oz	200–500 kcal for fish, poultry, meat (baked, boiled, roasted, broiled), all visible fat trimmed	If interested in eggs and shellfish, make calculations and replace.
Fruits	2–5	80–250 kcal, fruits or fruit juices, unsweetened	Make sure to include citrus fruits or a source of vitamin C.
Vegetables	2–5	20–250 kcal, with at least 1 serving of a dark green leafy vegetable	Many varieties have zero calories. Exclude peas, corn, beans, and potatoes.
Grain	2–4	50–350 kcal	Include potatoes, peas, beans, and corn.
Fats	1–3	100–300 kcal	
Free foods	No limit	Coffee, tea, lemon juice, celery, spice, condiments, consomme, bouillon and others. Very little calorie contribution.	

Table 20-5 uses the information in Tables 20-3 and 20-4 and the Appendix to develop a daily menu plan of approximately 1,400 kcal. Menu plans of any caloric level can be developed in a similar manner.

Collecting Meal Plans

A second simple procedure is to use menus preplanned for a certain caloric level. These weekly menu plans can be developed by the person seeking to lose weight or obtained free from nutrition textbooks, public health clinics, nutritionists and hospital dietitians, agricultural extension agents, state and federal health agencies, the U.S. Department of Agriculture, and many reputable commercial diet publications (see references for this chapter). The person follows the meal plans to the letter and repeats them weekly. With such preplanned menus, the person must also have emergency or specially-designed meal plans for situations such as dining out, hiking, or picnics.

Commercial Diet Plans

In the last few years, a number of reputable commercial diet plans have proved to be fairly successful in helping obese individuals lose weight. Two popular publications include the *Wise Woman's Diet* (by *Redbook* magazine) and *Weight Watchers Menu Plans* (by Weight Watchers Inter-

Table 20-4
Examples of Food Items Included in the Core Eating Plan

FOOD TYPE	SERVINGS PROVIDING EQUIVALENT AMOUNT OF CALORIES
Milk	1 c skim milk, ½ c whole milk, ⅔ c cheddar cheese
Meat	1 oz meat, 1 egg, ¼ c salmon, 3 sardines, 5 oysters
Fruits	½ c applesauce, 1 medium nectarine, ⅔ c blueberries, 1 small pear
Vegetables	½ c spinach, 1 medium artichoke, ½ c chard, ½ c cooked cabbage, 1 small cucumber, ½ c cooked mustard greens
Grain	1 sl bread, ½ c cooked cereal, ½ c cooked noodles or rice, 2 graham crackers, ½ c peas, ½ c cooked dried beans, ½ c mashed potato
Fats	½ T butter, margarine, or oil; 1 sl bacon; 1 T French dressing

Table 20-5
A 1,400-kcal Menu Plan

BREAKFAST	LUNCH	DINNER
½ pink grapefruit	½ c cottage cheese on lettuce and carrot sticks	3 oz breaded, baked haddock
½ c oatmeal		½ c asparagus spears
1 poached egg	1 c vegetable beef soup	1 baked potato
1 sl whole wheat toast	4 saltine crackers	1 sl French bread
1 t margarine	1 c sliced strawberries	1 t margarine
1 c skim milk	1 c skim milk	1 plum
Salt, pepper	Salt, pepper	10 grapes
Coffee or tea	Coffee or tea	1 c skim milk
		Salt, pepper
		Lemon
		Coffee or tea

national). An individual can purchase these diet plans and apply them conscientiously. Their menus do not differ greatly, since they are all low calorie and tasty. They do have drawbacks, however, such as high cost and time-consuming preparation.

The ADA "Food Exchange System"

Because many diabetics are obese and weight loss can eliminate some or all of their symptoms, the American Diabetes and American Dietetic Association have developed a "Food Exchange System" that deals in part with a weight reduction regimen (see Chapter 2). The system divides food products into six lists: (1) milk, (2) vegetables, (3) fruits, (4) bread, (5) meat, and (6) fats. Foods within each list have approximately the same caloric content and are thus interchangeable. (Refer to Chapter 2 for more information.) Table 20-6 presents meal plans using the Food Exchange System for twelve different caloric levels. One exchange in the table refers to a particular serving portion of the food. Table 20-7 translates the exchanges into a sample menu for 1,200 kcal.

THE BEST-LAID PLANS . . .

The regimens presented above show that planning a low-calorie diet is not all that difficult; the real catch is implementing it! Three basic problems interfere with compliance with a low-calorie regimen.

One is lack of time—plus being in a hurry for results. Most of us do not have leisure time to indulge in extensive food preparation. For a mother of two or three children, it is no small matter to assign specific blocks of time to cooking. An overweight salesman finds it equally

Table 20-6
Using the Food Exchange Lists to Prepare Menu Plans at 12 Different Levels

FOOD TYPE	FOOD EXCHANGE LIST	NUMBER OF EXCHANGES ASSIGNED TO THE DAILY PERMITTED NUMBER OF KILOCALORIES											
		600	800	900	1,000	1,100	1,200	1,300	1,400	1,500	1,600	1,700	1,800
Breakfast													
Meat (medium fat)	5	1	1	1	1	1	1	1	1	1	1	1	1
Vegetables	2	0	0	0	0	0	0	0	0	0	0	0	0
Fruits	3	1	1	1	1	1	1	1	1	1	1	1	1
Bread	4	½	1	1	1	1	1	1	1	1	1	1	1
Milk (nonfat)	1	½	½	½	1	1	1	1	1	1	1	1	1
Fats	6	0	0	0	0	0	1	1	1	1	1	1	1
Lunch													
Meat (medium fat)	5	2	2	2	2	2	2	2	2	2	2	2	2
Vegetables*	2	1	1	1	1	1	1	1	1	1	1	1	1
Fruits	3	1	1	1	1	2	2	2	1	2	2	2	1
Bread	4	½	0	1	1	1	2	1	2	2	2	2	2
Milk (nonfat)	1	0	½	½	½	½	½	½	½	½	½	½	½
Fats	6	0	0	0	0	0	0	1	1	2	2	2	2

*One of the two daily servings of vegetables must be raw and have few calories (see the exchange lists in Chapter 2). Adapted from A. Dean, Home and Family Series, Extension Bulletin E-782, Cooperative Extension Service, Michigan State University and the Food Exchange Lists of the American Diabetes Association. The exchange lists are based on material in the *Exchange Lists for Meal Planning* prepared by Committees of the American Diabetes Association, Inc. and The American Dietetic Association in cooperation with the National Institute of Arthritis, Metabolism and Digestive Diseases and the National Heart and Lung Institute, National Institutes of Health, Public Health Service, U.S. Department of Health, Education and Welfare.

Table 20-7
Sample Menu for a 1,200-kcal Diet Using the Exchanges in Table 12-16

BREAKFAST	LUNCH	DINNER
½ c orange juice	2 small boiled frankfurters	2 oz broiled hamburger
1 poached egg	½ c cooked green beans	½ c cooked summer squash
1 sl toast		Sliced tomato on lettuce
1 t margarine	1 sl whole wheat toast	½ c cooked rice
1 c skim milk	1 medium tangerine	1 small apple
Salt, pepper	1 small banana	12 grapes
Coffee or tea	½ c skim milk	½ c skim milk
	Salt, pepper	Salt, pepper
	Coffee or tea	Coffee or tea

difficult to prepare some of the menus. Even though some diet menus are easy to follow and prepare, losing just 4 to 8 lb will take about 1 to 2 months (1 to 2 lb weekly) of consistent effort.

The second problem is that we like to eat. Being forced to eat only 60 to 80 percent of one's normal intake for months or even years can be painful. Third, to lose weight many of us who are inactive must eat relatively little. Technical advances have made many routine tasks (doing laundry, fueling the furnace, traveling) almost effort free. Thus, routine activities are not likely to help a dieter get rid of excess calories. This problem is addressed in the second way of losing weight—exercising more.

Keep Moving!

The more active we are, the better the chance of losing weight. Exercise programs may be routine or systematic. All of us should make it a point to move more. We can park the car a few blocks from work and then walk, use stairs instead of elevators, garden, and mow the lawns. Every morning and evening, we should spend 10 to 15 minutes walking, bicycling, or jogging. Simple calisthenics can be performed for 10 to 15 minutes in the morning and before going to bed. During leisure time, we can enjoy vigorous sports, such as tennis or volleyball. We can adopt a more active lifestyle without getting hurt, exhausted, or frustrated.

On the other hand, recent trends show that many individuals—both thin and obese—are attempting rigid and strenuous exercise routines. If you are thinking of beginning such a program, consult a physician, an exercise physiologist, or another appropriate professional, especially if you are middle-aged or older.

About the same amount of energy is expended in performing any of the following activities: swimming 800 yards, running 1½ miles in 15 minutes, bicycling for 6 minutes, or walking 3 miles in 35 to 40 minutes. You can select a preferred suitable activity and do it every day of the week or a few days weekly. A vigorous exercise program can be obtained from professionals or reputable publications.

Any strenuous exercise program involves certain considerations. One controversial relationship is between heavy exercise and hunger. In some situations, a person's appetite increases immediately after expending a

THE "LITE" STUFF

The food industry has responded to our cries for weight reduction help. The supermarkets now have significant numbers of "light" or "lite" products ranging from beer to syrup. These products contain less fats, less sugars, or less alcohol, with the bottom line being fewer calories.

The Food and Drug Administration (FDA) requires that such products meet specific limits on caloric content. These rules apply to food products but not to alcoholic beverages. The latter are under the jurisdiction of the Bureau of Alcohol, Tobacco and Firearms. FDA rules provide that "low calorie" means a serving contains no more than 40 calories and no more than 0.4 calories per gram (28.4 equal 1 oz). To be called "reduced calorie," a food must be one-third lower in calories than a similar food in which calories are not reduced, but it also must be as nutritionally sound as the unmodified food.

The labeling requirements assure us that a food is truly "diet" or "dietetic," and you can rely on such labels to know both sugar content and other nutritional content necessary to your diet planning. We are fortunate as consumers, for we now have wider choices than ever before, and more "lightness" is on the way.

SOURCE: Adapted from L. Fenner. *FDA Consumer*, June 1982, p. 10.

moderate amount of energy. On the other hand, a person's appetite may actually decrease after strenuous work. This decrease has led to the suggestion that exhaustive exercise before a meal can actually cut down food intake. Although current thinking on this topic varies, it is generally agreed that jogging or running daily for 1 or 2 miles will not increase the appetite to the detriment of a person's dieting regimen.

Another consideration is the effect of the exercise on the individual. Some people tire quickly. Some become dizzy during weight loss because of hypotension. All obese individuals must pay careful attention to their backs. Backache is a common ailment among very fat people, and even a slight improper strain on the back can cause lifelong misery. Any activity chosen must be appropriate and must not harm the patient in any way. For example, a weak right hand is terribly tiring to a person engaging in tennis. Weight lifting can damage the fragile joints of many obese patients.

The physician or other health professional must tailor the exercise program to the patient after an intensive physical examination has established that any particular exercise program will not be harmful. With certain heart and circulatory problems, including uncontrolled hypertension, patients may be advised not to exert themselves—but losing weight is an important factor in controlling hypertension. Diseases such as severe anemia, varicose veins, and uncontrolled diabetes may prohibit the person from heavy exercise. Special tests can determine the patient's heart condition and the types and intensities of exercise to be prescribed.

The physician also serves as a model—good or bad. A doctor who maintains a good body weight, is physically fit, and enjoys wholesome sports will increase patient confidence. Encourage the patient. Remind him or her of the benefits of a good exercise program. For example, if the patient loses weight, many pains and aches may disappear. When fat is removed by exercise, skin will not be flabby, and the person will gain good muscle tone and a feeling of well-being.

Any exercise program must be started slowly and cautiously. Pick the type of exercise you like—games, competitive sports, or noncompetitive activities. And pick the best time of day for routine exercise, depending on your work and lifestyle.

Helping Patients Change Bad Eating Habits

Over the last few years, behavioral therapists have learned that obesity is related to bad eating habits learned throughout life. Once such "bad" behavior is identified and modified, the person will develop new eating habits. According to these experts, the key does not lie in a low-calorie diet but rather in the adjustment of behavior. It is assumed that after the behavior is corrected, the person will eat less. The assumptions behind this technique are described by Dr. M. J. Mahoney of Pennsylvania State University: (1) An obese individual is an overeater. (2) The obese and nonobese differ in eating style. (3) If the obese alter their eating styles, they will reduce. (4) The obese individual is stimulus bound. (5) Obesity is a learning disorder.

The procedures to reduce body weight by means of behavior modifications are composed of five parts (Hui): (1) Defining the problems and objectives, (2) compiling personal information about problems and objectives, (3) analyzing the data and clarifying the problem areas, (4) developing procedures to modify undesirable behavior, and (5) monitoring progress and changing strategy as necessary. How do these formal procedures translate into the client's language?

WHAT ARE THIS INDIVIDUAL'S PROBLEMS AND GOALS?
Initially, the client's life history is obtained, including the person's body weight history—past, present, and ideal (from both personal and medical viewpoints)—and changes during major points in life (such as military service, college, marriage, childbirth, divorce, and changes in drinking and smoking habits). The person's feelings toward food—likes, dislikes, and favored means of preparation are explored. The therapist then tries to determine the client's emotional well-being or lack of it—depression, anxiety, frustration, dissatisfaction, negative or positive attitude, and so on. Clients are encouraged to explore reasons for their actions and behavior: Why are they unhappy? Why do they eat so much? Why do they move or change jobs? Why do they have trouble with women or men friends? Why are they sexually frustrated? Finally, goals are set for the weight loss: how much to lose and the time needed for losing it. The goals are also planned in association with the need for weight loss before traveling, changing jobs, getting married, or any other special situation.

EACH CLIENT IS DIFFERENT
The clients are then asked to provide very detailed information on practically every aspect of their life. For example, they are asked to compile one week's eating record, day by day, hour by hour, minute by minute: when they eat, what, how, how much, where, with whom, and how they felt at the time. Other aspects of life to be recorded include time spent working, walking, running, moving, sleeping, using the bathroom, and exercising. Clients are also asked to recall the circumstances that they think have caused their overeating problem.

In compiling this personal record, the therapist and client should refrain from making value judgments. All the client's answers must be honest and accurate. The therapist is especially interested in factors that suggest why an eating episode occurred and the daily routines that surrounded the occurrence.

STUDY CAREFULLY WHAT IS LEARNED
The third step in behavior modification is to study the data and establish a clear profile of problem areas. Some questions the client and therapist might ask in analyzing the personal record are: Do you eat too much? How many calories do you eat? Do you get any exercise? Do you eat snacks between regular meals? Do you eat while watching television? Do you have morning and midafternoon coffee, doughnuts, or soft drinks? Do you eat snacks? At what specific times of day are these calories

consumed? What starts the eating? Is any behavior repeated every time something is eaten or drunk? Usually a pattern emerges showing the times, places, occasions, and emotional states when the person is most likely to overeat.

NOW, DEVELOP A PLAN OF ACTION

In developing procedures to modify a client's undesirable eating behaviors, the therapist and client first identify and agree on the list of eating behaviors to be changed. They also identify all external environmental factors that affect the client's eating habits.

Goals are set for modifying the behavior. A reasonable goal might be for the patient to lose 1 or 2 pounds weekly after some of the self-defeating behavior has been successfully modified. The therapist then proceeds to shape the client's behavior, one small step at a time, until the goals are reached. Any obvious, easy, and well-reinforced behavior change should be made to improve the client's expectation. The therapist should not suggest procedures that would be difficult or impossible for the client to perform, especially in the long term. Fad diets and devices should definitely be discouraged.

A set of rules regarding rewards, reprimands, and negative and positive reinforcements to be used should also be established. Measures should also be chosen so that the therapist and client both know how much the client has changed and how close he or she is to reaching the goals.

For example, one major kind of modification involves controlling the stimuli to eating, such as modifying the amount of foods eaten, the types of food consumed, and the frequency of eating. A special low-calorie diet is not necessarily involved. Some techniques used to reduce stimulus control of eating are shown in the box.

Rewards and Punishments

Weight reduction by behavior modification may involve both positive and negative reinforcement. For example, a contract may be made between the patient and therapist to the effect that if the patient fails to alter undesirable eating behavior and lose 1 to 2 lb a week, she or he will lose $5 per week, to be placed in the therapist's trust. This $5 will be used to buy more low-calorie cookbooks for the patient's reading or for other nonpersonal purposes. Positive reinforcement consists of some pleasurable reward—such as a movie or a concert—for any success on the patient's part. More information on methods of losing weight through behavior modification can be found in the references for this chapter.

Self-Help Dieters

Many overweight people have long recognized that the best help is helping themselves. Some therefore band together and help one another lose weight. Many self-help weight reduction group programs have developed all over the world. Some popular and fairly successful ones in this country include Weight Watchers, TOPS, and Overeaters Anony-

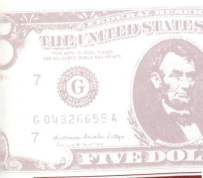

mous, all of which have a few things in common. The members meet either once a week or according to some schedule. During the meetings, there may be a lecture on food and nutrition, and the members talk to one another, exchange or study recipes and meal plans, or analyze

Some Techniques FOR CHANGING EATING BEHAVIOR

Modify the amount of food you eat.

Eat slowly, progressively lengthening the time allotted for the meal. For example, a meal should last 20 minutes or more. Delay tactics include such details as waiting 1 minute after sitting down before starting to eat.

Eat in small bites and count each mouthful.

Put food or eating utensils down between mouthfuls and chew the food completely. One suggestion is to chew each mouthful more than 10 times.

Do not eat without utensils.

Permit only one serving at a time.

Allow intervals between servings; for example, walk off to get a glass of water or use some other pretext for leaving the table.

Make servings of food look larger by using small plates and cups.

Finish one food item (such as meat) before starting the next (the vegetable, for example).

Leave all foods in the kitchen instead of putting them on the dining table. Another method is to place the serving plates on another table.

Make sure, if feasible, that something is left over on the plate after each meal. Discard these leftovers or save them for snacks or the next meal. Have containers available for putting away the foods.

Always keep foods in a covered container.

Eat only difficult-to-prepare foods.

Modify the types of food you consume

Do not buy favorite foods that are calorie dense and nutrient light, such as snacks and convenience items. These foods are also difficult to fit into a carefully planned diet regimen.

Avoid nibbling by preparing lunch after breakfast and dinner after lunch. It is not wise to prepare food when one is very hungry.

Shop for groceries on a full stomach; for example, immediately after breakfast, lunch, or dinner.

Nibble on "harmless" foods such as carrots and celery. Have low-calorie foods nearby.

Use a list when shopping and buy only the items on it.

Fill the stomach partially with some low-calorie foods before going to a party or feast.

Avoid eating when drinking coffee or alcohol, watching television, reading a magazine, and so on.

Reduce eating in restaurants, and at picnics, banquets, and parties as much as possible.

Spread out eating favorite foods over the different meals of the day.

Modify where and how often you eat

When eating, do nothing else. Concentrate on the eating process.

Confine eating to one place, preferably the same place every day.

Do not eat in the kitchen if you can avoid doing so.

Do not eat on the working table or in front of the television.

Eat sitting down.

If possible, eat at the same time each day.

Permit an interval between the desire to eat and the actual eating.

If possible, arrange a complete place setting before eating, especially for breakfast and dinner.

Kill the desire to eat during unplanned time by doing something that makes it impossible to eat (for example, have both hands occupied with knitting or playing cards).

If aware of a time when extra food is usually desired, arrange to be busy with some favorite work or activity that makes it difficult or inconvenient to eat.

exercise programs. To help members treat the program and its objectives more seriously, each member is required to pay a fee for attendance. In the nonprofit organizations, the money is used for expenses such as renting space, printing literature, mailing free brochures, and various other educational activities. During each meeting, the person who has succeeded in losing the most poundage is given overwhelming support, such as a standing ovation. This kind of encouragement lifts the individual's spirit.

The overweight persons essentially follow a special low-calorie diet designed by the organization, and they report the results during each gathering. They are also taught how to implement a workable and effective exercise program. Although there are no specific scientific data about the success rate of these self-help groups, scientists and physicians specializing in obesity generally agree that they probably have more success in helping people lose weight than most other approaches.

In addition to these self-help groups, many industrial corporations, community organizations, and other large institutions have started their own weight reduction programs, such as summer camps for obese children and teenagers, and physical fitness programs for firefighters, police officers, and automobile workers. Again, data on the success of these efforts are lacking, but it is felt that group programs of this nature can only help and will rarely hurt obese individuals in their continuing efforts to lose weight.

Is Hypnotism the Key?

In the last few years, some clinical hypnotists have claimed good success in helping people lose weight by means of hypnotism, although others have reported failure. A brief description of this technique is given below; for more information, consult a standard textbook.

A hypnotist may or may not be a medical doctor. However, in most states the person must be specially licensed. The procedure for weight reduction is very simple. The therapist first establishes a good relationship with the patient to earn the patient's trust, to develop confidence that hypnotism will help, and to establish familiarity with the practice, purposes, and effects of hypnotism. During the first few sessions, hypnosis is induced, the trance is deepened, and the patient is then awakened. The therapist and patient then explore the experience. Once the therapist is convinced that the patient responds favorably, specific posthypnotic suggestions are provided to the patient during the trance stage. Such suggestions, instructions, and commands vary and may be any of the following:

Substitution for overeating—The therapist suggests that the patient chew gum or eat carrots instead of eating ice cream, for example.

Transferring overeating habit—The patient is told to transfer the overeating activity to other activities such as riding a bicycle, physical exercise, or buying clothes.

Reduction of overeating—The patient is told that his or her present eating pattern is not normal and that he or she must eat less.

Aversion—The therapist suggests that the patient think he or she is eating, smelling, hearing, or feeling something bad and unpleasant every time he or she eats or wants to eat a doughnut or toast with butter.

Reliving childhood—The patient is told that he or she is very young and should participate in more physically demanding activities, spending all the calories he or she has been eating.

Health incentive—The therapist suggests that the patient is achieving superior health while losing weight by not eating too much.

Ego and image building—The therapist suggests how attractive the patient looks when he or she has lost weight and how there is promise of good social involvement.

After the patient has awakened from each trance, the total experience is again discussed. As the patient becomes more experienced, the hypnotic stage is made to last longer so that the suggestions can be repeated many times. Some patients are taught how to hypnotize themselves, repeating the same suggestions to themselves during the training ses-

AN EXAMPLE OF A POSTHYPNOTIC WEIGHT REDUCTION SUGGESTION

And now I want you to have a clear mental image in your mind, of yourself standing on the scales and the scales registering the weight you wish to be. See this very, very clearly for this is the weight you will be. See yourself looking the way you would like to look with the weight off those parts of the body you want the weight to be off. See this very, very vividly and summon this image into your mind many times during the day; particularly just after waking in the morning and before going to sleep at night, also have it vividly in your mind before eating meals. And this is the way you will look, and this is the weight you will be. As you believe this, so it will happen. When you have attained this weight, you will be able to maintain it, you will find yourself eating just enough to main-

tain your weight at the weight you would like to be. Until you *do* attain this weight you will find you have less, and less desire to eat between meals. In fact, very, very soon, you will have no desire at all, to eat between meals. You simply will not want to. Also you will find you will be content with smaller meals. There will be no sense of unhappiness or dissatisfaction, smaller meals will be quite satisfactory to you, and you will have no desire to eat large meals. Also you will have less, and less desire for high calorie, rich, unhealthy foods. Day by day, your desire for such foods will become less

and less, until very, very soon, you will have no desire at all for rich, high calorie, unhealthy foods. Instead, day by day, you will desire low calorie, healthy foods, and these will replace the high calorie foods, the rich foods, you have eaten in the past.

As you lose weight and approach closer and closer to the weight you wish to be you will find yourself growing stronger and stronger, healthier and healthier. Your resistance to illness and disease will increase, day by day. With less weight you will feel better and better, and your health will become better and better. Remember too, that your own suggestions will be just as effective as the suggestions I give you, either personally or by tape.

SOURCE: H. E. Stanton. *Am. J. Clin. Hypnotists* 18 (1975), p. 34.

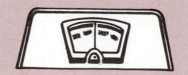

sions. Some physicians or therapists tape-record the suggestions so that the patient can take them home for repeated listening.

One Way Is to Lock a Patient's Jaw

Since December 1973, more than 100 obese patients have gone through the technique of having their jaws wired or locked to drastically reduce their consumption of foods (Stunkard). Physicians who have used the procedure have reported that some patients have lost nearly 100 lb in a few months. In these clinical reports, patients eligible for the procedure were specially selected—for instance, 50 percent overweight, free of health problems unrelated to the excess fat, and of acceptable oral and dental health. Under local anesthesia, their jaws were wired together near the canine and premolar regions. Patients resumed normal activity the next day and were able to speak normally two days later. The operation was uneventful and was described as "no worse than a tooth extraction."

The patients were sent home with the following instructions: (1) Eat a daily liquid diet of less than 1,000 kcal including milk, natural fruit juices, and vitamin and mineral supplements. (2) Use special procedures to maintain oral hygiene. Bad breath and dryness of mouth can be managed by dental aids such as mouthwashes and ointment. (3) As a precaution against aspiration (choking) and vomiting, keep a wire cutter with you. In case of emergency, use it as you were taught.

All patients underwent periodic checkups with special attention to oral health, infection, respiratory functions, and weight loss. Some common complaints included sore gums and monotony of the liquid diet. Some patients admitted noncompliance by using high-calorie fluids and blended food purees. Some attempts to squeeze solid foods between the teeth were also reported.

Some patients had unacceptable weight loss because of such reasons as infection, refusal to continue, and illness, but a substantial number did lose a large amount of body weight during the periods of jaw wiring. Aside from hair loss, there were no other ill effects.

Forced Exercise: The Prod

Physicians who have tried using forced exercise have also reported some success. Weekly or at some other interval, the patient comes to a clinic where he or she is required to perform a specified amount of exercise under medical supervision. Typical forced exercises include running on a treadmill and riding on a bicycle ergometer. Some clinicians claim that the patient loses weight, improves muscle tone, and develops strong respiratory functions. Some patients have lost up to 100 lb. However, experienced clinicians recommend special attention to the following factors when implementing forced exercises.

There should be appropriate medical supervision. Any forced regimen with the treadmill or ergometer should be implemented slowly, carefully, and with constant evaluation.

The patient should not fast. A diet of 700 to 1,000 kcal per day is advised. The patient's appetite must be monitored; for instance, those who exercise for only 15 minutes may eat an amount of food afterward that is equivalent to 2 hours of work.

Because coercion is involved in this technique, many patients undergo personality changes. These are important and should be monitored. For instance, a happy person may become quiet. Some change to an aggressive mood, whereas others become juvenile and refuse to exercise after they have come to the clinic. Each attending physician must decide whether such patients are appropriate for forced exercise.

Injury to the patient is not uncommon. Exhaustion, backaches, and joint pain or swelling are sometimes reported, and the patient should be warned about the possibility of back problems. Some clinicians suggest the use of protective covering for ankles, knees, joints, and wrists.

Can Drugs Help You Lose Weight?

Medical drugs have long been used to treat overweight individuals, although the recent attitude among the scientific community has not been encouraging (Stunkard). Table 20-8 summarizes substances that have been used in treating obesity (Hui).

One major group is anorectic drugs, which supposedly depress the appetite of the patient. In 1980 the FDA banned this class of chemicals in

Table 20-8
Characteristics of Drugs Used in Treating Obesity

DRUG	SIDE EFFECTS	MODE OF ACTION	EFFECTIVENESS
Morpholine, imidazoline, and phenylethylamines; e.g., amphetamines (no longer available for prescription)	Addiction, insomnia, dry mouth, hypertension, cardiac arrhythmias, impotence, constipation, allergy, blood disorders, paranoid reactions	Makes the person lose appetite and thus eat less	Not sure
Cellulose: sodium carboxymethyl, hydroxymethyl, methyl ethyl, and methyl derivatives; carrageenin, sodium alginate	Occasional laxative effects	Adsorbs water and expands stomach to produce satiety; slows down the passage of foods, making the person feel full	Not sure
Diuretics	Many; see Chapter 24	Loss of body water (weight loss is not fat)	None
Hormones			
Thyroid hormones	Hazardous: cardiovascular symptoms, including sweating and palpitation	Increases body metabolism	High doses and prolonged treatment effective; but effect transitory
Human chorionic gonadotropin hormone	Minimal	Unknown	Doubtful effect
Growth hormone	Increase in glucose tolerance; not enough data	Mobilizes body fat	May be effective; still being investigated
Progesterone	Not enough data	Reduces pulmonary complications of obesity	Doubtful effect

the treatment of obesity. Both their effectiveness and side effects have been questioned. In general, it is felt that this type of drug helps the patient starting a diet very low in calories overcome the difficult transition period (the first 2 to 6 weeks of dieting). However, the effectiveness of their long-term usage is questionable.

The use of thyroid hormones to treat obesity in patients with no thyroid dysfunction has also been very controversial for a number of years. One major criticism concerns the catabolic effect of the hormone on both fat and muscle protein. The weight lost by using this group of hormones is more muscle protein than fat. However, it is felt that using the hormone at the beginning of a weight reduction regimen has some scientific basis. The body responds to a low-calorie diet by lowering the basal metabolic rate, which obviously interferes with weight loss. An early, small dose of thyroid hormone raises the basal metabolic rate and provides the patient with the incentive of visible weight loss. The long-term usage of this hormone is questioned by authorities because it creates a negative nitrogen balance. Recently, the FDA has issued special warnings regarding the use of thyroid hormones in weight reduction.

Surgery—A Last Resort?

At present, **gastrointestinal bypass** is one surgical approach to treating obesity. The method carries high risks of morbidity and mortality (Stunkard). The technique involves either closing up the stomach partially (stomach stapling) or removing part of the small intestine. In either case, the operation reduces the amount of food digested and absorbed and thus effectively reduces caloric intake. Individuals going through this procedure may lose 100 lb within a few months to a year after the operation. At present, stomach stapling is preferred because of fewer complications. Figure 20-1 shows a patient before and after intestinal bypass surgery.

Some Doctors Starve Their Patients

Partial or total starvation—otherwise known as fasting—is one of the oldest methods of losing weight. In the last few years, it has been popular for two purposes: losing weight and achieving bodily and spiritual well-being. The following is concerned with losing weight (Hui).

As indicated earlier, if one reduces the caloric intake to less than 1,200 kcal per day, the person should be under a physician's supervision. Total or near-total starvation under medical supervision has proved successful in a number of cases, although a small number of patients have died. During the period without food, the doctor monitors a number of important clinical parameters: liver enzyme changes, body mineral balance, formation of the byproduct **ketone bodies**, dehydration, and psychiatric disturbances. These problems definitely require hospitalization, a generous supply of vitamins and minerals, and an occasional dose of sugar (glucose). Slow heart rate and pulse rate, hair loss, weakness, unpleasant taste and breath, low blood pressure, disturbed menstrual cycles, and occasional gum inflammation have been observed in fasting individuals, although none of these manifestations

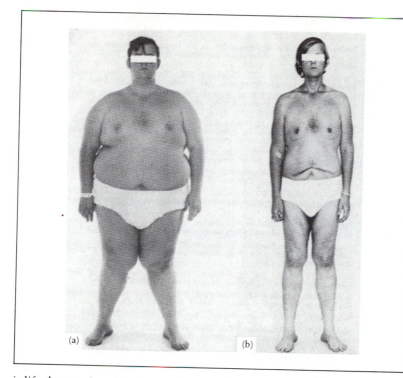

Figure 20-1: (a) A 20-year-old patient at 400 lb. (b) Same patient at 210 lb, 2 years after intestinal bypass.
SOURCE: H. W. Scott, et al. South. Med. J. 69 (1976): 789.

is life threatening. Further, patients under medical supervision are rarely starved completely; most receive about 500 kcal per day.

On the other hand, prolonged unsupervised fasting may result in fluid and electrolyte (mineral) imbalance, mineral and vitamin deficiency, and serious disorders of the heart and circulatory systems. Individuals who fast for more than 2 months develop dry, scaly skin and arrested hair and nail growth. The longer they fast, the more hair falls out. Other observations include abnormal heart rate, kidney damage, and central nervous system impairment; death may occur. At least in the beginning, the nonfatal symptoms are masked by high blood ketones (a body byproduct), which cross the brain barriers and create transient euphoria as a prelude to mental disturbance.

The weight loss created by starvation is a mixture of water, lean muscle, and fat loss with varying proportions of each. Experienced physicians use starvation to treat individuals who are 50 to 200 lb overweight, but not those who are only 5 to 20 lb overweight. As mentioned earlier, even under medical supervision, some patients die from food deprivation.

Some Doctors Make You Do Everything in the Book!

There are many well-run, authentic, reputable, and fairly successful weight reduction clinics in this country. They are staffed with physicians and nurses specializing in the treatment of or research on obesity. Some clinics also employ nutritionists, dietitians, behavioral therapists, and exercise physiologists. They normally provide comprehensive medical weight reduction programs. Well-organized programs may contain some or all of the following treatment procedures: (1) A comprehensive study of the patient's physical and mental condition and medical and weight history, (2) a carefully planned, slowly introduced diet tailored to the patient, (3) appropriate drug therapy for a defined period, (4) a well-designed, slowly introduced exercise program that may be composed of home activities as well as occasional forced exercises in the clinic, (5) intermittent or occasional fasting, and (6) systematic behavioral modifications of eating habits.

These programs can be successful if the patient is conscientious, but they have a number of basic problems. One is high cost. Since the patient has to visit the clinic frequently, the cost can be very high if the treatment period is long. Most insurance carriers do not cover this type of treatment unless health hazards are involved.

A second problem is that clinic programs are time consuming. If the patient has a job, attending the clinic weekly becomes difficult and sometimes impossible. And, no matter how well organized the program, all other nagging issues connected with losing weight are still there: the patience needed to lose weight, the willpower to eat less, unwillingness to change lifelong habits, psychological frustrations, and the difficulty of maintaining normal body weight after the excess is lost.

Don't Kid Yourself, Losing Weight Has Its Problems

When a person is on a diet, the weight loss, especially if rapid, is usually associated with a number of clinical problems. If under medical supervision, the patient will be forewarned. However, overweight individuals trying to lose weight on their own may not be aware of potential risks. Most of the problems are not serious or life threatening if the person follows a nonhazardous or acceptable dieting regimen, including an occasional 1 or 2 days of fasting. Some minor problems associated with weight loss are nervousness, trembling hands, coldness, and scaly and dry skin. The most common problems are briefly summarized below (Hui; Stunkard).

LOSS OF HAIR

Weight loss by reducing caloric intake or partial or total starvation is associated with hair loss. In some people, the hair falls off sparingly; in others, it falls out in chunks. The loss is usually not permanent, and hair grows back normally after dieting is stopped.

MENSTRUAL IRREGULARITIES

Dieting or weight loss in female patients frequently affects the menstrual cycle. Amenorrhea (cessation of menstruation) is most common. It is assumed that the starvation results in a lack of certain hormones to stimulate the uterus to slough its linings. Absence of uterine bleeding also characterizes *anorexia nervosa* (discussed in Chapter 19), a disorder identified mostly in young female patients who reject foods because of psychiatric problems. When such dieting women return to regular eating habits, their menstrual periods return within a short time.

DIETING AND ALCOHOL

Dieting and drinking alcohol are incompatible. A person on a very low calorie diet (for example, 1,000 kcal) for 2 or 3 days may develop hypoglycemia after drinking alcoholic beverages, even as little as 4 or 5 oz of whiskey. For example, within 1 hour after drinking, the person may suddenly feel tired, nervous, weak, nauseated, headachy, or ill, may sweat profusely, and may develop a fast pulse rate.

FAINTING

A person who has not eaten for a short while, such as 1 or 2 days, faints easily in situations such as being in a hot room, standing too long, or trying to stand from a sitting position. Low blood sugar, slow circulation, and low blood pressure have all been suspected to play a part. The popular warning "Don't fly on an empty stomach" makes sense in that the person who has been fasting for a while is more sensitive to a depressed oxygen supply. The hypotension developed will make the person faint.

Dr. Quickloss' New Book, *Losing Weight by Eating More*

The above title of a yet-to-be written book is eyecatching. But whether such a hypothetical book could deliver the goods is debatable. Dr. George V. Mann of Vanderbilt University once stated (*New England Journal of Medicine* 1974; 291: 178):

> *An endless succession of dietary regimens appear in the media, each purporting to be the ultimate solution. These permutations of fuel mixtures range from the impossible to the ridiculous. If they have any common feature it is that they make elaborate promises of success, they understate the rigors of adherence, and they try to place the decision for dietary restriction in the hands of the dieter. . . . The other common feature of reducing regimens is their commercialism—someone stands to make money from their promotion.*

Dieting is a good business for many publishers, authors, and merchants. In the United States, the fad diet market is a multimillion-dollar business. Practically all fad diets fall into one of the following three categories: (1) The dieter is asked to reduce the intake of one or two of the three major calorie-contributing nutrients—fat, carbohydrate, and protein. (2) The dieter is asked to consume daily the same one to three food products. (3) The dieter is asked to consume daily a nutrient (vitamin or mineral) or certain nonfood items.

The box on page 464 lists some once-popular fad diets.

FAD DIETS: DOOMED TO FAILURE

The diets listed in the box are similar in many respects (Hui; Stunkard). None of them teaches a person to eat a well-balanced and nutritious diet, and practically all of them are low in calories. For the first one or two weeks of a diet, there is always some weight loss. The dieter is pleased and word starts to circulate that the diet works. Actually, two facts can explain the weight loss: The diet is low in calories, and the dieter is losing a large amount of fluid, a loss that usually accompanies a reduction in food intake.

If a person is on a fad diet and can lose weight immediately or over a

PRESTO!
ANOTHER MIRACLE DIET!

The secret is a "magic" food
The Rice Diet
The Banana Diet
Candy Diet
Grapefruit Diet
Ice Cream Diet
"Nova Scotia" Diet
Vegetable and Fruit Diets
Eating with Wine
Yogurt Diet

The secret is high protein
Dr. Stillman's Quick Weight
Loss Diet
Dr. Stillman's Inches-Off Diet
New Diet Does It
Lazy Lady Diet
Ratio Diet

The secret is "low carbs"
Carbo-Calorie Diet
Carbo-Cal Diet
Dr. Yudkin's Diet
Drinking Man's Diet
Air Force Diet
Airline Pilots' Diet (Astronauts Diet)

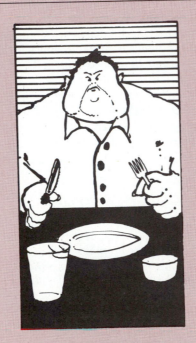

The secret is "low carbs/ high fats"
Dr. Atkin's Diet Revolution
Calories Don't Count
Eat, Drink and Get Thin
Eat and Become Slim

The secret is . . . a secret
The Miracle Diet
No Will Power Diet
McCall's Snack Diet
Zen Macrobiotic Diet
Nine-Day Wonder Diet
Olympia Diet
Magic Formula-Plus Diet
Miraculous Eggnog Diet
Fabulous Formula Diet
Counterweight Diet
Working Man's Diet
Amazing "New You" Diet
Hambletonian Wonder-Week Diet
Editor's Diet
North Pole Slenderizing Plan
Melon-Berry Diet
Vinegar/Lecithin/B_6/Kelp Diet

few months, why is the diet unacceptable? Let us assume that a person loses 5 lb in one week. This rapid loss is physiologically unsound, and in fact quite difficult even if a person is on total starvation. What the person has lost is mainly water with a small amount of protein and fat. When obese people who have "lost" 10 lb after 2 weeks on a fad diet start eating regularly again, they can regain 2 to 5 lb in 3 or 4 days, because they reaccumulate a large amount of water.

If a person can faithfully adhere to a low-calorie fad diet for 6 months, there will be a substantial weight loss. In this case, the loss is due to caloric expenditure exceeding intake. Some dieters claiming to have lost weight after being on a low-calorie fad diet for a long period in fact stay on the diet only initially, for example, for 3 or 4 weeks. After becoming bored with eating the same foods all the time, they randomly eat other foods but in small quantities to ensure a weight loss. Others may stay away from foods 2 or 3 days a week and eat some foods during other days. Extreme cases have been documented in which patients stay away from food completely and must be hospitalized (see Chapter 19).

From the situations above, two conclusions can be drawn. First, the individual will be receiving less than the RDA for a number of nutrients, since the low-calorie fad diet is basically imbalanced. Second, actual weight loss depends on the length of time a person can stay on the diet. A time will come, a week to a few months after starting the diet, when the person can no longer withstand the monotony of eating the same foods and will return to his or her regular eating habits, soon regaining as much or more than he or she had lost by dieting. Accumulating fat is much easier than losing it.

None of the fad diets provides adequate amounts of all essential nutrients. Some may actually be hazardous. For example, eating a large amount of fat and cholesterol may not be good for individuals predisposed to heart disease. Further, semistarvation without medical supervison is hazardous. Finally, what good is a diet if a person gets bored with it after a few days or weeks?

The Last Chance Diet

Recently, physicians at the Mount Sinai and New England Deaconess hospitals (Dr. Victor Vertes of Case Western Reserve University Medical School and Dr. George L. Blackburn of Harvard University Medical School, respectively) started the "modified fasting" program to lose weight (Hui; Stunkard). This program is based on the theory that if a fasting person is provided with essential amino acids (see Chapter 7), the body muscle protein mass will be rebuilt and maintained while the fat is being lost. Three high-quality protein mixtures have been tried by the physicians who started this technique: (1) a mixture of lean beef, chicken, skim milk, egg white, and cheese made from skim milk; (2) commercial nutrient liquid supplements made up of essential amino acids, electrolytes, minerals, vitamins, and a small amount of defined calories normally used for surgical and kidney patients; and (3) special protein solutions containing essential amino acids, such as Optifast, which are specially prepared for and ordered by the above physicians.

All patients on the modified fasting regimen are provided with adequate amounts of essential minerals and vitamins, and they are fully informed at the beginning that they must participate in a total approach to the obesity problem. In addition to the dietary and medical regimen, there is a personalized exercise program, instruction about foods and nutrition, counseling in behavioral modifications, and maintenance of their weight loss at all costs.

Some of the side effects of the modified fasting include: (1) postural hypotension (low blood pressure), at least at the beginning, because of diuresis (loss of water); (2) skin changes, dryness, and transient rash; (3)

fatigue, diarrhea, cold intolerance, hair loss, muscle cramps, amenor-rhea, decreased libido, euphoria (temporary), dry mouth, and bad breath; (4) inflammation of certain organs associated with the intestinal system; for example, the pancreas and gallbladder; (5) negative psychological reactions; and (6) constipation, nausea, vomiting, and a high blood level of a byproduct, uric acid. However, none of these effects is life threatening.

After the modified fasting program was reported in medical literature, some commercial enterprises started selling liquid and powder protein preparations, claiming that they help one to lose weight. Unfortunately, this unscrupulous practice has resulted in death. Some deaths followed the 1976 publication of the book *Last Chance Diet*, written by an osteopath, in which the author advocated fasting supplemented by liquid protein to lose weight. Although the book warns that medical supervision is necessary for such a dietary regimen, many individuals did not follow the advice. When sales of the book rose, commercial protein supplements began to appear in the market, such as Prolin (liquid), P-86 (powder), Ultrathin (powder), Naturslim (powder), and Slim-fast (powder). Within a short time, many individuals, from 5 to 200 lb overweight, tried the diet, some with medical supervision, others without. Since then, more than 20 individuals have died from this regimen, despite the fact that some were under medical supervision. At first the lack of potassium was blamed for the deaths. Later, this theory was refuted, and the reasons for death remain unknown. Almost all who died suffered heart abnormalities with arrhythmias.

Later the FDA (Food and Drug Administration) required a warning label on the products. Because of the adverse publicity caused by the deaths, many liquid products disappeared from the consumer market.

The Cambridge Diet

During the early 1980s, an extremely popular diet was the Cambridge Diet. The Cambridge Diet was nothing more than a liquid, oral formula. It contains about 44 g of carbohydrate, 33 g of protein, and 3 g of fat, providing a total of 330 kcal. The formula also contained RDAs of vitamins and minerals. In 1983, the reported death of a dieter following the Cambridge Diet led to collapse of the company selling this product. This company reportedly reached annual sales of hundreds of millions of dollars at the peak of the formula's popularity.

The Doctor's Quick Weight Loss Diet

Advocates of some diets claim that their plans make it possible to lose weight more quickly or at a higher caloric intake than other diets. This claim is often made for high-protein, low-carbohydrate diets. In "The Doctor's Quick Weight Loss Diet," Irwin Maxwell Stillman claims that his high-protein (virtually no carbohydrates) diet will cause the "system to burn more calories daily than with a diet of the same total caloric intake that includes other foods." He explains that fat is burned at a quicker rate on an "unbalanced" high-protein diet than on a balanced diet (Willis, March 1982).

The rationale for this claim is based on the concept of **ketosis**. Energy is obtained primarily from the breakdown of fat. Ketosis occurs when a person's diet is so low in carbohydrates that the fat deposits are broken down for energy faster than the body can use them. Ketone bodies are formed from the incomplete breakdown of fatty acids. In ketosis, the ketone bodies accumulate. This can lead to an acid/alkaline imbalance in the body. Because the excess ketones must be excreted into the urine, the dieter on a low-calorie, high-protein, low-carbohydrate diet gets rid of large amounts of water, leading to a quick and substantial weight loss. Ketogenic diets, therefore, require a large intake of fluid to wash out excess ketones; otherwise the dieter will become dangerously dehydrated. Because most of the loss is water, not body fat, many dieters regain most of the weight loss soon after normal eating is resumed.

Another physiological fact to consider before embarking on a ketogenic diet is that in ketosis the body's mode of burning calories may be similar to that of fasting. The body's fuel comes from glucose, which is most easily obtained from carbohydrates and less easily from protein. When the body lacks carbohydrates, as when a person is fasting or is on a low-calorie, very low carbohydrate diet, protein is degraded to supply the minimum level of glucose. This protein is taken from lean body mass—muscles and major organs such as the liver, heart, and kidneys. This is primarily the reason for the rather dramatic initial weight loss in low-calorie, high-protein diets. Whereas 3,500 calories are needed to burn a pound of body fat, it takes only 480 calories to eliminate a pound of "lean body mass."

Calories Don't Count

Originators of diets in the past few years seem to have kept in step with health concerns of their times. For example, in the early 1960s, the rising concern with the avoidance of saturated fat seems to have given credence to a ketogenic diet espoused by Dr. Herman Taller in the book *Calories Don't Count*. Taller theorized (Willis, March 1982) that the number of calories a person consumes doesn't matter, and that "the calories of carbohydrate and the calories of unsaturated vegetable oil work quite differently in the system." His unproven theories were based on the tenet that a person had to eat polyunsaturated fats to be slim. Because the book was being sold in stores alongside capsules of safflower oil, the FDA instituted proceedings charging violation of drug regulations against Taller, who was also convicted of mail fraud and conspiracy.

The Mayo Diet

A claim by some diets is that a certain food somehow burns calories to get rid of fat. One version of this is the grapefruit diet, in which dieters are instructed to eat grapefruit before each meal and then literally stuff themselves with as much bacon, eggs, meat, fish, and vegetables as they like (Willis, March 1982). The diet is based on the erroneous theory that grapefruit contains enzymes that somehow subtract calories by increasing the fat-burning process. The diet is often called the "Mayo Diet," although the famed Mayo Clinic in Rochester, Minnesota, steadfastly denies any association with it.

The Fabulous 14-day Fructose Diet

A recent entry into the weight loss sweepstakes is the fructose diet, which capitalizes on the current interest in fructose as an alternative to table sugar (sucrose—half fructose, half glucose) (Willis, March 1982). The Fabulous 14-day Fructose Diet is a ketogenic, low-carbohydrate, high-protein diet that provides approximately 700 to 1,000 calories a day. About 150 of those calories are from fructose.

The Beverly Hills Diet

Another recent and highly successful weight loss program is Judy Mazel's Beverly Hills Diet book, which was No. 1 on the New York Times nonfiction best-seller list for several weeks in the fall of 1981 (Willis, March 1982).

This diet combines sound health advice, such as limiting sodium, with trendy ideas such as the use of bran, sesame seeds, brewer's yeast, and raw butter. Basically, the Beverly Hills diet is a low-calorie fruit diet. For the first week the dieter eats only pineapples, bananas, papayas, mangos, strawberries, apricots, blueberries, watermelon, apples, and prunes.

It is not until the eleventh day of the diet that something other than fruit is allowed (bagels, butter, and corn on the cob), and it is not until the ninteenth day that a significant source of protein (steak or lobster) is permitted. Then, through the fifth week, protein foods are allowed only one day a week.

The Beverly Hills Diet is based on the false theory that protein and carbohydrate digestive enzymes cannot work together and that although protein enzymes are needed for digesting protein, and carbohydrate enzymes for carbohydrates, fruit does not need the body's enzymes for digestion because it has its own enzymes. Another unfounded claim made by Mazel is that the enzymes in fruit can render other foods less fattening.

"Fat," Mazel says, "means . . . undigested food. . . . When your body doesn't process food, doesn't digest it, the food turns to fat."

Mazel claims that to digest food properly, a process she calls "conscious combining" must be used. Her rules of conscious combining call for eating proteins only with other proteins, and fats and carbohydrates only with other carbohydrates and fats. Fruits are to be eaten alone. Because of the supposed enzymatic process, once a protein is eaten on a given day, the dieter must continue to eat only protein, with absolutely no carbohydrates or fruit, for the remainder of that day.

In an article in the November 15, 1981 issue of the *Journal of the American Medical Association*, Doctors G. B. Merkin and R. N. Shore wrote:

Not only is there no scientific evidence to support this diet plan, but it also contradicts established knowledge about nutrition. . . . Before a food can be absorbed into the bloodstream, it must be broken down by specific enzymes manufactured by the body. Enzymes in the food—the focus of Ms. Mazel's attention—are irrelevant to the absorption process. Food not broken down by enzymes will not be absorbed from the intestinal tract. It will pass out with the stool without supplying any calories whatever. Contrary to the main contention of the Beverly Hills Diet, then, it is the digested *food that has the potential to make you fat. Undigested food cannot possibly be fattening.*

Some potential and documented harmful effects from the Beverly Hills Diet include severe diarrhea, muscle weakness and dizziness, gout, kidney stones, heart problems, and perforated peptic ulcers. Other potential dangers include shock, strokes and even death, although there are no reports of deaths of persons following this diet.

More Weight Loss Wonders

Millions of Americans believe that somehow, as if by waving a magic wand, they will be thin and firm. Unwilling or unable to lose weight through diet and exercise, they turn to weight-loss gimmicks ranging from pills that supposedly let them eat unlimited pastas to rubber suits that make them sweat while they sleep. Most current diet gimmicks (Willis, November 1982) seem to fall into two categories: (1) Custom garments or body wraps that claim to "melt" away fat in a short time, and (2) pills that supposedly curb appetites without side effects, or allow dieters to eat as much as—or more than—normally and still lose weight. The pills are usually touted as the product of some previously undiscovered process.

BODY WRAPS

Who can resist ads for body wraps that promise "to burn away fat even while you sleep," to "lose 4–6 inches the first day"? Some of the plastic or rubber garments are worn around the waist; some cover the waist, hips, and thighs; others cover nearly the entire body. Some are to be worn while carrying out routine activities, others while exercising, and some while sleeping. One is inflated with air from a vacuum cleaner. Another uses an electric hair dryer to blow in warm air. Some are used after a cream, gel, or lotion is applied or after the wrap is soaked in a solution.

The FDA has investigated a number of these products and has taken action against several promoters of wrapping devices and latex exercise or sweat suits for making unsubstantiated medical or therapeutic claims.

The garments and wraps, with or without lotions and creams, reduce body dimensions by removing fluids. Most medical experts agree that such treatment will cause a loss of inches and perhaps pounds due to profuse perspiration, but the reductions are temporary. The fluid is soon replaced by drinking or eating. But rapid and excessive fluid loss is potentially dangerous because it can bring on severe dehydration and can upset the balance of important electrolytes in the body.

Wraps have no effect on fat deposits and will not dissolve fat, even temporarily. Fat is not broken down by perspiration. It is eliminated only when fewer calories are consumed than are needed to meet the body's energy requirements.

STARCH BLOCKERS

Starch blockers are an example of a product sold as a food but considered by the FDA to be a drug. Advertised and sold nationwide, starch blockers allegedly block or impede starch digestion and thus help in weight control and weight reduction (Willis, November 1982). One manufacturer touted the product as a "revolutionary new concept in natural weight control." Print and TV ads claimed people taking starch blocker pills could eat up to 600 kcal a day of foods such as bread, potatoes, and pasta without absorbing the calories.

Users of these products have complained to the FDA of nausea, vomiting, diarrhea, and stomach pains. The pills are considered to be particularly hazardous to diabetics, who may rely on their purported carbohydrate-blocking effect to calculate their diets.

According to the starch blocker theory, the pills contain a substance that inhibits the activity of the enzyme amylase, which digests carbohydrates (see Chapter 14).

Over 100 different starch blocker preparations have been widely sold by pharmacists and health food stores. Each starch blocker tablet is alleged to produce enough antiamylase activity to block the digestion and absorption of 100 to 150 g of starch (400 to 600 kcal). Thus, people who enjoy eating bread, spaghetti, and potatoes but who still want to lose weight have been urged in advertisements to take a starch blocker with their meals. This weight control concept has been so attractive to the public that over 1 million starch blocker tablets were consumed daily in the United States in the first part of 1982.

On October 31, 1983, the United States Postal Service charged (P.S. Docket No. 15/115) that General Nutrition Corporation (General Nutrition Centers, 418 Wood St., Pittsburgh, PA 15222-1878) was engaged in conducting a scheme for obtaining money through the mails by means of false representations in violation of 39 U.S. Code 3005 (formerly 39 U.S. Code 4005) with respect to the sale of the product Starch-Block. The company was forbidden to use the U.S. Postal Service to mail the product. In November 1983, the FDA was able to obtain permission from the court through further legal actions to destroy the remaining millions of tablets containing the substance. Some advertisements for the product are reproduced in the box on page 471.

SPIRULINA

Another natural substance promoted as a weight-loss wonder is spirulina (Willis, November 1982). It is sold as a food or food supplement in the form of a dark green powder or pill in many health food stores. Spirulina is one of about 1,500 known species of blue-green algae that grow in brackish ponds and lakes in mild and hot climates throughout the world. Pure spirulina is a source of protein and contains a number of vitamins and minerals. However, in the amounts normally consumed when taken according to label directions, the nutrients derived are insignificant. As a food, spirulina can be legally marketed so long as it is labeled accurately and contains no contaminated or adulterated substances.

Claims have been made that phenylalanine, an amino acid found in spirulina (and in most other protein sources), "acts on the brain's

Some Advertising Claims for Starch Blockers

Nearly 25% of the average American's calories come from starch (carbohydrates). Starch-Block was created in concentrated form to block calories from being absorbed in your system. This natural enzyme blocker prevents the breakdown of starch into simple sugars so that they are not absorbed as calories. With less calorie intake, you begin to lose weight . . . it's just that simple.

Starch-Block is not an appetite suppressant, dangerous fad diet, or chemically created drug. It's a natural enzyme that was lab tested. One group used Starch-Block and the other group did not. The group using Starch-Block lost more weight and with no undesirable side effects!

These exciting results were put to use in the development of STARCH BLOCK. Now you can put STARCH BLOCK to work for you!

Now! Eat the pasta, potatoes, cereals, and breads you want, and . . . *Block out up to 1800 Starch Calories a day with— Starch Block.* The revolutionary new concept in natural weight control is a pasta lover's dream come true! Think of it—a *single* Starch Block tablet can block the conversion of the starch in 1½ pounds of cooked spaghetti, for instance, into absorbable calories.

appetite center to switch off your hunger pangs." There is no scientific evidence for such claims.

Some nutritionists fear that consuming large amounts of spirulina might have an effect similar to that of the liquid protein diets that resulted in heart problems and even death for some dieters. As single-celled organisms, algae such as spirulina are rich in nucleic acids providing not only protein but also large amounts of uric acid which could result in kidney stones or gout.

"Cellulite"

Advertisements would convince us that "cellulite" is some special form of fat that women have, requiring special efforts to eliminate it (Fenner). Fat, however, is fat. Despite that fact, promoters have developed special methods for combating cellulite, and these methods sell well. "Loofah" sponges, cactus fiber washcloths, cellulite-dissolving creams, horsehair mitts, and bath lotions are among such products. Further, beauty salon treatments are available. The cellulite battles are curious in light of the lack of scientific evidence that cellulite even exists. The word does not appear in standard medical dictionaries, even those published since cellulite has become a battle cry of the weight wars, nor does it appear in the most recent Webster's dictionary. As you would expect, there is also no medical evidence that any of the special cellulite products have any effect on the loss of fat.

Promoters of cellulite products claim that tissues under the skin combine fat and other waste products not properly eliminated to yield a gel-like substance that bulges, a substance they call cellulite. The most common cellulite regions are thighs, buttocks, and hips. Medical experts have noted several facts that contradict cellulite theorists.

First, toxins are not held in the body in any one location. Second, if the liver or kidneys were not properly eliminating waste products, serious illness would result, such as toxemia. Third, there is no known link between waste products and connective tissue of the skin or fat cells.

What this contradictory information leads us to is the question: If cellulite doesn't exist, why do women have fat bulges with a wafflelike appearance whereas men do not? The answer rests in heredity and sex-linked characteristics. Men deposit fat in the abdomen. Women deposit it in the thighs, buttocks, hips, and breasts. Fat distribution is a hereditary characteristic, so you are likely to deposit fat in the same locations as your parents do.

The real key to the wafflelike appearance of women's skin versus men's skin is the difference between male and female cells. Women's skin has underlying fat cells that are large and round. Men's skin has small, polygonal cells that do not readily bulge. Further, women's skin is thinner, allowing subsurface structures to show more readily. With age, the skin becomes even thinner and more elastic.

In conclusion, the so-called cellulite is simple fat. Removing it requires diet and exercise, and it should be removed by age 35 to 40, while the skin is still elastic enough to return to its original shape. Special cellulite products bring no relief, and obesity experts agree that no treatment can result in fat elimination in a specific location of the body to the exclusion of other parts of the body. If an individual has excess weight, the loss of that excess weight will affect all body organs, including the so-called hot spots of cellulite theorists.

Some Diet Doctors' Advice

First, when using a diet to lose weight, check its authenticity and accuracy. Consult your physician, public health nutritionist, hospital dietitian, or an academic specializing in the field.

Second, when using any over-the-counter drugs, check their effectiveness and safety. Seek medical supervision if so advised on the label. Consult *Consumer Reports*, your physician, or an academic specialist in pharmacology and related fields. Any prescription drug that was not prescribed for *you* should not be taken without full awareness of its safety and effectiveness.

Third, do not believe any advertisement promoting a diet, drug, device, regimen, or other procedure that *guarantees* weight loss. At present, there is no known method that can guarantee weight loss with absolute safety.

Fourth, exercise—but take precautions. The exercise program must be appropriate for your individual age, sex, and medical conditions.

Proper professional advice must be sought, or a professionally written manual for physical activity must be followed.

Fifth, at present, avoid most mechanical devices for losing weight, which can be harmful. Body wrappings, for example, can impair circulation.

Finally, before adopting any diet or weight loss program, be sure that you are in normal health. Many diets, drugs, and exercise programs are all right for normal, healthy people. If at all feasible, inform your physician of what you are doing and ask him or her to help check your progress or check your health before beginning any program. If you are unable to consult your doctor, talk to other health professionals such as nutritionists. If they work in a health clinic, they will provide advice and assistance as a public service and will not charge a fee.

The most effecive way to lose weight is to combine at least a minimal amount of daily activity with learning the basics of good nutrition, retraining eating habits, and following a sensible and practical low-calorie diet.

STUDY QUESTIONS

1. What is the difference between the terms *overweight* and *obese*?

2. How many excess kilocalories (energy not spent) does it take to gain 1 lb of body fat?

3. Name at least six medical problems for which people more than 15 percent overweight run a higher-than-normal risk. What are some nonmedical problems associated with obesity?

4. What five considerations are essential to any successful weight loss program?

5. What assumptions underlie the behavioral modification approach to weight loss? Describe some techniques for reducing stimulus control of eating.

6. Discuss the techniques and potential hazards, if any, of hypnotism, jaw wiring, forced exercise, and surgical approaches to weight loss.

7. Is fasting recommended for those who are obese or only slightly overweight? What is a modified fasting program?

8. What physical problems tend to accompany weight loss, particularly if weight is lost quickly?

9. Compile a list of diet books that were popular during the last 2 years.

10. Compile a list of diet aids that were popular during the last 2 years.

REFERENCES

Fenner, L. "Cellulite: Hard to Budge Pudge." *FDA Consumer* 14 (May 1980): 4.

Hui, Y. H. *Human Nutrition and Diet Therapy.* Monterey, Calif.: Wadsworth Health Sciences, 1983.

Stunkard, A. J., ed. *Obesity.* Philadelphia: W. B. Sanders, 1980.

Willis, J. "Diet Books Sell Well but . . ." *FDA Consumer* 16 (March 1982): 14.

Willis, J. "About Body Wraps, Pills and Other Magic Wands for Losing Weight." *FDA Consumer* 16 (November 1982): 18.

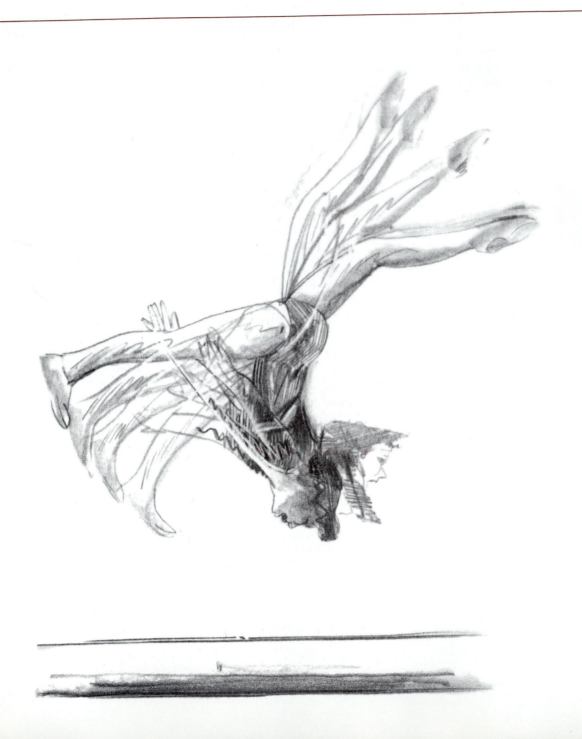

21

Nutrition AND Athletes

Luke
ENDANGERS HIS HEART

Luke, age 36, had practiced for the marathon for a year and wanted a competitive edge to enhance his first race. He had read that a technique called "carbohydrate loading" could improve endurance by building a maximum amount of glycogen in the muscles. He decided to try it.

One week before the marathon, Luke depleted his leg muscles by a fast 15-mile run. Then, for three days he ate mostly protein, consciously avoiding carbohydrate. He primarily ate meat, supplemented by several pounds of cheese.

For the next three days he began adding as much bread as he could hold, frequently eating a loaf at a sitting. Five days into this special diet, Luke felt a dull pain on the left side of his chest. The next day the pain became

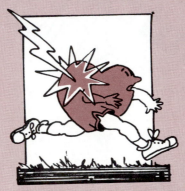

sharper and more severe. Light jogging did not increase the pain, but he did feel sporadic sharp pains while jogging. Luke skipped the marathon and consulted his physician. After confirming an abnormal electrocardiogram, the doctor advised Luke to switch to one small meal per day and to monitor his

pains. The pain subsided and disappeared in five days.

Two weeks later Luke ran for one and one-half minutes without pain, and the resulting EKG was normal. His physician advised him to avoid racing for four months and to greatly reduce his caloric intake.

Luke came dangerously close to demonstrating what clinicians have discovered about dietary manipulation and athletics. Although certain practices, especially carbohydrate loading, may increase endurance, heart trouble can be a high price to pay for trying to gain a competitive edge (Mirkin). Luke's heart trouble—*infarction*, the death of heart tissue—was precipitated by carbohydrate loading. The mechanism of the cause and effect relationship between the two is to date unknown.

Looking for the Magic Menu

Like Luke, many athletes try to increase their competitive edge with special diets. Researchers studying athletes have now come to some basic understandings regarding athletics and nutrition (Haskell et al.). First, the basic nutritional needs of an athlete differ little from those of the average healthy individual. Second, the RDAs used to plan optimal daily nutrient intakes for the general population apply equally to athletes, providing consideration is given to the increased physical activity of sports participants. Third, although most athletes nurture the idea that somewhere out there lurks that right combination of foods to improve performance, this is a myth. Fourth, if an athlete is healthy and well conditioned and eats a balanced diet, no dramatic improvements in nutritional state are possible. Finally, the relationship of a nutritious diet and physical conditioning to winning is in direct proportion to the athlete's desire and determination to win.

The one factor that makes the difference between champion athletes and other competitors is the psychology of winning. Thus, if an athlete believes a certain eating habit benefits performance, the habit should not be discouraged so long as the quantities consumed do not pose a hazard.

If an athlete decides to make a significant change in dietary habits, such as excessive consumption of a particular vitamin or drastic reduction of salt intake, or if an athlete anticipates undertaking a major weight loss or weight gain, he or she should do so only under the guidance of someone knowledgeable in the field of diet and nutrition.

Certain sports require large food intake, especially during the training stage and while the athlete is still growing. The need for meat, eggs, cheese, milk, bread, fresh fruits, vegetables, and juices in large quantities has caused many athletes, and their parents, to doubt they can afford training programs. Without adequate financial support, quantity and quality diets and intensive training can be weakened. In college sports, an attractive "training table" of large quantities of food has proved an effective recruiting device. Bill Ellington, Assistant Athletic Director, University of Texas, once stated: "The year-round training table is an important recruiting gimmick in this part of the country. We get a lot of boys from poor families who can't afford to pay for their food. The way prices are going, it is a strong selling point to middle-class families with big kids to feed."

The information contained in other chapters, especially Chapter 17, also applies in planning daily menus for an athlete. Generally, the athlete needs a substantial breakfast, a light lunch, and a satisfying dinner that is served one to two hours after daily practice is finished. The serving time of meals should be scheduled so that food digestion and absorption will not compete with the athlete's physical activity.

What *Should* Athletes Eat?

There is no "magic formula" for a winning combination of carbohydrate, protein, and fats, but a reasonable combination would be 15 percent of daily calories as protein, 55 percent as carbohydrate, and 30 percent as fats. Fats and carbohydrates serve as the major energy sources, with fats providing more calories than carbohydrates per unit weight. However, the body's physiology is such that carbohydrates are more efficiently utilized than fats. For example, our bodies release 5 kcal of energy from carbohydrates for each liter of oxygen consumed. Protein and fats are 4.5 and 4.6 kcal, respectively. Further, dietary fat intake must be considered in relation to the athlete's sensitivity to excessive cholesterol and saturated-fat consumption.

A significant concern to athletes is the relationship between protein and muscle mass. Generally, the belief that eating more eggs, meat, and cheese will enable an established adult athlete to develop more muscles and perform better in competition is erroneous. Later in this chapter we will, however, examine certain specific conditions in which high protein intake can be helpful.

The following section discusses the latest scientific and practical recommendations for the nutrition and dietary care of an athlete (Eiseman and Johnson; Haskell et al.; Williams).

CALORIES

Three factors influence an athlete's daily caloric need: personal criteria, type of sport, and environmental conditions. Caloric need varies according to such individual criteria as age, sex, type of body build, height, and weight (not only present weight but also ideal weight and past weight). Further variation relates to the particulars of the sport, such as conditioning regimens, practice frequency and duration, and type of sport. Finally, caloric need varies according to clothing required, temperatures encountered, and physical surroundings of practices and competition.

Obviously, the intensity and duration of training constitute the most significant variables. Depending on the circumstances, an athlete requires 3,000 to 7,000 kcal, compared with 2,500 to 3,000 for the nonathlete. The caloric need increases as conditioning and exercise increase, and the healthy athlete's appetite keeps pace. For example, estimates hold that an American college football player requires 4,000 kcal daily, about 15 percent more than a nonathlete undergraduate of the same age, sex, and so forth.

Although food carbohydrates and fats provide the major energy fuel for athletes, cultural differences can affect dietary habits. For example, calculations have shown that Italian athletes may derive as much as 5 percent of their caloric intake from alcoholic beverages such as wine.

PROTEIN

On the average, an athlete requires 0.8 g of protein per kg body weight. Since most athletes consume a high-calorie diet, adequate protein is available to them. Preference among athletes for high protein intake therefore lacks physiological justification and must be considered psychological.

In the case of a younger athlete, however, higher protein intake is necessary because the athlete is still growing and requires protein for the developing muscle mass. A second situation requiring higher protein intake involves contact sports and the need for protein in the repair of damaged tissue. For example, football and hockey players need extra protein. The greatest protein need would, therefore, occur for a young athlete in a contact sport. These athletes may require 1 to 2 g of protein per day per kg body weight.

It has been suggested that one can increase strength training by stimulating the muscles with more protein, but this has not been scientifically substantiated. For example, in an adult athlete, muscle mass is already established. Ordinary conditioning and exercising does not significantly break down or metabolize protein muscle, so no need for additional dietary protein is created. Although exercise does cause some of the amino acids to be released and metabolized after muscle glycogen has been depleted, even then no increased need for dietary protein exists.

Given the amount of food eaten by American athletes, protein deficiency would indeed be rare.

Red meat, poultry, fish, cheese, and eggs all provide good and complete protein. Provided an athlete makes a good selection of vegetables including beans, peas, and peanut butter, even a vegetarian diet is acceptable for athletes. A vegetarian diet for athletes has proved neither detrimental nor of special benefit to performance.

Athletes should realize that increased protein intake results in greater water consumption. Since muscle cells are 70 to 72 percent water, each gram of protein deposited accumulates 3 g of water. When protein intake is high, more waste products such as urea are produced, requiring more water for the excretion process. The kidneys must work harder to maintain the body's proper acid-base balance.

FATS AND CARBOHYDRATES

Many people believe that athletes and fats do not make good teammates, yet athletes often need fat. For example, in contact sports such as football, fat cushions the organs against damage. Cardiac muscle relies on fatty acids rather than carbohydrates as the preferred energy source. Extra fat in swimmers adds buoyancy, and higher flotation enables faster movement through water. This is especially helpful for long distance swimmers. Cold-water swimmers depend on fat as a thermal insulation. Because swimmers have an above average aerobic capacity, their muscular activity draws on fatty acids as well as glucose as fuel.

Usually, the greater the amount of body fat, the less oxygen the athlete can take in. Weight lifters and wrestlers seem to have successful performance despite fat, but their aerobic capacity is generally low. Fat constitutes an obvious handicap for certain sports. A high jumper, for example, will have decreased performance if he cannot easily lift his weight for the jump. The shot putter has no need for excess fat in comparison to muscle mass. Table 21-1 lists body fat approximations for athletes in various sports.

Whether body muscle draws energy from fats or carbohydrates depends on the athlete's maximum aerobic capacity. When sufficient oxygen is available, fat is used as fuel; this invariably involves low-intensity exercise. Carbohydrates serve as fuel sources during heavy physical exertion and endurance events. Thus, for light to prolonged aerobic work, 50 to 70 percent of energy for muscle activity comes from fats. Once 90% of maximum oxygen capacity is reached under strenuous exercise, exercise becomes anaerobic and uses carbohydrates. The carbohydrate use increases as oxygen availability decreases. Thus, a high-fat diet impairs performance in an endurance event, whereas a high-carbohydrate diet enhances it.

A small amount of body fat is always essential to athletes engaged in endurance exercise, since the fat contributes a "permanent" source of energy supply. The preference for fats or carbohydrates at any given time will, however, depend on variables including amount of oxygen available to muscles, intensity and duration of exercise, and personal health and conditioning.

Table 21-1
Approximate Body Fats in Players of Different Sports

PARTICIPANTS IN SPORTS	APPROX-IMATE % BODY FAT
Female gymnasts	2–4
Middle distance or long distance runners and skiers	3–5
Sprinters	6–8
Long distance swimmers	7–10
Heavy weight lifters and wrestlers	10–15
American football players	8–20
Sumo wrestlers	15–25

Figure 21-1 illustrates how fats and carbohydrates provide energy to the muscular activity. Muscular work receives support from glucose and fatty acids. Glucose can be obtained from the degradation of stored glycogen, and fatty acids are obtained from fat. The muscle and liver are the storage houses, respectively.

Maximum muscular activity is fueled by available glucose in muscle and by continuous breakdown of muscle and liver glycogen, as illustrated in Figure 21-1. For activities that last from a few seconds to a couple of hours, glycogen serves as an immediate and important source of energy. Simultaneously, muscle derives energy from free fatty acids. Although fats do contribute energy, muscles can become fatigued after their glycogen source is exhausted. Hence, after heavy training, the exhaustion of glycogen and the low blood glucose level may induce in the athlete a temporary hypoglycemic condition characterized by dizziness, headache, and nervousness. All available evidence confirms that the more glycogen we have in our muscles, the longer and better we can perform in such endurance events as long distance running.

Recent sports nutrition research has shown that an athlete can plan dietary intake so that maximum glycogen will be deposited in the body's muscles. The practice is variously known as glycogen loading, supersaturation, or supercompensation. To accomplish glycogen loading, about one week before an event an athlete exercises exhaustively to deplete glycogen. For the first three or four days, only fats and protein should be consumed. Exercise can be to any extent desired during this time. Then, for the next two days, the athlete should eat a high-carbohydrate diet and should exercise very little. At the end of the week of controlled dieting, muscles will be loaded with glycogen in preparation for the event. The training rule underlying the foregoing process is that conditioning and training should be curtailed for 30 to 45 hours prior to the event to permit muscle recovery of glycogen to maximum accumulation. Such glycogen maximization has proved of benefit in such

Figure 21-1: Interrelationship between liver and muscle in supplying muscular activity with glucose and fatty acids.

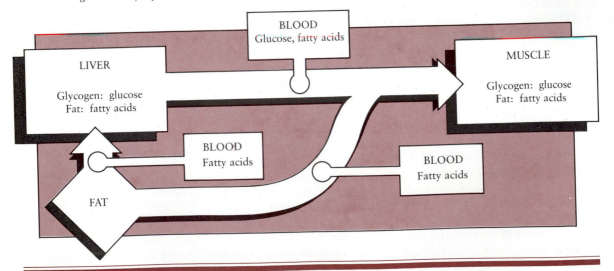

endurance events as marathon running, bicycling, and cross-country skiing, events in which performance is sustained for more than one hour and during which more than 70 percent of maximum oxygen consumption is sustained.

Some debate surrounds the choice of carbohydrates during the final two days of glycogen loading. The alternatives are mono- and disaccharides (juices and table sugar) or polysaccharides (starches). It appears that polysaccharides such as potatoes, bread, rice, and spaghetti are emptied slowly from the stomach. They may be expected to produce a slow, long-lasting insulin release from the pancreas, yielding a sustained high blood glucose level. The glucose is delivered to the muscle cells for glycogen formation that is slow, continuous, and lasting.

Water retention remains a concern relative to glycogen loading. Two to five pounds of weight gain may result from the loading period. Weighing daily after breakfast and after urination should show the progressive gain and confirm the glycogen deposition. The water will result in a feeling of heaviness and in stiffness of muscles. Hypoglycemia, which we discussed earlier in this section, will follow depletion of the large glycogen load. In addition to these drawbacks to glycogen loading, other adverse effects—effects that have not been examined for their seriousness—include potential heart trouble, possible **ketosis** during the noncarbohydrate period, and increased blood cholesterol and triglyceride levels.

Studies of the positive effects of glycogen loading have been performed. In a test of bicycle ergometer readings, glycogen-saturated athletes recorded 167 minutes, whereas balanced-diet athletes and high-protein-diet but otherwise balanced-diet athletes recorded 44 minutes and 57 minutes, respectively. In an 11-mile run test, glycogen "loaders" still had glycogen at the end of the race, whereas regular-diet athletes had depleted their glycogen. The higher the initial glycogen level of the runners in the test, the better the performance in terms of running ability and times. Among all subjects, running speed slowed as muscle glycogen levels decreased. To maintain a continuous and fast running pace, quadricep muscle glycogen should be 3 to 5 g per kg muscle.

Dr. Paul Slovic of the Oregon Research Institute in Behavioral Sciences, Eugene, Oregon, studied runners in the 1974 Trail's End Marathon at Seaside, Oregon (Slovic). Half the athletes finishing the race in less than 3 hours were glycogen loaders. Dr. Slovic found that for the first 10 miles of the race, there was no difference in pace between loaders and nonloaders. In the next 5 miles, glycogen loaders were 2 minutes faster. In the next 5 miles they were 2½ minutes faster. In the last leg of the 26-mile, 785-yard run, the glycogen-loaded runners had a much faster pace. The final time difference was a spread of 6 to 11.5 minutes. Though it was noted that glycogen loaders would have higher initial motivation and training ability, it still appears that carbohydrate saturation did not make a significant difference in the first half of the race but clearly did in the second half.

Some physicians have described unique benefits of fat to females in endurance events. They report that many women do not "hit the wall," a marathon term for glycogen depletion. One theory suggests that because women's bodies have a higher proportion of fat and are generally lighter than men's, they can derive more energy from fat than from carbohydrates. Another theory holds that female sex hormones may help in mobilizing and metabolizing the fat more efficiently. Such explanations have not yet been substantiated.

FLUIDS AND ELECTROLYTES

An athlete requires a high salt intake because body fluid is lost in perspiration. The 5 to 20 g of sodium chloride needed per day well exceeds normal need. Both too much or too little salt are harmful. For example, low blood sodium can cause heat cramps.

The normal replacement of salt occurs through consumption of salty foods. But if more than 5 to 7 pounds of sweat are lost, as through one to two weeks of heat exposure, salt tablets may be necessary. Salt therapy should be under a physician's guidance and should not be long-term. Usually, one seven-grain salt tablet is prescribed for each pound lost above a 6 to 7 pound weight or water loss.

Water compensation for sweat loss is more important than salt replacement, because the salt concentration in sweat is lower than in body fluids. When the athlete's body weight decreases by 4 to 5 percent owing to water loss, efficiency drops by 10 to 15 percent. A hockey player may consume 2.5 to 3 kg of body weight through sweating. The natural thirst response helps prevent the loss of body water beyond 5 percent, the danger level.

Through experience, we have learned the hard way that water is important to athletic health. It had been felt for many years that water created the likelihood of bloat. Then, in 1962, several southern high school and college football players died during practice as a result of dehydration, heat prostration, and rise in body temperature. Water is critical for both fluid balance and body temperature regulation. Since the tragedy, players stop every 30 minutes for water, and humidity machines warn when humidity is too low. Practice sometimes must begin as early as 4 to 6 A.M. to avoid the heat.

Various methods have been suggested for restoring fluid and electrolytes in an athlete: salt, water, salt and water, intravenous saline, glucose solution, salt and glucose solution, solution of electrolytes, and/or a mixture of potassium, sodium, water and carbohydrates. Some have claimed that giving electrolytes between games prevents cramps. No evidence recommends one therapy over another. Most assuredly, water or dilute salt solution should be freely accessible on the field for practice and games.

VITAMINS AND MINERALS

If an athlete consumes a well-balanced diet, no vitamin or mineral supplement will enhance performance. Studies have been undertaken to determine athlete behavior relating to supplements. The results of Dr. Ellington Darden's (Florida State University) interviews at the 1972 Munich Olympics are summarized in Table 21-2. Some of the athletes regularly took nutrient supplements.

Table 21-2
Some Olympic Athletes' Views on Nutrient Supplements

ATHLETE	SPECIALTY	VITAMINS AND MINERALS SUPPLEMENT	OTHER SUPPLEMENTS	SELECTED REMARKS FROM ATHLETE
Rod Milburn	Olympic champion, 110-meter high hurdles	None	None	
John Smith	World record holder, 440-yard run	Yes	Protein	To guard against possible insufficient intake.
Jim Ryan	Holder of world record in 1,500-meter run and mile run	None	None	
Steve Prefontaine	American record holder in the 3,000- and 5,000-meter runs	Yes	Breakfast drink with wheat germ oil	Practice will not hurt.
Jeff Galloway	American record holder for 10-mile run	None	None	
Frank Shorter	Olympic champion in the marathon	None	Carbohydrate loading	Training is more important than nutrition.
Deanne Wilson	American champion, women's high jump	12 different pills daily		The supplements may help.
Olga Connolly	Former Olympic champion, women's discus	None	None	
Mark Spitz	7 gold medals in swimming	None	None	
Doug Northway	Bronze medal winner in 1,500-meter freestyle swimming	1 multivitamin pill daily	Several salt tablets	
Tom Burleson	Tallest athlete at Olympics, 7'4", U.S. basketball team member	None	None	
Phil Grippaldi	Several times American champion, middle heavy weight class, U.S. weightlifting team member	7 individual vitamin pills at each meal	Liver protein supplement	Lag in endurance when not taking wheat germ oil.

SOURCE: Adapted from E. Darden. *J. Home Economics*, 65, (February 1973): p. 8.

Certain sports physicians occasionally inject calcium gluconate to relieve muscle cramps. This is a dangerous practice, since hypercalcemia (high blood calcium) may result (also see later discussion). Protection against muscle cramps should be achieved by consumption of fluid and electrolytes, including sodium, potassium, and calcium, well before contests occur. Muscle cramps will disappear after rest and fluid therapy. By the intake of good calcium food sources, such as milk and milk products, fluids, and vegetables, the well-conditioned athlete should never need calcium injections.

The term "sports anemia" refers to the lowering of blood hemoglobin and iron concentration during the early part of a strenuous training program, probably a result of the destruction of red blood cells. Some sports physicians suggest a need for more iron. Other sports physicians note that microscopic *hematuria* (blood in the urine) can develop and can escape detection. They propose hemoglobin monitoring every two weeks. Although some European swimmers develop anemia, long distance skiers do not. It has been theorized that higher altitudes may stimulate hemoglobin formation. Also refer to the later part of this chapter. The term "blood doping" has been ascribed to the reported practice of withdrawing blood from an athlete in peak condition, refrigerating it until just prior to performance, and then readministering it just prior to performance. Not only the ethics of such a practice but its benefit have been questioned.

Female athletes experience iron shortages, just as do female nonathletes. Studies have demonstrated that athletes can overburden the menstrual physiology. Pain, indisposition, and cessation of menses (periods) can result. It appears that such effects are influenced by a combination of training, changes in nutritional intake, and body composition changes. One study found that young girls undergoing intensive training had the onset of menstruation delayed by a few months in comparison with others not undergoing such intensive training.

From our discussion of the dietary nutrients relative to athletes, we can determine a daily food guide for an athlete. The diet should contain

3 to 5 servings of milk and milk products

3 to 5 servings of red meat, poultry, fish, eggs, cheese, peas, beans, and nuts

3 to 5 servings of vitamin C–rich fruits and juices (oranges, apples, etc.)

3 to 5 servings of colored vegetables (green and yellow)

3 to 5 servings of grain products (bread, cereal, rice, pasta)

The box shows meals served to American athletes during the 1968 and 1976 Olympics.

Body Weight Control

Body weight changes in an athlete are influenced by various factors. Athletes concern themselves with their body weight because of its competitive implications. Attempts to gain or lose weight should take into consideration the part of the body affected, as the weight may be fluid, muscle, and/or fat. The important question for weight control in athletes is: What is optimal body weight in relation to the best possible performance and to the anticipated energy expenditure?

Athletes regulate their own body weight (Eiseman and Johnson). If exercise uses more calories than consumed, weight loss results. Attempts to gain or lose can affect both health and performance and should therefore be under supervision. Attempts to gain or lose weight should follow certain basic health guidelines, and nutritious foods from all four food groups should be included. Supplements should not be necessary, except for female athletes, who may require iron and folic acid. The athlete should allow sufficient time to achieve the weight goal.

Each athlete should try to maintain optimal body weight. As we have seen, this will vary depending on the individual and the sport involved.

Foods Served American Athletes During 1968 and 1976 Olympics

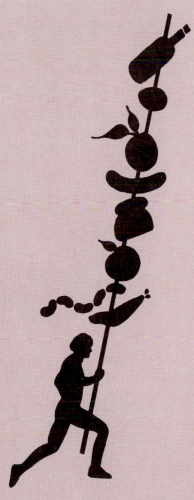

1968 Olympics

Breakfast

Bacon, ham, sausage links

Eggs in any typical American style

Cereals: hot oatmeals, dry cereals such as corn and wheat flakes

Toast, hard rolls

Butter, jam, honey

Drinks: milk, tea, coffee, fruit juice, Ovaltine, Postum

Fruits: prunes, other varieties

Lunch and dinner

Entrees: Broiled steaks, roast, pure beef hamburger (American style), fowl, roast lamb, fish (cocktail sauce for seafoods)

Salad: lettuce hearts, carrot sticks, celery, hard-boiled eggs

Soup: cream, vegetable, bouillon

Rice: boiled

Potatoes: mashed, boiled, baked

Vegetables: plain boiled; no cabbage, onions, or green peppers

Dessert: plain cakes, preserved fruits in syrup, ice cream

Beverage: coffee, tea, Ovaltine, Postum, milk

Fruits: fresh varieties daily

Juices: tomato, orange

Others: cola, soft drinks, fruit punch

1976 Olympics

Entrees

Poached Arctic char with parsley lemon butter, roast leg of lamb with mint sauce, grilled steak, chicken chop suey, baked breaded pork cutlet with barbecue sauce

Soups

Maritime clam chowder, bouillon

Vegetables

Green peas (buttered), eggplant (deep fried), kidney beans, corn, broccoli

Salads

Cole slaw, potato salad, seafood salad, tossed salad, lettuce wedges with tomato slices and green onions, marinated fiddleferns, deviled eggs, and cottage cheese

Bread and others

Potatoes (oven browned or boiled), noodles, rice, rolls, bread

Desserts

Maple syrup pie, fruit cup, fruit bowl, yogurt, ice cream and sherbet, apple crisp, cheese portions, cherry cheese cake, preserved apricots

Beverages

Coffee, black or green tea, buttermilk, milk, mineral water

Height, body build, body fat, lean body mass, and extent of hydration should all ideally be in optimal proportions. Refer to Table 21-1 for the percentage of fat found in various types of athletes. In general, the goal is lean body mass.

Most athletes will lose weight at the beginning of training. The loss will be water and fat. As training progresses, weight gain will occur, and this will be muscle. Athletes should periodically have body fat content estimated to alert them to drastic or adverse changes in body composition. Similarly, a rapid fluctuation of one or two pounds signals a change in fluid balance. Athletes should regularly monitor their weight. For contact sports, the ideal body weight is characterized by a heavy body frame with strong bones to cushion, buffer, and absorb constant impact. Despite the discussions emphasizing speed, strategy, and reaction time, contact sports have strength and bulk at their core.

When an athlete undertakes weight loss, certain health concerns should be considered. For example, the younger athlete should not sacrifice growth for weight loss. The adult athlete will lose about 2 lb per week if caloric intake is reduced by 500 kcal per day. If weight loss progresses faster, excessive energy expenditure, loss of body fluid, and loss of undigested food substances in the bowels will occur. Total starvation (fasting) is hazardous, since it entails fluid and tissue loss. The maximum recommended rate of loss can be 3 to 5 lb per week, providing it partly results from an increase in energy expenditure. A diet of 2,000 to 2,200 kcal per day should provide a reasonable rate of loss.

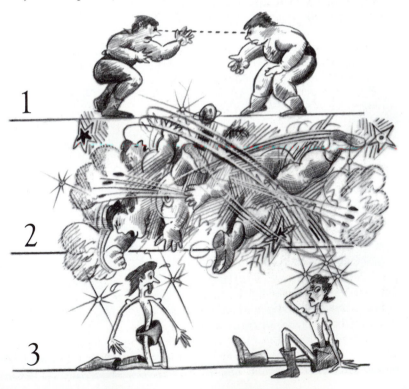

When an athlete undertakes weight gain, the goal is generally an increase in lean body mass, not body fat. Caloric increase coupled with regular conditioning is the only method of achieving this goal. To gain 0.5 kg lean body mass, the body would need 2,500 kcal. A gain of 1½ to 2 lb per week would require daily increase of 350 to 450 kcal. Excessive weight gain of the 15 to 25 lb range should be professionally evaluated. All weight gain should be achieved without drugs, hormones, or other supplements. The appropriate chapters in this book address daily menu designs.

The sport of wrestling provides insights into athlete weight control. A difference of 12 lb body weight is spread over three weight divisions in wrestling competition. A slight weight change can place a wrestler in another weight classification, and this can be advantageous to performance. Wrestlers have used semistarvation, starvation, and dehydration to lose weight. They have induced water loss by conditioning in a plastic suit and have utilized forced sweating, saunas, steam baths, diuretics, cathartics, and induced vomiting. Such techniques pose the hazard of excessive potassium loss in conjunction with the water loss. Since wrestlers who are not heavyweights usually have fairly low body fat storage, weight loss is loss of protein, glycogen, vitamins, minerals, and other body constituents. Resulting problems can include concentrated urine, defective body temperature regulation, and potential kidney stones, kidney inflammation, and even kidney failure (uremia).

Meals Before and During an Event

PREGAME MEAL

Any pregame meal should be 2 to 5 hours before the contest and should be savory. The foods served should be 500 to 1,500 kcal, be bland and easily digested, and be high in carbohydrate content. Greasy and fried foods should be avoided, as should gas-forming substances.

High-protein foods such as cheese, eggs, and steaks are retained in the stomach longer and are slowly released into the small intestine. Also, protein stimulates formation of gastric acid, which may lead to formation of other organic acids. Such acids, when absorbed, will not easily be disposed of by the kidneys, since less blood supply goes to the kidneys during a game. Much of the acid will be retained in the body and can influence the acid-base balances of the body fluids. Since fat is not rapidly released by the stomach, its absorption is slow. Very little energy from ingested fat will be available for body fuel during the game.

Carbohydrates are easily digested and may replenish the blood glucose level. Also, sugars are osmotically active; a certain amount of sugars will draw fluid from the stomach and give rise to satiety. All gas-forming foods such as cabbage, cucumbers, beans, radishes, peas, nuts, spices, oils, and raw fruits and vegetables should be avoided. The athlete should have plenty of fluid. Up to 4 or 5 cups of water will not result in ill effects and will provide good hydration.

The traditional heavy meal, emphasizing protein, before a football game has hung on as a habit. Sports medicine has labeled this practice invalid since the rate of muscle growth determines dietary protein need.

Thus the big pregame football meal, intended to stimulate muscle growth, reverses the true physiological progression. Though many players and coaches have rejected the practice, it is still found in the South.

Normally, ingested food remains in the stomach for 2 to 4 hours before moving to the small intestine for 1½ to 2 hours of digestion and absorption. Just before a game or similar athletic performance, tension will impede digestion. If there is food in the stomach or upper portion of the small intestine, nausea and vomiting are quite common, as are abdominal cramps. If digestion is still occurring during the athletic contest, blood supply to muscles will be reduced to accommodate digestion. Decreased circulation to muscles that are exercising accounts for swimmers' cramps, for example.

Pregame liquid meals have increased in popularity. They offer convenience to the mobile team and avoid the problems inherent in a solid meal. The liquid meal is easily digested, nutritionally sound, and eliminates vomiting, abdominal and localized cramps, and dryness of mouth in some athletes. The main advantage of the liquid pregame meal is its predigested status, which overcomes the indigestion potential of nervousness and tension. Such liquid meals are inexpensive and are commonly used for basketball, wrestling, and track and field sports. Many are manufactured expressly for athletes; others are simply high-density nutrient feeding designed for certain hospital patients. Most liquid meals provide 10 to 30 percent of the RDAs for an adult.

But pregame liquid meals may cause problems for the athlete. For example, if the preparation has a high fat content, nausea may result. For many athletes, the liquid meal lacks sufficiency, resulting in hunger pain. If carbohydrates are lacking, hypoglycemia may result after muscular activity. Irritability and impaired performance can be the by-products.

Some athletes, coaches, and sports physicians encourage drinking glucose or honey solutions a few hours before a game. They point to an improved blood glucose level, a potential energy source. Some scientists disagree with the practice. They explain that glucose and honey are osmotically active in the intestinal lumen, drawing fluid from blood plasma to the alimentary tract. This burdens the athlete's fight against dehydration. Some athletes develop intestinal cramps after drinking glucose, suggesting hypersensitivity to dietary glucose. Finally, the practice may impair endurance performance since the sudden influx of glucose triggers insulin release. That release of insulin hinders mobilization of fat for muscular exercise, putting greater demand on glucose and muscular glycogen. The speed with which glucose is driven into muscular cells can elicit a temporary hypoglycemia. The glucose meal actually shortens the time period during which muscular and liver glycogen can be exhausted.

EATING AND DRINKING DURING AN EVENT

Providing liquid meals during competition has become common practice for such endurance events as long distance running, cycling, and cross-country skiing, as well as for hockey, basketball, and similar fast-paced sports. Some athletes consume sugar solutions, such as 1 quart of water mixed with 3 tablespoons of sugar. Commercial drinks are similar in content.

The actual value of such drinks has not been ascertained. Nutritionally, the maximum amount an athlete can consume is about one liter, 800 to 1,000 kcal. The performance benefit of such a nutritional load remains unknown. Suggested benefits include fluid replacement, maintenance of blood glucose level, and psychological boost. The caloric boost of 800 to 1,000 kcal obviously cannot be ignored.

Occasionally, dextrose tablets, sugar-based candy bars, sugar-salt solution, watery rice puddings, fruit juices, and others are provided to athletes. The value of all these preparations remains unknown, but the practice of consuming them suggests that the psychological effect and perhaps the cooling effect have some benefit.

Use of Drugs and Hormones

Amphetamines, also known as "pep" pills, are among the most abused drugs on the athletic field. The chemical effects of amphetamine are lowered appetite, fatigue reduction, and increased alertness. A high dose is hallucinogenic, and the substance can be toxic to some individuals. Long-term use may lead to conditioning and addiction. Although the use of amphetamine may make the athlete feel that performance is improved, the value of such stimulation to athletic performance remains doubtful.

The hormones most familiar to athletes are anabolic and androgenic steroids. The term "anabolic" implies the ability to build up body mass. The term "androgenic" refers to the similarity to testosterone, a male sex hormone. Depending on the athlete's age, steroids can stimulate growth and body weight, induce early maturation of long bones, increase virility, damage liver function, lead to atrophy of testicles, or decrease fertility and sex drive.

An athlete of the junior high school age, for example, risks failure to reach ultimate height by using the hormone, since the long bones will mature earlier than normal. The young athlete's increased virility predisposes him to precocious puberty. An adult male athlete may suffer testicular atrophy, fertility decrease, and loss of sex drive. Liver damage may occur in any age group. Although steroids do increase weight, that benefit must be carefully weighed against the other effects. (This discussion applies to male athletes; however, female athletes are expected to face similar or related effects.)

As in the case of blood doping and similar techniques of artificially altering performance, the use of drugs and hormones to affect athletic performance creates a new set of concerns. Both athlete and coach must carefully consider the ethics and sportsmanship of the practice, but the most important consideration is health, for all such manipulations can affect the athlete's body in negative ways.

Clinical Problems

Like the clinical problem experienced by Luke at the beginning of this chapter, other athletic clinical problems surface with sufficient frequency to deserve special mention for the lessons they teach us (American Medical Association).

GASTROINTESTINAL DISCOMFORTS

Runners generally experience abdominal cramps or the need to have a bowel movement during running. This suggests that running has a positive effect on the bowels, perhaps causing an increase in certain blood hormones that can increase intestinal motility. Occasionally these symptoms can interfere with performance, creating troublesome abdominal cramping and/or diarrhea. A few runners have been known to experience severe nausea and vomiting under maximum stress.

Related to these effects is the phenomenon of esophageal reflux (regurgitation) and its attendant symptoms. Distance runners especially may experience heartburn, reflux symptoms, and regurgitation, but these effects are generally directly proportional to the quantity of food in the stomach. The fact that running generally results in cramping of the abdominal wall or in muscle spasm within the intestine itself only adds to such reflux problems. Such symptoms may dissipate or disappear with training. Antacids can provide some benefit, but experience has shown that such troublesome symptoms inexplicably persist with certain individuals.

ATHLETE'S ANEMIA

During exercise, hemoglobin (blood pigment) and hematocrit (red blood cell count) levels decrease. Studies of athletes have reached the following conclusion: During prolonged and intense exercise, the red blood cells "disintegrate" for unknown reasons, necessitating a recovery period; that is, for the regeneration of normal red blood cells. One suggested cause is the occurrence of mechanical damage to the red blood cells. This could help explain why iron therapy often fails to correct athlete's anemia. Other physiological explanations include state of hydration, posture, and environmental temperature.

BLOODY URINE

Runners may experience obviously bloody urine, a condition known as *hematuria*. This phenomenon generally occurs in men rather than women runners, leading investigators to suggest the source of blood loss as the lower urinary tract, rather than the kidneys, with friction between the prostate and bladder a likely cause of the bleeding. Dietary studies have not yielded consistent contributors to the malady, and clinical studies have demonstrated that the problem is not health endangering. Although debate surrounds the precise cause of bleeding, logic would suggest that the jarring of the organs during running, particularly the urinary bladder, results in the bleeding. Bleeding episodes typically remain unpredictable and are short-lived.

BLOCKAGE OF LUNG CIRCULATION (PULMONARY EMBOLISM)

A potentially fatal health hazard exists for athletes who undergo sudden weight loss to "make weight" for competition. This practice is most common for wrestlers but also occurs in young football players and among jockeys. Studies have shown that sudden weight loss through enforced dehydration, food and fluid restriction, and use of diuretics results in loss of muscle strength, decrease in blood volume, and reduction in kidney flow. The heart also pumps out less blood than normal.

These physiological changes, although not in themselves causal, predispose the athlete to suffer pulmonary embolism (blocking of blood supply to the lungs). Since blood coagulates more easily when the body is dehydrated, and since the trauma to blood vessels is quite likely in contact sports, a sequence of unfavorable events can occur, including blood vessel trauma, bleeding, blood clotting (or coagulation), movement of blood clots, and blocking of blood vessel(s) to lungs. Pulmonary embolism can be fatal. The highly dangerous practice of weight loss before competition should be avoided.

ELEVATED BLOOD CALCIUM (HYPERCALCEMIA)

Bone fractures among athletes engaged in certain sports are common. In most victims, proper medical attention permits uneventful recovery. Most such patients are mobile with the help of crutches, but others require confinement to bed for varying periods.

Bedridden patients, especially patients with bone fractures, have disturbed calcium metabolism. Calcium equilibrium in the body is determined by a number of factors: bone integrity, serum calcium, intestinal function, adequacy of active vitamin D, kidney function, and parathyroid (hormonal) activity. Prolonged immobilization may lead to such

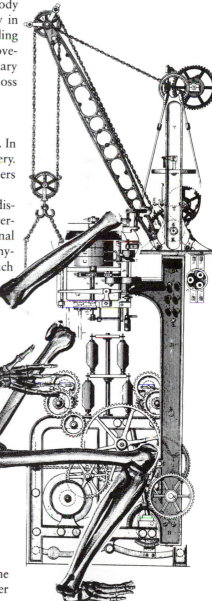

disorders as excess calcium in the blood (hypercalcemia); calcium stone formation (calculi) in the bladder, kidney, or urinary tract; and other abnormal conditions related to excessive calcium.

Characteristic symptoms of hypercalcemia are nausea, vomiting, loss of appetite, excessive thirst, excessive urination, headache, constipation, abdominal pain, listlessness, malaise, dehydration, psychosis, blunting of pain sensations, and coma. If untreated, hypercalcemia can lead to kidney failure, high blood pressure, seizures, and hearing loss.

Though hypercalcemia can progress to crisis level, the syndrome or disorder is readily treatable if it is recognized early. Treatment includes controlled movement of parts of the body, medications, and compliance with low-calcium diet by avoiding certain foods during the recovery period. All these require professional assistance.

Physical Fitness

Although recent polls show that well over half of adult Americans participate in some form of exercise, most people are not educated to physical fitness requirements. The key elements to physical fitness include frequency of activity, duration of activity, intensity of activity, and type of activity. The first step in beginning a quest for physical fitness involves program selection (Williams).

TESTING

If we want to become physically fit, we must first decide on the program we will follow to reach that goal. Program selection is an important process. Through counseling we can avoid unnecessary discomfort, pain, and even death.

Fortunately, the lifestyle changes of recent years, with emphasis on the importance of diet and exercise, have raised our consciousness about exercise testing. By measuring our performance on a treadmill or bicycle, trained professionals can, for example, determine whether we have signs of ischemic (reduction of oxygen supply) heart disease. Exercise testing can calculate the functional capacity of our cardiovascular system, a measurement important to exercise program selection. The goal in such testing is to determine predicted heart rate without causing chest pain. The level of treadmill or bicycle activity can then yield oxygen requirement values, enabling an "exercise prescription" that suits our medical condition, physical capabilities, and interests.

EXERCISE AND NUTRITIONAL FACTORS

The effects of controlled exercise are clearly beneficial. Experts have reasoned that the recent decline in cardiovascular mortality can be generally attributed to an increased health consciousness throughout our society, a consciousness characterized by over 20 million American joggers. As discussed in Chapter 6, exercise definitely helps modify known risk factors of coronary heart disease.

Most studies have shown that exercise decreases blood pressure in hypertensive patients, though such findings have not been conclusive. Similar studies have demonstrated that active men have blood pressure lower than inactive men. Exercise has been shown to decrease smoking. Numerous studies have confirmed that exercise lowers the levels of triglyceride in the blood. The blood levels of HDL cholesterol (see Chapter 6), thought to provide protection against heart disease, increase with exercise. In response to such findings, exercise has become a basic part of the rehabilitation program for patients who have undergone bypass surgery, as well as for those who have angina pectoris (heart-related chest pain) or who have suffered a myocardial infarction (heart attack). Except for patients with certain diseases—for example, congestive heart failure, acute myocarditis or acute infectious disease, or unstable angina pectoris—exercise programs can decrease morbidity and mortality.

AN IDEAL PROGRAM

The ideal physical fitness program must be suited to both your health considerations and your goals. For example, certain programs will yield increased strength; others will yield increased flexibility; yet others will yield cardiorespiratory endurance. Although all these goals are worthwhile and can be achieved simultaneously if desired, the most important goal is stimulating the heart and circulatory system. A physical fitness training session is characterized by a warm-up period, an endurance phase, occasional competition, and finally a cooling-down period. Typically the session will last up to an hour in total. Patients undergoing rehabilitation will normally be limited to about half that time.

Frequency and intensity vary according to the individual's medical and exercise history, but three sessions performed at 70 percent or greater of a person's maximal aerobic power will generally provide sufficient exercise. Three days per week allows ample time for recovery, so the body in general, and critical organs in particular, do not become stressed. The duration of physical fitness programs depends on our condition when we begin training. If we are "out of shape," it can take six months for us to gain our maximal aerobic power. For flexibility and strength programs, exercise must continue after the goal is attained to prevent loss of what has been achieved. An effective program includes dietary considerations.

CALORIC COST AND RUNNING

Exercise costs us calories. Using running as an example, studies have determined that pace has little effect on calorie expenditure (Harger et al.). That is, two men of equal body weight who run the same distance will expend about the same number of calories, regardless of whether one is in top physical condition and the other is a neophyte runner. To put it another way, a 150-pound man will utilize approximately 1 kcal per lb in running 1½ miles in 10 minutes. The same man would utilize about 140 calories in covering the same distance in 16 minutes.

Knowing such caloric costs, we can use exercise to control our weight. If we expend 100 extra calories per day, our weight loss would be 10 pounds in a year. Or, an individual who is following a 3,000-calorie diet and expending 200 calories per day through exercise can eat an additional 200 calories per day without gaining weight.

The key to physical fitness lies in tailoring a program to meet individual needs. In the beginning, low levels of energy expenditure are appropriate, since the body takes some time to adapt to exercise stress. Intensity, frequency, and duration are the variables through which we can adjust our exercise regimen in relation to our goals. The wisest approach to physical fitness training is one that begins with an evaluation of our exercise capabilities and results in an exercise prescription suited to us as individuals.

ATHLETIC ACTIVITY ARRESTS SEXUAL DEVELOPMENT

At the urging of a friend, Jack entered a cross-country race at the age of 14. He won by a significant margin and subsequently received a large amount of praise in the local paper. He then took up long-distance running with a passion.

Jack began a rigorous training program that included runs of 20 miles or bike rides of 50 miles and a daily program of calisthenics. He also followed a very restrictive diet.

Years laters, when Jack was a doctoral student in mathematics, he was admitted to a clinic for investigation of arrested sexual development. He was aware that his obsession with physical fitness and long distance running had slowed his maturation. His facial hair had not appeared, nor had his voice deepened. His genitals had remained small, and he rarely had an erection.

Jack's food habits had been unusual. He ate fruit, vegetables, cottage cheese, natural cereals, peanut butter, and honey. Sweets were excluded, and he ate very little meat. He ate irregularly, gorging at some meals or skipping meals altogether.

Clinical tests found that Jack's level of body fat was quite low due to chronic and acute weight loss. He was also in negative nitrogen balance (see Chapters 4 and 7). The clinic's diagnosis was anorexia nervosa, and Jack was placed on a program of physical restoration and behavioral modification (see Chapter 19) in order to restore his health.

Jack's case history illustrates that "all things in moderation" applies to physical activity, especially for younger athletes.

SOURCE: Adapted from R. A. Nelson, et al. *Mayo Clin. Proc.*, August 1973, p. 549.

STUDY QUESTIONS

1. Name the factors that influence an athlete's daily caloric need. Give two examples to illustrate each factor.

2. Discuss carbohydrate loading. Give rational advantages and disadvantages, and describe its current status.

3. Make a survey of different athletic teams in your college with reference to vitamin supplements, extent of usage, types of supplements, and belief in efficacy.

4. List the characteristics of an acceptable pregame meal.

5. Research and obtain information on some popular commercial beverages for athletes. Provide the name, cost, and recommended usage for each.

6. Explain the following terms: esophageal reflux, hematuria, pulmonary embolism, hypercalcemia. What is the relationship between each clinical condition and an athlete's health?

7. Ask the exercise physiologist in your school to explain the different requirements and goals of an exercise program for two different individuals.

REFERENCES

American Medical Association. *AMA: Medical Aspects of Sports.* Chicago: American Medical Association, 1983.

Darden, E. "Olympic Athletes View Vitamins and Victories." *J. Home Economics* 65 (February 1973): 8.

Eiseman, P., and D. Johnson. *Coaches' Guide to Nutrition and Weight Control.* Champaign, Ill.: Human Kinetics Publishers, 1982.

Harger, B. S., et al. "The Caloric Cost of Running: Its Impact on Weight Reduction." *J.A.M.A.* 228 (1974): 482.

Haskell, W., et al., eds. *Nutrition and Athletic Performance: Proceedings of the Conference on Nutritional Determinants in Athletic Performance, San Francisco, California, September 24–25, 1981.* Palo Alto, Calif.: Bull Publishing, 1982.

Mirkin, G. "Carbohydrate Loading: A Dangerous Practice." *J.A.M.A.* 223 (1973): 1511.

Slovic, P. "What Helps the Long Distance Runner Run?" *Nutrition Today* 10 (May/June 1975): 18.

Williams, M. *Nutrition for Fitness and Sport.* Dubuque, Iowa: William C. Brown, 1983.

Nutrition and Public Health

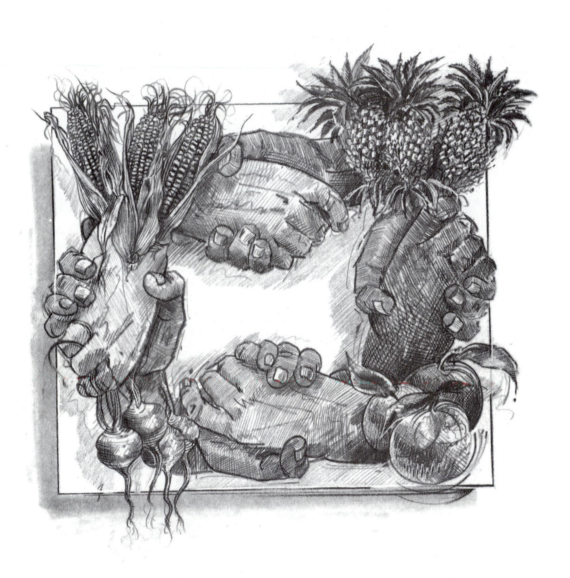

22

PUBLIC HEALTH
AND
COMMUNITY NUTRITION

A LOOK AT ONE COUNTY'S EFFORTS TO REACH THE BLIND

Lil Gyulveszy has been blind since childhood. For 3 years she has worked at the Cleveland Sight Center for the Blind, teaching and counseling visually impaired people who have personal problems or who want to participate in the center's rehabilitation program.

In 1977, she called the Cuyahoga County food stamp hotline. "I need to know more about the food stamp program so I can inform my clients about its availability," she said. "Could you send someone to my office so we can talk?"

That call prompted a meeting between staff members of the Cleveland Society for the Blind and the Cuyahoga County food stamp staff. After examining the hotline log and finding numerous calls from visually impaired people, the two agencies embarked on a joint venture to produce a food stamp brochure in braille. Their efforts have not only helped Cuyahoga County residents but have served as a model for other social service agencies preparing materials for the blind. . . .

Consider the case of Lucy Miller, the first person to receive food stamp information in braille in Cuyahoga County. Because of an accident, Miller has been visually impaired since childhood and is now totally blind.

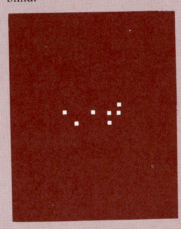

Miller has been using food stamps since 1964. She heard about the brochure in braille and contacted the food stamp staff and requested a copy. "Now I can read about the program and the income guidelines in my own home," she says. "This way I know that I am receiving the correct amount of stamps each month.". . .

Food stamp information in braille is helpful both to visually impaired people and to people who work with them.

As a caseworker and home rehabilitation teacher, Gyulveszy divides her work schedule between interviews at the center and working with clients in the community, "I go to the visually impaired person's home to teach braille and daily living skills," she says. "If the family I'm counseling is having financial problems, I tell them that food stamps can help supplement their food budget, and I encourage them to contact the food stamp office nearest their home.

"With this food stamp pamphlet in braille, I can direct them to the correct food stamp application center located in their part of town," she says. "Sometimes the people have heard of the food stamp program but do not understand how it works and where to apply. This brochure helps me help them.". . .

SOURCE: Adapted from E. Bowman. *Food and Nutrition*, June 1981, p. 3.

Senator Edward M. Kennedy delivered the following opening statement on June 21, 1974, the first day of the three-day National Nutrition Policy Study hearings:

Nutrition adequacy is a prerequisite for good health. No matter what conditions the body may be forced to suffer, the provision of adequate nutrition is the most fundamental requirement for survival. No internist can substitute for proteins. No surgeon can excise iron deficiencies, and no pediatrician can replace the nutrients lost in premature birth due to poor prenatal care. . . . The delivery of good nutritional care is, in the long run, the most important medicine that each of us can and must administer to ourselves.

Items concerning good and bad nutrition are in the news almost daily. Why the sudden interest? The intimate relationship between good health and wholesome dietary and nutritional habits is increasingly evident. Sophisticated technology and rapid communication are making the art and science of nutrition available to almost everyone. This chapter describes some formal routes by which nutrition services are reaching the public.

Preventive Nutrition

People want preventive nutrition. They want to know what they should eat, they want to enjoy what they eat, and most important, they want to eat to assure good health and a long life. The government has responded to such desires in several ways.

DIETARY GOALS: NOT EVERYONE AGREES

The United States Senate, through its Select Committee on Nutrition and Human Needs, has studied our nation's health from malnutrition to overnutrition. Using the studies of the 1960s and 1970s, the committee published *Dietary Goals for the United States* in 1977. A summary of the report is provided in Chapter 2. Here, we will briefly discuss the materials, assuming that you will refer to Chapter 2.

To meet Senate goals, certain changes in food selection and preparation are recommended. Consumption of fruits, vegetables, and whole grains should be increased, while consumption of refined and other processed sugars and foods high in such sugars should be decreased. The dietary goals report recommends decreased consumption of foods high in total fat and partial replacement of saturated fats, whether obtained from animal or vegetable sources, with polyunsaturated fats. The report advocates reduced consumption of animal fat and advises the public to eat meats, poultry, and fish that will reduce saturated fat intake. Except for young children, low-fat and nonfat milk should be substituted for whole milk, and low-fat dairy products for high-fat dairy products. Consumption of butterfat, eggs, and other high-cholesterol foods should be decreased. However, premenopausal women, young children, and the elderly should obtain the nutritional benefits of eggs. Finally, the report advises decreased consumption of salt and foods high in salt content.

In 1980, the federal government issued *Dietary Guidelines for Americans,* a publication that repeated the cautions about fat, sugar, cholesterol, and salt but also recommended a reduction in alcohol consumption and a loss of weight for those overweight.

Both federal publications stirred controversy among scientists and nutritionists. The National Academy of Sciences' National Research Council then issued *Toward Healthful Diets*, a publication that contradicted federal goals and guidelines. Such differences of opinion have left many consumers and professionals confused.

Dietary Advice Is Risky

Any dietary advice runs the risk of being based on inadequate information. In nutritional issues it proves difficult to determine when available facts warrant a final decision. For example, consider the traditional claim that persons slightly thinner than ideal weight tended to be healthier than those slightly above ideal weight. That position was widely accepted, but statistics now demonstrate that those slightly overweight have a life-span advantage.

Dietary advice also proves risky if its recommendations are too broad. For example, salt restriction is important for those with high blood pressure, but for others it may be unnecessary. Similarly, dietary advice may solve one problem but introduce another. Consider, for example, fats in meat. If you advise that fat correlates with heart disease and consumers consequently reduce meat intake, the consumers then may become iron deficient.

Despite the foregoing potential risks in giving dietary advice, there are various benefits to consider.

Benefits of Dietary Advice

When you look at the typical American diet of high fat, high salt, high sugar, and high cholesterol, you realize that those food patterns are only possible with a rather high standard of living. In that sense, they are not "normal." Since high consumption levels of those foods seem to correlate with obesity, diabetes, cancer, and heart disease, lowering consumption levels probably does more good than harm. Thus, advising reduction seems favorable to many nutritionists and medical practitioners.

Dietary advice that stresses more plant foods also stands as the wholesome approach to living, a positive outlook on health and nutrition that is hard to dispute and one that has growing appeal for a large number of consumers.

One trend within dietary advice has proved of significant benefit: the recommendation to maintain a balanced diet by consuming a wide variety of foods. Since that advice was first given through national guidelines, scientific evidence has continued to confirm its wisdom. Through a wide variety of foods we improve our chances of ingesting the various nutrients required for maintaining health.

Also, dietary goals demonstrate that legislators are genuinely concerned about the nutritional intakes of their constituents. Large-scale nutrition education and health care programs arise from this concern and from the belief that adequate health services are a right and a necessity, not just a luxury or a privilege.

The medical profession tends to consider health care and medical care as synonymous; they are not. Medical care centers on curing disease;

health care centers on the whole life span. Medical care is episodic; health care is continuous.

On the other hand, each person must contribute to his or her own health care, as clearly stated by Senator Kennedy. Furthermore, according to Dr. P. B. Peacock of the American Health Foundation, "Health maintenance refers to measures that will enable an individual to stay young and healthy in body and mind for as many years as possible. . . .

WEIGHT CONTROL AND NUTRITION EDUCATION PROGRAMS IN OCCUPATIONAL SETTINGS

The worksite offers a unique opportunity for implementing suggestions to improve the diet. Unfortunately, research has consistently shown that good advice on food consumption is rarely followed. Programs for weight loss, for example, have been notoriously ineffective. . . .

The few weight control programs in industry are part of general exercise programs. The weight loss effort may consist of a lecture or two by the company nurse. Some firms have contracted with organizations such as the local health department or a group like the American Diabetes Association or a commercial venture such as Weight Watchers. . . .

Kimberly-Clark Corporation, Neenah, Wisconsin: Weight control is one part of the Health Management Program of the Kimberly-Clark Corporation. Employees at the corporate offices and facilities near Neenah are invited to get a company-paid evaluation of their health risks, using an extensive 40-page medical history; laboratory tests including hemoglobin, blood sugar, cholesterol, triglycerides, liver function, urinalysis, chest X-ray, breathing, skinfold thickness, body density, electrocar-

diogram, hearing, vision, blood pressure, and temperature; complete physical examination; and tread-mill test. They then receive individualized health prescriptions that might include counseling and seminars on obesity. The company has spent $2.5 million to build an office for testing and a large physical fitness facility that includes a swimming pool, 100-meter track, exercise equipment, sauna, whirlpool, showers, and lockers.

The screening is offered annually to all employees. Physical examinations are given every 2 years for employees 40 and older and every 3 years for those under 40. More than 60 percent of Kimberly-Clark's 2,100 employees in Neenah have participated in the program. . . .

U.S. Air Force Hospital, Tinker Air Force Base, Oklahoma: An unusual nonvoluntary behavioral treatment program is being conducted at Tinker Air Force Base for personnel who meet the Air Force's criteria of obesity. Active duty personnel who have been identified at squadron level as being obese are referred to the treatment clinic at the hospital. Participants attend weekly classes, and progress reports are sent monthly

to each squadron's weight control monitor. Participants are dropped from the program when they achieve their goal. Maintenance sessions are offered to those who wish to attend. Average weight losses for these groups have ranged from 6 to 10 pounds, depending on the length of treatment (1 to 4 months).

According to its organizers, the program has met with enthusiastic endorsement by unit commanders, as well as the patients themselves, and has lent itself to easy adaptation to the military population. . . .

The potential for developing health promotion programs at the worksite has not yet been tapped. Nutrition education programs for weight reduction and attuned to cardiovascular risk factors related to diet offer particular promise because they can be put into practice so easily in company cafeterias. The combination of a prudent eating plan and the behavioral techniques which teach people how to adhere to such a diet have been developed and can be put into practice. As programs are developed, we hope that they will be designed so that their cost effectiveness can be evaluated.

SOURCE: Adapted from J. P. Foreyt, et al. *Public Health Reports*, 95 (1980): 127.

With our present knowledge, to achieve success in the control of these [cancer and heart] diseases we must directly influence those who are being protected and require that they take positive action on their own behalf. The development and maintenance of such programs is health maintenance."

PUBLIC HEALTH AND COMMUNITY NUTRITION SERVICES

Public health nutrition and community nutrition are important components of any health service program, since they educate the public about nutrition while they deliver the proper dietary and nutritional care to those who need it. The field of public-health nutrition is very similar to that of community nutrition. For convenience, this chapter assumes that the two fields have so much in common that their activities largely overlap. The following definitions are provided for reference purposes.

According to Dr. Cicely D. Williams, *community nutrition* is "the whole of the nutritional sciences applied to the consumer as groups or as individuals. It is the interface between food and people, and probably some 90 percent of all nutrition takes place in the home. Each culture has always had its especially preferred foods, food taboos, and food habits" (McLaren, D. J. [ed.], *Nutrition in the Community* [London: John Wiley & Sons, Inc., 1984,] p. xii).

According to the *Dictionary of Occupational Titles*, compiled by the U.S. Department of Labor, the *public health nutritionist* is defined as an individual who "organizes, plans and conducts programs concerning nutrition to assist in promotion of health and control of disease. Instructs auxiliary medical personnel and allied professional workers on food values and utilization of foods by the human body. Advises health and other agencies on nutritional phases of their food programs. Conducts in-service courses pertaining to nutrition in clinics and similar institutions. Interprets and evaluates food and nutrient information designed for public acceptance and use. Studies and analyzes scientific discoveries in nutrition for a public health agency and can be designated as Nutritionist, Public Health."

FOOD AND NUTRITION SURVEYS AND PLANNING

Public health and community nutritionists become involved in many types of activities and programs. One major activity of community nutritionists involves food and nutrition surveys and planning. A list of such projects with examples is provided below:

Food habits: Nutrition and dietary habits of ethnic populations; the elderly; rural and urban populations; and groups of low socioeconomic status.

Food prices: Rise in cost with reference to location, regional distribution, and other economic factors.

Nutritional status: Nutritional status of selected population groups including data such as weight, height, body build, and chemical analysis of blood and urine.

Nutrition education: Educating all segments of the population, especially children, the elderly, professionals, and individuals with illnesses; dissemination of relevant nutrition information.

Food safety: Family practices of safety in food preparation and preservation.

Food equipment usage: Extent of usage of some of the latest equipment including microwave ovens, electric pressure cookers, slow cookers, food processors, and freezers.

Oral hygiene: Health care of the mouth (teeth and gums) and effects of food, alcohol, and tobacco on the mouth.

Of these general subjects, both nutritional status and nutrition education require further elaboration.

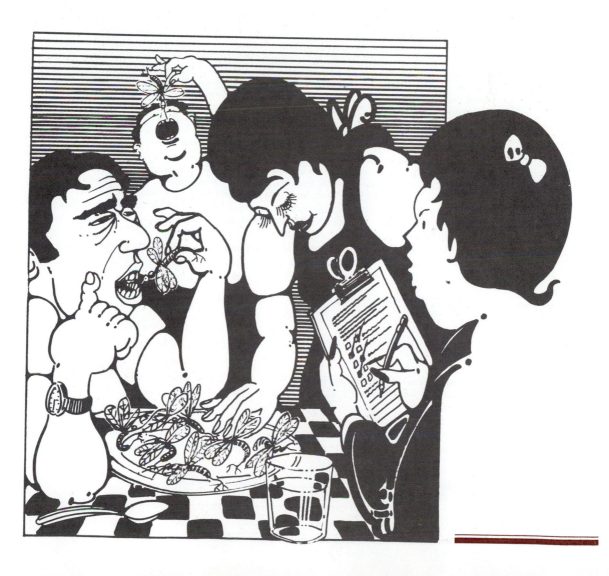

Nutritional Status Assessment

Table 22-1 summarizes methods of evaluating the nutritional status of an individual or individuals in a group. Nutritional assessment is especially important in evaluating children. The four major phases in assessing nutritional status are anthropometric measurements, clinical examinations, biochemical evaluation, and dietary evaluations. They are briefly discussed below (Symposium).

ANTHROPOMETRIC MEASUREMENT
Details of anthropometric measurements are provided in Chapter 3. The

Table 22-1
Methods of Evaluating Nutritional Status

PROCEDURE	PURPOSE AND BRIEF DESCRIPTION
Clinical assessment	To detect physical signs and symptoms of deviation from health due to malnutrition; to include medical history, physical examination, various anthropometric measurements such as height, weight, and subcutaneous fat, and X-ray measurement of bones.
Biochemical measurements	To obtain earliest evidence of deficient nutritional status. Depletion of body stores of nutrients is the first step in the development of nutritional-deficiency disease. Biochemical measurements of the levels of various substances in body tissue and fluids, e.g., blood and urine, can often provide preliminary information about the person's nutritional status. As the deficiency progresses, functional impairment develops, and finally the physical changes characteristic of a clinically manifest deficiency disease appear. Biochemical measurements, therefore, allow an identification of populations at risk, as well as populations with frank malnutrition.
Dental examination	To detect physical signs and symptoms of deviation from normal; to include an evaluation of dental health and the condition of the soft (periodontal) tissues of the mouth. While all dental findings cannot be claimed to result from inadequate nutrition, obvious relationship to dietary intake exists, e.g., the presence of caries may be associated with a low intake of fluoride.
Dietary evaluation	To assist in a complete interpretation of clinical and biochemical findings (see text). Information is basic to planning dietary changes, modifying existing programs, and initiating new ones that will have an influence on food habits and intake.
Collection of data on	To enable a complete assessment of possible causes underlying malnutrition to be made, and to provide a basis for future planning.
Level and distribution of income	(Monthly earnings, amount spent on food, clothes, etc.)
Income maintenance and other social service programs	(Length of period with or without a job, receiving welfare, etc.)
Government food and nutrition programs	(Participation in school lunch programs, food stamps, etc.)
General food availability and acceptance	(Distances from food stores, availability of ethnic foods, likes and dislikes for food purchased within short distances, etc.)
Health and educational facilities	(Hospital and colleges close by, etc.)
Socioeconomic, ethnic, and cultural characteristics	(Immigrants, Native-Americans, etc.)
Overall health status and disease factors	(Frequency of family members becoming sick, genetic diseases, etc.)

SOURCE: Adapted from *Ten-State Nutrition Survey, 1968–1970. I. Historical Development. II. Demographic Data.* U.S. Department of Health, Education, and Welfare Publication No. (HSM) 72-8130. Atlanta, Centers for Disease Control, 1972, p. 1–3.

techniques measure the following characteristics for a living person: height, weight, and body measurements (such as the thickness of triceps and subscapular skin folds). These data, together with knowledge of the race and sex of the individual, can be compared with standard tables to estimate the person's body fat, body water, and so forth.

CLINICAL EXAMINATIONS

Clinical examinations are not always possible because many subjects are involved. However, whenever feasible, the field physician or nurse should perform a complete physical examination of each subject, examining the hair, face, eyes, lips, tongue, teeth, gums, glands, skin, nails, subcutaneous tissues, muscular and skeletal systems, cardiovascular system, gastrointestinal system, genital system, and nervous system. The following examples of description of the physical signs and symptoms of malnutrition are adapted from U.S. Department of Health, Education and Welfare Publication No. (HSM) 72-8130, 1972 (pp. I-44-I-47).

Hair

Dry staring: Dry wirelike, unkempt, stiff hair, often brittle; sometimes may exhibit some bleaching of the normal color. . . .

 Abnormal texture or loss of curl (pediatric form only): Changes in texture of the hair to a soft, silk-like hair. Loss of curl self-explanatory.

Eyes

Thickened opaque bulbar conjunctivae (adult form only): All degrees of thickening may occur. The blueness of the sclera may disappear and the bulbar conjunctivae may develop a wrinkled appearance with increase in vascularity. The thickened conjunctivae may result in a glazed, porcelain-like appearance, obscuring the vascularity. Do not confuse with pterygium. . . .

Teeth

Visible caries 4+: For the purpose of the medical examination, caries refers to lesions readily visible. (This is in contrast to the usual definition that a tooth is considered carious when the enamel yields to underlying soft material with the explorer tip.) . . .

Skin

Follicular hyperkeratosis: This lesion has been likened to "gooseflesh" that is seen on chilling, but it is not generalized and does not disappear with brisk rubbing of the skin. Readily felt, as it presents a "nutmeg grater" feel. Follicular hyperkeratosis is more readily detected by the sense of touch than by the eye. The skin is rough, with papillae formed by keratotic plugs that project from the hair follicles. The surrounding skin is dry and lacks the usual amount of moisture or oiliness. Differentiation from adolescent folliculosis can usually be made through recognition of the normal skin between the follicles in the adolescent disorder. It is distinguished from perifolliculosis by the ring of capillary congestion that occurs about each follicle in scorbutic perifolliculosis. . . .

Abdomen

Potbelly (pediatric form only): Record if abdomen appears abnormally distended and enlarged, with due recognition of the usual contour of the young child.

Hepatomegaly: Record liver edges more than 2 cm below the costal margin.

Lower Extremeties

Pretibial edema: Record only if bilateral.

Calf tenderness (adult form only): Record when definite bilateral evidence of painful sensation occurs upon squeezing the calf muscles firmly between the thumb and finger. Record only if moderate or severe.

Absent knee/ankle jerk (adult form only): Record only if absent bilaterally with reinforcement.

Absent vibratory sense (adult form only): Test with tuning fork at 128 vibrations per minute over the lateral malleoli. Record as positive only if absent bilaterally.

Scrotum

Scrotal dermatitis (adult form only): The scrotum usually must be rotated to see the lesions. Differentiate from fungus infections, which usually extend onto the skin of the groin adjacent to the scrotum.

Pulse Rate and Blood

Pulse rate (adult form only): Count for a minimum of 30 seconds.

Blood pressure (adult form only): Take on right arm, with individual in sitting position. Make reading upon disappearance of sound. Record data to nearest even unit.

Skeletal (Pediatric Form Only)

Beading of ribs: Record when there is definitely palpable and visible enlargement of the costochondral junctions.

Bossing of skull: Record when there is abnormal prominence or protrusion of frontal or parietal areas.

Clinical manifestations of nutrient deficiencies will not be apparent unless malnutrition is in an advanced state. To diagnose the initial stages of malnutrition requires anthropometric, biochemical, and dietary data.

Signs of classic malnutrition are common in underdeveloped countries. Similar overt clinical symptoms from undernourishment are encountered less frequently in industrialized countries. On the other hand, malnutrition (see definition in Chapter 19) from excessive alcohol or calorie consumption is evident in the United States (also see Chapter 19). During a clinical examination, an American child with suspected or evident nutrient deficiencies should be given additional confirmatory studies. Examples of obvious poor nutrition signs in children are cavities, missing and decayed teeth, and gum hypertrophy. Overconsumption of sugary foods and poor oral hygiene are usually responsible for these clinical manifestations.

BIOCHEMICAL EVALUATION

A third important set of measurements indicating nutritional status are biochemical data—the levels of specific chemicals in major body fluids such as blood, urine, feces, tears, saliva, and mucus. From this information, actual or borderline deficiency of a particular nutrient can be determined. Chemical analyses of hair and skin can also be used to determine an individual's nutriture. Biochemical data are most valuable for identifying covert (subclinical) deficiencies before they progress to overt symptoms. Early detection enables early intervention.

The chemical substances analyzed are categorized into three groups: blood components, nutrients and their metabolites, and body waste products. Blood components include proteins such as albumin, hemoglobin, and fibrinogen; minerals such as **cations** (positively charged electrolytes such as sodium) and hydrogen ions; and special substances such as adenosine triphosphate and glutathione. Nutrients and their metabolites include protein (amino acids), fat (fatty acids, glycerol, phospholipids, cholesterol, and triglycerides), carbohydrate (glucose, fructose and galactose), vitamins, minerals, hormones, pyruvate and lactate, and creatinine. Body waste products include carbon dioxide, water, bilirubin, urea, and creatinine. Guidelines for classifying and interpreting blood group and urine data may be obtained from standard reference texts (Symposium).

DIETARY EVALUATION

The nutrient contribution or quality of an individual's diet is evaluated in accordance with the latest RDAs. If anthropometric measurements, biochemical data, and clinical observations are available to supplement the dietary evaluations, the nutritional status of an individual can be determined—a dietary study by itself cannot accomplish this. However, a properly conducted dietary survey serves as a focal point for developing government food and nutrition policies; designing health services and programs with an adequate food and nutrition component; implementing more intensive nutrition education programs; and counseling individuals, who can be encouraged to modify faulty eating habits that are unrelated to food availability.

To obtain accurate results in a dietary study is difficult. At present, five methods are available: the individual food history, the individual record of food intake, the individual recall of food intake, the household recollection of food intake, and individual and household food weighing.

Individual Food History

A qualitative and quantitative analysis of a person's past dietary practices is called a food history. It explores the patient's likes and dislikes for food, the type and quantity of food consumed, the locations and content of daily meals, the frequency of eating out, the use of alcoholic beverages, and the type and frequency of snacking. Obtaining a good history requires a willing and cooperative subject and a skillful interviewer. However, this procedure is usually very costly because it takes time.

Although commercial computer data enterprises can analyze the nutrient intakes of an individual if the diet history is provided on a standard form, computer analyses are not widely available. They are not recommended unless a qualified person such as a nutritionist interprets the results. The information derived from a dietary history is of little significance in determining a subject's present nutritional status. But it serves a useful purpose if it is interpreted along with other assessment data. If the patient shows overt signs of nutrient deficiencies, his or her diet history may confirm the specific nutrients involved.

Individual Record of Food Intake

In a second method, a nutritionist, dietitian, or nurse may ask a subject to keep a food record for 1 to 7 days. The information is valuable if the person records every item eaten and accurately lists portion sizes. Unfortunately, most people fail to meet both requirements.

Individual Recall of Food Intake

In a third method, the person is asked to recall what was eaten within the past 24 hours. Most people can recall their food intake over this time period with some accuracy. Meaningful results can be obtained if the interviewer is skillful. This method is probably the most common one used in a dietary survey.

Household Recollection of Food Intake

In the fourth method of dietary evaluation, the food preparer in the family is requested to recollect the type and amount of foods purchased and consumed by the entire family for the previous week. Other requested data include the number of family members and their ages, the food budget, the meals eaten away from home, and the number of guests eating in the house that week and their ages. An alternative is to find the difference in the weights of food available in the household at the beginning and at the end of each week. The amount of foods discarded after each meal must be taken into account as well. At present, these two techniques are the only convenient ways to estimate the amount of food consumed in a household, but they are not accurate.

Individual and Household Food Weighing

The most accurate way to estimate food intake is to ask a person or household to weigh foods served immediately before a meal and then subtract the weight of the leftovers. This method, however, is inconvenient and time consuming. Although most dietary studies do not require this procedure because of the large number of subjects involved, diet weighing is used in some situations.

In a human nutrition experiment with a controlled environment, such as a metabolic study or a study of the food intake of a diabetic or kidney patient, sometimes the exact amount of food consumed *must* be known. This knowledge may be part of the mandatory treatment of the disease, or it may be necessary because the patient has difficulty in complying with a prescribed diet either because of eating habits or job routines.

Major Nutrition Surveys

HOUSEHOLD FOOD CONSUMPTION, 1965–1966

Conducted by the U.S. Department of Agriculture (Beal and Laus), the Household Food Consumption Survey involved the general population. It obtained one day's food intake of over 14,000 individuals, providing the first information of its kind for the United States. The study recorded information by sex and by age.

All surveys have certain limitations, and findings must be understood and interpreted within those limitations. For example, the Household Food Consumption Survey sampled individual households; it did not survey such group living situations as boarding houses, rest homes, and medical institutions. Also, about two thirds of the households surveyed were located in the urban North. Finally, considerably more of the adults over 65 were in low-income households in comparison with adults under 65.

TEN STATE NUTRITION SURVEY, 1968–1970

The Ten-State Nutrition Survey was the first to clearly assess the problems of hunger and undernutrition. Groups such as the poor, migrants, Hispanics of the Southwest and inner city, and industrial-area dwellers were intentionally included in the survey since they were thought to be at risk for undernutrition. The states included in the survey were Washington, California, Texas, Louisiana, South Carolina, Kentucky, West Virginia, Michigan, New York, and Massachusetts. The survey covered more than 85,000 people.

This survey made clinical assessments, took medical histories, conducted physical examinations, took physical measurements, made dental examinations, tested blood and urine, assessed food intake and food consumption patterns, and gathered relevant social data. It used a somewhat complex analysis of income in relation to diet. Generally the survey found that those residing in the lower-income Southern states had lower intakes of protein, niacin, and iron.

HEALTH AND NUTRITION EXAMINATION SURVEY, 1971–1972

The Health and Nutrition Examination Survey, known as the HANES program, was conducted by the National Center for Health Statistics and was designed to assess nutrient intake adequacy. Factors evaluated were quite similar to those of the Ten-State Survey; however, dietary intake was compared to an adequacy index developed by a committee representing numerous national and international organizations.

Government Food and Nutrition Programs

Besides surveying the nutritional adequacy of the diet of varying population groups, the government and certain independent agencies offer nutritional assessment, nutrition education, and feeding programs to groups at high risk of being undernourished. A partial listing of currently available government food and nutrition programs is provided in the box on page 512 (Swenerton and Dunkley; Vermersch). Because funding for most programs listed has to be renewed periodically, their implementations are subject to the political and economic climate of the nation. Thus, they may or may not be in existence in any particular year.

FOOD STAMP PROGRAM
The food stamp program (Johnson et al.) was initially conceived in the early sixties to help people below the poverty line purchase food at a discount by means of stamps that the government redeemed. The face

EXAMPLES OF GOVERNMENT FOOD AND NUTRITION PROGRAMS

Department of Agriculture

School lunch program

School breakfast program

Special milk program

Summer food program

Supplemental food program for women, infants, and children

Family food assistance program

Food stamp program

Expanded food and nutrition education program (EFNEP)

Food distribution program

Department of Health and Human Services (Child Development Services Bureau)

Head Start program: parent and child centers

National Center for Child Abuse and Neglect

Programs for children with developmental disabilities as authorized by the Disabilities Act

Special projects for children authorized under Title XX of the Social Security Act

Special projects for certain members of families with dependent children as authorized under Title XIX of the Social Security Act

Early periodic screening, diagnosis, and treatment (EPSDT) as authorized under the Social Security Act

Department of Health and Human Services (Office of Human Development Services)

Title VII nutrition programs of the Older Americans Act administered by the Administration on Aging.

Department of Health and Human Services (Indian Health Services)

The Nutrition and Dietetics Branch attempts to provide comprehensive nutrition service for more than half a million American Indians and Alaskan natives

Independent Agencies

Various food and nutrition programs for the community sponsored by independent agencies such as the Community Services Administration

value of the stamps was that sufficient to obtain an adequate nutritional diet.

As the program operates now, an eligible household receives that number of stamps necessary to purchase a "Thrifty Food Plan" for the household's size. The Department of Agriculture designs Thrifty Food Plans to exceed by 5 percent the RDAs for calories, protein, iron, calcium, vitamin A, thiamine, riboflavin, niacin, and vitamin C. If, for example, the Thrifty Food Plan for a four-person household costs $180 and the family has $90 available, as determined by formula, toward that expense, the family is given the $90 difference in food stamps.

HEAD START PROGRAM
Sponsored by the Child Development Services Bureau of the Department of Health and Human Services, the Head Start program has one major objective (Swenerton & Dunkley; Vermersch): to provide education and

assistance to disadvantaged children so that they are better prepared for school and social interaction. The Bureau issues standards and guidelines for children enrolled in the program and employs physicians and other allied health personnel as consultants. All the children are required to achieve certain performance standards with respect to family participation, health screening, oral health, educational competency, social service benefits, and, most relevant to this discussion, dietary care. Health care received by a child and family in a Head Start program includes anthropometric measurements, screening for anemia, evaluation of family eating patterns, food for part of the day, and nutrition education.

To take anthropometric measurements in a Head Start program, the growth rate, weight, height, build, head circumference, and skinfold thickness of each child should be obtained. The child should be screened for anemia by such means as measuring hematocrit and hemoglobin levels. The eating practices and nutritional status of each member in the family should be ascertained, as should special dietary needs and feeding problems of the enrolled child as determined through interviews.

According to Head Start regulations, if children are enrolled in a part-day program, they should be supplied with one third of their RDAs; if full day, they should be fed one third to two thirds of their RDAs. Children are fed only the approved quantity and quality of any specific type of food product. The eating times and food preparation of all meals should be in accordance with the cultural backgrounds of the children. The eating environment—tables, chairs, utensils, and lighting—should also satisfy approved guidelines. Any modification of children's eating behavior must be accomplished without force or reward. For example, they should not be forced to eat all food given them or talked into eating a certain food with the promise of a reward afterwards. Every child should be given the opportunity or encouraged to participate in food preparation and cleanup after eating.

An attempt is also made to improve home feeding through nutrition education. Whenever feasible, the parents, the children, and the staff are educated in such matters as basic nutrition knowledge; food groups; menu planning; budgeting; and food buying, selection, and preparation. Each family should be considered for possible participation in other programs, such as the food stamp program, school lunch program, and supplemental food programs for women, infants, and children.

A public health or community nutritionist working with Head Start and other food- and nutrition-related programs should be competent in developing, conducting, implementing, and supervising program responsibilities.

Health Services with a Food and Nutrition Component

Public health and community nutritionists may be members of health teams that dispense health services with a food and nutrition component. The types of clinics or centers through which public health and community nutritionists should be qualified to deliver health services include:

Children's clinics

Day care centers

Dental health programs and clinics

Diabetic centers

Drug addiction rehabilitation centers

Family planning programs

Genetic counseling services

Handicapped children health service programs

Health intervention programs, such as those pertaining to smoking, alcoholism, and blood pressure

Health screening and testing services

Indian health and migrant health programs

Intensive infant care programs

Local community nutrition programs for individuals and families

Open-door (free) clinics

Pregnancy and prenatal clinics

School health services

Weight control clinics

Women's centers

Two of the services listed above bear further discussion.

PREGNANCY AND PRENATAL SERVICES

As a member of a health team, a nutritionist provides dietary and nutrition care for pregnant or nursing mothers and newborn infants. In this capacity, the nutritionist is responsible for the development and implementation of prenatal services such as basic medical care, childbirth classes, weight fluctuation evaluations, daily meal planning, counsel on nutrient supplements, evaluating dietary needs during trips, family assessment and counseling, and home and hospital visits. He or she consults and coordinates efforts with other health personnel, especially physicians and nurses, concerning special nutrition and dietary needs in both normal and complicated pregnancies and provides nutritional education for nontrained members of the health team, health aides, staff, and personnel.

The nutritionist also teaches nutrition and dietary concepts to special groups such as pregnant teenagers, expectant parents, illiterate mothers, poor migrant women, and other individuals who may be at high nutritional risk. He or she distributes information regarding all aspects of infant feeding and develops and prepares nutrition education materials for posting, distribution, and demonstration projects. The nutritionist also refers clients to other established health programs with a food and nutrition component from which the clients may benefit. Such programs include the food stamp program and special food and nutrient supplement programs for women, infants, and children.

Many young adults, minority groups, and poor people are not happy with established health and medical services such as health centers, local physicians, hospitals, and county health departments. Some parts of the country have free open-door clinics and drug rehabilitation and education centers that are maintained by activist health professionals (including doctors, nurses, and medical and nursing students). Some of the open-door clinics occasionally accept state and federal financial assistance, and most drug addiction rehabilitation centers now receive some form of government backing.

Such centers and clinics have several characteristics in common. They almost always provide multiple health services at little or no cost, and most are staffed by volunteers. They do not have any red tape or checks on eligibility—they serve all who come. They train and use paraprofessionals to provide health services. Many of these centers and clinics have benefited from the federal government's revenue sharing and other programs, and many have developed cooperative relationships with hospitals, medical schools, and health departments.

The multiple health services provided by these centers and clinics include:

Counseling on family and legal problems

Family planning and abortion referrals

Pregnancy and parental counseling

Crisis intervention

Genetic counseling

Disease care and prevention: sexually transmitted disease, clinical manifestations of drug abuse, hepatitis

Comprehensive care for patients with drug problems (prescription, over-the-counter, and illicit drugs)

Health education

Referral to medical clinics and other agencies

Counseling on food, nutrition, and diet

The clientele of these centers and clinics are often good candidates for nutrition education and counseling services. Many of them are vegetarians or practice other nontraditional food and dietary habits, and they tend to reject most conventional sources of nutrition and health advice. However, most of the young adults can be made aware of their own nutrition needs and dietary intakes and are receptive to useful information on nutrition-related medical problems. For example, vegetarians may receive valuable information from a qualified nutritionist. Malnourished drug addicts require significant help in rebuilding their bodies and may be very receptive to nutritional care. Young women can be informed of the intricate relationship between nutritional status and the use of oral contraceptive pills.

The one-to-one interaction between the clientele and the nutritionist

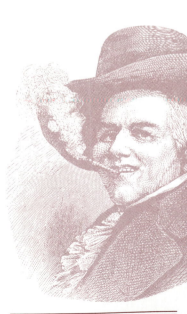

can be most productive. The centers or clinics can serve as information education centers by displaying food and nutrition literature. All health personnel in these places should emphasize the need for correct nutritional information and dietary care, and they should provide proper nutrition referral services. Unfortunately, many of these centers and clinics do not have qualified public health or community nutritionists or dietitians to provide the needed services, although many are staffed with nutrition aides who do seek advice from nutrition service centers. Qualified nutritionists should be sought to staff programs either part-time or full-time on a voluntary basis or with partial compensation. Many nutritionists are willing to donate their time to help such centers identify dietary and nutritional problems and to suggest solutions and means of obtaining qualified personnel.

In addition to the services discussed above, public health and community nutritionists perform many other activities. The references for this chapter provide additional information.

Important Issues in Nutrition and Public Health

One of the most difficult tasks of a nutritionist is to transfer information to the general public. This applies especially to controversial subjects. Many such subjects have been discussed throughout this book, and the index can be used to identify them. In the following, we will discuss one controversial and important topic in nutrition and public health.

CANCER AND DIET

When it comes to health, it is a rare person who will not immediately think of cancer. We will provide a brief discussion below (National Research Council; Roe).

The uncontrolled growth and spread of abnormal cells constitutes the various diseases known as cancer. The spreading cells, known as tumors or neoplasms, can be benign and simply create a crowding condition; or they can be malignant and move into other tissues via the blood or the lymph. Substances that cause tumors to become malignant more frequently than otherwise are known as *carcinogens*.

Cancer ranks as the second leading cause of death and will develop in one in every four Americans. One in every five American deaths can be classified as at least cancer related. Although any part of the body can be affected by cancer, lungs rank as the most vulnerable, followed by the large intestine and the breast. Of the various organs most commonly affected by cancer, only the death rate from lung cancer is on the increase.

Estimates place cancer that is related to environmental factors, and thus preventable, at the 80 to 90 percent level. Environmental factors that have been identified as carcinogenic include drugs, alcohol, air contaminants, water contaminants, tobacco smoking, radiation, hair dyes, and viruses. We do not know exactly how carcinogens promote cancer. They may genetically damage cells, or they may simply do outright damage to cells. What is known is that many years can pass between exposure to carcinogens and the ultimate development of cancer.

To test for carcinogens, laboratory animals are used. Since small animals such as rats and mice develop cancer characteristics similarly to humans, they are the experimental animals chosen. Since the lifespan of such animals is much shorter than the time needed for cancer development, high doses of suspected carcinogens are administered. High doses have been criticized as being of dubious worth, but those who criticize such tests are overlooking the fact that high doses of noncarcinogens do not produce cancers in laboratory animals. The fact that certain substances do produce cancer is important evidence, evidence we should not discount.

The changes that have occurred in recent years in scientific attitudes toward diet and cancer can be partially understood in light of difficulties in finding a cure for cancer. If cures for all forms of cancer had been found fairly soon after identification of the disease, attention might never have been focused on diet. However, the prolonged study of cancer produced some interesting insights. For example, the kinds of cancer predominant in the United States are different from those predominant in other countries. Once scientists began to ask why, attention was shifted to environmental factors, including diet.

The focus on diet and its relationship to cancer initially culminated in a report issued by the National Academy of Sciences stating that there was insufficient evidence of a diet-cancer link to enable dietary recommendations. Two years later, the picture changed. The National Research Council of the National Academy of Sciences issued another report that did make anticancer diet recommendations. The change in attitude resulted from scientific evidence that showed a relationship between diets high in fats and cancer of the breast, colon, and prostate.

The anticancer dietary recommendations do not differ significantly from those of the American Heart Association for prevention of heart disease. To be avoided are well-marbled steaks; rich ice cream and other high-fat dairy products; and smoked, salt-cured foods. Recommended are fruits, vegetables, and whole grain products. The anticancer dietary recommendations stress that they are based upon inconclusive findings; however, they also note that most forms of cancer are externally caused and should therefore be preventable.

Estimates have placed diet in association with about one third of the cancer in men and over half the cancer in women. This compares with smoking, which is estimated to cause one fourth of cancer incidence. The incidence of stomach and bowel cancer should be most affected by dietary modification, while breast and lung cancer would be less affected.

Included in the dietary recommendations is the reduction of alcohol consumption, especially for those who smoke. Excessive alcohol consumption has been linked with cancer of the mouth, throat, esophagus, and respiratory tract. The recommendations also encourage carcinogenicity testing of additives and care in avoiding contaminants.

The recommendation regarding fats is that fats of all types should not constitute more than 30 percent of caloric intake. Some studies indicate that eating patterns make this goal difficult to achieve; however, other studies suggest it is a reasonable goal. The concern with fats is that they increase hormonal levels and may therefore contribute to hormone-dependent cancer of reproductive organs, prostate, and breast.

The recommendation to increase fruit, vegetable, and grain intake indirectly addresses findings suggesting that certain vitamins may help prevent cancer. For example, dark-green and yellow vegetables contain vitamin A and retinoids, which inhibit carcinogenesis. As an antioxidant, vitamin C can prevent nitrates and nitrites from becoming carcinogenic nitrosamines (see Chapter 25). Such vegetables as turnips, broccoli, and cabbage are also thought to contain anticancer substances.

Though the anticancer dietary recommendations do not specially address fiber as beneficial to cancer prevention, the recommended dietary modifications would assure high fiber intake. Fiber has a scrubbing effect on the digestive tract and appears to reduce the risk of digestive tract cancer.

Alcohol recommendations suggest that the darker colored beverages may be a greater risk than the lighter colored ones. This suggests that alcohol itself may not be the cancer link but rather the contaminants (see below) in the alcoholic beverages, since they are what causes the darker coloring.

Other concerns regarding diet and cancer are not yet ready for recommendation. Protein intake cannot be clearly linked to cancer, since protein foods typically contain other nutrients such as fats. Since there are over 2,000 food additives, only a few have been thoroughly tested. Most additives occur in very small amounts, so it proves very difficult to determine the cancer risk of additives.

Accidental or involuntary additives, commonly known as contaminants, continue to undergo testing. Such contaminants as PCBs (polychlorinated biphenyls) and pesticides occur irregularly in our food (also see Chapter 25). Certainly it is possible that they could contribute to cancer risk; however, this cannot be proved as yet. The best course of action is to prevent such contaminants from entering our food supply.

Minerals are also undergoing further study relative to cancer. Some minerals, such as the antioxidant selenium, appear beneficial in preventing cancer. Iron deficiency and iodine deficiency can lead to upper respiratory and thyroid cancer, respectively. Lead is suspected of having cancer-causing potential, and arsenic is similarly suspected. Zinc has proved a paradoxical mineral. At some stages of cancer development it appears beneficial, while at other stages it appears harmful.

Obviously, far more research is needed into the relationship between diet and cancer. However, it appears that the direction is set. Certain foods have a role in preventing cancer. Other foods contribute to cancer. The general medical opinion on anticancer dietary recommendations is that it is in our own best interest to follow them.

STUDY QUESTIONS

1. What are at least five recommendations from the 1977 edition of *Dietary Goals for the United States?* What dietary changes are recommended to meet these goals? Are these suggestions followed by all nutritionists?

2. What four general methods are used in determining people's nutritional status? What is the best single method of determining adiposity?

3. Which areas and body systems should be examined for clues to nutritional status? Are these sufficient for diagnosing the early stages of malnutrition?

4. What is the most valuable contribution of biochemical analyses in evaluating nutritional status? What is analyzed?

5. What is dietary study? How is it used? Describe at least three methods of conducting dietary studies, and discuss their pros and cons.

6. Describe the work of drug addiction rehabilitation centers and open-door clinics. Why are they important? How do they help their clients?

7. Using library resource materials, write a report on the latest development of the relationship between cancer and diet.

8. What is the Head Start Program? Describe its origin and current status. Using library resource materials, analyze its accomplishments.

REFERENCES

Beal, V. A., and M. J. Laus. "Proceedings: Symposium on Dietary Data Collection, Analysis, and Significance. *Mass. Agric. Expt. Stat. Res. Bull.,* No. 675, 1982.

Johnson, S. R., et al. "The Food Stamp Program: Participation, Food Cost, and Diet Quality for Low-Income Households." *Food Tech.* 35 (1981): 58.

National Research Council. *Diet, Nutrition, and Cancer.* Washington, D.C.: National Academy Press, 1982.

Roe, D. A., ed. *Current Topics in Nutrition and Disease: Diet, Nutrition and Cancer: From Basic Research to Policy Implications.* New York: Alan R. Liss, 1983.

Swenerton, H., and W. L. Dunkley. "Recent Activities of Public Agencies to Assure Healthful Diets for Americans." *J. Dairy Sci.* 65 (1982): 484.

Symposium. "Assessment of Nutritional Status." *Am. J. Clin. Nutr.* 35 (1982, supplement): 1112.

Vermersch, J., ed. "Nutrition Services in State and Local Public Health Agencies." *Public Health Reports* 98 (1983): 7.

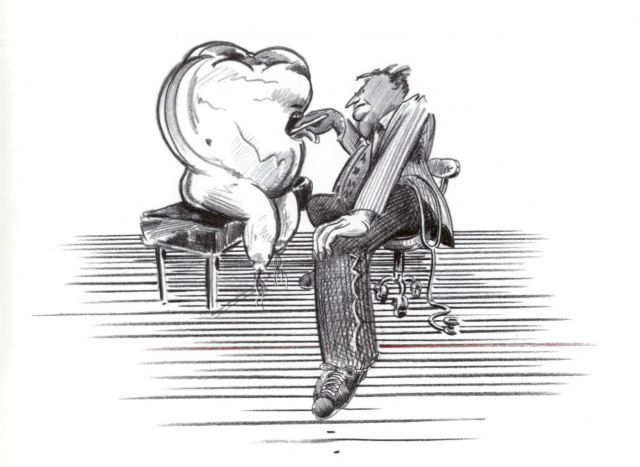

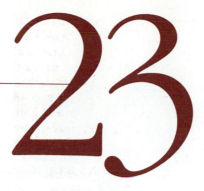

23

Nutrition
AND
Oral Health:

NOT JUST TEETH

Hal's teeth were eaten away

Hal sought dental assistance at age 54, complaining of pain in his upper front teeth whenever he drank either hot or cold liquids. The dentist found significant loss of tooth surfaces. Initially she suspected that Hal's teeth were being worn away by upper and lower teeth rubbing together, a problem known as malocclusion. However, tests did not confirm any malocclusion. When she asked about

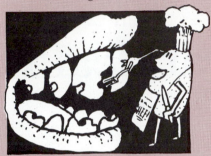

Hal's dietary habits, the dentist learned that almost every night before retiring Hal would drink

a cup of lemon tea and would subsequently suck the lemon. He had been doing this for over 30 years.

The dentist diagnosed that Hal's teeth had been gradually and painlessly worn away by erosion, a dissipation of tooth surface by nonbacterial chemical action. In Hal's case, the loss of tooth surface resulted from the long-term effect of citric acid from lemon.

Did you know that approximately 90 percent of all U.S. children have dental decay by the age of 4? Or that 10 percent of all Americans have lost *all* their natural teeth? These statistics tell us that an obvious pattern of oral health neglect exists in the United States—not simply neglect of proper brushing but neglect of nutrition and oral health. Not only the teeth but the gums are affected; gum (periodontal) disease, like dental caries, can cause loss of permanent teeth (Randolph). Oral health in the United States presents a disturbing picture—but one that has brightened in the last five years.

How Your Teeth Are Structured

As Figure 23-1 shows us, enamel, dentin, cementum, and pulp constitute the four layers of our teeth (Randolph). The outer layer, *enamel*, is the most durable of all our body tissues, yet enamel has a basic chemical composition that can, like bone, be decalcified by organic acids. Enamel is 96 percent inorganic, 3 percent water, and 1 percent organic and has the chemical name of hydroxyapatite. Like enamel, *dentin*, which composes the core of the hard portion of our teeth, primarily consists of calcium and phosphorus. Dentin is 70 percent inorganic, 20 percent organic, and 10 percent water and contains a high percentage of the insoluble protein **collagen**, which is a normal component of connective tissue (for example, gums and tendons). Collagen is highly susceptible to degeneration by bacterial action.

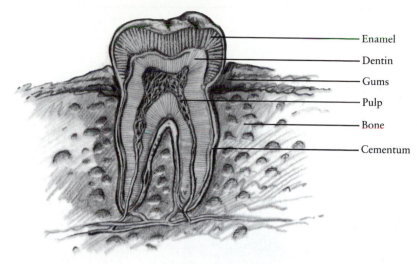

Enamel

Dentin

Gums

Pulp

Bone

Cementum

Figure 23-1: The anatomy of a tooth and the surrounding structures.

Cementum, also an inorganic (46 percent) calcified tissue, provides a surface for attachment of tooth and tissue. Cementum is 32 percent water and 22 percent organic and is the most bonelike portion of our teeth. *Pulp,* the soft center of teeth, is organic, containing nerves, blood vessels, lymphatic vessels, and fibrous tissue. Occupying approximately 75 percent of the tooth's length, pulp connects to both the body's nutritional system and its nervous system through tooth roots.

People tend to believe that deciduous teeth ("baby" teeth) cannot be too important since permanent teeth displace them, but they really do serve a vital function. The deciduous teeth maintain the alignment pattern for permanent teeth. If a deciduous tooth is lost before its permanent replacement is ready to fill the space, improper spacing may occur, leading to crowding and the danger of malocclusion. The presence of the deciduous teeth enables proper speech development as well. Figure 23-2 shows the permanent teeth.

Dental Health Begins Before Birth

In Chapter 16 we saw that tooth nutrition begins before birth. The pregnant mother's nutrient intake serves a vital role in the child's tooth development, and adequate supplies of calcium, iron, protein, and vitamins are essential to the process. For example, vitamin C enables dentin to calcify. Vitamin A also promotes calcification so that teeth develop normally. Vitamin D triggers the deposition of calcium and phosphorus in the developing teeth.

Maternal vitamin D deficiency has been found to result in significantly inadequate deciduous enamel, a condition known as *enamel hypoplasia* (see Figure 23-3). Studies in underdeveloped countries indicate that maternal malnutrition, especially protein deprivation, adversely affects deciduous dentition, resulting in both defective enamel and severe caries.

If a child's teeth are to develop properly, the pregnant mother must

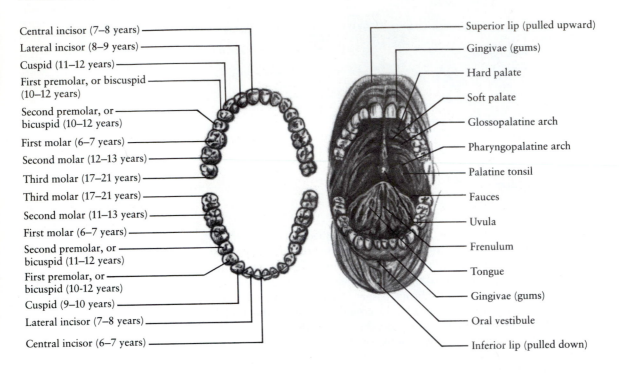

Central incisor (7–8 years)
Lateral incisor (8–9 years)
Cuspid (11–12 years)
First premolar, or biscuspid (10–12 years)
Second premolar, or bicuspid (10–12 years)
First molar (6–7 years)
Second molar (12–13 years)
Third molar (17–21 years)
Third molar (17–21 years)
Second molar (11–13 years)
First molar (6–7 years)
Second premolar, or bicuspid (11–12 years)
First premolar, or bicuspid (10-12 years)
Cuspid (9–10 years)
Lateral incisor (7–8 years)
Central incisor (6–7 years)

Superior lip (pulled upward)
Gingivae (gums)
Hard palate
Soft palate
Glossopalatine arch
Pharyngopalatine arch
Palatine tonsil
Fauces
Uvula
Frenulum
Tongue
Gingivae (gums)
Oral vestibule
Inferior lip (pulled down)

Figure 23-2: The permanent teeth.

eat a balanced and adequate diet, with special emphasis on the key nutrients mentioned above. Although it would seem logical that increased fluoride intake by the expectant mother would enhance infant dentition, this has not been found to be the case. The remainder of this chapter will therefore address oral health following birth.

Nutrient Deficiencies and Oral Structures

Oral tissues are continually changing and growing. A consistent supply of essential nutrients must be available to prevent bacterial and chemical damage of these sensitive tissues. Without adequate nutrition, infection readily occurs (see Chapter 19). The condition of the tongue is often the primary indicator of oral disorders and other health problems. Burning sensations and redness may be the initial signs. Physicians inquire about a burning sensation in the mouth (glossodynia) or look for a shiny surface on the tongue (glossitis) because these are signs of nutrient deficiency or other infections. Similarly, color changes of the tongue and mouth can signal metabolic disorders.

The effect of various nutrient deficiencies on oral structures has been discussed in detail in different chapters in Units I and II of this book. This section summarizes these materials for easy reference. Lip lesions can be indicative, for example, of protein, iron, folic acid, niacin, vita-

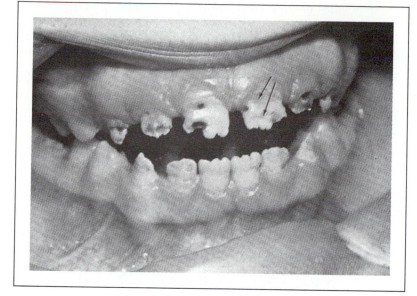

Figure 23-3: Typical enamel hypoplasia in the primary dentition of a child with hereditary vitamin D–dependency rickets. SOURCE: G. Nikiforuk and D. Fraser. "The Etiology of Enamel Hypoplasia: A Unifying Concept." J. Pediatr. 98 (1981): 888.

min B_{12}, or riboflavin deficiency. Lesions usually first appear in the corners of the mouth, then extend to surrounding tissues, and are followed by crusting and even scarring. Such conditions can, of course, occur from various nonnutritional causes as well, such as sunburn, licking of the lips, and poorly fitting dentures.

Inflammation of mucous membranes in the mouth can show niacin deficiency, a condition common among alcoholics. White ulcers on the oral mucous membranes, a painful condition, are related to folic acid or vitamin B_{12} deficiency. Changes in tongue color can range from pink pallor to purple. Pink pallor can indicate iron deficiency or vitamin A deficiency. Purpling of the tongue is seen in riboflavin deficiency. Reddening of the tongue, especially at the tip and sides, often signals niacin deficiency.

Changes in the papillae (protuberances) on the tongue's surface also are symptomatic of deficiencies. Riboflavin deficiency will result in a pebblelike tongue surface. Protein, iron, and B complex vitamin deficiency make the tongue appear red and slick. Excess sodium intake causes the tongue to swell. Dehydration causes it to shrink and become dry. Burning sensations can be related to folic acid or vitamin B_{12} deficiency and are often a precursor to the white ulcers mentioned earlier.

Gingivitis, inflammation of the gum tissue adjacent to the teeth, intensifies as a result of nutritional deficiency. For example, both vitamin C deficiency and niacin deficiency can cause gingivitis, which results from dental plaque irritating the tissue, to worsen and result in ulcerated gums.

Periodontitis—inflammation and breakdown of the supporting structures of the teeth—also intensifies from nutritional deficiency. Since bone loss characterizes periodontitis, calcium deficiency can contribute to the susceptibility of breakdown. Again, you should understand that the nutrient deficiency does not *cause* the periodontitis; it simply adds to its progress and its severity. Nutrition's most important role in gum disease is to provide for healthy oral tissues that will be less likely to break down.

Dental Caries

In the first 20 to 30 years of life, tooth loss generally occurs as a result of dental caries, or "cavities," as we commonly call them. The formation of the disease called dental caries requires a complex process dependent on the presence of susceptible teeth (called "the host"), bacterial action in the mouth, a dietary ingredient such as fermentable carbohydrate from table sugar (called "the substrate") to stimulate bacterial action, and time for the decay of the teeth to occur (Randolph).

HOW "CAVITIES" DEVELOP

Tooth decay begins when the enamel is decalcified by acids produced by bacteria interacting with plaque. Once the dentin is invaded by bacteria, a cavity occurs. When the bacteria reach the pulp, they destroy it, often creating the need for extraction. (Figure 23-4 shows classic dental decay.)

Since dental caries has plagued us throughout history, it would seem that we should be closer to eradicating the disease, yet we have seen that its statistical significance is astounding. The prevalence of dental caries can best be understood in terms of several dietary factors, including type of food consumed, clearance rate, frequency of eating, and "detergent" effects of food.

BACTERIA PLUS CARBOHYDRATES EQUALS PLAQUE

Foods have physical properties that affect tooth decay. For example, a sticky food slow to dissolve in saliva will contribute to decay, whereas

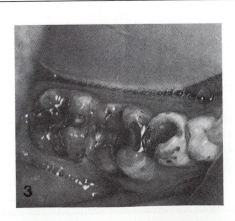

Figure 23-4: This 22-year-old patient had high caries frequency and severe degree of fluorosis. SOURCE: B. Forsman. Comm. Dent. Oral Epid. 2(1974): 132. Copyright 1974 Munkogaard International Publishers Ltd., Copenhagen, Denmark.

liquid foods that do not adhere to the teeth cause fewer cavities. Central to understanding the dietary factors influencing the health of our teeth is **plaque,** a sticky, gelatinlike material that adheres to teeth. Plaque contains colonies of bacteria and their acidic byproducts. The bacteria will be of two types, those causing caries (cariogenic) and noncariogenic. The primary cariogenic bacteria are streptococci, which ferment carbohydrates from our diet, producing organic acids that in turn demineralize enamel. Antibiotics reduce both the incidence and the severity of caries, suggesting that we may someday use a vaccine to prevent dental caries.

Until a vaccine is available, we must realize that our diet provides caries-causing bacteria with the food they need for growth, including essential amino acids, vitamins, minerals, and carbohydrates. These caries-causing bacteria convert sucrose, glucose, and fructose into dextran and amylopectin. **Dextran** is a complex, insoluble carbohydrate, a polysaccharide, that causes plaque to stick tenaciously to our teeth. **Amylopectin,** another polysaccharide, can be fermented by the bacteria to maintain acid production, even when the diet is sugar free. Using carbohydrates from our diet, especially sucrose, plaque bacteria primarily produce lactic acid, which in turn demineralizes the enamel.

SUCROSE PLAYS A ROLE

The role of sucrose, or table sugar, in dental decay has been well established (Acheinin). For example, there are individuals with a rare genetic disease who vomit if they consume sucrose or fructose. Such individuals, who must avoid both sucrose and fructose, have excellent dental health. In England and in various remote island countries, national increases in sugar use resulted in a parallel increase in dental caries. A classic Scandinavian study, the Vipeholm study, investigated the effect of diet on cariogenic bacteria. The Scandinavian study found, for example, that individuals who ate toffee several times each day had twelve times the cavities of those without frequent exposure to sugar. Even in poor countries with undernourished populations, low incidence of dental caries reflects an absence of sugar, despite less than optimal nutrition.

THE TIME FACTOR: WHEN AND HOW OFTEN YOU EAT

Another dietary factor affecting dental health concerns the frequency of eating and selected time factors. For example, the Vipeholm study found that those eating sweets between meals developed more caries than those eating sweets only at bedtime. Between-meal eaters expose their teeth to sugar for longer periods, even when the amount of sugar consumed daily is no greater than that of mealtime sugar eaters. Time factors also influence tooth susceptibility. Teeth develop caries more easily during the two- to four-year period after eruption than later, after enamel maturation occurs. This finding helps explain why young children and teenagers have more caries than other age groups. Finally, studies like Vipeholm demonstrate that caries development can be reduced if cariogenic stimulators, such as sucrose, are removed from the teeth as soon as possible after consumption.

Fluoride

Fluoride remains the only dietary element we know of that retards tooth decay (Andrus; Leverett). The positive effects of fluoride on dental health have been sufficiently publicized that hundreds of millions of the world's people now benefit from fluoridation programs. About half the United States population benefits from fluoride through fluoridated water.

SOME STATISTICS

Fluoride studies have demonstrated a reduction of tooth decay by over 50 percent in those who drink water containing 1 part per million (ppm) of fluoride during the years of tooth formation. Although fluoride benefit continues even in adults, its effectiveness lessens after the formative years of the teeth.

The manner in which fluoride affects teeth not only varies with the person's age but also varies between deciduous and permanent teeth. Deciduous teeth benefit from fluoride prior to their eruption, so fluoride's value for baby teeth occurs in the first year of life. The effect on permanent teeth is greater prior to their eruption than after eruption.

FOOD AND BEVERAGE SOURCES

Most foods contain very slight traces of fluoride, with about 0.2 to 0.5 mg per day being found in the average American diet (Clark and Corbin; Rao). If fluoridated water containing 1 ppm of fluoride is available, the daily intake approaches 1.5 to 2.0 mg. Dietary supplementation provides a source of fluoride that is especially beneficial to those who do not have access to fluoridated water.

FLUORIDATED WATER

Of the various means for providing fluoride, community water fluoridation costs the least (averaging 2 to 4 cents per person per year) and provides the greatest benefit (Andrus). Fluoride tablets have produced limited results, perhaps because the children studied did not take the pills regularly. The use of toothpaste and mouth rinses containing fluoride has yielded as high as a 50-percent reduction in new decay.

Despite the favorable findings regarding fluoride, the U.S. Public Health Service estimated in 1975 that only about half of the U.S. population received fluoridated water. Figure 23-5 depicts how fluoridation programs are distributed in the United States. The use of fluoridation has increased, partly because various states have passed legislation requiring that community water supplies be fluoridated. As mentioned earlier, fluoridation is used in various countries and may be the most widely recognized of preventive health measures. Such countries as Brazil, Canada, Czechoslovakia, New Zealand, and the Soviet Union join the United States in having fluoridation in a significant number of their communities.

The extent of and need for fluoridation varies according to several factors. For example, arid areas require less fluoride concentration, since more water is consumed there. Similarly, the benefit of fluoride varies in

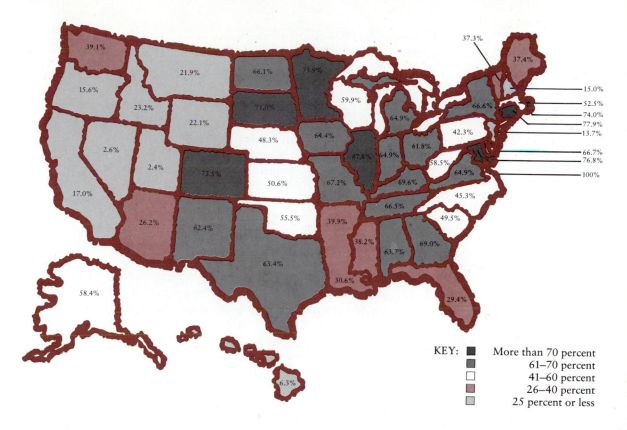

KEY:
- ■ More than 70 percent
- ■ 61–70 percent
- □ 41–60 percent
- ■ 26–40 percent
- ■ 25 percent or less

relation to an individual's age. Table 23-1 shows recommended fluoride supplementation for children at various ages, depending on the concentration of fluoridated water available. Some areas that lack community fluoridation have opted for fluoridated water in public schools. Such schools can have slightly higher levels of fluoride concentration since the children also consume nonfluoridated water.

Figure 23-5: Percent of state populations with fluoridated water supply.
SOURCE: Fluoridation Census 1980, U.S. Department of Health and Human Services, Public Health Service, Centers for Disease Control, Atlanta.

Table 23-1
Recommended Fluoride Supplementation

FLUORIDE CONCENTRATION OF WATER SUPPLY (ppm)	DESIRABLE FLUORIDE SUPPLEMENTATION (mg/day)				
	AGE 0–6 MO	AGE 6–18 MO	AGE 18–36 MO	AGE 3–6 YR	AGE > 6 YR
<0.2	0	0.25	0.5	0.75	1.0
0.2–0.4	0	0†	0.25	0.5	0.75
0.4–0.6	0	0†	0	0.25	0.5
0.6–0.8	0	0†	0	0	0.25
>0.8	0	0†	0	0	0‡

SOURCE: From Fomon, S.: *Nutritional Disorders of Children: Prevention, Screening and Follow-Up.* U.S. Dept. of Health, Education, and Welfare, 1976.

†0.25 for breast-fed infants between 6 and 12 months of age.

‡In this age group, the hazard of fluorosis is low, and some additional protection will probably be afforded by fluoride supplementation. However, fluoride supplementation is probably not desirable when drinking water provides more than 1.1 ppm. Most public health authorities use 1 ppm as the limit.

FLUORIDE SUPPLEMENTATION

Since fluoride ingestion in the first years of life may produce lifetime resistance to dental caries, and since most children first see a dentist after age 3, the family doctor can play a significant role in dental health during the first three years of life. As shown in Table 23-1, fluoridated water may be short of the fluoride needed to produce optimal protection. In such cases, daily fluoride supplements in keeping with age are recommended (American Academy of Pediatrics; Randolph).

Fluoride is generally supplemented by liquids or tablets and may be ingested or topically applied (Heifetz). It has been recommended that physicians not prescribe more than a three-month supply and that instructions for use should be provided. Liquid drops are especially suitable for infants while they are consuming only breast milk, cow's milk, or formula since all three contain almost no fluoride. If formula is diluted with fluoridated water, no supplement should be given. In tablet form, the content is from 0.5 to 1.0 mg of fluoride. Tablets are suitable for older children. Topical fluoride applications usually are performed by professionals and utilize high concentrations of fluoride.

Fluoride varnishes have been developed to keep fluoride in direct contact with the teeth for a longer time. Such topical applications serve three beneficial purposes. First, the presence of the fluoride reduces the solubility of the enamel. Second, the fluoride serves as a remineralizing agent. Finally, the fluoride negatively affects microbial activity.

Two types of fluoride used as cariostatic (caries prevention) agents are calcium fluoride and fluorapatite. Calcium fluoride, the more soluble of the two, is applied directly to the tooth surface to become a part of the enamel. Fluorapatite serves a more protective role, a barrier coating or sealant. Varnishes enable calcium fluoride to be held next to the teeth, thus facilitating the formation of fluorapatite.

Since the goal of topical applications is to stabilize the fluoride's protective ability, special instructions must accompany their use. For example, the teeth must be thoroughly brushed and flossed before the fluoride is applied. Varnish/enamel contact time can be increased by timing the application so that only a light meal is eaten afterward. The patient should be told not to brush for as long as 24 hours after application. Repeat applications should generally occur at six-month intervals.

Varnishes have proved the most effective of topical applications since they can be quickly applied. Children usually find them acceptable, thus eliminating a major drawback to other topical applications, the problem of children gagging on liquid fluoride washes. (Liquid washes must remain on the teeth for a certain period of time to be effective. Often the fear of swallowing or aspirating the substance during this time causes gagging, which diminishes the chance of a successful application.)

TOXICITY

Numerous studies of fluoridated water have demonstrated that no danger exists from the ingestion of fluoride at optimal levels (Leverett). Since dietary fluoride supplementation significantly benefits preschoolers, with

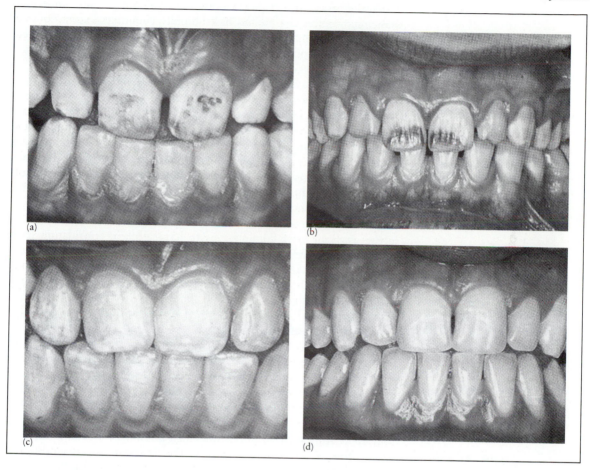

Figure 23-6: (a) Moderately severe mottling, showing staining and pitting of enamel, associated with 5–6 ppm F in water. (b) Moderate mottling with staining associated with 3–5 ppm F in water. Enamel surface is intact. (c) Mild mottling with white translucencies, but enamel surface is hard: 2 ppm F in water. (d) Teeth of child living in area with 0.9 ppm F in water; note excellent appearance of hard, shining enamel.
SOURCE: J. R. Forrest. "Mottled Enamel." Br. Dent J. 119 (1965): 316.

little risk of tooth staining or pitting (fluorosis), the practice is advisable as long as water concentrations are below 1 ppm. Fluorosis, the primary side effect of excessive fluoride ingestion, is characterized by the formation of white lines or patches on the teeth. In more advanced cases of fluorosis, brown staining and pitting can occur. Fluorosis should not occur if recommended dosages are followed. Fluoride levels in the 6- to 10-ppm ranges are considered excessive. It is well known that many sources of drinking water contribute fluoride naturally. Thus, occasional fluorosis occurs in areas where the drinking water contains excessive fluoride. Figure 23-6 illustrates fluorosis from too much fluoride in the drinking water.

Electrolyte disturbances (mineral imbalances) can result if too much fluoride supplement is accidentally ingested. This is why physicians are encouraged to prescribe no more than a three-month supply. Long-term ingestion of excessive quantities of fluoride can possibly lead to **osteoporosis** (a bone disease; also see Chapter 18). Normally, this condition would only occur if both malnutrition and an exceptionally high natural concentration of fluoridated water were present simultaneously.

Fluoride poisoning via ingestion remains unusual because under normal circumstances the human body rapidly eliminates excess fluorides by the kidneys and because calcified structures in the body rapidly utilize fluoride. Little fluoride has an opportunity to accumulate in the body.

FLUORIDE SHORTAGE

Community water supplies usually are fluoridated through the use of hydrofluosilicic acid (hereafter referred to as "the acid"), a byproduct of the manufacture of phosphate fertilizer. When an unfavorable farm economy exists, many farmers will significantly reduce or eliminate the purchase of chemical fertilizers, thereby causing a shortage of the acid.

When such shortages of the acid in liquid form occur, communities either lower the amount used or else switch to sodium fluoride, which is not a byproduct and is produced by a different manufacturing process. The cost of sodium fluoride is almost four times that of the acid. The higher cost can force communities to have a lower fluoridation level. Such economically imposed variations in community fluoridation programs can bring about a temporary need for dietary supplementation or topical application in localities where the need may not have previously existed or been as great.

Caries in the Nursing Infant

A particular form of dental caries can result from children nursing from bottles containing sweetened drinks. The damage will occur to the upper front four teeth (maxillary incisors).

It can become a common practice to allow a child to go to sleep while nursing on a bottle containing sweetened water, chocolate milk, soft drinks, fruit juices, or other sweet beverages. The practice subjects the four upper front teeth to a constant sugar bath and can lead to rampant caries. This is sometimes known as the "nursing bottle syndrome"; Figure 23-7 provides an example.

Nursing caries can also result from breast-feeding if the infant is permitted to nurse for a prolonged period. The disease will begin following tooth eruption and can result in abscesses. If the teeth are lost, speech impairment will result (Randolph).

Acidity and the Teeth

As was seen in the case of Hal at the beginning of this chapter, foods contain acids that can damage our teeth even though we do not have dental caries. Such chemical damage occurs by the acid eating away the enamel, dentin, and cementum over a long period of exposure.

ACIDITY FROM FOOD AND BEVERAGES

Tooth erosion can be caused by prolonged exposure to such citrus fruits as lime, lemon, orange, and grapefruit, or such other fruits as green

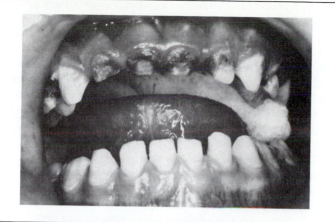

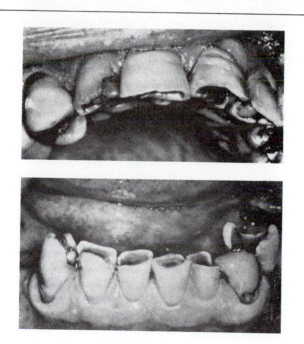

Figure 23-7: Rampant decay in primary dentition of 4-year-old boy with continuous history of bottle-feeding prior to sleeping. Lower anterior teeth are not carious because of protection from tongue during sucking and swallowing. SOURCE: T. E. Cone, Jr. J.A.M.A. 245 (1981): 2334. Copyright 1981, American Medical Association.

Figure 23-8: Loss of incisal tooth tissue in a patient who ate large quantities of fresh fruit. SOURCE: K. J. Lewis and B. G. N. Smith. Br. Dent. J. 135 (1973): 400.

apples, apricots, pineapples, peaches, and plums. The chemical damage results whether the long-term use is of the fruit itself or its juice.

Erosion also results from the carbon acid in carbonated beverages such as colas. Excessive use of vinegar can erode teeth as well. Products that could cause vinegar erosion are salad oils, pickled onions, and such Oriental foods as sweet and sour sauce. Figure 23-8 illustrates tooth erosion from acidic foods and beverages.

ACIDITY FROM NONFOOD SOURCES
Teeth can also be damaged by acidity that occurs in an environment over

a prolonged period. For example, competitive swimmers have experienced erosion due to high acidity in swimming pool water. It is common for large pools to be chlorinated with chlorine gas, which is less expensive than other products. Chlorine gas interacts with water to form hydrochloric acid. If adequate amounts of soda ash are not used to buffer the pool's acid, the resulting acidity will be high enough to damage teeth. Similarly, industrial workers can sustain tooth damage from prolonged and excessive exposure to acid fumes. (See also Figure 23-8.)

Periodontal Disease

When we reach middle age, the primary cause of the loss of teeth shifts from dental caries to periodontal disease—disease of the gums and other tissues, including bone, which surround the teeth (Randolph; Schoen and Freed). Inflammation of the gums, *gingivitis*, occurs as the initial phase of periodontal disease. *Periodontitis*, a more severe disease, involves the bone beneath the gums. If gingivitis goes untreated, it leads to weakening and destruction of the fibers that hold the teeth in place. In the final stage of periodontal disease, the alveolar (supporting) bone (see Figure 23-1) that contains the tooth sockets will recede, leading to tooth loss.

HOW PERIODONTAL DISEASE DEVELOPS

The major factor contributing to periodontal disease is inadequate oral cleanliness with its resultant bacterial growth. As would be expected, the incidence of periodontal disease is greatest in poor countries with few dentists and in areas, including parts of the United States, with limited access to dentists. Once gingivitis develops, sensitive gums can lead to consumption of soft foods, often perpetuating bacterial growth and hastening the spread of the disease.

When plaque amasses at the junction of gum and teeth, periodontal disease results. When a mixture of minerals known as *calculus* builds on the teeth under the gum tissue, the teeth are further loosened. What technically occurs in periodontal disease is that certain types of microorganisms (spirochetes, primarily) invade the crevices between teeth and gums and attach to roots of the teeth. The microorganisms create toxins, and the periodontal tissues recede from the toxins, resulting in loosened teeth that ultimately fall out if the condition remains uncorrected.

NUTRITION AND PERIODONTITIS

Specific nutritional relationships to periodontal disease are few. Vitamins A and E have proved beneficial. Niacin shortage often leads to diseased gums, and bleeding gums result from scurvy, a disease caused by deficiency of vitamin C. Both of the foregoing problems are, however, specialized periodontal problems. Protein deficiency adversely affects the endocrine system, a protector of gum tissue through hormonal secretions. Bone deterioration is also associated with protein shortage. Iron deficiency, especially in women, has been found to contribute to weakening of gingival tissue. Logically, calcium and phosphorus shortage would negatively affect the alveolar bone.

There are several actions available to the individual suffering from periodontal disease (Axelsson and Lindhe). Although oral hygiene and sufficient nutrient intake can stem such problems, dental experts also encourage the eating of firm fiber foods such as carrots, which have a cleansing or detergent action.

After eating, toothpick use is beneficial. Brushing and flossing, followed by irrigation (washing out), is recommended. Patients can carefully apply various salts to control bacterial activity of the type that affects tooth roots. Helpful products include table salt, baking soda, and Epsom salts. If gums have begun to recede, the patient can apply fluoride gel to the infected area. Such gels are available without prescription or in a stronger form by prescription.

The technique for patient self-treatment of periodontal disease especially focuses on washing out of the areas between teeth and gums, a process called *irrigation*. A warm brine solution is initially used in a water appliance (see further in this chapter). Following irrigation, an antibacterial solution (mixture of hydrogen peroxide, table salt, and baking soda) is worked into areas between teeth and gums by a pointed stimulator or by a brush with highly flexible bristles.

Oral Hygienic Aids

Although no particular products are recommended here, a general knowledge of the available oral hygienic aids can be valuable. Certainly the most widely recognized of such hygienic aids is toothpaste.

TOOTHPASTE

In 1982, the American Dental Association recommended use of only five brands of toothpaste: Aim, Aqua-fresh, Crest, Colgate and Macleans. (Crest contains sodium fluoride; the others contain sodium monofluorophosphate.) The dental association makes recommendations only after thorough research has been reviewed by the association's Council on Dental Therapeutics. Since the research cost must be borne by the toothpaste manufacturers, many toothpastes have not been studied.

Fluoride has been fully accepted by the Council on Dental Therapeutics as a toothpaste additive of proven worth as an anticavity agent. There are several toothpastes available, many of them by foreign manufacturers, with different additives. For example, vitamin C and calcium are additives that have not been proved to be of benefit in toothpaste. Foreign toothpaste manufacturers add antimicrobial agents, such as chlorhexidine digluconate, an agent not approved for use in toothpaste in the United States.

Abrasives are the next most common additives after fluoride. The history of abrasives goes back thousands of years and includes such products as sand, pumice, dyes, metals, and acids. Charcoal is currently used as an abrasive in some foreign toothpastes, though no American manufacturers use it. Such additives are intended to remove stain.

Most abrasive toothpastes are presented as smokers' toothpastes, with the claim that they remove both food stain and nicotine stain. Since toothpastes vary in their abrasive ability anyway, more frequent brushing with a less abrasive toothpaste should accomplish the same results.

The Council on Dental Therapeutics has recently accepted that potassium nitrate used as an additive can reduce sensitivity to hot and cold in teeth that are otherwise normal. Potassium nitrate has been shown effective in reducing pain in hypersensitive dentin. Studies found no adverse side effects. Such a product containing 5 percent potassium nitrate is being marketed as Denquel Sensitive Teeth Toothpaste. The council has also recognized Colgate's combination of two fluorides, sodium monofluorophosphate and sodium fluoride, as effective in remineralization. The theory behind the combination is that more complete remineralization of white spot lesions will occur before they can become carious.

OTHER DENTIFRICES

Although toothpaste is the most common dentifrice, mouthwashes, gels, tooth powders, and rinses also belong to the dentifrice group. Partially because of their granulated characteristic, tooth powders appear to be more abrasive, causing some manufacturers to advertise that their product is no more abrasive than commonly accepted pastes. An example of such a product is Arm and Hammer Baking Soda, which has been used as a dentifrice for many years.

Mouthwashes and rinses provide a benefit in oral hygiene because they can reach tooth surfaces not easily reached by brushing or flossing. Fluoride has become a mouthwash additive. Products such as Listermint with Fluoride, ACT Fluoride Dental Rinse, and Colgate's Fluorigard emphasize their ability to reduce cavities even beyond the level of reduction achieved in fluoridated water supply areas where regular brushing occurs with a fluoride dentifrice. Up to a 40 percent further reduction has been claimed.

As mentioned in regard to periodontal diseases, other fluoride rinses and brush-on fluoride gels can be obtained through prescription. Usually the brush-on gels are for daily use, whereas the stronger fluoride rinses are recommended for weekly use.

WATER APPLIANCES

An effective element in oral hygiene, one especially useful in the prevention and treatment of periodontal disease, is the water appliance. Studies have determined that some of the microorganisms involved in periodontal disease are free floating. A water appliance can wash these microorganisms out from the spaces between teeth and gums. A further benefit of such appliances is the ability to include additional cleansing agents in the water used by the appliance. Manufacturers of such appliances sometimes claim that stimulation of gums provide a further positive effect.

By mixing such materials as table salt, baking soda, and hydrogen peroxide in a water appliance, several beneficial aspects can be accomplished. The baking soda and salt dehydrate bacteria. The hydrogen peroxide brings oxygen into contact with anaerobic bacteria. The pulsating action of the water stream washes the bacteria out of the mouth. For individuals on salt-free diets, Epsom salts can be substituted for table salt in such antibacterial solutions.

Preventive Measures

As we saw at the beginning of this chapter, dental caries is a widespread disorder, ranking as the most common disease in the United States. Dental disease in general is the third most expensive disease in our nation, following only heart disease and cancer. For these reasons, dental disease undergoes frequent review.

THE GOOD NEWS

The National Center for Health Statistics and the National Caries Prevalence Study, conducted by the National Institute of Dental Research, have found that dental caries has been significantly reduced in the United States. Studies conducted as recently as 1981 show that the number of children found to be free of caries has increased from 28 percent to slightly over 36 percent. A measurement called the DMF index (D = untreated decay, M = missing teeth, and F = filled teeth), shows that a 50 percent reduction in DMF surfaces has been achieved for children between the ages of 6 and 17 (see Figure 23-9).

This encouraging news is related to several factors. Certainly fluori-

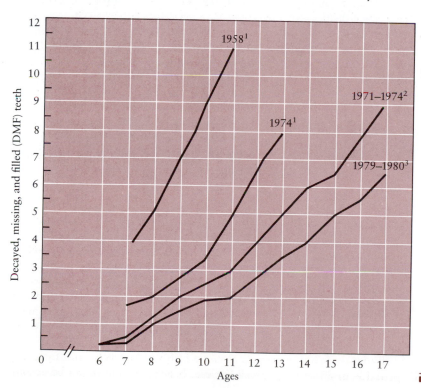

Figure 23-9: The decline in the average number of decayed, missing, and filled (DMF) teeth among U.S. children and youths 6 to 17 years of age from 1958 to 1980. SOURCE: J. Amer. Dent. Assoc. 105 (1982): 75. 1. R. L. Glass and S. Fleisch. No data available for 13-year-old children in 1958; water nonfluoridated. 2. PHS. Water fluoridated and nonfluoridated. 3. NIDR. Water fluoridated and nonfluoridated.

dated water supplies are a primary reason for the reduction, as are use of fluoride dentifrices and increased public awareness, which leads to improved oral hygiene. Similar improvement has been found in regard to periodontal disease, which affected 75 percent of the adult population. Reductions have also been accomplished in root surface caries and in edentulousness (tooth loss). New products promise further improvement, though decreases are not likely to be as dramatic as has been the case recently. Improved dentifrices will provide further dental health improvement. A new sugar-free sweetener, Aspartame (marketed as Nutra Sweet), may lower caries incidence. The product is a sweet compound of two amino acids (see Chapter 7), aspartate and phenylalanine, and is digested and utilized as protein. The product tastes sweet but provides only 0.10 calorie while delivering the same sweetness as a teaspoon of sugar (16 calories). Dieters are likely to respond quite favorably to the increased palatability of restricted diets. Also see Chapter 20.

RECOMMENDATIONS

We have seen that good nutrition, fluoridation, and oral hygiene to control plaque are key preventive measures. To such a list of preventive measures we must add education, since knowing what must be done provides the first step in doing it.

Effective oral hygiene involves not only proper brushing but also dental flossing. In combination, the two can remove plaque before it penetrates the enamel. Such cleansing is especially important prior to sleep, since the rubbing action of saliva decreases during sleep.

Preventive dietary measures include avoidance of bacteria-feeding foods, mainly fermentable carbohydrate such as pastries and candy. Fruits and vegetables should replace candy and cookies as snacks. Sticky candies should especially be avoided. Fluoride intake should be ensured, particularly during the early years of life, as should good general nutrition, characterized by a well-balanced and nutritious diet.

Many of us tend to neglect oral health. Yet improved oral health is available to us all, if we will only apply the preventive procedures we have discussed. We have the responsibility and the capability to continue to alter the discouraging statistics of dental and periodontal disease incidence.

STUDY QUESTIONS

1. Describe the basic structure of a tooth.

2. Describe the effect of deficiency of the following nutrients on adult oral structures: folic acid, vitamin B_{12}, niacin, riboflavin, protein, iron, vitamin C, and calcium.

3. What are the major factors contributing to dental caries? Briefly explain each factor.

4. Discuss the role of fluoride in cavity prevention. Research the fluoridation status of the town(s) in which you were raised.

5. Discuss the toxicity of fluoride.

6. Name ten foods and ten beverages whose acidity can erode the teeth.

7. Describe what a person can do to avoid periodontal disease.

8. Make a list of toothpastes available where you live and ascertain their fluoride and additive contents.

REFERENCES

Acheinin, A. "The Role of Dietary Carbohydrate in Plaque Formation and Oral Disease." In *Present Knowledge in Nutrition,* 5th ed. Washington, D.C.: The Nutrition Foundation, 1984.

American Academy of Pediatrics. "Fluoride Supplementation: Revised Dosage Schedule." *Pediatrics* 63 (1979): 150.

Andrus, P. L. "The Role of Fluoride in the Prevention of Dental Caries." *Texas Med. J.* 78 (1982): 57.

Axelsson, P., and J. Lindhe. "Effect of Controlled Oral Hygiene Procedures on Caries and Periodontal Disease in Adults: Results After 6 Years." *J. Clin. Periodontology* 8 (1981): 239.

Clark, N., and S. Corbin. "The Evolution of Standards for Naturally Occurring Fluorides." *Public Health Rept.* 98 (1983): 53.

Glass, R. L., and S. Fleisch. "Decreases in Caries Prevalence, School Children Ages 7–13, Denham, MA, 1958 and 1974 (Nonfluoridated). American Dental Association Health Foundation. Foods, Nutrition and Dental Health Foundation Fourth Annual Conference. Research Institute. Park Forest South, Ill.: Pathotox, 1981, pp. 181–188.

Heifetz, S. B. "Alternative Methods of Delivering Fluorides: An Update." In *Dental Caries Prevention in Public Health Programs,* edited by A. M. Horowitz and H. B. Thomas. *USDHHS,* NIH Publ. No. 81-2235 (1981): 25.

Leverett, D. S. Fluorides and Dental Caries." *Science* 220 (1983): 146.

NIDR. "Prevalence of Dental Caries in United States Children, 1979–1980." *National Dental Caries Prevalence Survey.* National Institute of Dental Research, 1981, pp. 1–12.

PHS. "Basic Data on Dental Examination Findings of Persons 1–74 Years, United States, 1971–1974. Public Health Services (PHS), National Center for Health Statistics, Series 11, 1981, p. 223.

Randolph, P. M. *Diet, Nutrition, and Dentistry.* St. Louis: C. V. Mosby, 1980.

Rao, G. S. "Dietary Intake and Bioavailability of Fluoride." *Ann. Rev. Nutr.* 4 (July 1984): 20.

Schoen, M. H., and J. R. Freed. "Prevention of Dental Disease: Caries and Periodontal Disease." *Ann. Rev. Public Health* 2 (1981): 43.

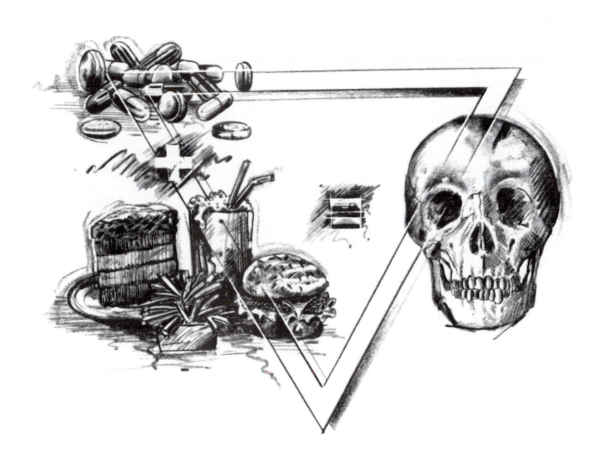

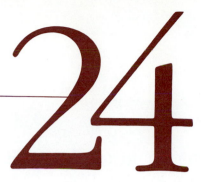

24

Nutrition AND Drugs:

DRUG-CAUSED DEFICIENCIES

Nutrition, Drugs, and Death: A Case History

MaryLou was 19 years old and had been dieting for seven years. A friend told her that diet pills known as "rainbow pills" would make her lose weight regardless of how much she ate. MaryLou obtained the pills by prescription and began the recommended dosage. She took one each of three different-colored pills before breakfast, a different-colored one before lunch, another different-colored one before dinner, and yet two more different-colored ones before bedtime.

MaryLou did not concern herself with what she was taking. Her weight loss was rapid, and she was tremendously encouraged. Just before her twentieth birthday, MaryLou's best friend found her dead in her bed.

A subsequent autopsy found only the early symptoms of bronchopneumonia. An examination of the rainbow pills showed that they contained amphetamines (a stimulant), barbiturates (a depressant), thyroid and other hormones, diuretics ("water pills"), laxatives, digitalis (a heart stimulant), antispasmodics (against spasms),

and hypotensives (drugs to lower blood pressure). But none of these were found by the coroner to be at a lethal level in MaryLou's body. It was the family doctor who, when consulted about MaryLou's medical

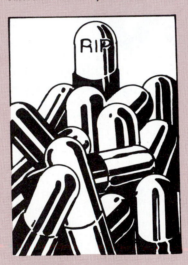

history, provided the key to understanding MaryLou's death.

The family doctor had another patient whose potassium levels were reduced by taking rainbow pills. That same

patient had the preliminary signs of digitalis poisoning. By putting the symptoms of the living patient together with the circumstances surrounding MaryLou's death, the physician and coroner theorized that MaryLou's death was caused by a combination of interactions. The amphetamines produced anorexia (loss of appetite), resulting in reduced potassium intake. The laxatives promoted excretion of what little potassium remained. Potassium is vital to the electrical functions of heart muscle. In the absence of potassium, the heart becomes sensitive to digitalis, which is normally nontoxic. Digitalis toxicity can cause irregular heart rhythms, including standstill.

It was theorized that MaryLou died from cardiac arrest occurring as the result of digitalis poisoning related to an extremely low potassium level. After MaryLou's death, rainbow pills were banned. Physicians are no longer permitted to prescribe drugs that reduce appetite for the purpose of weight loss.

SOURCES: FDA Fact Sheet #CSS D7-7-69; R. C. Henry, *Nutrition Today*, 3 (March 1968): 18.

Drugs Can Affect Your Nutritional Well-Being

Many people are tremendously concerned about the relationship between drug usage and nutrition. This concern involves not only prescription drugs but also such illicit drugs as hallucinogens and marijuana. The interest in the drug/nutrition connection has generated a wealth of information through research, clinical studies, and case reports. Instead of a detailed presentation of the numerous findings, this chapter concentrates on the six subject areas most regularly questioned by the general public: drugs and the body's well-being; the effect food can have on a drug's effectiveness; the difference in drug effectiveness in relation to the degree of nourishment; special dangers in certain food and drug combinations; the relationship between drugs and breast milk; and the preventive measures available to us.

BEWARE: A VITAMIN CAN BE A DRUG

As we saw in Chapter 8, nutrients such as vitamins can become drugs (at least can meet the definition of drugs) if the nutrients are used for pharmacological effects. For example, if a person has a bladder infection and a megadose of vitamin C is prescribed, the vitamin C is not being used for its characteristics as a vitamin but rather is being prescribed to acidify the urine. Such a usage of vitamin C is pharmacological rather than nutritional. Niacin, a B vitamin, is similarly used to lower blood cholesterol.

MOST IMPORTANT, DRUG EFFECTS VARY

As you can well imagine, the effects of drugs on the body can vary almost as much as our bodies vary. Numerous factors produce these varying results. Consider, for example, the usage differences that can occur. The drug can vary; the dosage can vary; time and frequency of consumption can vary. Reactions also vary according to the health status of the drug user. If, for example, you are malnourished, the drug's effects will generally be more profound than if you were well nourished. If your body nutrition is good, your body can effectively deal with a larger drug dose than you could otherwise handle. Conversely, a malnourished person may require a higher dosage to produce a desired therapeutic effect. We also vary in our general ability to adapt to ingested foreign substances such as drugs. Those with better adaptive abilities typically have fewer nutritional problems. Finally, our ability to absorb drugs and nutrients varies; for example, owing to age or differences in digestive-juice production, our drug response can vary.

Our nutritional status can be affected by single or multiple drug therapy. Effects may be short-term or long-term. In our digestive system, we can expect such pharmacological effects as diarrhea (laxative) or constipation, nausea and vomiting, altered taste and smell sensitivity, changing intestinal absorption ability, and fluctuation in bacterial growth in the intestine. Drugs thus affect appetite and feelings of fullness, digestion, absorption, utilization, storage, synthesis, and metabolism of nutrients. Of special concern is how drugs can affect the body's ability to manufacture and metabolize nutrients.

HOW DRUGS AFFECT NUTRIENT UTILIZATION

Many drugs, such as laxatives, antibiotics, and medications for diabetics, decrease absorption of nutrients. This can happen in various ways. For example, dietary vitamin A, or carotene, can dissolve in mineral oil, a popular laxative, and be lost in the bowel, since the oil is not absorbed. Drugs may simply damage intestinal walls so that fewer nutrients are absorbed. Drugs can damage small accessory organs along the digestive tract causing fewer nutrients to be digested or absorbed. Also, drugs can directly destroy, displace, or change nutrients themselves.

Inside the human body, a drug can join with a nutrient, rendering the nutrient incapable of being utilized normally. When this occurs, the nutrient will simply be excreted by the kidney.

Drugs affect all nutrients—carbohydrate, fat, protein, vitamins, minerals—to varying extent. For example, drugs can cause fat to be deposited in the liver, can cause blood insulin levels to fluctuate, can reduce body vitamin storage, and can increase excretion of minerals in the urine.

In the next section we will look at the specific drugs that affect our nutritional status (Hui; Spiller).

SPECIFIC DRUG EFFECTS
Table 24-1 presents both clinical usage and specific effects on nutritional status of a number of drug categories. Figure 24-1 depicts folic acid (a B vitamin) deficiency symptoms resulting from long-term therapy for epilepsy.

Food Can Make a Drug More or Less Effective

Just as drugs can interfere with our food utilization, so too can foods and nutrients affect the action of drugs (Lamy). Foods can change drug absorption, can neutralize drug effects, can interact with drugs, and can influence their excretion rate.

IN YOUR BODY, FOODS COMPETE WITH DRUGS
Doctors prescribe drugs for maximum therapeutic effect. Yet, it has long been assumed that the presence of food in the intestinal tract, the primary absorption site, affects the absorption of most drugs. The extent of this effect remains unclear. We know that food can increase or decrease acidity, digestive secretions, and intestinal motility. Such effects directly determine whether a drug will be easily destroyed, how long it will stay in the intestine, whether a drug will become crystals, whether a drug will be absorbed at all, and other technical changes.

SOME SPECIFIC EXAMPLES
Dietary minerals such as iron, magnesium, calcium, and aluminum salts demonstrate how food chemicals or nutrients can affect drug absorption. These minerals can chemically join with tetracycline, a commonly used antibiotic, to form tiny solid particles (insoluble precipitate). Simultaneous ingestion of these minerals and tetracycline causes the drug to lose its therapeutic value, requiring a large dose to offset the loss. This example shows that the common practice of taking such drugs with food or liquids to mask the drug taste may be questionable. Patients should be given specific directions about combining drugs with meals or snacks, including the rationale for them.

Another well-known example is the negative effect of a fatty diet on the absorption of griseofulvin, a drug that fights fungus infection. It is speculated that bile secretion, stimulated by fat, makes griseofulvin more water-soluble and, thus, less of the drug is absorbed.

Table 24-1

Examples of Common Drugs, Their Clinical Usages, and Their Specific Effects on Nutritional Status

DRUG	CLINICAL USAGE	POSSIBLE DIRECT AND INDIRECT EFFECTS ON NUTRITIONAL STATUS
Alcohol	A minor ingredient in medications*	An alcoholic shows the following: Thiamine and magnesium deficiencies most common; deficiencies of folic acid, niacin, and pyridoxine may also occur. May decrease absorption and utilization and increase excretion of affected nutrients.
Alkylating agents	Cancer chemotherapy	
Cyclophosphamide (Cytoxan)		Anorexia, vomiting, nausea, hemorrhagic cystitis and colitis, ulceration of intestinal mucosa.
Nitrogen mustard (Mustargen)		Anorexia, vomiting, nausea, diarrhea, and metallic taste.
Analgesics	Multiple uses	
Aspirin		May fluctuate blood glucose, deplete body folic acid and vitamin C. Stomach bleeding may result in iron-deficiency anemia. Potential hypernatremia, especially undesirable for heart or kidney patients.
Cocaine		Decreases sensitivity of taste, especially of bitterness and sweetness.
Phenylbutazone		May ulcerate stomach walls, decrease intestinal mucus secretion.
Antacids	Buffering stomach acids	
Aluminum hydroxide		Chronic ingestion results in hypophosphatemia, especially with low phosphate intake. Also causes constipation and potential vitamin malabsorption.
Calcium carbonate or too much milk		Milk-alkali syndrome. Hypercalcemia, which can be serious.
Sodium bicarbonate		Hypernatremia, especially undesirable for kidney and heart patients.
Antibiotics	Destruction of pathogenic organisms	Most drugs can irritate intestinal walls, causing diarrhea, thus fluid and electrolyte imbalance. Causes malabsorption of various nutrients to different extents. Decreases nutrient contribution by intestinal flora, for example, vitamins such as K, folic acid, biotin, and B_{12} and amino acids.
Bleomycin (Blenoxane)	Cancer chemotherapy	May cause stomatitis, anorexia, nausea, vomiting, fever, oral ulceration.
Cycloserine	Antituberculosis, treatment of urinary tract infection	Folic acid and pyridoxine deficiencies.
Dactinomycin (actinomycin D, Cosmegen)	Cancer chemotherapy	May cause stomatitis, anorexia, nausea, vomiting, diarrhea, oral ulceration.
Griseofulvin	Controlling growth of some dermatophytes	May cause loss of taste sensitivity; nausea.
Isoniazid	Antituberculosis	Niacin and pyridoxine deficiencies.

*Authority to prescribe this stype of medication is now "limited."
†Clinical usage of these drugs is uncommon in the United States.

Continued on page 546

Table 24-1 (*continued*)

DRUG	CLINICAL USAGE	POSSIBLE DIRECT AND INDIRECT EFFECTS ON NUTRITIONAL STATUS
Neomycin (and kanamycin)	Nonabsorbable; gut sterilization and prevention of coma from liver failure	May damage small intestine walls; malabsorption of various nutrients usually not significant because of short-term usage.
Paraaminosalicylic acid (PAS)	Antituberculosis	Decreases absorption of fat and vitamin B_{12}, especially if given at high dosage.
Tetracycline	Multiple uses (systemic effect)	May specifically affect bone growth, malabsorption of various nutrients. Usually not significant because of short-term usage.
Anticholinergics Belladonna Propantheline bromide	Treatment for peptic ulcer	May cause dry mouth, constipation, and urinary retention.
Anticoagulants Coumarin	Preventing blood clotting	Works by counteracting the function of vitamin K (the synthesis of prothrombin).
Phenindione		Steatorrhea. May bring about loss of fat-soluble vitamins and essential fatty acids in the stool.
Anticonvulsants (including sedatives) Barbiturates Phenytoin (Dilantin) Others	Sedation, tranquilizing, control of epilepsy	Folic acid and vitamin D deficiencies; sometimes vitamin K deficiency (see Figures 16-1 and 16-2).
Antihistamines Chlorpheniramine Promethazine	Multiple uses, e.g., antiallergy	Dry mouth, increased appetite; intestinal problems may cause malabsorption of nutrients.
Antihyperglycemic drugs (oral) Biguanides Metformin Phenformin Sulfonylureas	Lowering blood glucose; optional treatment for diabetes	May interfere with vitamin B_{12} absorption. May increase appetite.
Antihyperlipidemic drugs Cholestyramine Clofibrate	Lowering blood cholesterol	Both may interfere with the absorption of fat-soluble vitamins A, D, and K, fat, iron, and vitamin B_{12}. Clofibrate may also induce nausea and abnormal muscle metabolism.
Niacin		May interfere with glucose metabolism.
Antihypertensives Hydralazine	Lowering blood pressure	Vitamin B_6 deficiency by binding with B_6 and increasing its excretion.
Propranolol		Hypoglycemia.

*Authority to prescribe this stype of medication is now "limited."
†Clinical usage of these drugs is uncommon in the United States.

Table 24-1 (*continued*)

DRUG	CLINICAL USAGE	POSSIBLE DIRECT AND INDIRECT EFFECTS ON NUTRITIONAL STATUS
Anti-inflammatory drugs Colchicine	Treatment for gout	Maldigestion and malabsorption. Diarrhea and steatorrhea. Sodium, potassium, B_{12}, lipid, nitrogen, fat-soluble vitamins may be lost in stool. Decreases disaccharidases in intestine. Lowers blood carotene concentration. Damages the intestinal walls.
Antimanic depression agents Lithium carbonate	Treatment for mental disorders	Blocks release of thyroid hormone, which can cause hypothyroidism with possible goiter. Strange, unpleasant taste sensation. May affect renal function and fluid and electrolyte balance.
Antimetabolites Cytarabine (Cytosar) 5-Fluorouracil 6-Mercaptopurine Methotrexate	Cancer chemotherapy	Most produce nausea, vomiting, and diarrhea. Also anorexia, megaloblastic anemia. Antagonist to pyrimidine. Also stomatitis, gastrointestinal ulceration and bleeding. Also stomatitis, fever. Antagonist to purine and pantothenic acid. Also stomatitis, anorexia, abnormal liver function, and gastrointestinal ulceration.
Antipsychotic drugs Butyrophenone Phenothiazines Thioxanthenes	Treatment of psychiatric problems	Weight gain, hyperglycemia, lactation, temperature irregularities, and paralytic ileus.
Appetite depressants Amphetamine* Fenfluramine	For losing weight	Decreased food intake results both in decreased caloric and essential nutrient intake.
Bulking agents Guar gum Methylcellulose	For losing weight	These substances take up fluid and swell in the intestine. There may be decreased caloric and essential nutrient intake.
Cardiovascular drugs Digitalis and its glycosides Quinidine Procainamide	Treatment of heart problems Increasing the force and velocity of cardiac contraction Treatment of antiarrhythmias	Most can produce anorexia, nausea, and vomiting.
Chelating agents Deferoxamine Penicillamine	Treatment of poisoning with heavy metals; sometimes used for other diseases such as arthritis and Wilson's disease	May also chelate essential minerals such as calcium and iodine.

*Authority to prescribe this stype of medication is now "limited."
†Clinical usage of these drugs is uncommon in the United States.

Continued on page 548

Table 24-1 (*continued*)

DRUG	CLINICAL USAGE	POSSIBLE DIRECT AND INDIRECT EFFECTS ON NUTRITIONAL STATUS
Diuretics	Removing excess water from body	
Benzothiadiazine		Diabetogenic; increased urinary excretion of potassium, hypokalemia.
Thiazide		
Diazoxide		
Furosemide (Lasix)		Increased urinary potassium, hypokalemia.
Ethacrynic acid		Increased urinary calcium, hypocalcemia.
Spironolactone		Hyperkalemia; decreased urinary excretion of potassium.
Triamterene		Hyperkalemia; hypocalcemia, possible folic acid deficiency.
Chlorothiazide		Increased urinary potassium, hypokalemia.
Hydrochlorothiazide		Decreased urinary calcium, hypercalcemia.
Thiazides		
Chlorthalidone		Increased urinary excretion of zinc.
Furosemide (Lasix)		
Herbal medicines	Multiple uses in some countries†	Diarrhea may cause loss of fluid and electrolyte. Presence of oxalic acid in plant parts may cause some essential mineral elements to precipitate. Some plant parts, when ingested, may cause hypoglycemia.
Hormones		
Insulin	Lowering blood glucose	Increases appetite.
Oral contraceptive pills (mestranol, conjugated estrogens, ethynyl estradiol)	Contraception	Multiple and profound effects on the nutritional status of a woman. May produce vitamin B_6, B_{12}, and folic acid deficiencies. Affects the body metabolism of protein, fat, carbohydrate, calcium, phosphorus, magnesium, and zinc. Effects of the new "low-dose" contraceptive pills are unknown.
Steroids (cortico-steroids such as cortisone and prednisone)	Multiple uses	Diabetogenic; growth retardation; muscle protein catabolism; adipose tissue deposition; electrolyte imbalances, hypernatremia, hypokalemia, hypocalcemia, fluid retention; potential osteoporosis; increased excretion of zinc and iodine; peptic ulcer.
Purgatives	Laxatives (cathartics)	
Mineral oil		May result in loss of fat-soluble nutrients in the stool.
Phenolphthalein		May interfere with the absorption of calcium and vitamins.
Miscellaneous		
Marijuana (either smoked or ingested)		May increase appetite.

*Authority to prescribe this type of medication is now "limited."
†Clinical usage of these drugs is uncommon in the United States.

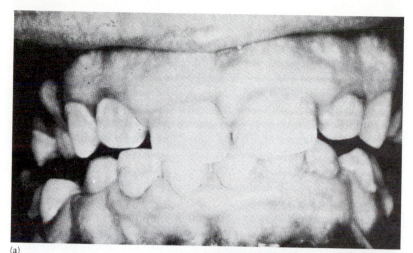
(a)

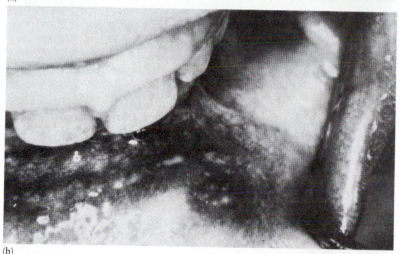
(b)

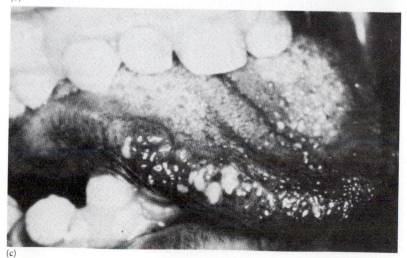
(c)

Figure 24-1: *Oral changes in a folic acid–deficient patient precipitated by anticonvulsant drug therapy. (a) Macrogingival pallor and gingival hyperplasia. (b) Ballooning and ulcerations of alveolar mucosa. (c) Ulcerative glossitis.*
SOURCE: *G. M. Stein and H. Lewis.* J. Peridontology 44 *(1973): 645.*

Nutritional Status Can Help or Harm

Nutritional imbalances are known to affect the metabolism of drugs. If the metabolic process fails, the substances may be toxic to the body. To handle a drug properly, the body requires many nutrients: niacin, riboflavin, pantothenic acid, ascorbic acid, folic acid, vitamin B_{12}, protein (amino acids), fat, glucose, iron, copper, calcium, zinc, and magnesium. If any nutrient is lacking, normal drug metabolism can be diminished. The toxicity of the drug may be increased or decreased by the metabolic alteration. In effect, the altered metabolism yields a change in the dosage's planned therapeutic effect, rendering the dosage either too high or too low under the circumstances. These consequences have been confirmed in animal studies and are presumed to hold true for humans as well (Hui; Spiller).

In humans, an extreme nutrient deficiency or an extreme nutrient excess can be expected to unbalance drug metabolism. For example, children in underdeveloped countries often have inadequate dietary protein and calories. Their malnourished bodies can affect drug metabolism in a unique fashion. When protein is lacking, manufacture of important enzymes involved in drug metabolism is reduced. For example, many protein-deficient children are infested with hookworms. The drug used to combat hookworms, tetrachloroethylene, is known to be toxic in high doses, yet undernourished children do not exhibit toxic effects when given large doses of the drug. It is thought that because of the depressed quality of the enzymes involved, the drug forms fewer of the usual toxic byproducts.

Disturbances of drug metabolism are all too likely when nutrition is unbalanced. In the case history of MaryLou, we saw that otherwise nontoxic levels of digitalis can become fatal if potassium is severely depleted. Similarly, the aged commonly have adverse reactions to many drugs, possibly because of deficiency of vitamin C, an important nutrient necessary for the normal process of drug metabolism.

Some Foods and Some Drugs Make Strange Bedfellows

A CHECKLIST FOR CAUTION

Certain foods and beverages are known to be incompatible with certain therapeutic drugs. These incompatible reactions occur as the result of certain pharmacologically active ingredients in the food, notably ethyl alcohol and various amines. These food ingredients especially react with drugs for treating psychiatric illness (monoamine oxidase inhibitors) and alcohol abuse (disulfiram). Table 24-2 summarizes the incompatible relationships. The case of cheese and tyramine illustrates the potential severity of food/drug incompatibility (Hui; Lamy; Spiller).

THE CASE OF CHEESE AND HEADACHE

Cheese and other foods contain the chemical tyramine (and its related amines; see Table 24-2). Drugs such as Marplan (phenelzine; see Table 24-2) are often prescribed for treating depression. Tyramine can react with phenelzine to create a "hypertensive crisis" in the patient. Reaction can occur within one-half to one hour of consuming the food if the drug was taken some time before eating. Extreme symptoms can include severe headache, brain stem hemorrhage, and even death.

Chemically, it appears that the drug raises blood levels of certain chemicals that help control our nervous system (for example, serotonin and norepinephrine). Such substances also reinforce the cardiovascular effects of tyramine. The severity of reaction depends on the drug dosage, amount of food ingested, patient susceptibility, and the interval between drug and food consumption.

The severity of the reaction can also be affected by the condition of the food. For example, when cheese matures, putrefaction from bacterial action yields a higher content of tyramine, which is produced from the amino acid tyrosine (see Chapter 7). Thus, cheeses with a strong flavor,

Table 24-2
Food/Drug Interactions: Some Examples

FOODS INVOLVED	PHARMA-COLOGICALLY ACTIVE INGREDIENTS	AFFECTED DRUGS		CLINICAL SYMPTOMS
		TYPE	THERAPY	
Major types:* cheese, Marmite (a hydrolyzed yeast product), chicken liver, pickled herring, meat extract (Bovril), broad beans, beer, wine	Phenylethylamine derivatives (pressor amines): tyramine, dopamine, and norepinephrine	Monoamine oxidase inhibitors, e.g., isocarboxazid, tranylcypromine, pargyline, phenelzine, nialamide, procarbazine	Treating depression	A marked rise in blood pressure and other cardiovascular changes; vomiting, nausea, headache, palpitations. Cerebral hemorrhage and death may result. Sometimes termed "hypertensive crisis."
Minor types:* canned figs, sour cream, aged meats, soy sauce, raisins, caffeine, chocolate				
Charcoal-broiled beef	Polycyclic hydrocarbon	Phenacetin	Analgesic	May increase degradation of drugs, thus decreasing their effectiveness.
Alcoholic beverages and any foods that use wine or other form of alcohol as a preparation ingredient, e.g., wine sauce or beef in wine.	Ethyl alcohol	Disulfiram (Antabuse)	Treating alcoholics	Low blood pressure, nausea, flushing, headache, vomiting, weakness, visual problems, convulsions
		Metronidazole (Flagyl)	Treating vaginitis from *Trichomonas vaginalis*	Same as above
		Sulfonylureas	Oral antihyperglycemic agents for diabetes	Headache, blurred or double vision, fine tremors, uncontrollable yawning, mental confusion and incoordination

*"Major types" refers to those foods that are more likely to cause the interaction; "minor types" are less likely because of either infrequent consumption or a low level of the active substances.

resulting from acidity and rancidity, and those aged a long time, have higher tyramine content. Cheddar cheeses rank high in tyramine content, followed by Roquefort, Camembert, and Stilton cheeses.

Use of the class of chemicals "monoamine oxidase inhibitors" (MOAs) in treating depression has declined, primarily because of hypertensive reactions. Some clinicians believe this to be an overreaction to a problem not fully understood. They point out that tyramine content varies from food sample to food sample, that MOA inhibitors help many patients, and that hypertensive reactions can be prevented.

Can Mother's Milk Be Bad for Babies?

For centuries, breast milk has been considered the perfect food for infants. But long-standing jokes about infants rejecting breast milk because the mother gorged on garlic, onion, or other strong foods are now gaining credence through clinical findings. Chemical ingredients in onions, garlic, and chocolate apparently produce an unpleasant reaction in nursing babies. A greater concern is that drugs can also appear in breast milk and affect nursing infants. Doctors are justifiably concerned about the possibility that therapeutic drugs and nondrug chemicals can make their way from mother to infant.

Several factors have contributed to the heightened concern in the medical community. First, breast-feeding has regained popularity and is steadily on the increase. Second, drug use is also on the increase. Numerous new drugs are available, and the number of over-the-counter (OTC) drugs has substantially increased. In addition, more women are taking oral contraceptives while nursing, and industrial and household chemicals have contaminated the environment. For example, pesticides have been found in breast milk.

No wonder the drugs that nursing mothers take and the chemicals they are exposed to have become important issues. Yet we know relatively little about the passage of chemicals from the mother's blood plasma via the milk to the infant. Mothers are understandably reluctant to allow experimental studies of chemical passage to their nursing infants, so most scientific literature on the subject relies on animal studies, which themselves are difficult to conduct.

WHEN DO DRUGS APPEAR IN BREAST MILK?

Evaluation of drug passage hinges on several factors. The amount appearing in the milk primarily depends on the type of drug consumed, the concentration of the drug, and the time elapsed between drug ingestion and breast-feeding. Contrary to popular belief, the quantity of milk secreted has little to do with the amount of the drug passing to breast milk. Method of drug administration does affect passage, since injected drugs appear faster than oral doses. The amount appearing in the milk may range from high to insignificant. For various reasons, the drug's presence may be harmless. For example, it may be nontoxic or ineffective, may be destroyed by the infant's system, or may not be absorbed by the infant. Certain drugs may be harmless unless they reach the infant in large quantities, whereas others may be harmful in small quantities.

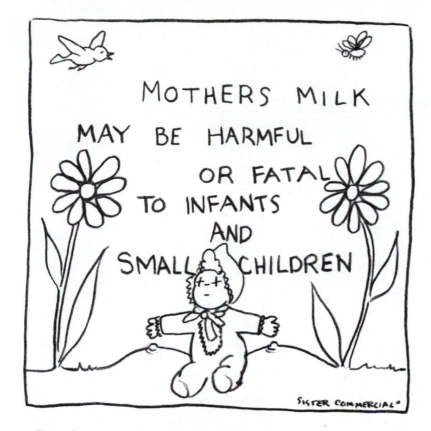

To make matters more complex, the same drug may be harmless or fatal. The difference in reaction varies: The infant's small size can heighten the drug's effectiveness, the infant's detoxification system may be immature, the drug may accumulate in the infant, or the infant may have hereditary problems that aggravate the drug's harmfulness.

For such reasons, physicians must be especially careful when prescribing drugs for a nursing mother. The physician must also determine whether the patient is using OTC drugs and whether environmental chemicals are inadvertently present. If the mother has a recognizable disease such as high blood pressure, edema, diabetes, and arthritis, she must be informed of the potential risk to the child. Of course, physicians can recommend interruption of breast-feeding if a drug that passes to breast milk must be used. Other professionals such as nurses, dietitians, and nutritionists should be equally familiar with the drugs that can pass to breast milk.

A REFERENCE CHART FOR A NURSING MOTHER
Table 24-3 relates various common drugs and chemicals to breast-feeding and lists possible reactions. The table also advises whether breast-feeding can be recommended in each case. The recommendation for most drugs is "monitoring needed." This means that both mother and doctor should be alert to the implications of taking the drug.

Table 24-3
Passage of Drugs and Chemicals into Breast Milk and Infant Reaction

DRUG	CLINICAL USAGE	SECRETED IN BREAST MILK			INFANT REACTION	BREAST-FEEDING OK?		
		YES	NO	MAYBE		YES	NO	MONITORING NEEDED*
Alcohol	Not used clinically but consumed individually	x			None†			x
Analgesics	Multiple uses							
Salicylates (aspirin)				x	None			x
Phenylbutazone			x		No information			x
Antibiotics	Destruction of pathological organisms							
Ampicillin		x			May cause diarrhea, candidiasis			x
Erythromycin		x			No information			x
Isoniazid	Antituberculosis	x			None			x
Metronidazole (Flagyl)	Antiprotozoal agent	x			May cause vomiting, loss of appetite, blood problems			x
Nalidixic acid		x			May cause hemolytic anemia if mother is uremic			x
Nitrofurantoin				x	None	x		
Oxacillin		x			None	x		
Penicillin		x			Usually no effects when taken in very small amount; may provoke antigenic response			x
Streptomycin		x			None if mother otherwise healthy; may cause ototoxicity if mother has renal failure			x
Sulfonamides				x	May cause neonatal jaundice, hemolytic anemia			x
Tetracycline		x			None			x
Anticancer agents	Treatment of cancer				Possibility of bone marrow depression			
Cyclophosphamide		x			No information			x
Methotrexate			x		No information			x

*As a precautionary measure, monitoring is recommended even if a drug is currently known not to be secreted in milk.
†Medical texts record one known case of mild intoxication of an infant breast-fed by a woman who had consumed a few glasses of wine (reported in 1936).

Table 24-3 (*continued*)

DRUG	CLINICAL USAGE	SECRETED IN BREAST MILK			INFANT REACTION	BREAST-FEEDING OK?		MONITORING NEEDED*
		YES	NO	MAYBE		YES	NO	
Anticoagulants	Preventing blood clotting							
Heparin			x		Destroyed in infant's intestinal system if ingested			x
Coumarins (some)		x			May cause hemorrhage			x
Pheninindione		x			Prothrombin time may increase; one case with postoperative hepatoma		x	
Warfarin		x			No information			x
Anticonvulsants	Sedatives and control of epilepsy				May reduce effectiveness of other therapeutic drugs			
Barbiturates				x	May cause depression of central nervous system			x
Phenytoin (Dilantin)		x			No information			x
Phenobarbitone		x			May develop methemoglobinemia if large dose			x
Antihistamines	Multiple uses	x			No information			x
Antihyperglycemic drugs	Used orally to lower blood glucose				Possible hypoglycemia			
Phenformin HCl (DBl)		x			No information			x
Tolbutamide (Orinase)		x			No information			x
Antihypertensives	Lowering blood pressure							
Propranolol		x			No information, although suspected to cause cardiovascular and hypoglycemic problems			x

*As a precautionary measure, monitoring is recommended even if a drug is currently known not to be secreted in milk.

†Medical texts record one known case of mild intoxication of an infant breast-fed by a woman who had consumed a few glasses of wine (reported in 1936).

Continued on page 556

Table 24-3 (*continued*)

DRUG	CLINICAL USAGE	SECRETED IN BREAST MILK			INFANT REACTION	BREAST-FEEDING OK?		
		YES	NO	MAYBE		YES	NO	MONI-TORING NEEDED*
Anti-inflammatory drugs	Treatment of arthritis							
Colchicine		x			No information			x
Antipsychotic drugs	Treatment of psychiatric problems							
Chloral hydrate		x			Sedation			x
Chlorpromazine				x	No information			x
Diazem		x			Sedation			x
Diazepam (Valium)		x			Weight loss, lethargy			x
Dichloralphenazone		x			Sedation			x
Lithium carbonate		x			No information, suspected to cause flaccid muscles			x
Propoxyphene HCl (Darvon)		x			No information			x
Cardiovascular drugs	Treatment of heart problems							
Reserpine		x			May produce galactorrhea in the mother, diarrhea, lethargy, and sucking difficulties such as respiratory blockage			x
Diuretics	Eliminating body water							
Cyclopenthiazide			x		No information			x
Furosemide			x		No information			x
Hydrochlorothiazide		x			No information			x
Environmental chemicals and related substances	Rare				May produce undesirable effects, depending on the substance			
Chlorobenzene		x			Multiple, extreme, adverse effects, e.g., coma, death			x
Chlorophenothane (DDT)		x			No information			x
Mercury		x			May produce adverse effects, e.g., nerve damage			x

*As a precautionary measure, monitoring is recommended even if a drug is currently known not to be secreted in milk.

†Medical texts record one known case of mild intoxication of an infant breast-fed by a woman who had consumed a few glasses of wine (reported in 1936).

Table 24-3 (*continued*)

DRUG	CLINICAL USAGE	SECRETED IN BREAST MILK: YES	SECRETED IN BREAST MILK: NO	SECRETED IN BREAST MILK: MAYBE	INFANT REACTION	BREAST-FEEDING OK?: YES	BREAST-FEEDING OK?: NO	BREAST-FEEDING OK?: MONITORING NEEDED*
Polychlorinated biphenyls		x			May produce adverse effects, e.g., discoloration of skin			x
Hormones and related substances	Multiple uses							
Insulin, adrenaline, corticotropin		x			Destroyed in infant's intestine	x		
Oral contraceptive pills	Contraception	x			Male infants may develop gynecomastia; female vaginal linings may proliferate; may decrease milk supply		x	
Thyroxine, corticosteroids			x		No information			x
Laxatives	Purgatives, cathartics							
Aloe		x			May be laxative			x
Anthraquinone derivatives		x			As above			x
Cascara		x			As above		x	
Phenolphthaleine (in nonprescription items)		x			No information			x
Rhubarb		x			No information			x
Senna		x			May cause diarrhea			x
Narcotics	Multiple uses							
Heroin		x			Addiction, withdrawal symptoms		x	
Methadone		x			None			x
Morphine, codeine		x			None			x
Miscellaneous	Variable							
Allergens (milk, fish, cheese)	None	x			Destroyed in infant's intestine	x		
Minerals	As supplement							
Iodide		x			May produce thyroid goiter and cancer if large dose			x

*As a precautionary measure, monitoring is recommended even if a drug is currently known not to be secreted in milk.

†Medical texts record one known case of mild intoxication of an infant breast-fed by a woman who had consumed a few glasses of wine (reported in 1936).

Continued on page 558

Table 24-3 (*continued*)

DRUG	CLINICAL USAGE	SECRETED IN BREAST MILK			INFANT REACTION	BREAST-FEEDING OK?		MONITORING NEEDED*
		YES	NO	MAYBE		YES	NO	
Fluoride		x			May mottle teeth if large dose			x
Nicotine (smoking)	None	x			No known immediate health hazard to infants if maternal smoking is less than 1½ packs of cigarettes a day; more than this may reduce milk supply and disrupt infant feeding schedule and response	x		
Radioactive materials, e.g., ^{125}I, ^{131}I	Thyroid diagnosis and therapy	x			May destroy infant thyroid	x		
Theophylline	Multiple uses	x			May cause irritability			x
Vitamins	As supplement							
D		x			May cause hypercalcemia if large dose			x
Carotene (A)		x			May cause yellowing of skin if large dose			x

*As a precautionary measure, monitoring is recommended even if a drug is currently known not to be secreted in milk.

†Medical texts record one known case of mild intoxication of an infant breast-fed by a woman who had consumed a few glasses of wine (reported in 1936).

Nutrition and "The Pill"

As mentioned earlier, the increased use of oral contraceptives, popularly known as "the Pill," places a new emphasis on this issue. Oral contraceptives are known to affect the metabolism of virtually all nutrients. Such effects are subject to the variables we have already examined, such as dosage, length of time used, prior nutritional status, nutrient intake, and individual susceptibility.

We know that serum albumin, a blood protein, may be reduced in those taking the pill. Blood fatty chemicals such as triglycerides, fatty acids, and cholesterol (see Chapter 6) have been found to increase. The pill can affect blood levels of certain amino acids.

The primary ingredient in oral contraceptives, estrogen, has been reported to cause increased calcium absorption. Because of this effect, and because less blood is lost when the menstrual period is regulated by the pill, iron requirement may be lowered in pill users, as can copper and zinc requirements.

Oral contraceptive effects on vitamins have been studied rather thoroughly. Lower levels of ascorbic acid, thiamine, riboflavin, and B_{12} have

Pamela's Pills
DO NOT AGREE WITH HER DIET

At age forty, Pamela decided to have a hysterectomy, and standard blood tests were ordered prior to her surgery. The laboratory results showed that her red blood cells were reduced in count and enlarged in size, confirming megaloblastic anemia. Because this clinical abnormality is related to various conditions, Pamela's surgery was postponed, and numerous other tests were performed to determine the cause of her anemia.

Pamela had been a vegetarian throughout her life. She had also taken oral contraceptives for eight years. Her only complaints

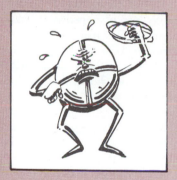

had been painful menstruation, fatigue, sudden weight loss, and ankle swelling—all of which had started in the six months prior to her decision to have a

hysterectomy. Tests showed that Pamela's plasma folic acid (a vitamin) level was low, and she was placed on 8 mg daily of the vitamin. One month later, the hysterectomy was performed without complications.

Pamela's condition was concluded to be the result of her vegetarian diet, which prevented a normal intake of folic acid, in addition to the action of her oral contraceptives, which further prevented the conversion of dietary folic acid (inactive) into the active vitamin her body needed.

SOURCE: J. D. Green. *South. Med. J.* 68: (1975): 249.

been found, but deficiency manifestations usually do not occur. Vitamin K need may be reduced, as may vitamin A need. Folic acid and vitamin B_6 have been cause for special concern.

Folic acid deficiency symptoms occur in a small number of women taking the pill. Often other factors, such as alcoholism, low dietary intake, and reduced absorption are also present to account for the vitamin lack. Some reports have indicated that abnormal changes in the cells lining the genitourinary tract could be related to inadequate levels of folic acid in pill users. Although it has not been determined whether oral contraceptives directly interfere with folic acid absorption, some clinicians recommend supplementation of folic acid.

It is now firmly established that oral contraceptives definitely result in a deficiency of vitamin B_6 in about 10 to 30 percent of pill users. The high incidence of headache and depression among these patients is now traced to a lack of this vitamin. Apparently, reduction of vitamin B_6 participation in body metabolism of brain chemicals indirectly causes the depression and headache.

Various efforts have been made to remedy the situation of adverse effects of the pill on the patient's nutritional status. Including vitamins and minerals in the pill has been suggested. Regular blood and urine checking for the levels of vitamins and minerals is another alternative. However, medical politics, clinical philosophies, technical uncertainties, and other factors have prevented any major health policy from being adopted.

Marijuana and Nutrition

Because more people are using it and clinicians are interested in its potential pharmacological applications, marijuana has become a subject of nutritional study. Long-term clinical trials have not occurred, but the abiding scientific view is that marijuana is an unsafe collection of chemical compounds. Despite that overall view, certain medical possibilities have been confirmed, and certain effects on general nutrition have been determined (Green; Hollister).

Historically, marijuana has been used in such countries as Vietnam, Cambodia, China, and India for various treatments ranging from hair loss to loss of appetite. Primarily it has served as a masking agent, providing relief from such discomfort as toothache, menstrual pain, and other types of severe pain. Numerous studies are underway in the United States, and potential benefits for therapeutic use appear in three areas.

Tests have shown that synthetic THC, the most active ingredient in marijuana, reduces eye pressure associated with glaucoma. It has reduced muscle spasms associated with multiple sclerosis and cerebral palsy. More related to nutrition, it has shown promising results in relieving nausea, vomiting, and loss of appetite in cancer patients undergoing chemotherapy.

Marijuana's effect on appetite has been established; it increases hunger, especially for sweets. There are, however, some qualifications in regard to this finding. Because so many people believe marijuana increases hunger and appetite, test subjects may be biased. It has also been noted that the use of marijuana often involves social settings where food ingestion can be stimulated by peer pressure. Because of such variables, few researchers make unqualified claims regarding marijuana's effect on hunger and appetite.

An Ounce of Prevention

Both preventive and corrective measures are needed to ensure that therapeutic drug use will not harm a patient's nutritional status. More clinical studies are needed, as are long-range programs, since the complexities regarding the relationship between drugs and nutrition require careful study. Further study is especially needed among populations who take drugs for long periods; for example, women taking oral contraceptives and older Americans need further study.

Practicing physicians are encouraged to be familiar with drug-nutrition relationships. They are also encouraged to be at the forefront of efforts to reduce drug-induced malnutrition. Such efforts include legislation to bring certain nonprescription drugs under tighter control, constraints on excessive use of prescription drugs, and educational efforts. Although nurses, nutritionists, dietitians, and other allied health professionals do not prescribe drugs, their concerned participation in these efforts is obviously important.

STUDY QUESTIONS

1. Discuss at least five ways in which drugs may alter the amount of nutrients actually available for use by the body. Give examples of specific drugs that may have these effects.

2. Why is it important to monitor the foods or liquids taken with drugs? Give two examples.

3. What factors could render drugs passing into breast milk harmless to the nursing baby? What factors could exaggerate their effects?

4. Discuss the relationship between cheese and headache.

5. Name the nutrients most likely affected by oral contraceptive pills.

6. Give at least five examples of drugs thought to reach infants through breast milk and their possible effects on the baby. What precautions should be taken to minimize dangers of infant reaction to chemicals in breast milk?

REFERENCES

Green, J. "Marijuana: Hints of Medicinal Value." *FDA Consumer* 13 (March 1979): 19.

Hollister, L. E. "Hunger and Appetite After Single Doses of Marijuana, Alcohol, and Dextroamphetamine." *Clin. Pharm. Therap.* 23 (1971): 44.

Hui, Y. H. *Human Nutrition and Diet Therapy.* Monterey, Calif.: Wadsworth Health Sciences, 1983.

Lamy, P. P. "How Your Patient's Diet Can Affect Drug Response." *Drug Therapy* 10 (1980): 82.

Spiller, G. A., ed. "Nutritional Pharmacology." In *Current Topics in Nutrition and Disease*, Vol 4. New York: Alan R. Liss, 1981.

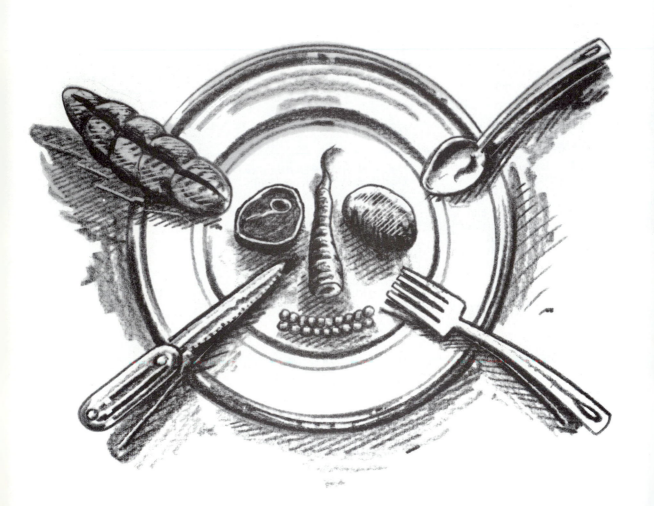

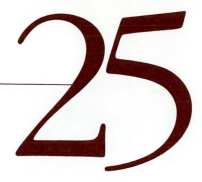

FOOD SAFETY:

ARE FOOD CHEMICALS SAFE?

NIACIN POISONING FROM BAGELS

On April 27, 1983, 14 of 69 persons attending a brunch had acute onset of rash, pruritis, and sensation of warmth. The illness was of relatively short duration, with an incubation period of approximately 30 minutes after consumption of one or more of the pumpernickel bagels served at the brunch.

Because the bagels were uncharacteristically light in color, ingredients were suspected and investigated. The local factory that produced the bagels had attempted to enrich the pumpernickel flour by adding niacin (see Chapter 9). A large quantity of the B vitamin had been added, apparently from an improperly labeled container. Laboratory studies revealed 60 times the normal level of niacin in the pumpernickel flour—each bagel contained approximately 190 mg (the RDA for niacin is

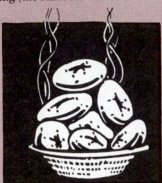

6.6 mg/1000 calories or about 13 mg/day for the average adult). Measures were taken to assure proper labeling of all ingredient containers in the bagel factory.

Ingestion of excessive amounts of niacin (nicotinic acid) all at once can produce an acute syndrome of cutaneous vasodilation of the face and trunk, itching, and sensation of heat. Gastrointestinal distress has also been noted. Although alarming, these symptoms usually resolve spontaneously over several hours without sequelae. Outbreaks of this syndrome have previously been reported in association with inappropriate use of food additives or with mislabeled food containers. The unusual color of the implicated food was also noted in these outbreaks. (See *Morbidity and Mortality Weekly Report*, June 17, 1983.)

Types of Food Hazards

According to Dr. V. O. Wodicka, former head of the Bureau of Foods of the Food and Drug Administration (FDA), the risks posed to us by our food supply and our ways of eating are, in decreasing order of severity: (1) microbiological hazards, (2) nutritional hazards, (3) environmental pollutants, (4) natural toxicants, (5) pesticide residues, and (6) food additives.

Dr. Wodicka's priorities are based on four important premises. First, a hazard must be scientifically measurable and applicable to humans. Second, a hazard from a high-risk source is assumed to occur more frequently than that of a low-risk one. Third, a high-risk hazard is one that has been clinically documented to hurt more people than a low-risk one. Fourth, it is assumed that the usage of any food chemicals complies with *all* legally applicable regulations.

Microbiological hazards are the most dangerous for the safety of our food supply and will be our first discussion topic. In brief, when people eat a food product containing a harmful number of bacteria or harmful amount of bacterial toxin, they become ill. There may be vomiting, abdominal cramps, vision trouble, and even death, all of which are clinically measurable. Food poisoning has harmed many people, and hardly a day goes by without someone in this country suffering from it.

As discussed throughout this book, there are many documented nutritional hazards. For example, many alcoholics do not eat the right quantity and quality of food and may suffer severe nutritional imbalances and hazards. A middle-aged person who eats a large amount of salt may be predisposed to high blood pressure. Although these hazards occur frequently, their clinical manifestations are not so acute and severe as microbiological hazards, which can pose immediate danger.

Although environmental pollution is widespread, situations that severely endanger health are uncommon. Many instances of environmental contamination started years ago; such instances are expected to occur less frequently in the future because of tighter federal regulations. However, two notorious instances of accidental environmental pollution have involved human foods. One was the well-publicized mercury contamination of seafood that resulted in the poisoning of many Japanese villagers in the 1950s. In this instance a chemical firm dumped large quantities of mercury into a nearby river from which many of the victims and their families fished.

The accidental contamination of animal feeds with the fire retardant polybrominated biphenyl in Michigan during the early 1970s forced the government to destroy contaminated milk cows, cattle, beef, poultry, eggs, cheese, and milk. The risk to human health of this incident is still unknown.

The fourth most dangerous hazard in the food supply is natural toxicants. Probably all of us have heard of wild mushroom poisoning. Pesticide residues and food additives rank the lowest on the hazard list because, when used in accordance with federal regulations, they have not produced any adverse clinical effects that are *measurable*. Documented cases of poisoning due to food additives are so far the result of noncompliance with federal regulations.

In this chapter we will cite various documented cases of food hazards (biological, chemical, and so forth), but you should always remember that the cases cited can occur tomorrow, even if the precise example we use is from last year, or ten years ago.

Bacteria and the Like

Spoiled food may cause illness. The contamination usually results from bacteria introduced during preparation, serving, or storage. Since the illness is limited to individuals rather than a large number of families or households, it is not epidemic. In general, illness from eating spoiled food is usually moderate and may occasionally be mild. Each of us during our lifetimes will probably suffer from food contamination to some degree (Gilchrist).

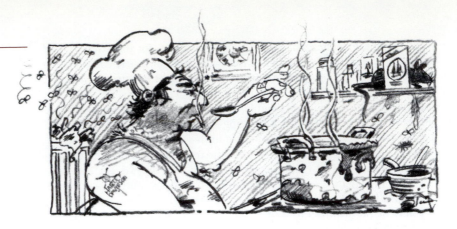

FOOD POISONING

Food poisoning by biological agents may cause abdominal pain, diarrhea, nausea, vomiting, and general discomfort and malaise. Severe symptoms are fever and nervous disorders. The instability of vital signs (pulse and respiration), tiredness, and dehydration suffered by the victim are due mainly to a loss of fluid and electrolytes (minerals). Individuals who are most susceptible to moderate and severe reactions are the sick, the very young, and the elderly. Most adults can tolerate the discomfort and intestinal upset of food poisoning.

Food poisoning by biological agents is classified into two types. *Food-borne infection* results from the consumption of food containing a large number of live bacteria capable of producing enough toxin in the intestine to poison the host. Incubation for this type of poisoning is about 36 to 48 hours. *Food-borne intoxication* results from the consumption of a food in which the pathogenic bacteria have already released the toxin capable of poisoning the host. The incubation period for this type of poisoning is about 1 to 12 hours.

The growth of bacteria is determined by the type of food, the presence or absence of oxygen, moisture content, acidity or alkalinity, time, and temperature. However, given sufficient time, bacteria can frequently adapt to all types of foods and all conditions of moisture, acidity, oxygen, and temperature; in fact, most bacteria can adapt to a new environment within about 4 hours and start multiplying thereafter. For this reason, foods should not be left at room temperature for more than 4 hours. Figure 25-1 presents a temperature guide to food safety.

SANITATION IN COOKING

To avoid food poisoning, personal hygiene is very important. Hands should always be clean whenever food is handled. Hot water and soap should be used to wash hands after going to the bathroom, and hands should also be washed before handling cooked foods, and after handling raw foods. A person who is ill should not prepare food. During food preparation, contact between hands and the mouth, nose, or hair should be avoided, as should coughing and sneezing over foods. Tissues or handkerchiefs should be used to prevent contamination. Food tasting

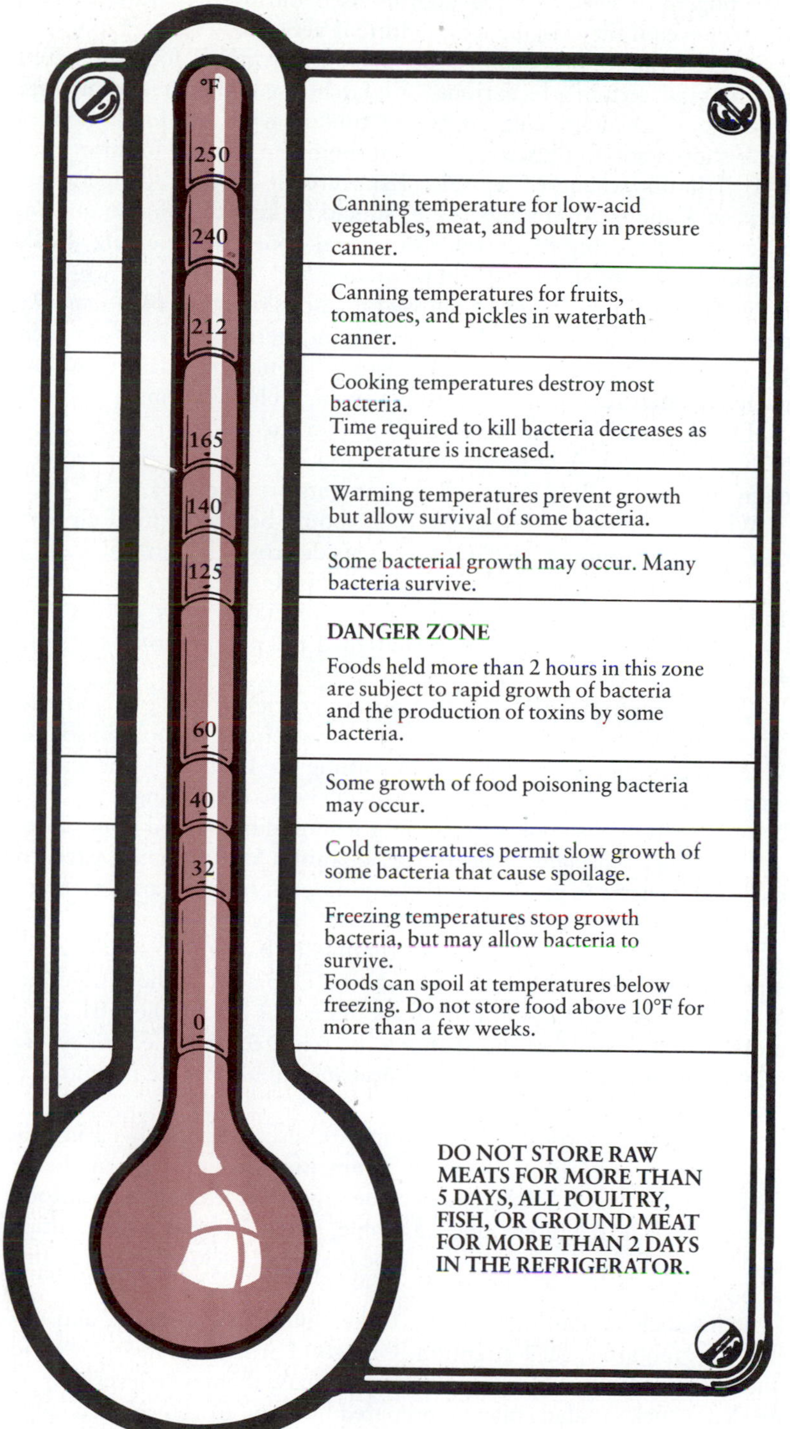

°F

250

240 — Canning temperature for low-acid vegetables, meat, and poultry in pressure canner.

212 — Canning temperatures for fruits, tomatoes, and pickles in waterbath canner.

165 — Cooking temperatures destroy most bacteria.
Time required to kill bacteria decreases as temperature is increased.

140 — Warming temperatures prevent growth but allow survival of some bacteria.

125 — Some bacterial growth may occur. Many bacteria survive.

DANGER ZONE

Foods held more than 2 hours in this zone are subject to rapid growth of bacteria and the production of toxins by some bacteria.

60 — Some growth of food poisoning bacteria may occur.

40 — Cold temperatures permit slow growth of some bacteria that cause spoilage.

32 — Freezing temperatures stop growth bacteria, but may allow bacteria to survive.
Foods can spoil at temperatures below freezing. Do not store food above 10°F for more than a few weeks.

0

DO NOT STORE RAW MEATS FOR MORE THAN 5 DAYS, ALL POULTRY, FISH, OR GROUND MEAT FOR MORE THAN 2 DAYS IN THE REFRIGERATOR.

Figure 25-1: *Temperature guide to food safety. Distributed by the U.S. Department of Agriculture.*

with fingers or with cooking utensils used during preparation is not advised, even if the cooking temperature is very hot.

In addition to practicing good personal hygiene, food preparers should take certain precautions. All kitchen equipment and utensils should be thoroughly cleaned before contact with any food. Cooked foods should not be allowed to stand at room temperature for more than 2 to 3 hours whenever feasible. Exposure of food to temperatures between 5 and 60°C (40 and 140°F) should be kept to a minimum. The practice of preparing foods a day or several hours before eating should be done with care and avoided if possible.

Hot foods should never be allowed to cool slowly to room temperature before refrigerating. The slow cooling period provides an ideal growth temperature for bacteria. Foods should be refrigerated immediately after removing them from a steam table or warming oven. To cool foods rapidly for storage, a shallow pan, cold running water, or ice bath can be used. A large amount of food in a big container requires many hours of cooling before all the contents are below 75°C (45°F).

When leftovers are served, the food should be heated until all parts reach a temperature of 74°C (165°F). This destroys all *vegetable cells of bacteria*. Whenever possible, food should be chopped into small pieces and boiled to destroy any susceptible vegetable cells of the bacteria. No cooling should be permitted after preparation—the food should be served hot.

Certain popular foods—stuffed turkey, gravies, cream pies and puddings, sandwiches, and salads—are frequent culprits in food poisoning. When preparing roast turkey, avoid stuffing the bird; cook the stuffing separately. If turkey is stuffed with raw fillers, avoid stuffing it the night before. If stuffing is cooked separately, it should be cooked immediately after mixing, especially if in a large quantity. Stuffing is an excellent place for bacteria to grow, and if a large amount of lukewarm stuffing is permitted to stand at room temperature, the organisms will multiply.

Gravies and broths are quite susceptible to bacterial contamination, especially as leftovers. These foods should be placed in the refrigerator as soon as possible. Gravy or broth should not be held in the refrigerator more than 1 or 2 days, and it should be reheated or boiled for several minutes before serving. A reheated dressing should not be permitted to stay at room temperature.

Cream pies, pastries, and puddings are also often involved in food poisoning. People dislike keeping cream pies and pastries in the refrigerator, because the crust can become soggy. But leaving them at room temperature is definitely not advisable, since bacteria will multiply rapidly. Ideally, such pastries should be prepared as close to serving time as possible.

Items such as ham sandwiches, turkey and chicken salads, and deviled eggs require special attention. One good practice is to freeze sandwiches immediately after preparation and thaw them whenever they are needed. Chicken salads may be prepared by using frozen chicken cubes, which will thaw as the salad stands; the entire salad dish should be kept cool.

For reference purposes, Table 25-1 presents some known food-borne diseases, including the causative organisms, symptoms, and preventive methods. Every household should have such a chart handy—just in case.

Table 25-1
Characteristics of Different Food-Borne Diseases

DISEASE AND ORGANISM THAT CAUSES IT	SOURCE OF ILLNESS	SYMPTOMS	PREVENTION METHODS
Salmonellosis *Salmonella* (bacteria; more than 1,700 kinds)	May be found in raw meats, poultry, eggs, fish, milk, and products made with them. Multiplies rapidly at room temperature.	Onset: 12–48 hours after eating. Nausea, fever, headache, abdominal cramps, diarrhea, and sometimes vomiting. Can be fatal in infants, the elderly, and the infirm.	Handling food in a sanitary manner Thorough cooking of foods Prompt and proper refrigeration of foods
Staphylococcal food poisoning Staphylococcal enterotoxin (produced by *Staphylococcus aureus* bacteria)	The toxin is produced when food contaminated with the bacteria is left too long at room temperature. Meats, poultry, egg products; tuna, potato, and macaroni salads; and cream-filled pastries are good environments for these bacteria to produce toxin.	Onset: 1–8 hours after eating. Diarrhea, vomiting, nausea, abdominal cramps, and prostration. Mimics flu. Lasts 24–28 hours. Rarely fatal.	Sanitary food handling practices Prompt and proper refrigeration of foods
Botulism Botulinum toxin (produced by *Clostridium botulinum* bacteria)	Bacteria are widespread in the environment. However, bacteria produce toxin only in an anaerobic (oxygenless) environment of little acidity. Types A, B, and F may result from inadequate processing of low-acid canned foods, such as green beans, mushrooms, spinach, olives, and beef. Type E normally occurs in fish.	Onset: 8–36 hours after eating. Neurotoxic symptoms, including double vision, inability to swallow, speech difficulty, and progressive paralysis of the respiratory system. **Obtain medical help immediately. Botulism can be fatal.**	Using proper methods for canning low-acid foods Avoidance of commercially canned low-acid foods with leaky seals or with bent, bulging or broken cans Toxin can be destroyed after a can is opened by boiling contents hard for 10 minutes—**not recommended**
Perfringens food poisoning *Clostridium perfringens* (rod-shaped bacteria)	Bacteria are widespread in environment. Generally found in meat and poultry and dishes made with them. Multiply rapidly when foods are left at room temperature too long. Destroyed by cooking.	Onset: 8–22 hours after eating (usually 12). Abdominal pain and diarrhea. Sometimes nausea and vomiting. Symptoms last a day or less and are usually mild. Can be more serious in older or debilitated people.	Sanitary handling of foods, especially meat and meat dishes and gravies Thorough cooking of foods Prompt and proper refrigeration
Shigellosis (bacillary dysentery) *Shigella* (bacteria)	Food becomes contaminated when a human carrier with poor sanitary habits handles liquid or moist food that is then not cooked thoroughly. Organisms multiply in food stored above room temperature. Found in milk and dairy products, poultry, and potato salad.	Onset: 1–7 days after eating. Abdominal pain, cramps, diarrhea, fever, sometimes vomiting, and blood, pus, or mucus in stools. Can be serious in infants, the elderly or debilitated people.	Handling food in a sanitary manner Proper sewage disposal Proper refrigeration of foods

Continued on page 570

Table 25-1 (*continued*)

DISEASE AND ORGANISM THAT CAUSES IT	SOURCE OF ILLNESS	SYMPTOMS	PREVENTION METHODS
Campylobacteriosis *Campylobacter jejuni* (rod-shaped bacteria)	Bacteria found on poultry, cattle, and sheep and can contaminate the meat and milk of these animals. Chief food sources: raw poultry and meat and unpasteurized milk.	Onset: 2–5 days after eating. Diarrhea, abdominal cramping, fever, and sometimes bloody stools. Lasts 2–7 days.	Thorough cooking of foods Handling food in a sanitary manner Avoiding unpasteurized milk
Gastroenteritis *Yersinia enterocolitica* (nonspore-forming bacteria)	Ubiquitous in nature; carried in food and water. Bacteria multiply rapidly at room temperature, *as well as* at refrigerator temperatures (4° to 9° C). Generally found in raw vegetables, meats, water, and unpasteurized milk.	Onset: 2–5 days after eating. Fever, headache, nausea, diarrhea, and general malaise. Mimics flu. An important cause of gastroenteritis in children. Can also infect other age groups and, if not treated, can lead to more serious diseases (such as lymphadenitis, arthritis, and Reiter's syndrome).	Thorough cooking of foods Sanitizing cutting instruments and cutting boards before preparing foods that are eaten raw Avoidance of unpasteurized milk and unchlorinated water
Cereus food poisoning *Bacillus cereus* (bacteria and possibly their toxin)	Illness may be caused by the bacteria, which are widespread in the environment, or by an enterotoxin created by the bacteria. Found in raw foods. Bacteria multiply rapidly in foods stored at room temperature.	Onset: 1–18 hours after eating. Two types of illness: (1) abdominal pain and diarrhea, and (2) nausea and vomiting. Lasts less than a day.	Sanitary handling of foods Thorough cooking of foods Prompt and adequate refrigeration
Cholera *Vibrio cholera* (bacteria)	Found in fish and shellfish harvested from waters contaminated by human sewage. (Bacteria may also occur naturally in Gulf Coast waters.) Chief food sources: seafood, especially types eaten raw (such as oysters).	Onset: 1–3 days. Can range from "subclinical" (a mild uncomplicated bout with diarrhea) to fatal (intense diarrhea with dehydration). Severe cases require hospitalization.	Sanitary handling of foods Thorough cooking of seafood
Parahaemolyticus food poisoning *Vibrio parahaemolyticus* (bacteria)	Organism lives in salt water and can contaminate fish and shellfish. Thrives in warm weather.	Onset: 15–24 hours after eating. Abdominal pain, nausea, vomiting, and diarrhea. Sometimes fever, headache, chills, and mucus and blood in the stools. Lasts 1—2 days. Rarely fatal.	Sanitary handling of foods Thorough cooking of seafood
Gastrointestinal disease Enteroviruses, rotaviruses, parvoviruses	Viruses exist in the intestinal tract of humans and are expelled in feces. Contamination of foods can occur in three ways: (1) when sewage is used to enrich garden/farm soil, (2) by direct hand-to-food contact during the preparation of meals, and (3) when shellfish-growing waters are contaminated by sewage.	Onset: After 24 hours. Severe diarrhea, nausea, and vomiting. Respiratory symptoms. Usually lasts 4–5 days but may last for weeks.	Sanitary handling of foods Use of pure drinking water Adequate sewage disposal Adequate cooking of foods

Table 25-1 (*continued*)

DISEASE AND ORGANISM THAT CAUSES IT	SOURCE OF ILLNESS	SYMPTOMS	PREVENTION METHODS
Hepatitis Hepatitis A virus	Chief food sources: shellfish harvested from contaminated areas, and foods that are handled a lot during preparation and then eaten raw (such as vegetables).	Jaundice, fatigue. May cause liver damage and death.	Sanitary handling of foods Use of pure drinking water Adequate sewage disposal Adequate cooking of foods
Mycotoxicosis Mycotoxins (from molds)	Produced in foods that are relatively high in moisture. Chief food sources: beans and grains that have been stored in a moist place.	May cause liver and/or kidney disease.	Checking foods for visible mold and discarding those that are contaminated Proper storage of susceptible foods
Giardiasis *Giardia lamblia* (flagellated protozoa)	Protozoa exist in the intestinal tract of humans and are expelled in feces. Contamination of foods can occur in two ways: (1) when sewage is used to enrich garden/farm soil, and (2) by direct hand-to-food contact during the preparation of meals. Chief food sources: foods that are handled a lot during preparation.	Diarrhea, abdominal pain, flatulence, abdominal distention, nutritional disturbances, "nervous" symptoms, anorexia, nausea, and vomiting.	Sanitary handling of foods Avoidance of raw fruits and vegetables in areas where the protozoa is endemic Proper sewage disposal
Amebiasis *Entamoeba histolytica* (amoebic protozoa)		Tenderness over the colon or liver, loose morning stools, recurrent diarrhea, change in bowel habits, "nervous" symptoms, loss of weight and fatigue. Anemia may be present.	Sanitary handling of foods Avoidance of raw fruits and vegetables in areas where the protozoa is endemic Proper sewage disposal

SOURCE: C. L. Ballentine and M. L. Herndon, *FDA Consumer*, July–August 1982, pp. 25–28.

BOTULISM, DESPITE THE USE OF A PRESSURE COOKER
On November 7, 1982, a Humboldt County, California family of four ate a noon meal of lasagna containing home-canned swiss chard. The same evening the 32-year-old mother in the family became ill with nausea, vomiting, diarrhea, double vision, and headache. She was seen briefly at a local hospital emergency room on November 8, and on November 9 she was admitted to another local hospital with progressive weakness. She had fever and pneumonia on x-ray, but weakness and respiratory failure seemed out of proportion to her pneumonia. Short-

ness of breath progressed to frank respiratory failure. She was transferred on the evening of November 10 to a larger community hospital.

Between November 7 and 12 her 34-year-old husband, 10-year-old daughter, and 5-year-old son had onset of similar but milder neurologic illness. When these additional cases came to medical attention on November 11, the diagnosis of botulism was entertained for the first time. After treatment with antitoxin, all recovered.

The family lived in a trailer in a rural area. The mother had home canned produce for years without incident (about 500 jars a year) and regularly used a pressure cooker for low-acid vegetables. The mother had noted that the swiss chard for the meal had had a peculiar taste. She put most of it in the center of the baking dish; she had eaten mostly from the center; and her daughter—who dislikes greens and was least affected—had selected portions from the sides of the baking dish. The lasagna was baked at 350°F for just 30 minutes.

The mother "followed the book" in home canning: she used a pressure cooker and followed recommendations of the manufacturer whose jars she used. Tests at the county health department laboratory showed that the pressure cooker operated satisfactorily. However, authorities disagree on whether greens such as spinach, swiss chard, and beet greens should ever be home canned.

Both the mother's canning brochure *and* the USDA (in the Home and Garden Bulletin, No. 8, "slightly revised" June 1977) approve the home canning of greens, but with one big difference: her brochure called for heating quart jars in a pressure cooker for 70 minutes, whereas the USDA recommended 90 minutes. In contrast, the University of California, Davis, in its leaflet (#2270) *Home Canning of Vegetables*, revised May 1976, reports that "home canning (of greens) is not recommended." Presumably, the reason for the university's position relates to heavy soil contamination of these particular vegetables and the fact that many layers of greens, packed tight, could resist heat penetration. The ultimate safety factor for home-canned vegetables is that, after opening jars, the contents should be brought to a boil over direct heat, the clumps broken up, and the food simmered at least 10 minutes (at sea level to 3,000 feet) *before* such food is used. (The lasagna, evidently, did *not* get hot enough.) Also, evidence of improper home canning at the family's premises included a few half-filled jars, rusted and deformed screw bands, and improper seals. Except for jams and jellies, virtually all home-canned products were confiscated and disposed of by the county health department. (See *Morbidity and Mortality Weekly Report*, Jan. 28, 1983.)

DRINKING RAW MILK

During May 1983, two outbreaks of gastrointestinal illness following consumption of raw milk occurred in Pennsylvania. A total of 57 people became ill.

The first outbreak occurred following a visit by 60 first-grade students and three teachers to a dairy farm in south-central Pennsylvania. Symptoms included fever, abdominal pain, vomiting, diarrhea, headache, and bloody stools. Onset of illness ranged from 1 to 8 days. Illness lasted from 5 hours to 12 days. Cookies and small cups of raw milk were served at the farm.

The second outbreak occurred on May 20 when 43 kindergarten children and two teachers visited a dairy farm in central Pennsylvania. Raw milk and cookies were also served at the second farm.

Illness was associated with the quantity of milk consumed, not with eating cookies or touching farm animals.

Raw milk is an important vehicle in the transmission of the harmful bacteria *Campylobacter*. In 1981 and 1982, five of ten and six of eleven food-borne *Campylobacter* outbreaks reported to the Centers for Disease Control were traced to raw milk consumption. Outbreaks of campylobacteriosis have followed consumption of raw milk on school-sponsored trips in Michigan, Minnesota, and Vermont; a field trip in Maryland resulted in an outbreak of salmonellosis and campylobacteriosis. These, and similar occurrences in England, point out the necessity of protecting schoolchildren from exposure to unpasteurized dairy products while on outings. (See *Morbidity and Mortality Weekly Report*, July 8, 1983.)

Natural Food Toxicants: You Can't Always Trust Mother Nature

Poisoning by natural toxicants in food is not common in the United States, although it is in underdeveloped countries. Table 25-2 summarizes the characteristics of some common natural food toxicants. The following sections provide brief discussions of plant toxins and fish poisoning (Ory).

YOU'VE HEARD ABOUT POISONOUS MUSHROOMS

Many edible plants contain natural toxic substances. Mushroom poisoning is well known. When deaths from eating mushrooms have occurred in the United States, the victims were usually amateur collectors who ate either *Gyromitra esculenta* or *Amanita* species. Preventing mushroom poisoning is still very difficult because, despite all the literature on mushroom identification, classifying these fungi is still a problem.

Different individuals have highly variable responses to mushroom toxicity. Some people are very susceptible; others are not. Also, a person can become accustomed, or "conditioned," to mushroom poisoning.

In the United States, the major toxic mushrooms are *Amanita phalloides* and *A. muscaria*, whose toxins are cyclopeptides and alkaloid-like compounds, respectively. *A. phalloides* have been responsible for the most serious mushroom intoxication, and the antidote currently available is not 100 percent effective.

In *A. phalloides* poisoning, the victim suffers diarrhea, vomiting, abdominal pain, and intense thirst. The victim often screams from the intense pain, although the pain occasionally subsides. If a large quantity of the mushroom is eaten, the victim rapidly weakens and may die within 48 hours. If poisoning is less severe, cold skin, jaundice, and cyanosis develop in 2 or 3 days, and the patient may die 6 to 8 days after

Table 25-2
Natural Toxicants in Food

TOXICANT	FOOD SOURCE	EFFECTS	DESTROYED BY HEAT		
			YES	NO	UNKNOWN
Antitrypsin	Soybeans, lima beans	Destroys trypsin in digestive tract	x		
Aglycone of methylazoxy-methanol-β-glucoside	Cycad	Unknown			x
Ascorbic acid oxidase	Vegetables, fruits	Destroys vitamin C	x		
Avidin	Egg white	Antagonizes biotin	x		
Goitrogen	Cabbage, rutabagas	Goiter	x		
Hemagglutinins	Soybeans, lima beans	Retards animal growth	x		
Lipoxidase	Soybeans, lima beans	Destroys vitamin A	x		
Mushroom toxins	Mushrooms	Many		x	
Oxalic acid	Rhubarb, spinach	Binds calcium and zinc		x	
Phytic acid	Oatmeal	Binds calcium and iron		x	
(β-N-oxal)-amino-1alamine*	Vetches (lathyrus plants)	Lathyrism		x	
Solanine	Immature or sprouting potatoes	Vomiting, diarrhea		x	
Sterculic acid	Cottonseed oil	Interference with digestion and reproduction	x		
Thiaminase	Fern, fish, clams	Antagonizes thiamine	x		
Unknown	Fava or broad beans	Favism		x	

*This is one suspected toxin. The exact chemical compound responsible for human poisoning is still unknown.

eating the poison if there is no medical attention. Coma and convulsion may precede death. Autopsy of the victim usually shows a fatty liver with necrosis, kidney degeneration, and hemorrhage of some organs.

SPINACH: WAS POPEYE WRONG?
Many common vegetables—rhubarb, spinach, Swiss chard, beet tops, lamb's-quarters, purslane, and poke—contain **oxalic acid** (also see Chapter 12). The oxalates exist as insoluble calcium oxalate crystals, which can be observed in the leaves under a microscope. They can decrease calcium absorption from foods, thus rendering calcium—which occurs in spinach, for example—unavailable. Rhubarb leaves contain three to four times as much oxalic acid as the stalks. Acute oxalic acid poisoning occurs in children who have eaten the raw leaves and stalks of rhubarb. These children develop gastroenteritis with abdominal pain, vomiting, and diarrhea. If the poisoning is severe, there can be convulsions, failure of the blood to clot, and coma. Since a number of house plants contain oxalic acid, care is needed to prevent children from

accidently ingesting them. Sheep poisoning by oxalic acid is not uncommon, since the coarse plants found on their ranges contain about 35 to 40 percent oxalic acid by dry weight.

Though bracken fern has been listed as a natural food available in the wild, cooking and eating the fiddlehead-shaped fronds has been linked with stomach cancer in Japan. Fresh, canned, and cooked bracken fern have been linked with cancer of the gastrointestinal tract and with cancer of the bladder. Tests indicate that metabolic conversion of bracken fern results in a carcinogenic metabolite. Since the fern occurs worldwide in pine woodlands and since its use occurs in many recipes, the potential danger is significant.

POISON IVY FROM CASHEW NUTS?

During April 1982, a poison ivy–like dermatitis (skin irritation) affected 54 persons who consumed cashew nut pieces sold by a Little League organization in a south-central Pennsylvania community. The cashew pieces, sold in 7-oz bags, were imported from Mozambique and processed for distribution by a Pittsburgh company. The league had purchased the bags of cashew nuts from a local distributor.

About 20 percent of those who ate cashews developed pruritic (itching) rash of the extremities, trunk, groin, and buttocks. Some who were affected reported blistering of the mouth. None of those who did not eat cashews developed rash.

Local, state, and federal food inspectors reported no obvious violations in manufacturing plants that had processed the cashews.

The cashew tree, *Anacardium occidentale*, belongs to the same family of plants (Anacardiaceae) as the *Rhus* species, which can cause poison ivy, poison oak, and poison sumac. This tree bears a pear-shaped fruit called the cashew apple. On one end of the fruit is the cashew nut, which is not encased in the pulp of the fruit. It is composed of an inner kernel and a double-layered outer shell. Between the layers of shell is an oil containing 12 chemically distinct antigens, including cardol and anacardic acid, which are immunochemically related to certain oils found in the *Rhus* species. These oils have irritant and allergenic properties. Cashew nuts are partially processed to remove shells and oil before importation into the United States, and then they are cooked and packaged before distribution.

This report documents what may be the largest outbreak of cashew nut-related dermatitis among persons not working directly with the raw nuts or its oil. A previous report described six cases of dermatitis among dock workers who unloaded whole, unprocessed nuts; one case in a person who shelled and ate raw cashews; and one case in a chemist who prepared an ether extract of cashew nut oil. A second report described four cases of vesicular dermatitis among children who played with souvenir toy burros made of cashew nuts and beads wired together. A third report described five cases of generalized skin inflammation among persons who ate raw cashew nuts; all five were also exquisitely sensitive to *Rhus* antigen.

Health authorities concluded that incompletely processed cashew nuts may pose a health risk to persons sensitive to poison ivy, poison oak, or poison sumac. (See *Morbidity and Mortality Weekly Report,* March 11, 1983.)

PLEASE BE CAREFUL WITH HERBAL TEAS

Perhaps no nonalcoholic beverage has enjoyed as great a popularity in recent years as has tea. Nearly four hundred spices, herbs, and combinations of same are used to produce the myriad of flavors collectively known as herbal tea. Some of these teas contain psychoactive agents, and cases of clinical intoxication have resulted (Bryson et al; Segal).

In one case, a 30-year-old man entered the hospital with loss of appetite, diarrhea, and an intoxicated feeling. His skin had yellowed, and his nails had yellow bands. His body looked emaciated, and his eyes failed to focus.

Six months before, he had started drinking Kavakava tea. Initially, his mouth and throat had numbed, followed by an intoxicated feeling. To obtain that feeling, he drank the tea six times per day for six months. After he discontinued its use, the symptoms disappeared.

The tea, made from the crushed roots of the kava plant from the South Pacific islands, turns skin yellow from what is suspected to be kava-pyrones deposited in keratin (the skin). The relevant effects are believed to result from dihydromethysticin, a mildly anticonvulsant substance.

In another case a 40-year-old woman experienced nausea, sweating, dryness of mouth and throat, and an intoxicated feeling after drinking tea made from two ground nutmegs. Four hours later her vision was disturbed; she had hallucinations, headache, and a loss of balance. After one day, the symptoms disappeared.

Nutmeg poisoning results from myristicin, which produces depression of the central nervous system alternating with periods of stimulation. Nutmeg poisoning also causes respiratory and cardiovascular difficulties.

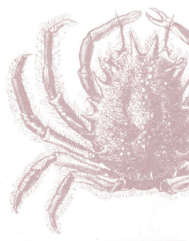

In yet another case, a 20-year-old man entered the hospital with jimson weed tea intoxication. Shortly after ingestion, he experienced flushing, restlessness, blurred vision, and thirst. He would collapse and then recover, with recovery accompanied by hallucinations. The symptoms lasted several days. The jimson weed plant contains atropine and scopolamine, and the man had thus ingested 10 to 15 mg of alkaloids.

A woman arrived at the hospital's emergency room complaining of blurred vision, a dry mouth, inability to urinate, and bizarre behavior. The initial examination showed elevated blood pressure, rapid pulse, and pupil dilation. This 26-year-old patient had been making tea for the last three days from burdock root purchased in a health food store. An examination of the tea showed it contained atropine, an alkaloid known to be a respiratory and circulatory stimulant. The toxic effects, known as anticholinergic syndrome because they impede the parasympathetic nerves, were offset by administration of physostigmine.

Burdocks occur widely in nature and must be used with caution. They have historically been used as coffee and tea substitutes without reported complaints; however, this case shows that the danger is present.

Because so many different herbs are used, herbal tea can bring you into contact with plants that you would probably never encounter in any other way. In addition to the potential risk of allergic reactions to such plant extracts, reaction to psychoactive agents as seen in the above cases is not uncommon.

BEWARE OF POISONOUS SEAFOODS

Seafood poisoning may be caused by shellfish toxins or poisonous fish. Paralytic shellfish poisoning is a significant problem in the United States (Ory). Mussels, clams, and sometimes scallops and oysters from both seacoasts and other locations can cause poisoning in humans. The one-celled organisms responsible are *dinoflagellates*, (including *Gonyaulax catanella* and perhaps *G. tamarensis* and *Pyrodinium phoneus*), which grow in the water and serve as food for shellfish. Once consumed, a poison from the dinoflagellate—*saxitoxin*—is retained in the host's tissues. The shellfish themselves are not susceptible to the chemical compound, but when they are ingested by a human, poisoning symptoms appear in 30 minutes to 3 hours. If poisonous dinoflagellates are suspected to be in the water, authorities can quarantine the area. However, this precaution is sometimes considered useless; the presence of toxic shellfish in one location does not mean that its immediate neighborhood is unsafe, nor does their absence guarantee its safety. At present, shellfish from Alaska are under constant observation, since they are widely distributed to other locations for sale.

Cooking can reduce the toxicity of saxitoxin but does not guarantee safety. Most toxin occurs in dark meat—very little is ever found in white meat. The symptoms of paralytic shellfish poisoning are very severe. The

CIGUATERA FISH POISONING, ST. CROIX, VIRGIN ISLANDS

An outbreak of ciguatera (a toxin) fish poisoning involving at least 69 persons, including three tourists, occurred at St. Croix, Virgin Islands, from February 25 through March 20, 1981.

Investigation by health authorities revealed that 20 of 21 patients were found to have eaten red snapper in the 48-hour period before onset of illness. The fish was traced to a fisher-man who had landed catches of approximately 1,500 pounds which were distributed to local restaurants and retailers. An embargo was placed on the sale of any snapper remaining from this catch. Red snapper is one species of fish that sometimes carries the ciguatera toxin.

Symptoms of ill persons who ate red snapper included diarrhea, pain and weakness in the lower extremities, abdominal pain, itching, vomiting and other clinical signs.

Ciguatera fish poisoning is endemic in many areas of the Caribbean and South Pacific; cases are also frequently reported from south Florida and Hawaii.

SOURCE: Adapted from *Morbidity and Mortality Weekly Report*, April 3, 1981.

patient develops numbness of the fingertips and lips, and the paralysis gradually moves toward the chest. Death can result from respiratory paralysis. Although about 5 to 10 percent of the victims die within 3 to 20 hours after eating the shellfish, those who survive the first 24 hours are considered to have a good chance of recovery.

There are many poisonous fish, most of which are found in tropical waters in areas around coral reefs. Many poisoning outbreaks occur in Japan, where neurological symptoms occur for which there are no antidotes. For more information on poisonous fish, consult the references at the end of this chapter or standard textbooks on poisonous fish.

Food Additives: A Question of Trade-offs

The safety of food additives is a hot topic. Few days now pass without the appearance of a newspaper article on the safety of chemicals used in food processing. Colleges across the nation offer courses about the issues involved. Unfortunately, it is extremely difficult to convince the general public—including college students—that there is no such thing as absolute safety in foods. The hazards and degrees of safety of food chemicals are best evaluated by considering their risks, benefits, and costs, as the government is doing. Such comparisons will be the primary means of evaluation until there are new scientific data.

As we indicated at the beginning of this chapter, as a food hazard, food additives (preceded by pesticides) rank the lowest. Yet most of us ingest some pesticide residues and food additives with our food. Today, some 3,000 substances are intentionally added to foods (as additives) to produce desired effects, such as keeping bread longer and improving the texture of ice cream. As many as 10,000 other compounds or combinations of compounds unintentionally find their way into various foods during processing, packaging, and storage. Unintentional additives include infinitesimal residues of pesticides used to treat crops, minute amounts of drugs fed to animals, and chemical substances that migrate from plastic packaging materials.

Since small amounts of food additives, pesticide residues, and other chemicals are so common in our food supply, consumer groups and concerned citizens have questioned their safety. Some of the risks mentioned by these individuals or groups are difficult to substantiate with current scientific knowledge.

One frequently asked question is, Can pesticide residues and food additives cause such nonspecific manifestations as headache, nervousness, tiredness, depression, and irritability? Although these symptoms are important, they are very difficult to define and categorize. Unless medical science improves, it will be some time before the concrete relationship can be established between these symptoms and the usage of the chemicals.

Another common question is, Can pesticide residues and food additives be responsible for human cancer, birth defects, and mutations? Legally, if such substances are permitted in food, they are not supposed to produce such clinical problems, at least in animals. However, in humans, there is still no satisfactory way to indicate whether they produce the effects in question. More scientific data are needed.

A third question is, Can pesticide residues and food additives accumulate in our bodies and produce some future harm that is not apparent now, such as shortened life span? Again, information is difficult to obtain, and there is no way to know what will happen to a person 20 years from now.

FIRST, A FRAME OF REFERENCE

To help the public understand food and color additives, the FDA provided a group of reference tables in April, May, and June issues of *FDA Consumer*, 1979. Such tables are described below.

Major Functions of Intentional Food and Color Additives

An additive is intentionally used in foods for one or more of the following purposes: to maintain or improve nutritional value, to maintain freshness, to help in processing or preparation, or to make food more appealing. Table 25-3 describes the major functions of food and color additives and provides some examples. Table 25-4 describes examples and food sources of food additives according to their functions. Table 25-5 lists natural and synthetic colors legally permitted to increase the appeal of foods.

Table 25-3
Major Functions of Food Additives and Food Colors

MAJOR FUNCTION	EXAMPLES	SPECIFIC USES
To maintain or improve nutritional quality	Nutrients	Enriching (replacing vitamins and minerals lost in processing); fortifying (adding nutrients that may be lacking in the diet)
To maintain product quality	Preservatives (antimicrobials)	Preventing food spoilage from bacteria, molds, fungi, and yeast; extending shelf life; protecting natural color and flavor
	Antioxidants	Delaying or preventing rancidity or enzymatic browning
To facilitate processing or preparation	Emulsifiers	Helping to distribute evenly tiny particles of one liquid throughout another; improving homogeneity, consistency, stability, and texture
	Stabilizers, thickeners, texturizers	Imparting body or improving consistency or texture; stabilizing emulsions; affecting "mouth feel"
	pH agents	Regulating acidity or alkalinity
	Anticaking agents	Preventing caking, lumping, or clustering of a finely powdered or crystalline substance
	Dough conditioners, maturing and bleaching agents	Accelerating the aging process; improving baking qualities
	Leavening agents	Affecting cooking results such as texture and volume
	Humectants	Permitting retention of moisture
To maintain or improve appeal or sensory characteristics	Flavor enhancers	Supplementing, magnifying, or modifying the original taste and/or aroma without imparting a characteristic flavor
	Flavors	Heightening natural flavor; restoring flavors lost in processing
	Colors	Providing appetizing, desired, or characteristic color
	Sweeteners	Making the aroma or taste more agreeable or pleasurable

Table 25-4

Examples and Food Sources of Food Additives According to Their Functions

FUNCTION	FOOD ADDITIVE	FOODS IN WHICH USED	PURPOSE(S)
To improve or maintain nutritional value	β-carotene	Margarine	Fortification
	Iodine, potassium iodide	Salt	Fortification
	Iron	Grain products	Enrichment, fortification
	Vitamin A	Milk, margarine, cereals	Fortification
	Vitamin B_1, vitamin B_2, niacin	Flour, breads, cereals, rice, macaroni products	Enrichment
	Vitamin C	Beverages, beverage mixes, processed fruit	Fortification
	Vitamin D, vitamin D_2, vitamin D_3	Milk, cereals	Fortification
	Vitamin E	Cereals, grain products	Fortification
To maintain product quality (antioxidants)	BHA (butylated hydroxyanisole), BHT (butylated hydroxytoluene)	Bakery products, cereals, snack foods, fats and oils	Delay or prevention of undesirable changes in color, flavor, or texture, such as enzymatic browning or discoloration due to oxidation; delay or prevention of rancidity in foods with unstable oils
	Citric acid	Fruits, snack foods, cereals, instant potatoes	
	EDTA (ethylenediaminetetraacetic acid)	Dressings, sauces, margarine	
	Propyl gallate	Cereals, snack foods, pastries	
	TBHQ (tertiary butylhydroquinone)	Snack foods, fats and oils	
	Tocopherols (vitamin E)	Oils and shortening	
	Vitamin C (ascorbic acid)	Processed fruits, baked goods	
To maintain product quality (antimicrobials)	Benzoic acid, sodium benzoate	Fruit products, acidic foods, margarine	Prevention of food spoilage from bacteria, molds, fungi and yeast; extension of shelf life; protection of natural color or flavor
	Citric acid	Acidic foods	
	Lactic acid, calcium lactate	Olives, cheese, frozen desserts, some beverages	
	Parabens (butylparaben, hyptylparaben, methylparaben propylparaben)	Beverages, caketype pastries, salad dressings, relishes	
	Propionic acid (calcium propionate, potassium propionate, sodium propionate)	Breads and other baked goods	
	Sodium diacetate	Baked goods	
	Sodium erythorbate	Cured meats	
	Sodium nitrate, sodium nitrite	Cured meats, fish, poultry	

Table 25-4 (*continued*)

FUNCTION	FOOD ADDITIVE	FOODS IN WHICH USED	PURPOSE(S)
	Sorbic acid (calcium sorbate, potassium sorbate, sodium sorbate)	Cheese, syrups, cakes, fruit products, beverages, mayonnaise, processed meats	
To aid in processing or preparation (pH control agents)	Acetic acid and sodium acetate	Candles, sauces, dressings, relishes	Controlling (changing and maintaining) acidity or alkalinity; affecting texture, taste, and wholesomeness
	Adipic acid	Beverages and gelatin bases, bottled drinks	
	Calcium lactate	Fruits and vegetables, dry and condensed milk	
	Citric acid and sodium citrate	Fruit products, candles, beverages, frozen desserts	
	Fumaric acid	Dry dessert bases, confections, powdered soft drinks	
	Lactic acid	Cheese, beverages, frozen desserts	
	Phosphoric acid and phosphates	Fruit products, beverages, oils, ices and sherbets, soft drinks, baked goods	
	Tartaric acid and tartrates	Confections, some dairy desserts, baked goods, beverages	
To aid in processing or preparation (anticaking agents)	Calcium silicate	Table salt, baking powder, other powdered foods	Helping keep salts and powders free-flowing; prevention of caking, lumping, or clustering of a finely powdered or crystalline substance
	Iron ammonium citrate	Salt	
	Silicon dioxide	Table salt, baking powder, other powdered foods	
	Yellow prussiate of soda	Salt	
To aid in processing or preparation (maturing and bleaching agents, dough conditioners)	Acetone peroxide, benzoyl peroxide, hydrogen peroxide	Flour, breads, and rolls	Acceleration of aging process (oxidation) to develop the gluten characteristics of flour; improving baking qualities
	Azodicarbonamide	Cereal flour, breads	
	Calcium bromate and potassium bromate	Breads	
	Sodium stearyl fumarate	Yeast-leavened breads, instant potatoes, processed cereals	

Continued on page 582

Table 25-4 (*continued*)

FUNCTION	FOOD ADDITIVE	FOODS IN WHICH USED	PURPOSE(S)
To aid in processing or preparation (leavening agents)	Baking powder, double-acting (sodium bicarbonate, sodium aluminum sulfate, calcium phosphate)	Quick breads, caketype baked goods	Affecting cooking results; improving texture and increasing volume; some flavor effects
	Baking soda (sodium bicarbonate)	Quick breads, caketype baked goods	
	Yeast	Bread, baked goods	
	Vitamin C (ascorbic acid)	Fruit products, acidic foods	
To aid in processing or preparation (emulsifiers)	Carrageenan	Chocolate milk, canned milk drinks, whipped toppings	Helping to evenly distribute tiny particles of one liquid throughout another, e.g., oil and water; modification of surface tension of liquid to establish a uniform dispersion or emulsion; improvement of homogeneity, stability, consistency, and texture
	Dioctyl sodium sulfosuccinate	Cocoa	
	Lecithin	Margarine, dressings, frozen desserts, chocolate, baked goods	
	Monoglycerides, diglycerides	Baked goods, peanut butter, cereals	
	Polysorbate 60, polysorbate 65, polysorbate 80	Gelatin and pudding desserts, ice cream, dressings, baked goods, nondairy creams	
	Sorbitan monostearate	Cakes, toppings, chocolate	
To aid in processing or preparation (stabilizers, thickeners, texturizers)	Ammonium alginate, calcium alginate, potassium alginate, sodium alginate	Dessert type dairy products, confections	Imparting body, improving consistency, texture; stabilizing emulsions; affecting appearance and mouth feel of the food; many are natural carbohydrates that absorb water in the food
	Carrageenan	Frozen desserts, puddings, syrups, jellies	
	Cellulose derivatives	Breads, ice cream, confections, diet foods	
	Flour	Sauces, gravies, canned foods	
	Furcelleran	Frozen desserts, puddings, syrups	
	Modified food starch	Sauces, soups, pie fillings, canned meals, snack foods	
	Pectin	Jams and jellies, fruit products, frozen desserts	

Table 25-4 (*continued*)

FUNCTION	FOOD ADDITIVE	FOODS IN WHICH USED	PURPOSE(S)
	Propylene glycol	Baked goods, frozen desserts, dairy spreads	
	Vegetable gums, guar gum, gum arabic, gum ghatti, karaya gum, locust (carob) bean gum, tragacanth gum, larch gum (arabogalactan)	Chewing gum, sauces, desserts, dressings, syrups, beverages, fabricated foods, cheese, baked goods	
To aid in processing or preparation (humectants)	Glycerine	Flaked coconut	Retention of moisture
	Glycerol monostearate	Marshmallow	
	Propylene glycol	Confections, pet foods	
	Sorbitol	Soft candies, gum	
To affect appeal characteristics (flavor enhancers)	Disodium guanylate	Canned vegetables	Supplementation, enhancement, or modification of original taste and/or aroma of a food without imparting a foreign taste or aroma
	Disodium inosinate	Canned vegetables	
	Hydrolyzed vegetable protein	Processed meats, gravy and sauce mixes, fabricated foods	
	MSG (monosodium glutamate)	Oriental foods, soups, foods with animal protein	
To affect appeal characteristics (flavors)	Vanilla (natural)	Baked goods	Making foods taste better; improvement of natural flavor; restoration of flavors lost in processing
	Vanillin (synthetic)	Baked goods	
	Spices and other natural seasonings and flavorings	Many products	
To affect appeal characteristics (sweeteners)	Corn syrup, corn syrup solids, invert sugar	Cereals, baked goods, candies, processed foods, processed meats	Making aroma or taste of a food more agreeable or pleasurable
	Dextrose, fructose, glucose, sucrose (table sugar)	Cereals, baked goods, candies, processed foods, processed meats	
	Nonnutritive sweeteners (saccharin)	Special dietary foods, beverages	
	Nutritive sweeteners (mannitol [sugar alcohol], sorbitol [sugar alcohol])	Candies, gum, confections, baked goods	

Table 25-5
Colors Legally Permitted to Increase the Appeal of Foods

COLOR ADDITIVE	ORIGIN		FOODS IN WHICH COLOR IS PERMITTED
	NATU-RAL	SYN-THETIC	
Annatto extract (yellow-red)	x		No restrictions
Dehydrated beets, beet powder	x		No restrictions
Ultramarine blue		x	Animal feed only, 0.5% by weight
Canthaxanthin (orange-red)	x	x	Limit = 30 mg/lb food
Carmel (brown)	x		No restrictions
β-apo-8′-carotenal (yellow-red)	x	x	Limit = 15 mg/lb food
β-carotene (yellow)	x	x	No restrictions
Citrus red no. 2		x	Orange skins of mature green eating oranges limit = 2 ppm
Cochineal extract, carmine (red)	x		No restrictions
Toasted, partially defatted, cooked cottonseed flour (brown shades)	x		No restrictions
FD&C blue no. 1		x	No restrictions
FD&C red no. 3		x	No restrictions
FD&C red no. 40		x	No restrictions
FD&C yellow no. 5		x	No restrictions
Ferrous gluconate (black)		x	Ripe olives
Grape skin extract (purple-red)	x		Beverages only
Iron oxide (red-brown)		x	Pet foods only, 0.25% or less by weight
Fruit juice, vegetable juice	x		No restrictions
Dried algae meal (yellow)	x		Chicken feed only
Tagetes (Aztec marigold)	x		Chicken feed only
Carrot oil (orange)	x		No restrictions
Corn endosperm (red-brown)	x		Chicken feed only
Paprika, paprika oleoresin (red-orange)	x		No restrictions
Riboflavin (yellow)	x	x	No restrictions
Saffron (orange)	x		No restrictions
Titanium dioxide (white)		x	Limit = 1% by weight
Turmeric, turmeric oleoresin (yellow)	x		No restrictions

Note: Usage of this list must be supplemented with the latest legal developments.

Legally, food colors are divided into two major categories: uncertified and certified. Uncertified colors consist of those mainly from natural sources, and certified colors of those synthesized from organic petroleum products. Table 25-5 indicates these two groups of chemicals. The procedure for obtaining legal permission to use a new food color additive is nearly the same as that for a food additive (see discussion later), with one additional important requirement: all legally permitted synthetic food colors must be certified. This means that each batch of the chemical sold for food processing must be sampled by the government to ensure that it complies with specifications concerning chemical purity and other qualities.

Synthetic food colors are not derived from food sources, and their long chemical names have caused some trouble. For simple identification, the colors are assigned initials, the shade, and a number; for example, FD&C red no. 2 ("FD&C" stands for Food, Drug, and Cosmetics).

FOOD ADDITIVES AND THE DELANEY AMENDMENT

By broad definition, a *food additive* is any substance that becomes part of a food product when added either directly or indirectly. In 1958, New York Congressman James G. Delaney sponsored a part of the Federal Food, Drug, and Cosmetic Act, which stated: ". . . no additive shall be deemed to be safe if it is found to induce cancer when ingested by men or animals, or if it is found, after tests which are appropriate for the evaluation of the safety of food additives, to induce cancer in man or animals. . . ." This clause has caused considerable upheaval in food regulations (Nutrition Foundation).

Critics of the clause argue that it has several weaknesses. Essentially, they claim that it does not consider that a high dose could be carcinogenic (cancer-causing), while a low dose may not be. They argue that it unfairly overlooks naturally occurring nutrients that can be carcinogenic—nutrients such as selenium. They also argue that the test procedures are overly sensitive.

Advocates of the clause argue that there is no such thing as a safe level for carcinogens. They point out that the Delaney clause prevents special interest groups from gaining approval for questionable additives. They further argue that the additives that cannot meet the tests of the Delaney clause are not essential products anyway.

The Delaney clause has been reviewed in light of food law controversies. For example, saccharin was to be banned, but consumer and industry pressure brought a moratorium on the ban. Nitrites have also been the subject of controversy.

When nitrites combine with amines, byproducts of protein digestion, nitrosamines result. Nitrosamines cause cancer in test animals, but nitrosamines are never added to foods, whereas nitrites are. Yet nitrites naturally occur in carrots, celery leaves, lettuce, drinking water, and human saliva. Further, nitrites are used as additives to combat botulism in processed foods. Botulism is often fatal. There are, of course, other methods of preserving foods besides using nitrites, but the point of the example of nitrites in regard to the Delaney clause is that additive issues can be complex.

Some advocates of a change in the Delaney clause have argued that a risk:benefit analysis should be the deciding factor. Diabetics, for example, felt that saccharin's value to them outweighed the cancer risk. Such debates will not easily be resolved.

SAFETY TESTING

The testing of an additive is very complicated, comprehensive, expensive, and time consuming (Nutrition Foundation). There are two major aspects of this testing: (1) ascertaining the substance's efficacy and levels of consumption and (2) testing for toxicity.

In the first step, the company ensures that the chemical will perform the expected function. For example, if a chemical is supposed to thicken a certain type of spaghetti sauce, it must be able to do so. Next the company determines, for an average person, the approximate quantity and frequency of consumption of the sauce. Finally, the company determines the quantity of chemical to be added and its approximate intake by the average consumer.

Despite the expense and the time involved, toxicity safety testing for chemical additives is necessary for human health. Federal legislation also requires it. Seven kinds of tests must be undertaken.

Metabolism of the Additives

To determine the metabolic fate of chemical additives in the body, their radioactive forms are fed or injected into animals and the subsequent metabolism studied. Occasionally, paid human volunteers are given small doses of radioactive chemicals to study their metabolic paths.

Acute Test

Second, federal regulations require that an acute toxicity test of the chemicals be carried out in at least two or three species of animals, such as rats, mice, and dogs. The chemicals are fed or injected into the animals at different dosage levels. The lowest dosage that can kill half of the animal test population is known as the LD_{50}. A number of variables are involved: animal species, administration routes, lethal dose, number of animals, and time elements. Data from the most sensitive animals are compared with the expected levels of usage. If the expected usage levels are higher than the lethal dose, the chemicals obviously cannot be used, although this is unlikely since the lethal dose is usually very large.

Subacute Test

Federal regulations further require that a subacute test be carried out in at least two or three animal species, such as rats, mice, and dogs. These animals are fed the chemicals in their feeds and/or drinking water over 2 to 3 months. During the feeding period, the animals are observed, weighed, and studied before and after they are killed. The lowest dose that produces no harm is then used to estimate a safe human consumption level. The criteria of harm are important. Observable signs of harm include weight loss, hair loss, hemorrhage, diarrhea, infection, and early death. The lowest harmless dose is not expected to cause any of these manifestations. However, problems such as headache, depression, lassitude, and sleeplessness are impossible to detect in an animal.

A common term used to describe the highest dose that produces no adverse effect in the animals is NED ("no effect dose"); sometimes it is also known as the MED ("minimum effect dose"). The dose is usually expressed in terms of milligrams additive per kilogram body weight of animal. The NED or MED is divided by 100, and the new figure is known as the acceptable daily intake, of ADI, for humans. The actual level of use of the chemical is expected to be lower than the ADI. Currently, there is much discussion regarding this factor of 0.01 or one-hundredth of the no effect dose—some consider it high, others low.

Chronic Testing

Chronic testing is probably the most expensive and time-consuming test required, lasting as long as 3 to 4 years. Again, two or three species of animals are required, and the number of animals tested must be statistically significant. The animals are fed the chemicals daily and permitted to die from natural causes. The doses fed the animals vary, usually ranging from low to as high as 100 to 1,000 times the amount normally consumed by humans. The clinical status of the animals is monitored throughout the study. There are three controversial arguments against chronic testing with animals. One is the prohibitive cost; another is uncertainty about the accuracy in applying the results to humans. There is also a growing tendency to view animal testing as cruel.

Carcinogenicity Testing

Perhaps one of the most troublesome aspects of the safety testing of food additives is carcinogenicity (cancer-causing properties). One technique involves feeding animals a high dosage of a chemical compound for their natural lifetimes and determining whether any of them develop cancer. One must be careful to distinguish between the carcinogenicity of a substance and its ability to produce other overt clinical symptoms.

There are many controversial arguments regarding carcinogenicity testing in animals. The basic mechanism of how cancer develops in humans is still unknown. A chemical compound that is harmless or carcinogenic to animals may not be so in humans. Furthermore, cancer usually does not develop at the moment of exposure to a lethal chemical, but months and even years later. Suspicion that a substance may cause cancer 10 to 20 years later is much different from proof that it will do so. Also, the routes of administering a chemical to the animals—oral (in feed or water), injection (intravenous, intramuscular, subcutaneous, or intraperitoneal), implantation in capsules, inhalation, or topical application—may give different results. Test results will also vary according to experimental design, interpretation, evaluation, and extrapolation. Clearly, we need a more reliable method to detect carcinogenicity.

Mutagenicity Testing

The term *mutagenicity* refers to an alteration of genetic material so that a change is passed on to offspring. Mutations usually have adverse effects, such as mental retardation, susceptibility to diseases, defective reproductive functions, shortened life span, and possible susceptibility to developing cancer. At present, there are a number of tests to determine the mutagenicity of chemicals. The tests are controversial, expensive, time consuming, and uncertain. The old method of feeding animals with the chemical and studying the chromosomal changes of the second generation is still used, although the validity of its extrapolation to humans is uncertain.

Teratogenicity Testing

The potential of substances to cause birth defects in newborns is called *teratogenicity*. A teratogen can also be a mutagen, although the reverse is not necessarily true. In testing for teratogenicity, pregnant animals are fed a substance, and the effect of the chemical on the newborns is studied. At present, it is possible to detect gross birth defects such as missing toes and tails and abnormal kidney and heart sizes. But there is no method of ascertaining less obvious changes, such as an abnormal hormonal system, the early detection of which is important since it may not only affect the newborn immediately but also may affect the child's future development. At present, sophisticated methods are being developed to study teratogenicity, especially very subtle changes.

NITRATES, NITRITES, NITROSAMINES

We have discussed nitrates briefly earlier. Both nitrates and nitrites are naturally occurring salts that are also used as additives (Foster). Nitrosamines are compounds in which the nitrite *ion* has combined with an amine, a process that occurs naturally in the environment.

In nature, nitrates occur in water, and nitrites occur in many vegetables. You may have also heard of nitrates in fertilizers. What you may not have heard is that nitrates and nitrites can both be converted to nitrosamines during cooking or in your stomach.

A concern exists in regard to nitrates and nitrites as additives, since they can convert to nitrosamines—and nitrosamines are known carcinogens. What is not known is whether consuming nitrates or nitrites as additives can create a risk of cancer.

Presently, nitrites are added to such food products as bacon, hot dogs, processed poultry, and ham. While the amount added is not very high, consumers have expressed concern and have considered what they can do to minimize the risk.

The solution to minimizing risk lies in eating a balanced diet from a variety of food sources. If, for example, a person ate bacon at every meal, that would not be healthy, but bacon can certainly be eaten occasionally without fear. Bacon fat should not be reused. It is additionally wise to consume vitamin C when consuming nitrite, since vitamin C has been reported to prevent nitrosamine formation in the stomach. However, some scientists believe this move is premature. Avoiding extra crispy bacon is also beneficial, since nitrosamines are formed near the burning stage in the cooking of bacon. With these few precautions, risk will be considerably minimized.

Acute *methemoglobinemia*—a blood disorder—is caused by exposure to certain drugs or chemicals that oxidize hemoglobin to a form that is capable of binding oxygen. Methemoglobinemia results in decreased oxygen delivery to the tissues, with subsequent symptoms of cyanosis, weakness, dizziness, and headaches. Agents that can cause this syndrome include nitrites, nitrates, and other oxidizing chemicals. In

CASES OF THE BLUES— NITRITE POISONING

On March 19, 1975, 16 of 30 people were hospitalized with nausea, vomiting, headache, weakness, collapse, and cyanosis, beginning about 2 hours after the group had shared a common lunch prepared by a Filipino family. One dish served was mushrooms. An initial diagnosis of mushroom poisoning was made, and investigators began tracing the source of the commercial mushrooms used in the food. On March 23, all three members of another Filipino family became ill with nausea, vomiting, acute weakness, headache, and cyanosis (blue lips and other discoloration of face) 1 to 1½ hours after eating a common lunch. All three were hospitalized, and a clinical diagnosis of nitrite poisoning was

made. The lunch had consisted of various ethnic dishes seasoned with spices and monsodium glutamate (MSG). No mushrooms had been used in this meal.

The symptoms of all hospitalized persons were consistent with nitrite poisoning. Investigation revealed that both families had purchased food at the same Filipino market and that MSG purchased recently at this store had been used to season food involved in both incidents. Further investigation in the kitchen of the second family revealed a clear polyethylene bag nearly full of white crystalline powder and labeled "MSG." Powder samples were found to contain sodium nitrite.

Questioning revealed that the

store purchased the MSG in 100-lb sacks and repackaged it into 11-oz plastic bags for sale at the store's two branches. The store also purchased sodium nitrite in similar sacks and sold it repackaged for use in curing meats. Sacks of sodium nitrite and MSG were stored side by side in the storeroom of the market. Apparently, one sack of sodium nitrite had been repackaged and then mislabeled as MSG.

All but approximately twelve of the small mislabeled bags were recovered, and no further cases of nitrite poisoning were reported. All patients were released from the hospital without serious after-effects.

SOURCE: Adapted from *Morbidity and Mortality Weekly Report*, May 31, 1975.

addition to methemoglobinemia symptoms, these agents may also cause nausea and vomiting. Although mushroom poisoning has symptoms similar to those described, it has not been associated with methemoglobinemia.

Sodium nitrite, a white crystalline powder physically similar to salt or MSG, has been responsible for several outbreaks of food-borne methemoglobinemia besides those in the case study. Symptoms have occurred within one hour of the meals and have often been attributed initially to other disease entities.

LEAD IN FOOD

Although you obtain much of your food from "tin" cans, those cans are in fact steel that has been *coated* with tin. Tin is used because it resists both oxidation and acids. To seal or solder the cans, lead is used, and approximately one third of the lead we ingest comes from such solder. The remainder of our unintentional lead ingestion comes from water pipes, pesticides, vehicle emissions, and paint.

"POT LUCK" WITH A VENGEANCE

In July 1981, the San Bernardino County Health Department was notified about a possible food-borne outbreak associated with a "pot-luck" brunch served at a local college office party. The number at risk was not known but of 15 people interviewed, 9 reported symptoms. Five of the 9 were 40 years of age, or older. Symptoms included dry mouth, dizziness, tachycardia, blurred vision, memory lapse, tingling, anxiety, confusion and/or drowsiness, nausea, and headache. Each victim showed some or all of these symptoms.

Three were hospitalized for overnight observation. The incubation period ranged from 50 minutes to 2 hours, and the me-

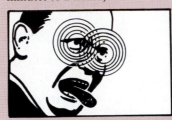

dian duration of illness was 3 hours.

Food histories implicated "zucchini cake" and the symp-

toms suggested an intoxication. The woman who prepared the cake reported that she was under the influence of alcohol when she prepared the cake and that she might have "possibly put marijuana into it." Laboratory tests confirmed the presence of cannabinoids in the implicated cake, but quantitation was not done. The cake reportedly could serve 25. Law enforcement authorities indicated that no legal action would be taken unless charges were filed. No one has done so.

SOURCE: *California Morbidity*, October 16, 1981.

The toxic effects of lead are well known and include anemia, kidney damage, and damage to the nervous system. Risks to the young are much greater since they absorb almost half of the lead they ingest, whereas adult absorption is generally about 5 to 10 percent of the amount ingested. The significant difference between child and adult absorption has brought the focus on minimizing lead contamination in children's food.

The FDA's initial efforts were with evaporated milk, a product then widely used in the preparation of infant formula. The FDA established a limit of 0.5 ppm of lead in evaporated milk cans. With the cooperation of industry, the lead content of the cans was reduced by 85 percent in the early seventies. The lead level in other infant formula products was similarly reduced. Manufacturers also switched from cans to glass jars as a further precaution against lead ingestion by children.

After the dramatic reduction in the lead content of children's foods, attention shifted to adult foods, especially those commonly eaten by children. The goal of the FDA has been a 50-percent reduction of lead levels, and various manufacturing changes promise that achievement, or more. For example, canners have begun to use seamless cans, thereby reducing the amount of lead needed to seal the can. The canners who still use seams have gone to a process of electrical welding of seams, eliminating the need for lead solder. Survey emphasis will continue to focus on apple juice, orange juice, fruit punch, applesauce, tuna, string

LEAD POISONING
FROM MEXICAN FOLK REMEDIES

In summer 1981, the first cases of lead poisoning associated with the Mexican food remedy *azarcon* were identified in Los Angeles, California, and in Colorado. Since that time, nine additional confirmed cases associated with the ingestion of azarcon or the related remedy, *greta*, have been reported in California, and five cases have been reported from Michigan and Wisconsin.

Greta and azarcon are powders with total lead contents varying from 70 percent to greater than 90 percent. Being powders, they provide a large

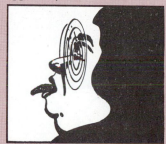

surface area for potential absorption. These remedies apparently are most often administered to infants and children with diarrhea or similar problems, who are the most susceptible in terms of clinical im-

pact and the capacity to absorb lead.

With the identification of multiple cases of lead poisoning and indication of significant exposure, major media efforts publicizing the dangers of azarcon and greta have been directed at Hispanic communities in California. Until recently, these substances were available at herb shops and from folk healers on both sides of the Mexican-American border. The FDA has initiated a national recall of greta.

SOURCE: Adapted from *Morbidity and Morality Weekly Report*, October 28, 1983.

beans, baked beans, tomatoes, chicken noodle soup, and vegetable soup. These ten products have been identified as adult products often consumed by children.

The cooperation between the government and industry in reducing lead contamination of food has been a remarkable success story, one that continues to promise a significant improvement in food safety.

COOKWARE: UNINTENTIONAL ADDITIVES

A concern of nutritionists, health practitioners, and consumers has been the potential of food contamination resulting from cooking and storage. Although we tend to think of cookware as fixed and unchanging, in fact metals may migrate from cookware to food, and to your body (Henderson).

The possibility that you may be unintentionally adding aluminum, copper, or lead to your meals has resulted in several investigations into leaching, the means by which one substance dissolves into another, and into possible connections between cookware substances and disease. It is known, for example, that aluminum can migrate into foods, especially salty or acidic foods. For this reason, acidic foods such as tomato juice, sauerkraut, citrus juices and carbonated drinks should not be stored in aluminum. Similarly, copper can migrate to any food, especially those high in acid.

Both aluminum and copper are naturally present in foods and reach

ZINC POISONING AND FRUIT PUNCH

On November 19, 1982, a group of students in a Grant County, New Mexico, junior high school became ill, with symptoms of headache, chills, dizziness, nausea, and vomiting. Illness was confined to students who attended a home economics class that day where fruit punch and cookies, prepared the previous evening, were served.

Onset of illness ranged from 5 minutes to 2 hours after the punch—a mixture of two brands of commercial fruit punch, lemonade, and ginger ale—was consumed. The mixture was stored overnight in three 5-gallon water containers that had galvanized metal linings, with large areas of corrosion. The punch was transferred to plastic pitchers immediately before it was served.

Analyses showed elevated levels of zinc and slightly elevated levels of iron in the punch. No other metals, including cadmium, showed elevated levels.

Zinc is a major constituent of

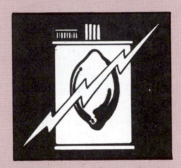

galvanized metal. On contact with acidic foods and beverages, it is converted to zinc salts, which are readily absorbed by the body.

Outbreaks of illness manifested by fever, nausea, vomiting, abdominal cramps, and diarrhea have been reported after consumption of foods or beverages prepared or stored in galvanized containers. In previously reported outbreaks, zinc levels found in contaminated foods or beverages have exceeded 1,000 parts per million. In adults, 225 to 450 mg of zinc can cause vomiting (the *emetic* dose), but the dosage may be lower for teenagers with lower body weights.

The FDA considers galvanized metal an unacceptable surface material for equipment and utensils used with food and beverages (other than water).

SOURCE: Adapted from *Morbidity and Mortality Weekly Report*, May 20, 1983.

our bodies in minimal amounts. Aluminum compounds are also approved for use in antacids, cheeses, and bread. Copper is considered an essential nutrient (see Chapter 12) and aids in the absorption and metabolism of iron. The health concerns regarding these two metals thus lie in the quantities we ingest.

Harmful levels of copper result in nausea, vomiting, and diarrhea. For this reason, the FDA recommends that you use only tin-lined copper cooking utensils. Aluminum can be tolerated by our bodies at higher levels than copper, and excess aluminum is excreted as waste material. Aluminum has, however, been investigated relative to Alzheimer's disease, a progressive brain disorder characterized by learning difficulties and memory loss. Some Alzheimer's victims have been found to have increased levels of aluminum in the brain, but it is not known whether the disease preceded the aluminum retention or vice versa. Corrosive aluminum cookware has been implicated in the occurrence of *dialysis dementia,* a form of mental deterioration from aluminum poisoning in kidney patients.

Cadmium and lead are metals used in ceramic glazes. Both can be leached from enamel and are potentially hazardous. Again, acidic foods present the greatest concern. Correcting mixing and firing procedures can guard against lead and cadmium migration, and the FDA maintains a surveillance program in that regard. There are, however, increasing numbers of local industry cooking utensils that may not have been properly mixed and fired. Accordingly, consumers should avoid cooking and storing in such utensils.

SULFITES: POTENTIALLY DANGEROUS

Especially if you have asthma, restaurant salad bars can be fatal. Sulfites are preservatives used to keep fruits and vegetables fresh and flavorful. They also occur in dried fruits, beer, wine, and baked goods and are additionally used in restaurants for potatoes and seafood. The danger in sulfites is that many people have allergic reactions to them. Such reactions have included nausea, diarrhea, anaphylactic shock, acute asthma attacks, and loss of consciousness. One death has also been reported (Hecht and Willis).

Six sulfiting agents have been approved by the FDA for use as preservatives: sodium sulfite, sulfur dioxide, sodium bisulfite, potassium bisulfite, sodium metabisulfite, and potassium metabisulfite. Sulfiting agents also occur in such medications as cardiovascular drugs, antiemetics (nausea prevention), antibiotics, anesthetics, intravenous solution, and analgesics (pain relievers). Though it may seem ironic, they are also used in nebulized bronchodilator solutions for the treatment of asthma. Their use in treating asthma has caused some confusion, because an asthmatic who fails to respond to bronchodilator treatment may be reacting to the sulfite rather than failing to respond to the medication.

In response to the numerous cases of allergic reaction to sulfites, alternatives to their use as food preservatives and in medications are being explored. Consumers should be aware of their own potential sensitivity to sulfites. Initial symptoms of an anaphylactic reaction can include flushing, itching, hives or welts, wheezing, and swelling of skin and mucous membranes. Advanced symptoms can include low blood pressure, throat closure, cyanosis (skin turning blue), loss of consciousness, and respiratory arrest. Those who suspect they may be allergic to sulfites should always inquire about their use in restaurants.

TANNING FROM A BOTTLE

Food coloring is now available for you too, as a method of obtaining a tan without exposure to the sun. You should, however, give careful consideration to using such products, since the potential side effects can be unpleasant (Fenner). Further, the long-range effects are not known.

Tanning pills have not been tested for their safety and therefore do not have the approval of the FDA. They contain synthetic versions of natural coloring substances that give the color to vegetables and fruits such as carrots and apricots, and to marine life such as brine shrimp and algae. The two naturally occurring substances are beta-carotene and canthaxanthin.

Beta-carotene gives color to carrots, apricots, peaches, and other yellow fruits and vegetables. Since it is a dietary substance, it has been tested extensively. Consuming significant amounts of dietary beta-carotene will turn the skin yellow, a condition known as *carotenemia*. This side effect also occurs through use of a medication containing beta-carotene that is prescribed for individuals whose skin is highly sensitive to sunlight. Beta-carotene also has use in that your body converts it to vitamin A (see Chapter 10). Since beta-carotene studies have shown it to be a safe substance, it has been approved as an additive to give coloring to processed foods and as an ingredient in cosmetics.

Canthaxanthin gives the reddish-orange color to brine shrimp. It also occurs in sea trout and mushrooms and in such waterbirds as flamingos. It has no known use in our bodies but is often the primary ingredient in tanning pills. Canthaxanthin has also been approved for use as a food color and occurs in pizza, spaghetti sauce, barbecue sauce, and catsup. Canthaxanthin has not, however, been studied to the extent that beta-carotene has.

The use of beta-carotene and canthaxanthin in tanning pills poses potential problems. First, canthaxanthin occurs in such pills at levels far above those approved for its use as a food additive. Its potential toxicity is not known. Second, cases of adverse side effects such as diarrhea, cramps, and hepatitis have been reported. Third, consumers often mistakenly believe that tanning pills will prevent sunburn.

The tan resulting from the pills containing synthetic food coloring is simply the skin taking on a dye. The excessive levels of the chemicals dye the liver, skin, and fatty tissues. If you stop taking the pills, the yellow-orange tan will fade. During the time you are taking them, your stools will likely be bright red, and your blood plasma will be bright orange rather than pale yellow. Individuals taking the pills have had side effects ranging from dry skin and welts to drug-induced hepatitis; however, the symptoms could not be positively blamed on the tanning pills.

Since the toxicity of such products is not known, consumers would be well advised to avoid them. Pregnant women especially should not use them, because their effects on the fetus are not known.

FOOD CHEMICALS THAT HAVE BEEN BANNED FROM USE
The FDA prohibited the use of a number of chemicals in foods for human consumption because they either present a risk to the public health or have not been shown safe by adequate scientific data (Hui). Table 25-6 lists the food additives that manufacturers are presently prohibited from adding to food; it is preceded by a list of prohibited synthetic food colors. For easy reference, the table and list include only *some* of the substances prohibited from use in food for human consumption.

Prohibited synthetic food colors:

Butter yellow	FD&C green no. 1
Sudan 1	FD&C green no. 2
FD&C red no. 1	FD&C yellow no. 1
FD&C red no. 2	FD&C yellow no. 2
FD&C red no. 4	FD&C yellow no. 3
FD&C red no. 32	FD&C yellow no. 4
FD&C orange no. 1	FD&C violet no. 1
FD&C orange no. 2	Orange B

Table 25-6
Additives Prohibited from Use in Foods for Human Consumption

FOOD ADDITIVE	USAGE
Agene (nitrogen trichloride)	Bleaching and aging substance for flour
Cobalt salts	Stabilizer in beer permitting foam formation
Coumarin	Flavoring agent
Cyclamate	Artificial sweetener
Diethyl pyrocarbonate (DEPC)	Preservative, especially for alcoholic beverages
Dulcin (p-ethoxyphenyl urea)	Artificial sweetener
Ethylene glycol	Humectant, solvent
Monochloroacetic acid	Preservative
Nordihydroguaiaretic acid (NDGA)	Antioxidant
Oil of calamus	Flavoring agent
Polyoxyethylene-8-stearate (Myrj 45)	Emulsifier
P-4000	Proposed artificial sweetener
Safrole	Flavoring agent
Thiourea	Preservative

PUBLIC CONFIDENCE

Public confidence in the use of chemical additives in food is currently low, mainly because of uncertainty about the health hazards that they pose. Public confidence might increase if consumers had more information about food chemicals, government regulations governing their use, and the differences between measurable and nonmeasurable health hazards. The public mistrusts the government when they believe that the government is not releasing everything known about food chemicals. Unfortunately, the knowledge of scientists (in and out of government) about the safety of food additives is limited, and the public must recognize this. People should seek a balance between the relative risks and benefits of food and color additives.

As a consumer, you should become informed. Start by reading labels to find out what is in the foods you buy. Additives must be listed with the ingredients, although the law permits colors and flavors to be described in general terms like "artificially flavored" and "artificially colored."

Learn what the various additives do and decide which ones are of most concern to you. If you have questions, contact the consumer affairs officer at your nearest FDA office, listed in the telephone directory under U.S. Department of Health and Human Services, or write to the manufacturer.

Exercise your right to choose. Once you are informed, you can select foods on the basis of which characteristics—convenience, appeal, storage characteristics, or ease of preparation—mean the most to you. You might want to continue buying bread with sodium propionate if you know it prevents mold, but you may not want to buy cookies that are artificially colored. The choice is yours.

Finally, make your views known. Let manufacturers and your representatives in Congress know what you want and do not want in your food. Discuss the problems with academicians in foods and nutrition.

Food additives, like most things in life, involve a trade-off. Scientists will never be able to guarantee that anything added to foods is absolutely safe. Ultimately, the consumer must decide what degree of risk is acceptable for foods that keep well and are appealing, nutritious, convenient, and readily available year-round.

Food Radiation: A New Process

For years a chemical known as ethylene dibromide (EDB) has been used as a fruit and grain fumigant to extend shelf life of foods and to kill insects and microorganisms that damage foods. Research showing that EDB is a carcinogen has brought about the need for an alternative method of delaying food spoilage. The FDA's answer to the problem is low-dose radiation (Lecos).

Radiation technology experts claimed for years that radiation could revolutionize the food processing industry by delaying the spoilage of fresh produce. They have explained that radiation can enable meat to remain fresh for over a week in a home refrigerator and that radiated strawberries can stay red and firm for up to two weeks beyond when nonradiated strawberries would be moldy.

The concern about the radiation of food lies with its safety, especially its safety in the eyes of the consumer. The medical x-rays you receive require one rad of energy, with a rad defined as a unit of absorbed radiant energy. The recommended radiation for fruit and vegetables is 100,000 rads.

Just as dental x-rays do not make teeth radioactive, so too the radiation of food does not make it radioactive. The process of radiating food involves a conveyor belt passing through a concrete room. In the room, the food is exposed to such materials as cobalt 60 or cesium 137, both very powerful radioactive isotopes.

The potential for significant impact on food processing has been compared to the impacts of canning or freezing. Proponents also point to added benefits. For example, radiation could virtually eliminate such dangerous organisms as trichinae in pork or salmonella in chicken. It has been considered that such preservatives as nitrites, suspected of causing cancer, can be eliminated.

Food industry spokesmen have been encouraged by the potential that radiation has for preventing the 25 to 30 percent spoilage rate that now exists for nonradiated fresh foods. The use of the process in over 25 countries resulted in a United Nations recommendation in 1980 that up to one million rads could safely be used for food radiation. At that time, the process was used in the United States only for controlling bacteria in spices, for preparing foods for hospital cancer patients, for preparing food for the space program, and for sterilizing medical instruments.

Tests of the effects of radiation on nutrient content show no loss of nutrient values. Radiation of food can cause minute chemical changes known as unique radiolytic products (URPs). Although available research shows these to be safe, long-term tests will be necessary before final conclusions can be reached. Until that research is in, the process of food irradiation will be considered comparable to cooking in microwave ovens.

At present, the FDA is in the process of proposing regulations that would allow the use of low-dose radiation to process and preserve fruits and vegetables. According to standard FDA procedures, there will be a waiting time before the actual use of radiation is implemented.

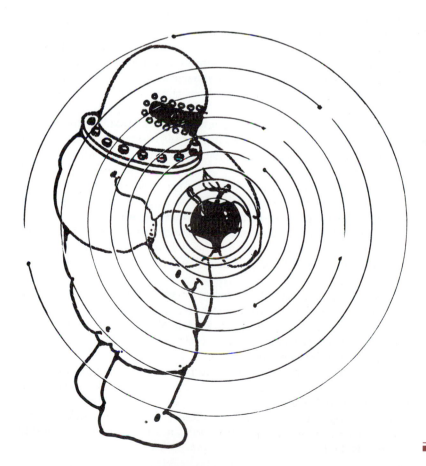

And Then There Was PCB

PCBs AND OIL DISEASE

Yusho is Japanese for oil disease. The word comes from a contamination case in the late sixties when heat-exchange fluid in a Japanese manufacturing plant leaked into rice oil. The fluid contained PCBs (polychlorinated biphenyls, powerful environmental contaminants; see below) and affected over 1,000 people who used the contaminated product.

The most common early symptom of exposure to halogenated aromatic hydrocarbons such as PCBs is *chloracne*. Since the turn of the century, this form of acne has been recognized as an occupational hazard associated with chlorinated chemicals. As chlorinated hydrocarbons were increasingly used for electrical insulation, such terms as "electrician's rash" and "cable rash" became common. Trade names for the chemicals gave rise to such terms as Aroclor acne and Halowax acne.

The Japanese who were exposed in the Yusho incident had chloracne of the face and genitals. Black pigmentation of face, lips, eyelids, and gums also developed. Infants were born with brown pigmentation over their entire bodies, though the condition disappeared in a few months.

Over ten years after the exposure, Yusho patients had numbness and pain in extremities, swelling and pain in joints, headache, coughing, and symptoms similar to bronchitis. Studies of employees in a capacitor manufacturing plant show that employees have chloracne, pigmentation changes, headaches, eye swelling and discharge, and respiratory problems. One of the most disquieting concerns regarding PCB exposure is that general symptoms persist and worsen with time, giving rise to the possibility that cancer may result.

Since the Yusho case, PCBs have been recognized as common environmental contaminants that represent a safety hazard (Nicholson and Moore). Along with dioxin and PBBs (see below), they belong to a chemical group called halogenated aromatic hydrocarbons.

PCBs—FREQUENCY AS POLLUTANT

Once the concern in regard to PCBs as a health threat had arisen, scientists began to study them to determine to what extent they had contaminated the environment. They have been found in both freshwater fish and saltwater fish, in whales and seals, in polar bears, in North American and European birds, and in various predators such as mink and fox.

Human tissue studies have found PCBs in Americans, Europeans, Japanese, and Israelis. Germans had the highest content, 7 to 10 parts per million (ppm). Over 90 percent of Americans have detectable levels, and 40 percent of them are above 1 ppm. That PCBs are so widespread environmentally seems surprising since the chemicals are used in sealed systems such as transformers, capacitors, and heat exchangers.

Sources of Contamination

Part of the reason for PCBs being widespread is their tenacity. They are extremely stable, resisting heat to 800°C and resisting other chemicals. When transformers burn, they rupture, releasing PCBs. About one fourth of PCB use is in paint and ink, plastics, adhesives, and copying paper. When these products are burned, PCBs are released. Recycling of paper products can place PCBs into paper products such as food wrappings. In backtracking PCBs found in cow's milk, the source was traced to paint inside silos in which cattle feed had been stored.

Since their danger has been recognized, PCBs are banned in Japan. In the United States they are used only in closed systems, but products manufactured prior to the 1970s contain them and are still in use.

Extent of Pollution

It is estimated that over a half million tons of PCBs were manufactured in the United States through 1970. Another one million tons were probably manufactured in other countries. In North America, estimates place 300,000 tons in dumps and landfills, where it can leak to air and water. The 30,000 tons released to the air probably returned in rain and snow. Another 60,000 tons were released to fresh and coastal waters as industrial waste.

PBBs IN MICHIGAN

In Michigan in the fall of 1973, herds of dairy cattle lost their appetites, became thin and weak, developed open sores, and gave birth to stillborn calves. Careful investigation found that cattle feed had been contaminated with toxic chemicals.

The contamination occurred after polybrominated biphenyls (PBBs), ingredients in fire retardants, became accidentally substituted for magnesium oxide, a feed supplement for dairy cattle. Both products came from the same manufacturer. A farm cooperative then mixed the supposed feed supplement with other feed and distributed it to dairy farms.

By 1976, almost 30,000 of Michigan's dairy cattle had died or were destroyed. Sheep, pigs, and chickens also had to be destroyed, as did milk, eggs, butter, and cheese. Consumers of the Michigan products had ingested elevated levels of PBBs for almost one year.

Michigan farmers exposed to the PBB contamination of dairy cattle and their milk complained of headache, rashes, loss of appetite, and numbness. Laboratory tests showed elevated PBB levels in the blood of the farmers.

A comparison of Michigan farmers likely to have been contaminated and Wisconsin farmers who were not affected showed obvious differences. Skin problems, arthritis-like symptoms, and fatigue occurred in the Michigan farmers. A random sampling of Michigan residents found PBBs in 90 percent of the blood samples and 100 percent of the fat tissue samples, whereas PBBs were not found in those who had recently moved to Michigan. This finding suggests that the initial PBB contamination is no longer in the food supply.

Ten Common Food Allergies

Although food allergy is a problem of the person and not the food, there is sufficient common complaint among the public to include a section on this topic under the chapter of food safety.

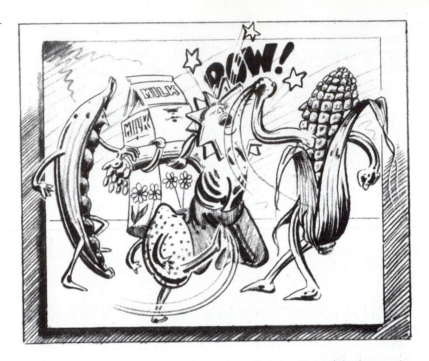

Although food allergy rarely constitutes a serious, life-threatening concern, it results in chronic illness for many sufferers. This problem can be significantly eliminated if you are alert to the most common **allergens** and the manifestations of allergic reaction (Atkins and Metcalfe).

Cow's Milk. The allergen in cow's milk is probably the most common. A susceptible person may be allergic to whole, skim, evaporated, or dried milk, as well as to milk-containing products such as ice cream, cheese, custard, cream and creamed foods, and yogurt. If exquisite milk allergy exists, even butter and bread can create a reaction.

Symptoms can include either or both constipation and diarrhea, abdominal pain, nasal and bronchial congestion, asthma, headache, foul breath, sweating, fatigue, and tension.

Kola Nut Products. Chocolate (cocoa) and cola are products obtained from the kola nut. An allergy to one almost always means an allergy to the other as well.

Symptoms most commonly include headache, asthma, gastrointestinal allergy, nasal allergy, and eczema.

Corn. Because corn syrup is widely used commercially, corn allergy can result from a wide variety of foods. Candy, chewing gum, prepared meats, cookies, rolls, doughnuts, some breads, canned fruits, jams, jellies, some fruit juices, ice cream, and sweetened cereals all utilize corn syrup. Additionally, whole corn, cornstarch, corn flour, corn oil, and cornmeal can cause allergic reactions to such foods as cereals, tortillas, tamales, enchiladas, soups, beer, whiskey, fish sticks, and pancake or waffle mixes.

Symptoms can be bizarre, ranging from allergic tension to allergic fatigue. Headache can take the form of migraine.

Eggs. Those with severe allergy to eggs can react to even their odor. Egg allergy can also cause reaction to vaccines, since they are often grown on chicken embryo. Allergic reactions are generally to such foods as eggs themselves, baked goods, candies, mayonnaise, creamy dressings, meat loaf, breaded foods, and noodles.

Symptoms can be widely varied, as with milk. Egg allergy often results in urticaria (hives) though, like chocolate, larger amounts are usually necessary to produce that symptom. Other symptoms include headache, gastrointestinal allergy, eczema, and asthma.

Peas (legumes). The larger family of plants that are collectively known as peas include peanuts, soybeans, beans, and peas. Peanuts tend to be the greatest offender, and dried beans and peas cause more difficulties than fresh ones. Products that can cause selected allergy reaction are honey (made from the offending plants) and licorice, a legume. Soybean allergy presents a problem similar to corn owing to its widespread use in the form of soybean concentrate or soybean oil.

Legume allergies can be quite severe, even resulting in shock. They commonly cause headache and can be especially troublesome for asthma patients, urticaria patients, and angioedema sufferers (blood vessel swelling and spasm).

Citrus fruits. Oranges, lemons, limes, grapefruit, and tangerines can cause eczema and hives and often cause asthma. They commonly cause canker sores (*aphthous stomatitis*). Although citrus fruit allergy does not cause allergy to artificial orange and lemon-lime drinks, if patients are allergic to citric acid in the fruits then they will also react to tart artificial drinks and may also react to pineapple.

Tomatoes. This fruit, commonly called a vegetable, can cause hives, eczema, and canker sores. It also causes asthma. In addition to its natural form, it can be encountered in soups, pizza, catsup, salads, meat loaf, and tomato paste or tomato juice.

Wheat and other grains. Wheat, rice, barley, oats, millet, and rye are known allergens, with wheat the commonest of the group. Wheat occurs in many dietary products. All common baked goods, cream sauce, macaroni, noodles, pie crust, cereals, chili, and breaded foods contain wheat.

Reaction to wheat and its related grains can be severe. Asthma and gastrointestinal disturbances are the most common reactions.

Cinnamon. Of various spices that can cause allergic reaction, cinnamon is generally the most potent. It occurs in catsup, chewing gum, candy, cookies, cakes, rolls, prepared meats, and pies. Bay leaf allergy generally occurs as well, since this spice is related to cinnamon. Pumpkin pie reactions are also common owing to the high cinnamon content in them.

Other spices most frequently mentioned as allergens are black pepper, white pepper, oregano, the mints, paprika, and cumin.

Artificial food colors. Although various artificial food colors have been implicated in such problems as hyperactive syndrome in children, as allergens the two most common offenders are amaranth (red dye) and tartrazine (yellow dye). Amaranth is most often encountered, but reactions to tartrazine tend to be more severe.

Food colors occur in carbonated beverages, some breakfast drinks, bubble gum, flavored ice foods, gelatin desserts, and such medications as antibiotic syrups.

Other Food Allergens. Any food is capable of producing an allergic reaction. However, those offenders often mentioned after the top ten are pork and beef, onion and garlic, white potatoes, fish, coffee, shrimp, bananas, and walnuts and pecans.

Vegetables, other than those already mentioned, rarely cause allergic reactions. Fruits that usually are safe include cranberries, blueberries, figs, cherries, apricots, and plums. Chicken, turkey, lamb, and rabbit prove the safest meats. Tea, olives, sugar, and tapioca are also relatively safe foods, although some herbal teas can cause unique difficulties (see earlier discussion).

Diagnosis Is Important

Food allergies can generally be determined by diet control. The suspected offender or offenders can be removed from the diet until all symptoms disappear. Then, the suspected foods can be reintroduced to the list one at a time. This process, known as elimination and challenges, can lead to identification of an offender. Treatment consists of avoiding the offender.

STUDY QUESTIONS

1. What are the symptoms of bacterial food poisoning? In whom are these conditions most likely to be severe?

2. Briefly explain the potential health risks in foods. Which is thought to be the most serious hazard? What general questions about food safety are yet unanswered?

3. Distinguish between food-borne infection and food-borne intoxication. What are the two most important kinds of food-borne intoxication discussed in the text?

4. What are some common sources of staphylococcal bacteria in foods? Under what conditions do they grow best? Give at least five foods in which they may be found. What preventive measures should the cook take?

5. What are some sources of *Clostridium perfringens*? Under what conditions do they grow best?

6. What is the main source of botulism? What are the symptoms of poisoning by *Clostridium botulinum*? How can death be averted? How can the toxin be destroyed in foods?

7. Describe at least eight measures that help prevent food poisoning.

8. Define: acute test, subacute test, chronic testing; carcinogenicity; mutagenicity; and teratogenicity.

9. Using library resource materials, list the current *legal* status of nitrites/nitrates, lead, saccharin, aspartame, and the Delaney amendment.

10. What are antioxidants? Give some examples.

11. Describe at least five ways in which chemicals are used in food processing and give examples of each.

12. How many synthetic and natural colors are legally permitted as food additives?

REFERENCES

Atkins, F. M., and D. D. Metcalfe. "The Diagnosis and Treatment of Food Allergy." *Ann. Rev. Nutr.* 4 (July 1984): 22.

Bryson, P. D., et al. "Burdock Root Tea Poisoning: Case Report Involving a Commercial Preparation." *J.A.M.A.* 239 (1978): 2157.

Fenner, L. "The Tanning Pill: A Questionable Inside Dye Job." *FDA Consumer* 16 (February 1982): 23.

Foster, E. M. "Food Safety: Problems of the Past and Perspectives of the Future." *J. Food Protect.* 45 (1982): 658.

Gilchrist, A. *Foodborne Disease and Food Safety.* Chicago: American Medical Association, 1981.

Hecht, A., and J. Willis. "Sulfites: Preservatives That Can Go Wrong." *FDA Consumer* 17 (September 1983): 11.

Henderson, D. "Cookware as a Source of Additives." *FDA Consumer* 16 (March 1982): 11.

Hui, Y. H. *Human Nutrition and Diet Therapy.* Monterey, Calif.: Wadsworth Health Sciences, 1983.

Lecos, C. "Irradiation Proposed to Treat Food." *FDA Consumer* 18 (May 1984): 11.

Nicholson, W. J., and J. A. Moore, eds. "Health Effects of Halogenated Aromatic Hydrocarbons." *Ann. N.Y. Acad. Sci.* 320 (1979).

Nutrition Foundation. *A Proposed Food Safety Evaluation Process: Final Report of Board of Trustees, Food Safety Council.* Washington, D.C.: Nutrition Foundation, 1982.

Ory, R. L. *Antinutrients and Natural Toxicants in Foods.* Westport, Conn.: Food and Nutrition Press, 1981.

Segal, R. K. "Herbal Intoxication: Psychoactive Effects from Herbal Cigarettes, Tea, and Capsules." *J.A.M.A.* 236 (1976): 473.

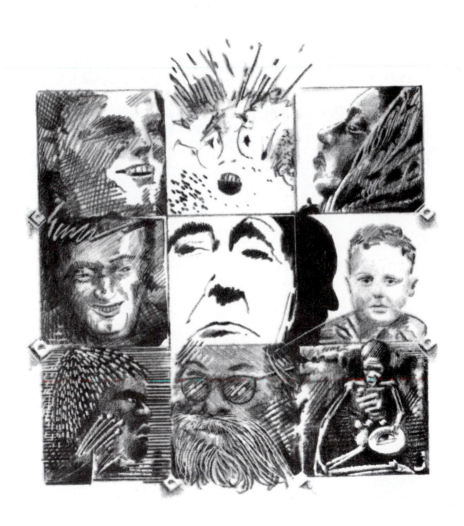

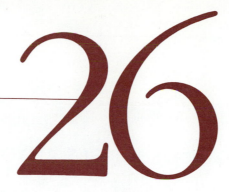

26

Culture AND Nutrition:

WE EAT WHERE WE ARE

Sautéed Grasshoppers, Anyone?

Carol Miller, a home economics major in the California State University system, made national news by promoting the eating of insects, a practice known as entomophagy. She acknowledged that Americans have a cultural aversion to insects, but noted that insects are rich in nutritional values, and plentiful. Beef is 15 to 20 percent protein, and chicken reaches 20 percent, but termites have 40 percent protein, and grasshoppers have 60 percent.

As a protein source, insects can supplement such incomplete foods as bread, grain, beans, rice, and pastas. You can boil, steam, simmer, and bake insects. They can be used in salads, soups, and stews, and they are easily included in breads and cookies. They are not just crop-damaging pests: they may someday help combat malnutrition.

A significant number of people, from Arctic Eskimos to South American Indians, eat maggots, and insects are bred for human consumption in Asian countries. For various Central Australian tribes, insects occupy

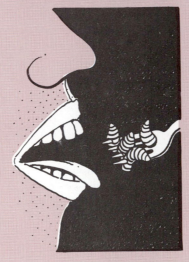

a basic food category. In Papua New Guinea, insect-eating is common enough to require careful use of pesticides. Studies have shown that insects can be more nutritious than the vegetables they eat.

Increasingly, nutritionists and food research specialists are discussing the potential that insects may hold for nutrition. It has been suggested that insect farming may stimulate economics, increase nutritional value of insects, and help control food distribution inequities. Collection of wild insects, by light at night, for example, could help reduce crop damage. Given the increase of protein deficiency in many developing countries, insects stand as a resource that bears further investigation.

SOURCE: Adapted from J. R. Gorham. *Bull. Soc. Vector. Ecol.* 3 (1976):11; and C. Hillinger, *Philadelphia Inquirer*, Dec. 14, 1975.

Hunger is one reason why some people in the world eat insects. Anthropologists have long confirmed that people in different parts of the world eat (or do not eat) certain foods for various reasons. This is explored in the next section.

Food Taboos versus Nutrition

Food taboos often develop around the belief that you can assume the characteristics of what you eat (Barker). For example, Native Americans favored venison for the deer's qualities of speed and stealth. Conversely, the lumbering bear was less favored. When a tribe especially honored a particular animal, their "totem" animal, that animal might be consumed only on special occasions, or not at all. The Omaha Indians, for example, had the elk as their totem animal and believed they would break out in boils if they ate elk meat.

Dietary laws can have social and economic significance. In the Hindu religion, which is characterized by a caste system, the Brahmins, the highest caste, are strict vegetarians. Their avoidance of meat is based on their belief that everyone was once an animal; hence, every animal will one day be a human being. A lower caste can eat meat if the animal is killed in a certain manner. The lowest caste, the "untouchables," can eat anything obtained in virtually any manner.

Fasting is a dietary custom of mixed origins. Among certain religions, specific foods may be avoided at certain times. Among Catholics, for example, all meat was once avoided during Lent and on Fridays. While that proscription has changed, the Muslim Ramadan—a month of fasting—continues. In remembrance of the handing down of the sacred scriptures, the Koran, Ramadan involves abstaining from food, water, and tobacco from sunrise to sunset. The nutritional impact of fasting for a short period is generally negligible. But when Ramadan occurs during the heat of summer, dehydration can become a concern for field workers.

Nutritionists are also concerned that bans against meat and animal products may contribute to infant mortality among some sects. Nevertheless, food taboos will persist, and nutritionists must plan to accommodate them.

Food behavior, a fascinating and complex subject, is an individual's response to stimuli related to the selection, procurement, distribution, manipulation, storage, consumption, and disposal of food. Food behavior in the United States is complex and diversified because people of many cultural origins are living in proximity, and the country is making rapid advances in technology. In this chapter, we will explore the relationship between culture and nutrition, with special emphasis on the nutritional adequacy of the diets of different cultures.

A Literal Melting Pot

Most of us can easily answer the question, What are your favorite foods? Generally, we respond with tastes developed during childhood. Basic food habits usually prove resistant to change.

Despite their food habits, Americans have a wide variety of food tastes. This variety is due partially to the significant mobility of Americans, partially to a wide variety of choices, and partially to such trends as eating at restaurants and eating "ethnic." It is considered stylish to sample the cuisines of other countries.

At home, though, we usually prefer less variation. Our food patterns tend to follow family history—and especially what our parents liked and disliked. Where an ethnic community is established, food habits can become readily apparent. Especially in major cities, it is not uncommon to find neighborhood grocery stores that have shelves of food catering to ethnic tastes of a significant segment of the surrounding community.

Personal food patterns become especially important when we are old and when we are ill. Success in encouraging such patients to eat often depends on including their special preferences in their diets. Other chapters, such as 17 and 18, address meal planning for specific groups. This chapter addresses food patterns of people in the United States of different regions, ethnic origins, cultural backgrounds, religious backgrounds, and lifestyles (Baker; Root and DeRochement; Sanjur).

THE HISTORY OF CHICKEN SOUP AS MEDICATION

In Egypt, several thousand years ago, an epidemic that killed many young Egyptian males had no effect on a minority population living in the same area. The unafflicted population had a diet that included soup made of boiled chicken and herbs and vegetables. This case gave rise to the accepted medicinal value of chicken soup.

The *Bible* does not contain explicit references to chicken soup's healing properties, but it has been noted that the dietary guidance received by Moses on Mount Sinai contained no limitations on chicken, despite prohibitions regarding most all food. Some scholars believe that the recipe for chicken soup was transmitted to Moses on the same occasion but was relegated to the oral tradition.

For centuries chicken soup was widely used in Europe and was once commercially pro-

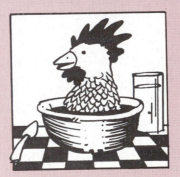

duced. The soup has been employed for thousands of years in the treatment of viral and bacterial illnesses. Chicken soup is still widely used to treat a variety of disorders, but its use occurs mainly among faithful followers in the general public.

Although the product has not been standardized, it has been studied. Scientific findings include rapid absorption following oral administration, wide distribution throughout body tissues, and the conversion to byproducts that have antibacterial power.

SOURCE: Adapted from N. L. Caroline and H. Schwartz. *Chest* 67 (1975): 215.

REGIONAL DIFFERENCES

For many years, obvious regional food patterns could be found in the United States. Those pronounced differences have faded considerably as techniques for processing, storing, and transporting foods have advanced. National advertising has had its effects, as has the mobility of our population.

In certain parts of the country, though, remnants of regional food preference persist. Such preferences often reflect availability that has spawned popularity. For example, seafood enjoys popularity in coastal areas because of ready availability, lower cost that reflects lower transportation expense, and local industry advertising. Preference is thus influenced by climate, geography, and economics.

In California, the state's agricultural richness affects preference, as do ethnic demographics—characteristics of human populations. California's large quantities of fruits and vegetables, the popularization of the salad as a part of the meal, and the large numbers of Mexican-Americans,

Orientals, and Italians all combine to give California its distinct cuisine.

In the southern states, corn, fish, and rice are often used. Hot breads, such as biscuits or corn bread, accompany meals. Green leafy vegetables are cooked with a piece of "fatback" (pork back fat), a regional practice that yields a consumable liquid known as pot liquor. Before mechanical refrigeration was developed, milk and cheese were consumed only in

Dwight Experienced Chicken Soup Withdrawal

Dwight, a 45-year-old businessman, went to his physician with complaints of fever, chest tightness, and general weakness. His temperature was 105°. Examination showed that he was suffering acute lung trouble and was in a severely weakened state. After x-rays and other tests, pneumonia was diagnosed.

The doctor prescribed chicken soup for Dwight. Within 36 hours he began to improve. By the fifth day his chest x-ray was normal. Due to his significant improvement, Dwight declined further chicken soup.

Three days after discontinuing his soup "medication," Dwight experienced sharp chest pain,

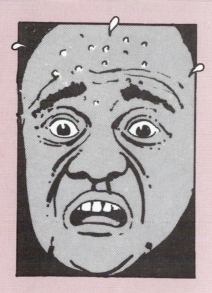

nausea, and vomiting, and he was subsequently hospitalized. The hospital found that he had a temperature of 104°, was suffering from severe respiratory distress, and could only be classified as acutely ill. Laboratory tests confirmed pneumonia.

Unfortunately, chicken soup was unavailable. With massive amounts of intravenous penicillin, Dwight recovered and was dischargd from the hospital 24 hours after admission. This case can be understood as an example of too abrupt a withdrawl from chicken soup.

SOURCE: Adapted from N. L. Caroline and H. Schwartz. *Chest* 67 (1975): 215.

small quantities; storage and shipping were not possible. The national consumption of dairy products has shown an increase since the 1940s and 1950s.

ETHNIC, CULTURAL, AND RELIGIOUS INFLUENCES

Each ethnic, cultural, and religious group has certain characteristic food patterns or preferences. Sometimes these characteristics remain unique to the group, but more often they become a part of our nation. In that regard the United States can be described as a melting pot, both figuratively and literally. The remaining part of this chapter will explore such influences.

Europeans

Many of the foods we have come to think of as typically American were in fact brought to us from European countries. Norwegian, Swedish, and Danish immigrants brought a greater use of milk, numerous cheeses, cream, and butter. In their native countries, Western Europeans relied on fish, shellfish, and vegetables. Especially popular were potatoes, dark breads, eggs, cheese, beef, pork, and poultry.

Central Europeans favored potatoes, rye flour, wheat, pork, sausage, and cabbage. Cabbage was especially favored and was eaten raw, cooked, or salted as sauerkraut. Common vegetables included turnips, carrots, squash, onion, beans, and greens.

Italian families in the United States have perpetuated many favorite foods of their ancestors and have concurrently made them basics of the American diet. The huge sale of pizza and pasta products and the number of Italian restaurants confirm this fact. There are nearly as many pizza stands in the United States as there are hamburger and fried chicken businesses. Daily the typical Italian diet features pasta made from hard-wheat dough. Its innumerable forms are seasoned with sauces, onions, tomatoes, cheese, peppers, and meat. Bread usually accompanies the meal.

Differences exist between northern and southern Italian foods. The northern area of Italy is more industrialized, and meat, root vegetables, and dairy products are more popular there. Southern Italy's preference tends toward fish, spices, and olive oil. The southern Italian diet can benefit from more green vegetables, eggs, fruits, meat, and milk. The latter two food items can especially benefit the nutrient intake of children.

Experienced dietitians and nurses know that hospitalization can be especially difficult for Italians, who have a strong sense of family and a strong preference for traditional foods. Institutional diets that cater to Italian patients can both reduce feelings of isolation and increase nutritional intake.

Native Americans

It may come as a surprise that over half the plant foods you eat—including corn, potatoes, squash, pumpkin, tomatoes, peppers, beans, wild rice, cranberries, and cocoa—come from North, Central, and South American Indians. The Native American diet also utilized acorns, wild fruit, fish, wild fowl, small and large game, and seafood. The food preservation methods that produce jerky and pemmican were introduced to the frontier Americans by the Native Americans. Corn, which has become a world staple, is a significant example of their culture's contribution.

Diet varies from tribe to tribe depending on geographical location. Historically, the natural resources of the tribe's home area determined such occupations as hunting, fishing, agriculture, and herding. Native Americans who lived near the coast used large amounts of seafood. Those in the Northwest were and still are great fishermen, and from Alaska to the Columbia River one of the most prized items is salmon. A favorite method of preserving fish and meat is smoking; racks of drying fish can be seen along the river banks where Native Americans live. Along the New England coast, shellfish is a favorite, especially clams. A favored method of cooking is open-air baking of clams and fish over hot coals. Sometimes seafood is baked in the sand. The item is wrapped in seaweed or similar materials and placed in sand kept hot by a fire.

In the past, the Plains Indians depended more on game, fowl, and freshwater fish. Native vegetables and fruits were generously used and cultivated if the group was a stationary, agricultural one. Many vegetables that originated in North and South America have become part of the American and world diet. Since little food storage was possible, nutritional life was characterized by the extremes of bounty and scarcity. Despite such fluctuations in availability, the historical Native American diet was undoubtedly more nutritional than is their diet today.

With the introduction of trading-post products such as lard, sugar, coffee, and canned meat and canned milk, the American Indian diet began to assimilate European food customs, leaving little today that can be distinguished as a Native American food pattern.

Native American food specialties that can be found today include the clambakes, fry bread (biscuit dough fried in fat), and wajupi, a pudding made from berries, sugars, and cornstarch. Northern California Indians have revived the use of acorns in preparing soup and flour, methods of preparing eels, and stews combining meat, vegetables, and berries. Often these traditional foods play a part in tribal ceremonies. As cultural renewal has taken place among Native Americans, and as the Native American heritage is becoming better understood, interest in traditional Native American foods is being revived.

The nutritional weakness of the Native American diet is a low intake of milk by children after weaning. Vitamin C intake is also low, and the greater use of fruits, vegetables, and lean meat will improve the diet.

The present generation of Native Americans may be consuming too much sugar and soft drinks. Sound nutritional education is needed. Extensive alcohol abuse among some adult males has also hurt the nutritional status of these people.

Black Americans

Among middle- and upper-income blacks, food selections are similar to those of their white counterparts. Among poor families, many of whom have come from or still live in the southern states, the traditional eating pattern is determined to a large extent by the cost and availability of foods. However, there are many food items preferred by black families, rich or poor.

The popularization of the term "soul food" indicates the effort to recognize the uniqueness of black American food habits. One characteristic black food habit is the use of hominy grits, especially for breakfast with some form of pork. Cornbread, muffins, or biscuits are preferred to yeast bread. There are differences between the dietary habits of southern blacks and northern blacks, and one of these differences is in the customary use of greens.

Among southern blacks, fresh greens such as mustard, turnip, and collard are popular and are usually served with pork such as fatback or salt pork. In the north, fresh greens are less available, and a much wider variety of frozen greens are used. Other vegetable favorites include fresh corn, lima beans, cabbage, sweet potatoes, and squash. The use of fresh fruit emphasizes oranges, watermelon, and peaches.

Black-eyed peas and corn are well liked, as indicated earlier; a mixture of black-eyed peas and rice called "Hoppin' John" is a favorite southern dish. A favorite method of preparing green vegetables is to boil them with a small amount of fat pork; the resultant juice (pot liquor) is also used in the meal. Potatoes (white and sweet) and yams are popular, and sweet potatoes are often made into pies.

Carbohydrate is generally obtained from grits, potatoes, and rice, though black-eyed peas and dried beans are also used. The latter provide some protein, as does fried fish, especially when locally caught. Other meats frequently used include poultry, pork (both cured and fresh), and wild game. All parts of an animal are used, especially among poor families. Dishes made from a slaughtered pig, for instance, include chitlings (the small intestines, cleaned and fried crisp); hog maws (the stomach lining); boiled pig's feet; and the neckbone, jaws, snout, and head, which are cooked and made into scrapple. Frying, stewing, and barbecuing are the favored methods of preparation. Sweets such as molasses, pastries, cakes, and candy are especially popular.

Milk consumption, which is often low, should be encouraged, especially among children. Buttermilk and ice cream are well liked by black Americans, although there is little use of cheeses. The use of more citrus fruits should be encouraged.

As the economic status of black people improves, they eat more meat and their diet improves generally. Since their typical diet is high in fat and carbohydrate and low in protein, iron, and vitamin C, an increased consumption of lean meat, milk, and citrus fruits will help balance their nutrient intake. Table 26-1 lists popular foods among blacks.

It is in preparation that the essence of the term "soul food" can be found. It is not necessarily the unique foods but rather the care in preparation that is emphasized. Food preparation offers the opportunity to minister to the physical health and well-being of those who will consume the food. The opportunity to bring happiness, health, and love through food preparation lies at the figurative and literal heart of the customary black dietary habits.

Jews

Orthodox Jews follow Old Testament and rabbinical dietary laws; Conservative Jews distinguish between meals served in the home and those outside it; Reformed Jews do not observe dietary regulations. The country of origin can further influence a Jewish family's dietary practices.

Foods used according to strict Jewish laws are referred to as "Kosher." Those who follow those dietary laws eat only animals that are designated as clean and are killed in a ritualistic manner. The method of slaughter minimizes pain and maximizes blood drainage. Blood, the symbol of life, is strictly avoided by soaking the meat in cold water, draining it, salting it, and rinsing it three times. Permitted meats include poultry, fish with fins and scales, and quadruped animals that chew the cud and have divided hooves. (Thus, pork cannot be eaten.) The hindquarter of quadruped animals must have the hip sinew or the thigh vein removed.

Kosher laws additionally require separation of meat and milk. Milk and its products must be excluded from meals involving meat but can be consumed prior to the meat meal. If a milk meal is to be consumed, meat and its products are excluded from the milk meal and for six hours thereafter. Usually two milk meals and one meat meal are eaten each day. A Kosher household will maintain two sets of dishes, utensils, and cooking supplies, one for meat meals and one for milk meals.

Certain foods, viewed as neutral, are referred to as *pareve*. Fruits, uncooked vegetables, eggs, and "clean" fish, since they are recognized as neutral, can be consumed with either meat or milk meals.

No food can be cooked or heated on Saturday, the Sabbath, so the evening meal preceding the Sabbath tends to be the most substantial of

Table 26-1
Characteristic Black Food Choices

PROTEIN FOODS	MILK AND MILK PRODUCTS	GRAIN PRODUCTS	VEGETABLES	FRUITS	OTHER
Meat	Milk	Rice	Broccoli	Apples	Salt pork
Beef	Fluid	Cornbread	Cabbage	Bananas	Carbonated
Pork and ham	Evaporated,	Hominy grits	Carrots	Grapefruit	beverages
Sausage	in coffee	Biscuits	Corn	Grapes	Fruit drinks
Pig's feet, ears, etc.	Buttermilk	Muffins	Green beans	Nectarines	Gravies
Bacon	Cheese	White bread	Greens	Oranges	
Luncheon meat	Cheddar	Dry cereal	Mustard	Plums	
Organ meats	Cottage	Cooked cereal	Collard	Tangerines	
Poultry	Ice cream	Macaroni	Kale	Watermelons	
Chicken		Spaghetti	Spinach		
Turkey		Crackers	Turnips, etc.		
Fish			Lima beans		
Catfish			Okra		
Perch			Peas		
Red snapper			Potatoes		
Tuna			Pumpkins		
Salmon			Sweet potatoes		
Sardines			Tomatoes		
Shrimp			Yams		
Eggs					
Legumes					
Kidney beans					
Red beans					
Pinto beans					
Black-eyed peas					
Nuts					
Peanuts					
Peanut butter					

SOURCE: "Nutrition During Pregnancy and Lactation." California Department of Health, 1975 (revised).

the week. Both chicken and fish are served at that meal. Any foods eaten on the Sabbath must be cooked on a preceding day.

On Jewish holidays, symbolic foods are eaten. For example, Passover, a spring festival, commemorates the flight of the Jews from Egypt.

JEWISH TRADITIONS
SOMETIMES CREATE MEDICAL PROBLEMS

Jewish law governs food practices that are ideally designed to promote health; however, cases have been reported in which medical conditions resulted from the practices.

In one case, a Jewish family was found to be suffering from salmonellosis. The family was following the practice of *Shmito*, which calls for abstaining from Jewish farm produce so that the poor and animals may eat it. Instead, the family ate produce from non-Jewish farms, and those farms used raw sewage for fertilizer. The sewage was the source of the pathogen sal-

monella. Being Orthodox Jews, they complied with the strict Rabbinic law and washed their hands meticulously before every meal and after going to the toilet. Repeated salmonella infection is uncommon under such careful hygenic practice.

In a second case, during the festival of Purim, an 8-year-old boy was admitted to a hospital after eating two dozen freshly baked Haman-Tashen, three-cornered cookies traditional with that feast. In addition to jam, the cookies contained poppy seeds, and it was suspected that opium alkaloids had

contaminated the cookies. Normally, poppy seeds are virtually opium alkaloid-free and do not possess any narcotic properties. However, laboratory analysis showed that opiates were present in the capsules containing the seeds used in the cookies. The symptoms of opium poisoning included vomiting, sweating, hallucinations, and abdominal pain. This accident could have been avoided if the poppy seeds had been bought from commercial sources.

SOURCE: Adapted from M. Berant. *JAMA* 250 (1983): 2469.

Passover celebration lasts eight days, and only unleavened bread, called matzo, is permitted. An Orthodox household will, therefore, use separate utensils for preparing unleavened bread to avoid any contact with leavening. Other holidays include Rosh Hashanah (Jewish New Year), Sukkoth (fall harvest), Chanukkah (the festival of lights), Purim (the arrival of spring), and Yom Kippur (the day of atonement), when fasting occurs.

Mexican-Americans

People of Mexican descent make up a large part of the population of the Southwest. They therefore reside close to their native country and maintain a close tie to traditional Mexican foods. A lack of refrigeration in such warmer climates creates a scarcity of meat, milk, eggs, vegetables, and fruits. For lower-income families, the expense of these nutrient-rich foods can be prohibitive.

Items basic to the Mexican diet include dry beans, chili peppers, tomatoes, and corn. The corn is ground, soaked in lime water, and baked on a griddle to make tortillas, the popular flat breads that can be rolled and filled with ground beef and vegetables to make tacos. Tacos provide nutrients from all four food groups, although the user of wheat tortillas reduces the calcium obtained from lime-soaked corn tortillas. Many foods are fried, and beans are even refried until they absorb all the fat.

Nutritionists encourage retention of the basic Mexican diet with only minor modifications. Because of iron, vitamin A, and calcium deficiencies, use of lean meat is recommended in taco fillings. Dark green and yellow vegetables, fruits, and milk—dried if fresh milk is too expensive—are also recommended. The milk is especially important for children. One Mexican dietary practice that is particularly encouraged is the practice of limiting the amount of sweets consumed.

Table 26-2 shows the characteristic Mexican-American food choices.

Puerto Ricans

The Puerto Rican diet has similarities to the dietary patterns of other Caribbean Islands but is noteworthy because so many Puerto Ricans emigrate to the United States.

Traditional emphasis is on beans, rice, and starchy root vegetables (and plantains) known as *viandas*. Rice and beans eaten together are a high-quality, complementary protein combination. The beans are often boiled and then cooked with *sofrito*, a mixture made from tomatoes, green peppers, onions, garlic, salt pork, lard, and herbs. *Viandas* are

Table 26-2
Characteristic Mexican-American Food Choices

PROTEIN FOODS	MILK AND MILK PRODUCTS	GRAIN PRODUCTS	VEGETABLES	FRUITS	OTHER
Meat	Milk	Rice	Avocados	Apples	Salsa (tomato-pepper-onion relish)
Beef	Fluid	Tortillas	Cabbage	Apricots	
Pork	Flavored	Corn	Carrots	Bananas	Chili sauce
Lamb	Evaporated	Flour	Chilies	Guavas	Guacamole
Tripe	Condensed	Oatmeal	Corn	Lemons	Lard (manteca)
Sausage (chorizo)	Cheese	Dry cereals	Green beans	Mangos	Pork cracklings
Bologna	American	Cornflakes	Lettuce	Melons	Fruit drinks
Bacon	Monterey jack	Sugar coated	Onions	Oranges	Kool-aid
Poultry	Hoop	Noodles	Peas	Peaches	Carbonated beverages
Chicken	Ice cream	Spaghetti	Potatoes	Pears	
Eggs		White bread	Prickly pear cactus leaf (nopales)	Prickly pear cactus fruit (tuna)	Beer
Legumes		Sweet bread (pan dulce)			Coffee
Pinto beans			Spinach	Zapote (or sapote)	
Pink beans			Sweet potatoes		
Garbanzo beans			Tomatoes		
Lentils			Zucchini		
Nuts					
Peanuts					
Peanut butter					

SOURCE: "Nutrition During Pregnancy and Lactation." California Department of Health, 1975 (revised).

good sources of B vitamins, iron, calories, and in some cases, vitamin C. Salt codfish is more popular than fresh fish. Chicken, beef, and pork are favored. Coffee with 2 to 5 oz of milk per cup—*café con leche*—is drunk several times a day, contributing to an otherwise low consumption of milk. Fruits prove an especially popular food due to availability, with such native fruits as papaya, mango, and acerola (the West Indian cherry, which is extremely high in vitamin C) being joined by bananas, oranges, and pineapple.

The mainstays of the Puerto Rican diet may be hard to find or expensive in the United States. And since Puerto Ricans come from an agrarian background and thus often lack the job skills for a highly industrialized society, they often find themselves in the lowest socioeconomic classes in the United States, living in crowded urban conditions with poor cooking and refrigeration facilities and unable to feed their families as well as they did in Puerto Rico. Consequently, malnutrition is not uncommon among their children. Also, Puerto Rican children born in the United States may have adopted favorite mainland foods such as hamburgers, hot dogs, canned spaghetti, and cold cereals instead of the traditional Puerto Rican food prepared by their mothers. If these children have picked up the mainland habit of snacking on nutrient-light foods, they may be more poorly nourished than people adhering to the relatively inexpensive but nutritionally adequate traditional diet of Puerto Rico.

Nutritionists encourage Puerto Ricans living in northern mainland cities to become familiar with different fruits, which are inexpensive when they are in season or canned; to use more milk, cheese, and inexpensive cuts of meat; and to substitute canned tomatoes for fresh tomatoes, which are expensive when not in season.

Middle Eastern People

Middle East peoples—Greeks, Iranians, Arabs, Turks, Armenians, and Lebanese—tend to be farmers. Dietary emphasis is on crops and animals raised—cattle, sheep, goats, chickens, ducks, geese, grains, fruits, and vegetables. Lamb holds the position of the favored meat, and wheat products, grains, and rice are the major energy sources. Popular dairy foods, derived from sheep, goats, and camels, are sour milk, including yogurt, fermented milk, and sour cream.

Lentils and beans may be boiled or stewed with tomatoes, onions, and olive oil; they may be eaten alone or mixed with other foods. A favorite combination is seasoned chick-peas mixed with bulgur (wheat that has been steamed, cracked and fried) and spices and then fried in fat.

Traditional vegetables include okra, squash, tomatoes, onions, leeks, peppers, spinach, brussels sprouts, cabbage, peas, green beans, dandelion greens, eggplant, artichokes, and olives. Grape leaves, used either fresh or canned, are stuffed with rice, bulgur, meat, and seasonings.

Fruits grown in these warm climates are used extensively. Some common ones are dates, figs, melons, cherries, oranges, apricots, and raisins.

Common Middle Eastern cereals include rice, wheat, and barley. Typical breads are flat, thin, and round and may be baked outdoors. Olive oil and butter from sheep's and goat's milk are used generously. Turkish coffee, a favorite beverage in the Middle East, is a strong, dark drink containing the crushed coffee bean and is served with a generous amount of sugar.

The Middle Eastern diet is a good one, contributing adequate nutrients. But Middle Eastern people in the United States may have difficulty obtaining the foods if they cannot afford them, since they are usually expensive.

Orientals

The United States is also home to many people of Asian heritage. The diets of the Chinese, Japanese, and Filipino are discussed below.

CHINESE

China is a vast country with many different regional foods. In the United States, most of the Chinese on the West Coast come from southern China and adhere to a Cantonese diet. This type of cookery uses little fat and subtle seasonings. Beef, pork, poultry, and all kinds of seafoods are well liked. In Chinese cooking, all parts of the animal are utilized, including organs, blood, and skin. Rice is the predominant cereal used by the Cantonese, both at home and in the United States. Northern Chinese use more bread, noodles, and dumplings, which are prepared from wheat, corn, and millet.

The Chinese diet is varied, containing eggs, fish, meat, soybeans, and a great variety of vegetables. Many green, leafy vegetables unfamiliar to

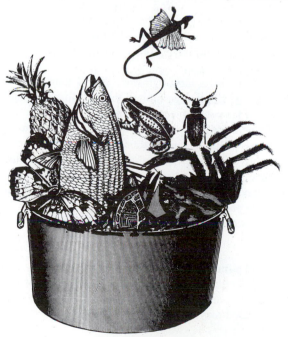

Americans, such as leaves of the radish and shepherd's purse, are enjoyed. Sprouts of bamboo and beans are incorporated into some dishes, giving a distinctive flavor and texture. Many Chinese recipes call for mushrooms and nuts. Eggs from ducks, hens, and pigeons are widely used—fresh, preserved, and pickled. Soy sauce is used both in preparation and serving. The high salt content of this flavorable condiment is a problem for Chinese patients whose salt intake may be restricted by the physician.

Chinese cookery is unique in many ways. Food is quickly cooked over the heat source, usually cut into small pieces so that the short cooking period is adequate. Vegetables retain their crispness, flavor, and practically all their nutrients: this method of cookery, which has been widely adopted, is quite beneficial. When vegetables are cooked in water, the liquid is also consumed.

Probably the greatest weakness in the Chinese diet is a low intake of milk and milk products, a consequence of lactose intolerance. However, a higher consumption of meat and the frequent use of soybeans prevent calcium and protein deficiency. In addition, for undefined reasons Chinese children born in the United States have a higher tolerance for milk.

Table 26-3 lists the characteristic Chinese foods.

JAPANESE
Japanese people who have emigrated to the United States, especially the older people, tend to follow the food habits of their homeland rather closely. Typical of the Japanese food pattern is much use of fish, both fresh and saltwater. Methods of preparation vary. Fish may be eaten raw or deep-fat fried, dried, or salted. Many kinds of vegetables may be prepared with meat or eaten separately. Protein intake comes from meat, fish, eggs, legumes, nuts, and, most popular of all, soybean curd (tofu), which is sold in many American grocery stores. Eggs are prepared in many ways and are well liked.

The basic cereal is rice, although since World War II wheat has been consumed. Milk and cheese are limited in the traditional Japanese diet, mainly because of lactose intolerance. Japanese born in the United States have a greater tolerance for dairy products such as milk and cheeses, and they also eat more fruits. It is important that the Japanese in this country eat enriched, converted, or whole-grain rice, which contains more nutrients than unenriched rice with the husks removed. To avoid excessive nutrient loss, they should also be told to refrain from washing the rice repeatedly before preparing it.

Table 26-4 lists characteristic Japanese foods.

FILIPINOS
The Filipino food pattern is similar to those of the Chinese and Japanese. The basic cereal is rice, and the principal sources of protein are fish, meat, eggs, legumes, and nuts. Meat is prepared by roasting, frying, or boiling; the fish used may be fresh or dried.

A large variety of vegetables and fruits is found in the diet. Vegetables are usually boiled or pan-fried, and some are used as salad dishes. Most fruits are eaten raw, but they are sometimes used in cooking.

Again, because of lactose intolerance, Filipinos have a low intake of milk and milk products. The consumption of good calcium and protein sources should be encouraged, especially among the young. Growing children may also have a problem with low caloric intake. Larger servings of food should be encouraged, especially more meat; food preparers

Table 26-3
Characteristic Chinese Food Choices

PROTEIN FOODS	MILK AND MILK PRODUCTS	GRAIN PRODUCTS	VEGETABLES	FRUITS	OTHER
Meat	Flavored milk	Rice	Bamboo shoots	Apples	Soy sauce
Pork	Milk (cooking)	Noodles	Beans	Bananas	Sweet and
Beef	Ice cream	White bread	Green	Figs	sour sauce
Organ meats		Barley	Yellow	Grapes	Mustard sauce
Poultry		Millet	Bean sprouts	Kumquats	Ginger
Chicken			Bok choy	Loquats	Plum sauce
Duck			Broccoli	Mangos	Red bean paste
Fish			Cabbage	Melons	Tea
White fish			Carrots	Oranges	Coffee
Shrimp			Celery	Peaches	
Lobster			Chinese cabbage	Pears	
Oyster			Corn	Persimmons	
Sardines			Cucumbers	Pineapples	
Eggs			Eggplant	Plums	
Legumes			Greens	Tangerines	
Soybeans			Collard		
Soybean curd (tofu)			Chinese broccoli		
Black beans			Mustard		
Nuts			Kale		
Peanuts			Spinach		
Almonds			Leeks		
Cashews			Lettuce		
			Mushrooms		
			Peppers		
			Potatoes		
			Scallions		
			Snow peas		
			Sweet potatoes		
			Taro		
			Tomatoes		
			Waterchestnuts		
			White radishes		
			White turnips		
			Winter melons		

SOURCE: "Nutrition During Pregnancy and Lactation." California Department of Health, 1975 (revised).

should also be instructed about the use of enriched rice without pre-washing.

Table 26-5 lists the characteristics of Filipino food choices.

The Eskimos: Meeting of Two Cultures

For years, the Eskimos of the far north have maintained their culture on a diet consisting almost entirely of meat and fish. This culture has fascinated nutritionists, since it runs counter to all that is known about the necessity of a balanced diet.

Caribou, whale, and seals form the staples of the traditional diet, with walrus, fish, and birds being of minor importance. Edible plants

Table 26-4
Characteristic Japanese Food Choices

PROTEIN FOODS	MILK AND MILK PRODUCTS	GRAIN PRODUCTS	VEGETABLES	FRUITS	OTHER
Meat	Milk	Rice	Bamboo shoots	Apples	Soy sauce
Beef	Ice cream	Rice crackers	Bok choy	Apricots	Nori paste
Pork	Cheese	Noodles (whole	Broccoli	Bananas	(used to
Poultry		wheat noodle	Burdock root	Cherries	season rice)
Chicken		called soba)	Cabbage	Grapefruits	Bean thread
Turkey		Spaghetti	Carrots	Grapes	(konyaku)
Fish		White bread	Cauliflower	Lemons	Ginger (shoga;
Tuna		Oatmeal	Celery	Limes	dried form
Mackerel		Dry cereals*	Cucumbers	Melons	called deni-
Sardines			Eggplants	Oranges	shoga)
(dried form			Green beans	Peaches	Tea
called mezashi)			Gourd (kampyo)	Pears	Coffee
Sea bass			Mushrooms	Persimmons	
Shrimp			Mustard greens	Pineapples	
Abalone			Napa cabbage	Pomegranates	
Squid			Peas	Plums (dried	
Octopus			Peppers	pickled plums	
Eggs			Radishes (white	called umeboshi)	
Legumes			radish called	Strawberries	
Soybean curd			daikon; pickled	Tangerines	
(tofu)			white radish		
Soybean paste			called takawan)		
(miso)			Snow peas		
Soybeans			Spinach		
Red beans			Squash		
(azuki)			Sweet potatoes		
Lima beans			Taro (Japanese		
Nuts			sweet potato)		
Chestnuts			Tomatoes		
(kuri)			Turnips		
			Waterchestnuts		
			Yams		

*Nisei only.
SOURCE: "Nutrition During Pregnancy and Lactation." California Department of Health, 1975 (revised).

and berries are scarce. Although it had been believed that Eskimos consumed the stomach contents of the animals, that assumption is debatable. There is agreement that the Eskimo diet is very high in protein and fat, and very low in carbohydrate.

The high protein content provides calories essential to an active life and additionally contributes to blood glucose, an essential metabolic fuel for the nervous system. What carbohydrate has been available has been obtained through synthesis of glycogen from muscles. A byproduct of the traditional diet has been the virtual nonexistence of diabetes. This disease has, however, been on the increase since the introduction of sugar to the culture.

Table 26-5
Characteristic Filipino Food Choices

PROTEIN FOODS	MILK AND MILK PRODUCTS	GRAIN PRODUCTS	VEGETABLES	FRUITS	OTHER
Meat	Milk	Rice	Bamboo shoots	Apples	Soy sauce
Pork	Flavored	Cooked cereals	Beets	Bananas	Coffee
Beef	Evaporated	Farina	Cabbage	Grapes	Tea
Goat	Cheese	Oatmeal	Carrots	Guavas	
Deer	Gouda	Dry cereals	Cauliflower	Lemons	
Rabbit	Cheddar	Pastas	Celery	Limes	
Variety meats		Rice noodles	Chinese celery	Mangos	
Poultry		Wheat noodles	Eggplants	Melons	
Chicken		Macaroni	Endive	Oranges	
Fish		Spaghetti	Green beans	Papayas	
Sole			Leeks	Pears	
Bonito			Lettuce	Pineapples	
Herring			Mushrooms	Plums	
Tuna			Okra	Pomegranates	
Mackerel			Onions	Rhubarb	
Crab			Peppers	Strawberries	
Mussels			Potatoes	Tangerines	
Shrimp			Pumpkins		
Squid			Radishes		
Eggs			Snow peas		
Legumes			Spinach		
Black beans			Sweet potatoes		
Chick peas			Tomatoes		
Black-eyed peas			Water chestnuts		
Lentils			Watercress		
Mung beans			Yams		
Lima beans					
White kidney beans					
Nuts					
Peanuts					
Pili nuts					

SOURCE: "Nutrition During Pregnancy and Lactation." California Department of Health, 1975 (revised).

A unique characteristic of Eskimo nutrition is the utilization of fatty acids from oils as energy. Tissues can adapt to the utilization of **ketone bodies** instead of glucose as energy source. The ketone bodies form in the liver and are characteristic of high-fat, low-carbohydrate diets. Eskimos thus provide a human example of a unique metabolic phenomenon.

As we saw in the discussion of vitamins, we should expect scurvy among Eskimos. But their culture has escaped scurvy because they eat fish and meat either raw or only slightly cooked. What little vitamin C is available is not destroyed by oxidation in the cooking process.

Vitamins A, D, E, and K are obtained in sufficient quantities from the traditional Eskimo diet, as are B vitamins. The diet is low in calcium, a problem that surfaces in bone fragility among Eskimos. Children are somewhat protected by a traditionally long nursing period.

As nontraditional dietary habits have gained popularity in the Eskimo culture, our problems have become theirs. Heart disease, diabetes, tooth decay, and hypertension are now on the increase.

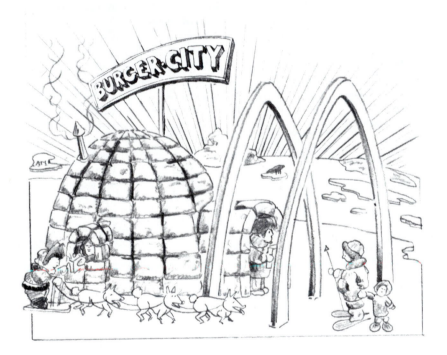

People and Their Land

As you have probably determined from these discussions of culture and nutrition, our food habits are very much influenced by our geographical location. Relationships between people and their land can be profound, and they have given rise to fields of knowledge ranging from cultural geography to literary analysis focusing on agrarian mythology. Although it has been said that we are what we eat, perhaps we should also say that we eat where we are.

STUDY QUESTIONS

1. What factors have weakened regional and ethnic food traditions?

2. Name some now-common American foods used by settlers from various parts of Europe.

3. What are some Kosher food regulations? What is the significance of pareve foods in Kosher meal planning?

4. How adequate is the traditional Mexican diet? Which foods are little used and why?

5. Describe Chinese cookery. What is the nutritional advantage of its food preparation methods? What food is notably lacking in the Chinese diet? Why?

6. Discuss the nutritional adequacy of the Eskimo diet.

7. Using library resources, select an area in which Native Americans reside and compare the dietary intake of the residents with those described in the text.

8. Discuss the nutritional adequacy of the diets of the following using research materials: Australian aborigines, Brazilians, and Jamaicans.

REFERENCES

Baker, L., ed. *The Psychobiology of Human Food Selection*. Westport, Conn.: AVI Publishing, 1982.

Root, W., and R. DeRochement. *Eating in America: A History*. New York: Eco Press, 1976.

Sanjur, D. *Social and Cultural Perspectives in Nutrition*. Englewood Cliffs, N.J.: Prentice-Hall, 1982.

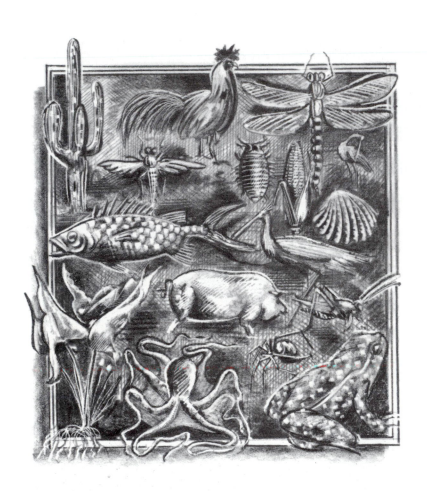

27

INTERNATIONAL NUTRITION:

OUR BATTLE WITH WORLD HUNGER

IN THE NEXT 60 SECONDS . . .

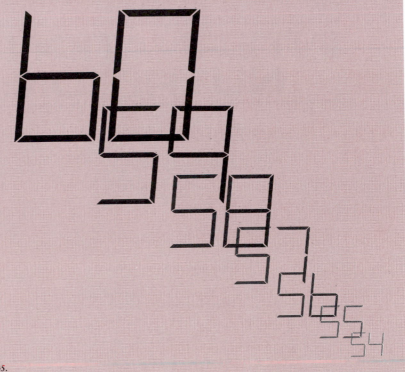

233 babies will be born
  136 in Asia
  39 in Africa
  23 in Latin America
  35 in the rest of the world

26 of these 233 will die before age 1
  19 in Africa vs. 1 in North America
  5 in Latin America versus 1 in Europe

34 more will die before age 15

50 to 75 percent of these deaths can be attributed to a combination of malnutrition and infectious diseases.

Many who do survive beyond age 15 will be stunted in growth and will suffer brain damage that can incapacitate them for life.

SOURCE: From "Overcoming World Hunger: The Challenge Ahead," a report of The Presidential Commission on World Hunger, March 1980, p. 45.

The Global Perspective

A familiar maxim is inherent in the issues surrounding international nutrition: "Give me a fish and I will eat for a day; teach me to fish and I will eat forever." From the perspective of international nutrition, we cannot help but be overwhelmed—overwhelmed by the wonder of people's tenacity for life, the nutritional needs they face, and the inequities of life. How many children in the world are malnourished? Where will we find the food to feed them? How do you provide them with clean water? What can anyone do about the terrible drought affecting some parts of the world? Such questions seem almost imponderable, but we cannot be human without confronting them (Berg). We feel a human obligation to battle world hunger.

We know the problems that surround issues of international nutrition and world hunger. We know certain nations have food surpluses, while others have shortages. We know that the economic principle of supply and demand has certain effects on nutrition. We have seen that, in a country with food shortages and starving people, food supplies can be brought in, increasing the supply. When the supply increases, prices drop. Then it becomes the farmers in that country who are suffering. These complexities make world hunger and international nutrition much more difficult problems than either might initially appear to be.

There may be no better perspectives on world hunger than those expressed by the World Food Conference of 1974 and the Presidential Commission on World Hunger of 1980. The former conference expressed its views in the following:

Large numbers of people, particularly the less advantaged in many countries, lack adequate and appropriate food resulting in adverse effects on their health, their development and their ability to learn and work for basic livelihood. Overconsumption among the affluent not only impairs their health but also contributes to reducing the food availability for less advantaged groups and furthermore using large food resources to feed animals. Malnutrition is closely linked to widespread poverty and inadequate social and institutional structures, and its effects are aggravated by infectious diseases and the lack of environmental sanitation. Increased agricultural production and increased incomes may not by themselves lead to improved nutrition. To this end a more just and equitable distribution of food and incomes is essential, among nations as well as within countries among their various social categories.

Information on food consumption patterns and on their consequences for the nutrition and health status of the majority of the population in developing countries is insufficient and inadequate. Improved knowledge about how to prevent malnutrition through better use of available food resources, including human milk, is essential.

The 1980 report of the Presidential Commission on World Hunger issued its statements after looking at the nature, extent, and causes of world hunger through the rest of this century. The commission's views are expressed in the following:

There are no physical or natural reasons why all the men, women and children in the world cannot have enough food to eat. With careful management of the world's natural resource base, it should be possible to maintain the global balance between population and food supply. Distressing as the problem of hunger is today, it will become much worse in an increasingly interdependent world, with fewer possibilities for easy adjustment, more people to feed and greater economic and political uncertainties, unless the indifference of many national leaders is replaced by concern and commitment.

The prospects for eliminating world hunger will depend in large measure on the attainment of greater economic growth and increased food production in the developing countries. However, unless the programs for achieving growth and producing more food are designed specifically to benefit poor and malnourished people in ways that enable them to help themselves, neither hunger nor poverty can be overcome in the foreseeable future.

In the end, the issue of ending world hunger comes down to a question of political choice—a factor that is no more predictable than the weather, but far more susceptible to human control. The quantities of food and money needed to wipe out hunger are remarkably small in relation to available global resources. The necessary human ingenuity also abounds in all nations of the world, although that quality is too often harnessed to different and often conflicting goals. The Commission agrees with other studies that if the appropriate political choices are made, the world can overcome the worst aspects of hunger and malnutrition by the year 2000. This end can be accomplished through the alleviation of malnutrition in the world of today, in tandem with more fundamental efforts to build a future world in which hunger will be unknown.

Multiple Causes of World Hunger

The complex and interrelated issues of food supply, population, poverty, culture, food preference, and politics have dominated history. There are many causes of world hunger and malnutrition, especially in underdeveloped countries (Brown, 1977; Caliendo; Levinson). Primary causes include natural and man-made disasters (such as accidents, sickness, drought, war, floods, and civil disorders), poverty and unequal distribution of wealth, lack of natural resources, culturally ingrained food habits, food contamination and unsanitary living conditions, malabsorption from all causes, ill-prepared pregnancy and lactation, infection, and ignorance and lack of education. For example, thousands of people died of starvation and disease in Mauritania during 1968 through 1973 because of the great Sahelian drought, as symbolized by the dead livestock and parched grazing grounds shown in Figure 27-1.

To illustrate the ecological nature of malnutrition, Doctors J. Cravioto and E. R. Delicardie of the United Nations developed a series of flow diagrams constructed with data obtained from their studies of communities in Mexico, Central America, South America, and Africa. Factors such as limited technology, resources, education, health knowledge, and large families in an underdeveloped or developing country can be associated with childhood undernutrition. These factors are not necessarily the causes of childhood malnutrition, but they are at least contributory factors.

The following analysis of the causes of world hunger combines some of the arguments presented by Doctors Cravioto and Delicardie with the reasoning of other experts.

Poverty lies at the root of hunger, both land poverty and financial poverty. If people have neither the money to buy food nor the land to

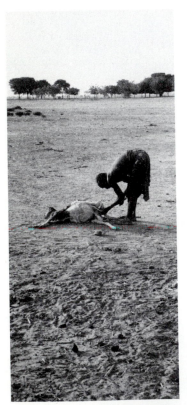

Figure 27-1: Drought in Mauritania. SOURCE: UNICEF photo by Davico.

grow it, we could double the world's food supply and still have 800 million people below the level of a minimally adequate diet.

Coupled with basic poverty is the problem of insecure food supply. In many nations, poor weather, political instability, or natural disaster can cause famine where it did not previously exist. Too many countries simply are not self-reliant.

We know that a group of poor living conditions contributes to malnutrition. Poor health, high unemployment, illiteracy, crowded housing, and contaminated water are all common to both poverty and malnutrition. Also common is unequal distribution. Two countries can be equal in both population and food production, yet the incidence of malnutrition in one country can be double the incidence of that of the other, simply because the available food in one country is not accessible to a large number of the country's population.

Land ownership is generally unequal, and the person with a large farm has food available, whereas the person without land does not. Unequal land ownership concentrates food in the hands of a few. Unequal food distribution can be offset only by efficient transportation systems, something often lacking in developing countries. Inequitable distribution proves a very difficult problem to resolve.

Similarly, low productivity characterizes many developing nations. Poor countries simply produce far less than industrialized ones. Such low productivity results from a combination of causes such as inadequate equipment, untrained workers, unequal land ownership, and unequal distribution of other assets necessary to food production. If a country cannot provide incentives to farmers to produce more, malnutrition is guaranteed to continue. If you further consider the inequities of such natural resources as rainfall, the uneven picture for malnutrition becomes clearer.

Given the foregoing restraints, you can then appreciate the difficulties that face a country seeking to become self-reliant in food production. Although the natural solution to inadequate agricultural land is to expand the agricultural land, such expansion can seem an insurmountable problem to untrained farmers who lack equipment, have only the

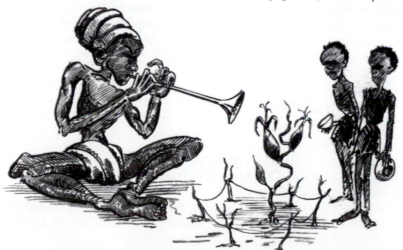

crudest of irrigation systems, and lack the physical energy to carry out large-scale projects.

The West African word "kwashiorkor" (also see Chapter 19) describes a serious form of protein deprivation that often results in death. The word literally means "the disease of the deposed baby when the next one is born." We mention this word here since it clearly illustrates that the West Africans understand one of the basic principles of world hunger, the direct link between high population density, high birth rates, and malnutrition. This link is another way of looking at a problem we mentioned earlier in this section, the problem of uneven distribution. Stated most simply, if there are a large number of people in one place but the food supply is in another place, there will be malnutrition. Consider how this principle applies to migration.

In many developing countries, population congregates in large cities. It has been estimated that by the year 2000 developing countries will have 40 cities with populations in excess of five million, whereas industrialized nations will have only twelve such cities. The malnutrition problem inherent in that projection is that the food is in the rural areas, and the developing countries lack adequate transportation and adequate food storage. Accordingly, those countries are, and will continue to be, forced to spend the country's resources for importing food to the population centers. This prevents the expenditures necessary to improve transportation, expand agricultural lands, improve storage, and build national food reserves, steps that are necessary for a country to become self-reliant in food production.

In summary then, human actions lie at the root of hunger. Poor countries must control population, invest in their country's development, and redistribute income-producing assets if hunger is to be defeated. For the battle against world hunger to be effective, the economic and political power of all nations must work in concert. That is indeed a large order.

Determining a Nation's Nutritional Status

Before we can combat undernutrition in the world, we must be able to identify those population groups that are at risk. Chapter 22 describes various ways of accomplishing this and should be consulted for more details. The methods of evaluating the nutritional status or well-being of a population group include:

Clinical assessment.

Biochemical measurements.

Dental examination.

Dietary evaluation.

Collection of data on: level and distribution of income; income maintenance and other social service programs; government food and nutrition programs; general food availability and acceptance; health and educational facilities; socioeconomic, ethnic, and cultural characteristics; and overall health status and disease factors.

As discussed in Chapter 22, only a combination of the above methods will provide useful information about the nutritional well-being of a population group. Each method by itself has weaknesses, some of which have already been discussed. Also, some of the techniques such as blood and urine testing cannot be effectively administered for large population segments. One method widely used is dietary evaluation. Let us examine this.

Although a record of 24-hour food intake remains a basic tool of nutrition study, this tool falls quite short for large groups. Since not everyone in a large group can be surveyed, conclusions must be based on a sampling of the population under study. As you have probably guessed, the very people with whom such studies are most concerned—the poor, the ill, the elderly—are usually poorly represented in such samples.

Assume for a moment though, that you have sampled 15 percent of your own town's population. Further assume that those responding to the survey have accurately recorded their 24-hour food intake. Further assume that what was eaten in that 24-hour period was representative of what is generally eaten. After that series of assumptions, what conclusions can you draw? If you found that one third of those sampled were below dietary standards, would it be safe to assume that one third of your household is undernourished? Could it be that the dietary standard is too high?

Given such difficulties regarding sampling, other assessment measures are sometimes considered. For example, the amount of food production can be divided by the population to yield availability per capita. Or, the amount of food production can be divided by what the per capita need should be, and the result can then be compared to dietary standards. Such measurements have been used by the Food and Agriculture Organization (FAO) of the United Nations to publish "Food Balance Sheets" for various nations. Although such measurements can give some indication of a country's nutritional status, what if the food was not evenly distributed? Could it be possible that 50 percent of the population actually consumed 80 percent of the available food? To put it another way, is it believable that all members of a country get an equal share of the available food? Obviously, you have concluded that food is not distributed equally.

Despite the difficulties of nutritional assessment of large population groups, efforts to find the malnourished go forward. We know that certain groups are subject to malnutrition, and we can seek out those groups. For example, when a natural disaster occurs, malnutrition can be expected to increase. The prevalence of disease can signal malnutrition. We know that countries without food shortages will have more deaths from heart disease, whereas those with food shortages will have more deaths from infectious diseases. A country's mortality statistics can thus tell us about food supply. In some countries, weather can signal malnutrition. For example, if severe winters are experienced, food transportation can be slowed or stopped, growing seasons can be shortened, and so on.

The battle against world hunger is thus a twofold battle. The goal is not only to bring nutrients to the malnourished but also to reduce the number of people in danger of malnutrition. The second half of this battle is a very real one. A country has only so much food available. If more of that food is provided to those suffering from malnutrition, those who were borderline may receive less food and may slip into the malnourished category.

Yet another technique for determining a country's nutritional status involves economic analysis. If, for example, income levels can be determined within a country, and food prices can be analyzed on a calorie basis, then the population's economic ability to obtain caloric need is known. There are some obvious weaknesses to this method as well; for example, there are differences of opinion among nutritional experts about how many calories can be considered adequate. Further, is a person adequately nourished if caloric intake is sufficient but comes solely from a single food such as rice?

When economic estimates are made of nutritional status of large population groups, staggering numbers result. Current economic estimates place the world's malnourished at nearly 500 million. Worse still, the trend in world hunger demonstrates that the number continues to increase.

Policies and Programs
INCREASING FOOD SUPPLY AND INCOME

Whatever the method of estimation used, if a country has significant malnutrition, what happens when food supply is increased? Consider what happens when a large amount of food is given to a poor country by a wealthier country (Caliendo). First, farm sales drop. Second, farmers must reduce their farm labor force when their sales are lower. The results of this chain of events can be no net reduction of malnutrition.

Experiences with increasing food supply have demonstrated that another element must be addressed. Malnutrition can be more effectively fought if the economic status of the poor can be improved. Where people have sufficient income to meet their basic needs, they expend any extra income on food. This increases demand, causing farmers to produce more food. Producing more food requires more farm labor. As meat consumption increases, grain production must increase for animal feed. The stimulation of the economy thus provides a cycle that battles malnutrition.

The effect of increasing income has caused some world hunger experts to conclude that malnutrition is not a problem of food production. For example, it does little good to help a country double its food production if the amount of income available to purchase food remains constant.

NUTRITION PLANNING FOR NATIONAL DEVELOPMENT

Since developing countries have been estimated to contain over a billion people who suffer from malnutrition ranging from mild to severe, nutrition planning is at the heart of national development (Berg; Caliendo). It does little good to stimulate manufacturing, if the potential work force lacks the energy to work. Nor can a country develop toward its potential when child and infant mortality stands at a high level due to malnutrition, with the attendant high susceptibility to infectious disease. Those nations that cannot raise the nutritional status of their people must pay the price in low national productivity, high medical costs, and poor quality of life. Nutrition intervention programs thus are economically wise, as well as humanitarian.

Forecasts of the world food supply show that sufficient food is available; however, it is unevenly distributed. The uneven distribution becomes a matter of concern for government planners whose food policies can determine the availability of surplus or the need for importation. Such policies should attempt to provide adequate nutrition for the country's population, to improve purchasing power for those with low incomes, and to prevent diseases that characterize malnutrition.

Nations once viewed protein shortage as the leading world food problem, but general malnutrition, which is basically inadequate food intake, now holds that position. For almost a half million people, increases in cereal grains, vegetables, and legumes are necessary to reduce the incidence of malnutrition and provide sufficient calories to give basic energy. To accomplish such goals, national projects that are labor intensive can enable the poor to have more to spend for food.

The Helping Hand

HIGH-PROTEIN FOODS

At the national and international levels, many efforts have been made to increase the availability of high-protein foods in underdeveloped countries. These include programs of supplementation and fortification and the "green revolution"—a highly technological approach to intensified food production. A simpler but perhaps more successful approach is supplying infants and children with special cheap and semisynthetic high-protein foods made of locally available food products. Many governments are issuing products that contain all the essential amino acids as well as other essential nutrients (Brown, 1977; Caliendo). Table 27-1 presents a partial list of those products and their major ingredients.

Figure 27-2 shows a severely malnourished child in the Provincial Hospital in Kuito, Angola, drinking K-Mix II (a high protein food mixture developed by UNICEF). Figure 27-3 shows children in Tchin Tabaraden (Niger) being fed a meal of milk and cooked grain. Figure 27-4 shows children in Dacca (Bangladesh) sharing a bowl of CSM (Corn-Soya-Milk plus sugar, a high protein food supplied by UNICEF).

SOME WORKABLE PROGRAMS

Many children are potential victims of hunger—and potential beneficiaries of programs to end malnutrition. The information discussed throughout this chapter indicates many of the complex problems involved and the vulnerability of young children. To overcome all the causes of world hunger and the specific at-risk factors affecting the life and health of so many of the world's children will be very difficult.

Underfeeding in underdeveloped countries will continue. But health workers who care for malnourished children continue to look for ways to rehabilitate as many children as possible (Levinson). Other simple, economical, practicable, and successful ways include the following:

Use of Local Food

One way of combating persistent malnutrition has been to promote the use of local foods that are inexpensive but nutrient rich. This method has been successful in ending moderate undernutrition among the children of Nepal (Bomgaars).

A large number of children under 4 years old in some districts of Nepal were labeled as *runche* ("the crying one") because of their miserable behavior, such as whining and refusing to eat or cooperate with family members and household activities. The natives believed that the children had been cast under a spell when they were touched by pregnant women. The local "cure" for the condition was a series of morning baths.

A nearby modern health project that provided medical care to more than 50,000 people was able to diagnose these children as being mildly

Table 27-1

Special High-protein Products Used by Different Countries to Combat Protein-Calorie Malnutrition*

COUNTRY OR AREA	PRODUCT	MAJOR INGREDIENTS
Algeria	Superamine	Dried skim milk, chick-peas, legumes, wheat
Brazil	Incaparina	Soya, maize
Chile	Lache alim	Soya, fish protein concentrate, dried skim milk
Colombia	Duryea	Soya, dried skim milk, maize
Central America	Incaparina	Cottonseed, maize
Egypt	Weaning food	Dried skim milk, chick-peas, broad beans, wheat
Ethiopia	Faffa	Soya, dried skim milk
India	Bal-Amul	Soya, dried skim milk, legumes, wheat
Kenya	Simba	Dried skim milk, maize
Madagascar	Weaning food	Soya, dried skim milk, rice
Mexico	Conasupo products	Soya, kidney bean
Mozambique	Super Maeu	Soya, dried skim milk, maize, malt
Nigeria	Arlac	Groundnut, dried skim milk
Peru	Peruvita	Cottonseed, dried skim milk, quinoa
Senegal	Ladylac	Groundnut, dried skim milk, millet
South Africa	Pronutro	Soya, groundnut, dried skim milk, maize, yeast, wheat germ
Taiwan	Weaning food	Soya, dried skim milk, rice
Thailand	Noodles	Soya, wheat
Turkey	Weaning food	Soya, dried skim milk, chick-peas, wheat
Uganda	Soya porridge	Soya, dried skim milk, maize
United States	WSB (wheat and soy blend)	Soya, wheat
Venezuela	Incaparina	Soya, cottonseed, maize
Zambia	Milk biscuit	Soya, casein, wheat

*Though some products have existed for many years, others change constantly. Current references should be used to supplement this list.

to moderately underfed. The health workers carried out a very successful management program that cured the malnourishment and prevented its recurrence. Instead of spending time, money, and personnel to "scientifically" identify the affected children, the project made use of the natives' traditional recognition and isolation of those children. Treatment was then administered to the young patients. Knowledge of local food availability and dietary practices permitted the health personnel to concoct a nutritious, cheap food product for the children. All activities were conducted in a way that minimally disturbed the native beliefs and practices.

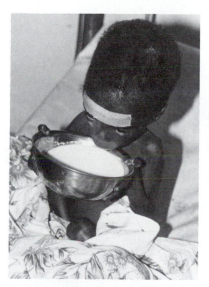

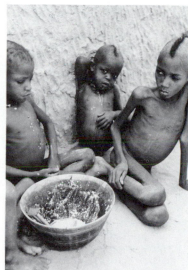

Figure 27-2: Rehabilitating an Angolan child.
SOURCE: UNICEF photo by Horst Ulax Cerni.

Figure 27-3: Rehabilitating children in Niger.
SOURCE: Agency for International Development.

Figure 27-4: Rehabilitating children in Bangladesh.
SOURCE: UNICEF photo by Jacques Danois.

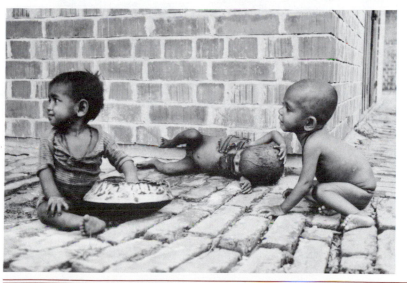

For example, the local people traditionally roasted corn and soybeans for adults as a snack and served the edentulous (no teeth) elderly a porridge made of roasted and ground grains. Grinding stones and grains (including wheat) were thus available and cheap. The health workers instructed the local residents to prepare a high-protein, high-calorie gruel by mixing and grinding roast corn, soybeans, and wheat. The

Somali Food Shelters in the Ogaden Famine and Their Impact on Health

The Ogaden is rough savannah country varying from red earth and sand to rock, lying south of the Ahmar Mountains east of the central southern highlands, west of Somalia, and north of Kenya. . . . Water is normally not abundant, and it had become acutely short after three unusually brief rainy seasons. The population, which is variously estimated between 300,000 and a million, consists largely of Somali nomads subsisting almost exclusively on the products of their herds of cows, camels, and goats. . . . The nomads live in transportable huts or dessas consisting of tightly woven grass mats fixed over semicircular frames. . . .

Drought and succeeding famine reached their peak in the savannah country of eastern Ethiopia in March and April of 1975. During a working visit to the Ogaden in July and August of 1975 we were able to observe the consequence of feeding large numbers of starving nomads in the "shelter" system. The effect was sixfold: the containment of starvation, the outbreak of

camp diseases, the activation of chronic disease by refeeding after starvation, the effects of a radical change in diet, the development of psychosomatic illnesses, and the disruption of social and family structure.

The shelter system, which was introduced because of the difficulties in distributing food to small groups of nomads on the move, provided us with a unique opportunity of examining the health problems of nomads ordinarily inaccessible for medical studies. . . . The nomads arrived, erected their huts, and appeared to be remaining indefinitely or until the program was closed down. Food distribution programs included twice-daily rations to adults as well as supplementary and intensive feeding for malnourished children and infants. . . .

All the observations reported were made during the provision of acute medical care by a mobile team consisting of the authors. . . . On arrival at a shelter, clinics were set up in any available building—usually a schoolhouse. In addition a scout

was sent to search in the shelters for severely ill and handicapped patients who were unable to attend the clinic. The feeding programs were examined, the incidence and degree of malnutrition and associated illnesses were observed, and as many sick as possible were examined and treated during each visit. . . .

Containment of starvation. The feeding program was highly effective. Whole wheat was boiled in half drums over small fires, soused liberally with liquid butter from cans, and distributed twice daily to adults and older children. Younger children received from 3 to 6 feeds daily of a variety of combinations of milk powder and cereals, a common one being a mixture of corn, soya-bean protein, and milk powder. We saw no signs of malnutrition in established members of the shelters except in those either acutely or chronically ill with infections. Newcomers to the camp, however, were invariably malnourished but usually showed few signs of active infection.

Camp diseases. These were

concoction was called *sarbottam pitho* (or "super flour") and was certified to be nutritious by chemical analyses. The children ate it, and their nutriture improved. The mothers were taught to supplement their breast-fed babies with this product as a preventive measure. *Runche* children were fed the product and were eventually rehabilitated. No attempt was made to stop the baths given the children.

common but varied from shelter to shelter. Bacillary dysentery and acute infectious hepatitis were the most common, the latter occurring predominantly in shelters where dishes were provided as part of the feeding program. There were never enough dishes to feed everyone at one sitting, so they were rinsed in warm water at the end of the first sitting and then refilled. Where the shelters did not provide eating utensils and the nomads had to provide their own, hepatitis was much less frequent. . . .

Refeeding disease. We were immediately impressed by the obvious recrudescence of infections following refeeding. . . . The local villagers had had no malarial attacks, but attacks were common in nomads shortly after arrival in the shelters. . . . Two other chronic infections were noted as likely to have been activated by refeeding—brucellosis and tuberculosis. . . .

Most impressive, was the reactivation of scrofula and bone and joint tuberculosis. We were often in the position to see

nomads on arrival at camp and over the succeeding weeks. Tuberculous lesions which had long been thought inactive by the patient and looked so on initial clinical examination began to break down and form sinuses or abscesses within two or three weeks. . . .

The nomads themselves observed spontaneously that they were getting worse in camp despite the food. . . . It is commonly, perhaps universally believed that infections so common in malnourished patients being treated in institutions are precipitated or aggravated by starvation itself. While we cannot deny this possibility we believe that severe and disabling infections are frequent on refeeding and that previous studies have not taken this possibility into account in describing the effect of complications of starvation.

Effect of the change of diet. The effect of changing the diet from virtually all milk and milk products with occasional meat to an all-wheat diet was severe constipation and abdominal

bloating in children and adults alike. There was a frequent demand for laxatives, which rarely appeared to be effective. The wheat was whole grain and should have provided enough residue but unfortunately it was not always eaten directly. Nomads would collect their ration, dry it in the sun, and pound it with a mortar and pestle to a crude flour which was then boiled with a little water into an edible paste. Often part of the ration was exchanged in the nearby village for beloved shai or tea, which was frequently preferred to food.

Conclusions

Shelters are a highly effective system of dealing with starvation in nomads but they create many problems yet to be solved. Important immediate needs are clothing, blankets, and preventive medical facilities for the eradication of acute infectious disease and tuberculosis. There is no simple means of long-term rehabilitation.

SOURCE: Adapted from M. J. Murray, et al. *Lancet*, June 12, 1976, p. 1283. Courtesy of the authors and *Lancet*. (Note that only a small section of the original article has been reproduced here.)

Promotion of Relactation

One means of combating protein calorie malnutrition involves the promotion of relactation in some women (Brown, 1978). The three essential factors for successful lactation in a woman are (1) a healthy baby with proper suckling reflexes, (2) an adequately nourished woman who is interested in nursing, and (3) conscientious support and encouragement from individuals close to the woman. The last criterion applies especially to women in underdeveloped countries. The same principles apply to *relactation*—stimulation of milk production in women who have not been breast-feeding. Recently, the use of relactation as a solution to malnutrition in young infants has received attention.

Breast-feeding by Female Relatives

In many underdeveloped countries and in certain modern societies, it is a custom that when a mother dies from childbirth, the surviving infant is assigned to a female relative (or even friend) for breast-feeding and care. If this woman is not making milk, she is given some local herbs and medicines and told to let the baby suckle on her as frequently as possible. It is unknown whether the native medications have any physiological or psychological effects. The baby is initially given a locally available porridge as a supplement, but many babies have been able to induce an adequate flow of milk in the woman after a brief interval of suckling without receiving milk. Modern drugs may be used to induce lactation if a nurse, physician, or knowledgeable health worker is present. However, support and encouragement by family and friends play a very important role.

Interrupted Breast-Feeding by the Mother

A second form of relactation is the renewal of breast milk in the baby's own mother. During the war in Bangladesh, many young infants suffered intestinal disorders, infection, body inflammation, diarrhea, and vomiting. These babies were given medical treatment when clinics became available. The period of treatment and recovery interrupted breast-feeding, and the mother's milk dried up. The lack of breast milk made it necessary to feed the babies with reconstituted dry milk. Unfortunately, the contaminated water used for diluting the dry milk invariably caused a recurrence of gastroenteritis.

Health workers found that these mothers' breasts could easily be induced to produce a normal flow of milk by letting the baby suckle as frequently as possible, especially if relatives and friends encouraged the women. During the wartime period of uncertainty and worry, this relactation process saved many infants from infection by contaminated water and assured proper nutrient intake. In a refugee camp, after one woman was shown how lactation could be reestablished to benefit the baby, other nursing mothers were willing to follow the procedure. No drug was used to induce lactation, and the practice prevented malnutrition. Government officials in Bangladesh and India are now aware of this practice and realize the convenience and economy of feeding the mothers well instead of paying for medicine and formula milk for the infants.

Wet-Nursing of Orphans

A third form of relactation involves hiring women to wet-nurse orphaned babies. At the end of the Vietnam war, South Vietnam had to deal with about 100,000 orphans, many of whom were infants. The task of feeding so many babies was very demanding, both in time and money. Health workers therefore began a large-scale employment of nearby women to wet-nurse the babies. Most of these women were not lactating. Again, interest, practice, and support enabled them to achieve a normal milk flow. Occasionally modern drugs were used to accomplish the purpose. These women benefited from this arrangement: they had income, meals, lodging, and supportive friends. The babies definitely benefited because, in addition to breast milk, each baby also had the personal care of an adult female who served as a mother.

Relactation has served a very useful purpose in the three circumstances cited. Whether it can be applied to a whole population of malnourished infants and children is being debated. However, under certain conditions, this process is cheap and conveniently workable.

Nutrition Rehabilitation Units

In the last 30 years, the art and science of using local nutrition units to rehabilitate malnourished children has been widespread and successful in many impoverished countries (Editorial). These units have three major functions: (1) to provide low-cost nutrition and dietary care to all individuals, (2) to rehabilitate malnourished children who have survived the emergency phase of underfeeding, and (3) to serve as major nutrition educational centers where natives (mainly women) can learn about proper dietary practices for the entire family, especially children.

These units have been organized and established according to the limitations and needs of the local people. At present, they are usually initiated by foreign and local health workers and local governments. Such units have been given many names such as mothercraft centers, family centers, nutrition rehabilitation villages, and other labels taken from local proverbs. Nutrition education is taught by a variety of methods including native songs, artwork, dances, and customs. Such units are usually started close to a hospital, health center, school, church organization, or farming area.

A number of significant health benefits have resulted from such units. The family, especially the mother, is no longer threatened by the authoritarian atmosphere of a hospital and its doctors and nurses. Thus, it is much easier to encourage the natives to follow health guidelines. The local residents accumulate a vast amount of knowledge concerning hygiene, economy, food preparation, feedings, and other nutritional information. As the underfed child becomes rehabilitated and well, the mother is especially pleased because she herself has brought about the recovery. Her attitude and behavior are influenced by her knowledge and observations. More people are willing to come and learn because satisfied mothers spread the news. The community is brought closer together and becomes exposed to some elements of medical care, education, agriculture, and community development.

A Call to Arms

These realizations and recommendations bring us back to the maxim about the giving of a fish and the teaching of fishing. It is not simply that self-sufficiency prevents dependence. Self-sufficiency also offers the opportunity for livelihood, and livelihood, economic capability, is a key factor in the battle against world hunger. We know that the problem of world hunger is the toughest one we face on earth, but we cannot abandon our resolve to confront it with determination.

STUDY QUESTIONS

1. Name ten factors responsible for world hunger. Discuss how to overcome each.

2. Using library resources, research and list twenty programs in which the United States contributes directly to the food supply of underdeveloped countries.

3. Research and identify ten high-protein products that are used in poor countries but are not listed in this book.

4. Research and identify other workable programs similar to those presented in this chapter (for example, relactation, rehabilitation units, and so forth).

5. Research and list government (state and federal) programs that help to feed the poor in this country.

REFERENCES

Berg, A., ed. *Malnourished People: A Policy View.* Washington, D.C.: World Bank, 1981.

Bomgaars, M. R. "Undernutrition: A Cultural Diagnosis and Treatment of 'Runche'." *J.A.M.A.* 236 (1976): 2513.

Brown, R. E. *Starving Children: The Tyranny of Hunger.* New York: Springer, 1977.

Brown, R. E. "Relactation with Reference to Applications in Developing Countries." *Clin. Ped.* 17 (1978): 333.

Caliendo, A. *Nutrition and the World Food Crisis.* New York: Macmillan, 1979.

Editorial. "Nutrition Rehabilitation Units." *Brit. Med. J.* 2 (1975): 246.

Levinson, F. J. "Toward Success in Combating Malnutrition: An Assessment of What Works." *Food Nutr. Bull.* 4 (1982): 23.

Appendixes

Table A-1
Recommended Daily Dietary Allowances (RDA) for the United States

AGE (YEARS)	WEIGHT (kg)	WEIGHT (lb)	HEIGHT (cm)	HEIGHT (in)	PROTEIN (g)	VITAMIN A (μg RE)*	VITAMIN D (μg)†	VITAMIN E (mg α-TE)‡
Infants								
0.0–0.5	6	13	60	24	kg x 2.2	420	10	3
0.5–1.0	9	20	71	28	kg x 2.0	400	10	4
Children								
1–3	13	29	90	35	23	400	10	5
4–6	20	44	112	44	30	500	10	6
7–10	28	62	132	52	34	700	10	7
Males								
11–14	45	99	157	62	45	1,000	10	8
15–18	66	145	176	69	56	1,000	10	10
19–22	70	154	177	70	56	1,000	7.5	10
23–50	70	154	178	70	56	1,000	5	10
>51	70	154	178	70	56	1,000	5	10
Females								
11–14	46	101	157	62	46	800	10	8
15–18	55	120	163	64	46	800	10	8
19–22	55	120	163	64	44	800	7.5	8
23–50	50	120	163	64	44	800	5	8
>51	55	120	163	64	44	800	5	8
Pregnant						+30	+200	+5	+2
Lactating						+20	+400	+5	+3

SOURCE: *Recommended Dietary Allowances*, 9th ed. (Washington, D.C.: National Academy of Sciences, 1980).

NOTE: The allowances are intended to provide for individual variations among most normal persons as they live in the United States under usual environmental stresses. Diets should be based on a variety of common foods in order to provide other nutrients for which human requirements have been less well defined. See text for detailed discussion of allowances and of nutrients not tabulated.

*Retinol equivalents. 1 retinol equivalent = 1 μg of retinol or 6 μg of β-carotene.

†As cholecalciferol. 10 μg of cholecalciferol = 400 IU of vitamin D.

‡α-tocopherol equivalents. 1 mg of d-α-tocopherol = 1 α-TE.

§1 NE (niacin equivalent) is equal to 1 mg of niacin or 60 mg of dietary tryptophan.

| | WATER-SOLUBLE VITAMINS | | | | | | MINERALS | | | | | |
VITAMIN C (mg)	THIA-MINE (mg)	RIBO-FLAVIN (mg)	NIACIN (mg NE)§	VITAMIN B_6 (mg)	FOLACIN‖ (µg)	VITAMIN B_{12} (µg)	CAL-CIUM (mg)	PHOS-PHORUS (mg)	MAG-NESIUM (mg)	IRON (mg)	ZINC (mg)	IODINE (µg)
35	0.3	0.4	6	0.3	30	0.5¶	360	240	50	10	3	40
35	0.5	0.6	8	0.6	45	1.5	540	360	70	15	5	50
45	0.7	0.8	9	0.9	100	2.0	800	800	150	15	10	70
45	0.9	1.0	11	1.3	200	2.5	800	800	200	10	10	90
45	1.2	1.4	16	1.6	300	3.0	800	800	250	10	10	120
50	1.4	1.6	18	1.8	400	3.0	1,200	1,200	350	18	15	150
60	1.4	1.7	18	2.0	400	3.0	1,200	1,200	400	18	15	150
60	1.5	1.7	19	2.2	400	3.0	800	800	350	10	15	150
60	1.4	1.6	18	2.2	400	3.0	800	800	350	10	15	150
60	1.2	1.4	16	2.2	400	3.0	800	800	350	18	15	150
50	1.1	1.3	15	1.8	400	3.0	1,200	1,200	300	18	15	150
60	1.1	1.3	14	2.0	400	3.0	1,200	1,200	300	18	15	150
60	1.1	1.3	14	2.0	400	3.0	800	800	300	18	15	150
60	1.0	1.2	13	2.0	400	3.0	800	800	300	10	15	150
60	1.0	1.2	13	2.0	400	3.0	800	800	300	10	15	150
+20	+0.4	+0.3	+2	+0.6	+400	+1.0	+400	+400	+150	#	+5	+25
+40	+0.5	+0.5	+5	+0.5	+100	+1.0	+400	+400	+150	#	+10	+50

‖The folacin allowances refer to dietary sources as determined by *Lactobacillus casei* assay after treatment with enzymes (conjugases) to make polyglutamyl forms of the vitamin available to the test organism.

¶The recommended dietary allowance for vitamin B_{12} in infants is based on average concentration of the vitamin in human milk. The allowances after weaning are based on energy intake (as recommended by the American Academy of Pediatrics) and consideration of other factors, such as intestinal absorption.

#The increased requirement during pregnancy cannot be met by the iron content of habitual American diets nor by the existing iron stores of many women; therefore the use of 30 to 60 mg of supplemental iron is recommended. Iron needs during lactation are not substantially different from those of nonpregnant women, but continued supplementation of the mother for 2 to 3 months after parturition is advisable in order to replenish stores depleted by pregnancy.

Table A-2
Estimated Safe and Adequate Daily Intakes of Additional Selected Vitamins and Minerals for the United States

| | AGE (YEARS) | VITAMINS | | |
		VITAMIN K (μg)	BIOTIN (μg)	PANTOTHENIC ACID (mg)
Infants	0–0.5	12	35	2
	0.5–1	10–20	50	3
Children and adolescents	1–3	15–30	65	3
	4–6	20–40	85	3–4
	7–10	30–60	120	4–5
	>11	50–100	100–200	4–7
Adults		70–140	100–200	4–7

SOURCE: *Recommended Dietary Allowances*, 9th ed. (Washington, D.C.: National Academy of Sciences, 1980).

NOTE: Because there is less information on which to base allowances, these figures are not given in the main table of the RDAs and are provided here in the form of ranges of recommended intakes.

Table A-3
Mean Heights and Weights and Recommended Energy Intakes for the United States

CATEGORY	AGE (YEARS)	WEIGHT		HEIGHT		ENERGY NEEDS (WITH RANGE)	
		(kg)	(lb)	(cm)	(in.)	(kcal)	(MJ)
Infants	0.0–0.5	6	13	60	24	kg × 115 (95–145)	kg × .48
	0.5–1.0	9	20	71	28	kg × 105 (80–135)	kg × .44
Children	1– 3	13	29	90	35	1,300 (900–1,800)	5.5
	4– 6	20	44	112	44	1,700 (1,300–2,300)	7.1
	7–10	28	62	132	52	2,400 (1,650–3,300)	10.1
Males	11–14	45	99	157	62	2,700 (2,000–3,700)	11.3
	15–18	66	145	176	69	2,800 (2,100–3,900)	11.8
	19–22	70	154	177	70	2,900 (2,500–3,300)	12.2
	23–50	70	154	178	70	2,700 (2,300–3,100)	11.3
	51–75	70	154	178	70	2,400 (2,000–2,800)	10.1
	>76	70	154	178	70	2,050 (1,650–2,450)	8.6
Females	11–14	46	101	157	62	2,200 (1,500–3,000)	9.2
	15–18	55	120	163	64	2,100 (1,200–3,000)	8.8
	19–22	55	120	163	64	2,100 (1,700–2,500)	8.8
	23–50	55	120	163	64	2,000 (1,600–2,400)	8.4
	51–75	55	120	163	64	1,800 (1,400–2,200)	7.6
	>76	55	120	163	64	1,600 (1,200–2,000)	6.7
Pregnancy						+300	
Lactation						+500	

SOURCE: *Recommended Dietary Allowances*, 9th ed. (Washington, D.C.: National Academy of Sciences, 1980).

NOTES: The data in this table have been assembled from the observed median heights and weights of children together with desirable weights for adults for the mean heights of men (70 in.) and women (64 in.) between the ages of 18 and 34 years as surveyed in the U.S. population (Health, Education and Welfare/National Center for Health Statistics data).

The energy allowances for the young adults are for men and women doing light work. The allowances for the two older age groups represent mean energy needs over these age spans, allowing for a 2% decrease in basal (resting) metabolic rate per decade and a reduction in activity of 200 kcal/d for men and women between 51 and 75 years, 500 kcal for men over 75 years, and 400 kcal for women over 75. The customary range of daily energy output is shown for adults in parentheses, and is based on a variation in energy needs of ± 400 kcal at any one age emphasizing the wide range of energy intakes appropriate for any group of people.

Energy allowances for children through age 18 are based on median energy intakes of children these ages followed in longitudinal growth studies. The values in parentheses are 10th and 90th percentiles of energy intake, to indicate the range of energy consumption among children of these ages.

	TRACE ELEMENTS*						ELECTROLYTES		
COPPER (mg)	MANGANESE (mg)	FLUORIDE (mg)	CHROMIUM (mg)	SELENIUM (mg)	MOLYBDENUM (mg)		SODIUM (mg)	POTASSIUM (mg)	CHLORIDE (mg)
0.5–0.7	0.5–0.7	0.1–0.5	0.01–0.04	0.01–0.04	0.03–0.06		115– 350	350– 925	275– 700
0.7–1.0	0.7–1.0	0.2–1.0	0.02–0.06	0.02–0.06	0.04–0.08		250– 750	425–1,275	400–1,200
1.0–1.5	1.0–1.5	0.5–1.5	0.02–0.08	0.02–0.08	0.05–0.1		325– 975	550–1,650	500–1,500
1.5–2.0	1.5–2.0	1.0–2.5	0.03–0.12	0.03–0.12	0.06–0.15		450–1,350	775–2,325	700–2,100
2.0–2.5	2.0–3.0	1.5–2.5	0.05–0.2	0.05–0.2	0.1 –0.3		600–1,800	1,000–3,000	925–2,775
2.0–3.0	2.5–5.0	1.5–2.5	0.05–0.2	0.05–0.2	0.15–0.5		900–2,700	1,525–4,575	1,400–4,200
2.0–3.0	2.5–5.0	1.5–4.0	0.05–0.2	0.05–0.2	0.15–0.5		1,100–3,300	1,875–5,625	1,700–5,100

*Since the toxic levels for many trace elements may be only several times usual intakes, the upper levels for the trace elements given in this table should not be habitually exceeded.

Table A-4
U.S. Recommended Daily Allowance (U.S. RDA)

NUTRIENT	ADULTS AND CHILDREN (4 YEARS OR OLDER)	INFANTS (BIRTH TO 1 YEAR)	CHILDREN (UNDER 4 YEARS)	PREGNANT OR LACTATING WOMEN
Required				
Protein (g)	45 or 65*	18 or 25*	20 or 28*	45 or 65*
Vitamin A (IU)	5,000	1,500	2,500	8,000
Vitamin C (mg)	60	35	40	60
Thiamin (mg)	1.5	0.5	0.7	1.7
Riboflavin (mg)	1.7	0.6	0.8	2.0
Niacin (mg)	20	8	9	20
Calcium (mg)	1,000	600	800	1,300
Iron (mg)	18	15	10	18
Optional				
Vitamin D (IU)	400	400	400	400
Vitamin E (IU)	30	5	10	30
Vitamin B_6 (mg)	2.0	0.4	0.7	2.5
Folic acid (mg)	0.4	0.1	0.2	0.8
Vitamin B_{12} (μg)	6	2	3	8
Phosphorus (mg)	1,000	500	800	1,300
Iodine (μg)	150	45	70	150
Magnesium (mg)	400	70	200	450
Zinc (mg)	15	5	8	15
Copper (mg)	2	0.6	1	2
Biotin (mg)	0.3	0.05	0.15	0.3
Pantothenic acid (mg)	10	3	5	10

*Lower value if protein efficiency ratio is equal to or greater than that of casein; higher value if protein efficiency ratio is less than that of casein, but greater than 20%.

Table A-5
Recommended Nutrient Intakes for Canadians, 1983

AGE	SEX	WEIGHT (kg)	PROTEIN (g/DAY)*	FAT-SOLUBLE VITAMINS		
				VITAMIN A (RE/DAY)[†]	VITAMIN D (μg/DAY)[‡]	VITAMIN E (mg/DAY)[§]
Months						
0–2	Both	4.5	11[¶]	400	10	3
3–5	Both	7.0	14[¶]	400	10	3
6–8	Both	8.5	16[¶]	400	10	3
9–11	Both	9.5	18	400	10	3
Years						
1	Both	11	18	400	10	3
2–3	Both	14	20	400	5	4
4–6	Both	18	25	500	5	5
7–9	M	25	31	700	2.5	7
	F	25	29	700	2.5	6
10–12	M	34	38	800	2.5	8
	F	36	39	800	2.5	7
13–15	M	50	49	900	2.5	9
	F	48	43	800	2.5	7
16–18	M	62	54	1,000	2.5	10
	F	53	47	800	2.5	7
19–24	M	71	57	1,000	2.5	10
	F	58	41	800	2.5	7
25–49	M	74	57	1,000	2.5	9
	F	59	41	800	2.5	6
50–74	M	73	57	1,000	2.5	7
	F	63	41	800	2.5	6
75 +	M	69	57	1,000	2.5	6
	F	64	41	800	2.5	5
Pregnancy (additional)						
1st Trimester			15	100	2.5	2
2nd Trimester			20	100	2.5	2
3rd Trimester			25	100	2.5	2
Lactation (additional)			20	400	2.5	3

SOURCE: *Recommended Nutrient Intakes for Canadians*, Health and Welfare Canada (Ottawa: Canadian Government Publishing Centre, 1983), Table X.1, pp. 179–180. Reproduced with permission.

NOTES: Recommended intakes of energy are provided in Table A-6 in which the figures for energy are estimates of average requirements for expected patterns of activity. For nutrients not shown, the following amounts are recommended: thiamine, 0.4 mg/1,000 kcal (0.48/5,000 kJ); riboflavin, 0.5 mg/1,000 kcal (0.6 mg/5,000 kJ); niacin, 7.2 NE/1,000 kcal (8.6 NE/5,000 kJ); vitamin B6, 15 μg, as pyridoxine, per gram of protein; phosphorus, same as calcium.

Recommended intakes during periods of growth are taken as appropriate for individuals representative of the mid-point in each age group. All recommended intakes are designed to cover individual variations in essentially all of a healthy population subsisting upon a variety of common foods available in Canada.

WATER-SOLUBLE VITAMINS			MINERALS				
VITAMIN C (mg/DAY)	FOLACIN (µg/DAY)‖	VITAMIN B$_{12}$ (µg/DAY)	CALCIUM (mg/DAY)	MAGNESIUM (mg/DAY)	IRON (mg/DAY)	IODINE (µg/DAY)	ZINC (mg/DAY)
20	50	0.3	350	30	0.4#	25	2**
20	50	0.3	350	40	5	35	3
20	50	0.3	400	45	7	40	3
20	55	0.3	400	50	7	45	3
20	65	0.3	500	55	6	55	4
20	80	0.4	500	65	6	65	4
25	90	0.5	600	90	6	85	5
35	125	0.8	700	110	7	110	6
30	125	0.8	700	110	7	95	6
40	170	1.0	900	150	10	125	7
40	170	1.0	1,000	160	10	110	7
50	160	1.5	1,100	220	12	160	9
45	160	1.5	800	190	13	160	8
55	190	1.9	900	240	10	160	9
45	160	1.9	700	220	14	160	8
60	210	2.0	800	240	8	160	9
45	165	2.0	700	190	14	160	8
60	210	2.0	800	240	8	160	9
45	165	2.0	700	190	14††	160	8
60	210	2.0	800	240	8	160	9
45	165	2.0	800	190	7	160	8
60	210	2.0	800	240	8	160	9
45	165	2.0	800	190	7	160	8
0	305	1.0	500	15	6	25	0
20	305	1.0	500	20	6	25	1
20	305	1.0	500	25	6	25	2
30	120	0.5	500	80	0	50	6

*The primary units are grams per kilogram of body weight. The figures shown here are examples.

†One retinol equivalent (RE) corresponds to the biological activity of 1 µg of retinol, 6 µg of β-carotene or 12 µg of other carotenes.

‡Expressed as cholecalciferol or ergocalciferol.

§Expressed as d-α-tocopherol equivalents, relative to which β- and γ-tocopherol and α-tocotrienol have activities of 0.5, 0.1 and 0.3 respectively.

‖Expressed as total folate.

¶Assumption that the protein is from breast milk or is of the same biological value as that of breast milk and that between 3 and 9 months adjustment for the quality of the protein is made.

#It is assumed that breast milk is the source of iron up to 2 months of age.

**Based on the assumption that breast milk is the source of zinc for the first 2 months.

††After the menopause the recommended intake is 7 mg/day.

Table A-6
Average Energy Requirements (Canada)

AGE	SEX	AVERAGE HEIGHT (cm)	AVERAGE WEIGHT (kg)	REQUIREMENTS*					
				kcal/kg[†]	MJ/kg[†]	kcal/DAY	MJ/DAY	kcal/cm	MJ/cm
Months									
0–2	Both	55	4.5	120–100	0.50–0.42	500	2.0	9	0.04
3–5	Both	63	7.0	100– 95	0.42–0.40	700	2.8	11	0.05
6–8	Both	69	8.5	95– 97	0.40–0.41	800	3.4	11.5	0.05
9–11	Both	73	9.5	97– 99	0.41	950	3.8	12.5	0.05
Years									
1	Both	82	11	101	0.42	1,100	4.8	13.5	0.06
2–3	Both	95	14	94	0.39	1,300	5.6	13.5	0.06
4–6	Both	107	18	100	0.42	1,800	7.6	17	0.07
7–9	M	126	25	88	0.37	2,200	9.2	17.5	0.07
	F	125	25	76	0.32	1,900	8.0	15	0.06
10–12	M	141	34	73	0.30	2,500	10.4	17.5	0.07
	F	143	36	61	0.25	2,200	9.2	15.5	0.06
13–15	M	159	50	57	0.24	2,800	12.0	17.5	0.07
	F	157	48	46	0.19	2,200	9.2	14	0.06
16–18	M	172	62	51	0.21	3,200	13.2	18.5	0.08
	F	160	53	40	0.17	2,100	8.8	13	0.05
19–24	M	175	71	42	0.18	3,000	12.4		
	F	160	58	36	0.15	2,100	8.8		
25–49	M	172	74	36	0.15	2,700	11.2		
	F	160	59	32	0.13	1,900	8.0		
50–74	M	170	73	31	0.13	2,300	9.6		
	F	158	63	29	0.12	1,800	7.6		
75 +	M	168	69	29	0.12	2,000	8.4		
	F	155	64	23	0.10	1,500	6.0		

SOURCE: *Recommended Nutrient Intakes for Canadians*, 1983, Table II.1, pp. 22–23. Reproduced by permission.

*Requirements can be expected to vary within a range of ± 30 percent.

[†]First and last figures are averages at the beginning and at the end of the 3-month period.

Appendix B: Food Composition Tables

Table B-1 shows the food values in selected foods. Foods are grouped under the following headings: dairy products; eggs; fats and oils; fish, shellfish, meat, and poultry; fruits and fruit products; grain products; legumes (dry), nuts, and seeds; sugars and sweets; vegetables and vegetable products; and miscellaneous items.

Most of the foods listed are in ready-to-eat form. Some are basic products widely used in food preparation, such as flour, fat, and cornmeal. The weight in grams for an approximate measure of each food is shown. A footnote indicates if inedible parts are included in the description and the weight.

The values for food energy (kcal) and nutrients shown are the amounts present in the edible part of the item, that is, that portion customarily eaten—corn without the cob, meat without bone, potatoes without skins, and European-type grapes without seeds. If additional parts are eaten—the potato skin, for example—the amounts obtained of some nutrients will be somewhat greater than those shown.

Values for thiamine, riboflavin, and niacin in white flours and white bread and rolls are based on the increased enrichment levels put into effect for those products by the Food and Drug Administration in 1974. Iron values for those products and the values for enriched cornmeal, pasta, farina, and rice (except the value of riboflavin) represent the minimum levels of enrichment promulgated under the Federal Food,

Drug, and Cosmetic Act of 1955. Riboflavin values of rice are for unenriched rice, as the levels for added riboflavin have not been approved. Thiamine, riboflavin, and niacin values for products prepared with white flour represent the use of flour enriched at the 1974 levels; values for iron for such products represent the use of flour enriched at the 1955 level.

Niacin values are for preformed niacin occurring naturally in foods. The values do not include additional niacin that the body may form from tryptophan, an essential amino acid in the protein of most foods. Among the better sources of tryptophan are milk, meats, eggs, legumes, and nuts.

Values have been calculated from the ingredients called for in typical recipes for many of the prepared items, such as biscuits, corn muffins, macaroni and cheese, custard, and many desserts. Values for toast and cooked vegetables are without fat added, either during preparation or at the table. Some vitamins, especially ascorbic acid, may be destroyed when vegetables are cut or shredded. Since such losses vary, no deduction has been made. For meat, values are for meat cooked and drained of the drippings.

A variety of manufactured items—some of the milk products, ready-to-eat breakfast cereals, imitation cream products, fruit drinks, and various mixes—are included. Frequently those foods are fortified with one or more nutrients. If nutrients are added, this information is on the label. Values shown here for those foods are usually based on products from several manufacturers and may differ somewhat from the values provided by any one source.

SOURCE: Adapted from Table 2 of Science and Education Administration, U.S. Department of Agriculture, *Nutritive Value of Foods*, Home and Garden Bulletin no. 72, rev. (Washington, D.C., April 1981); and published results in scientific journals by other investigators.

Table B-1
Nutritive Values of the Edible Part of Foods

FOOD	APPROXIMATE MEASURES, UNITS, OR WEIGHT	WEIGHT (g)	WATER (%)	FOOD ENERGY (kcal)	PROTEIN (g)	FAT (g)
Dairy products (cheese, cream, imitation cream, milk; related products)						
Butter. See Fats, oils; related products.						
Cheese:						
Natural:						
Blue	1 oz	28	42	100	6	8
Camembert (3 wedges per 4-oz container)	1 wedge	38	52	115	8	9
Cheddar:						
Cut pieces	1 oz	28	37	115	7	9
	1 cu. in.	17.2	37	70	4	6
Shredded	1 c	113	37	455	28	37
Cottage (curd not pressed down):						
Creamed (cottage cheese, 4% fat):						
Large curd	1 c	225	79	235	28	10
Small curd	1 c	210	79	220	26	9
Low fat (2%)	1 c	226	79	205	31	4
Low fat (1%)	1 c	226	82	165	28	2
Uncreamed (dry curd, less than ½% fat)	1 c	145	80	125	25	1
Cream	1 oz	28	54	100	2	10
Mozzarella, made with—						
Whole milk	1 oz	28	48	90	6	7
Part skim milk	1 oz	28	49	80	8	5
Parmesan, grated						
Cup, not pressed down	1 c	100	18	455	42	30
Tablespoon	1 T	5	18	25	2	2
Ounce	1 oz	28	18	130	12	9
Provolone	1 oz	28	41	100	7	8
Ricotta, made with—						
Whole milk	1 c	246	72	430	28	32
Part skim milk	1 c	246	74	340	28	19
Romano	1 oz	28	31	110	9	8
Swiss	1 oz	28	37	105	8	8
Pasteurized process cheese:						
American	1 oz	28	39	105	6	9
Swiss	1 oz	28	42	95	7	7
Pasteurized process cheese food, American	1 oz	28	43	95	6	7
Pasteurized process cheese spread, American	1 oz	28	48	80	5	6
Cream, sour	1 c	230	71	495	7	48
	1 T	12	71	25	Trace	3
Cream, sweet:						
Half-and-half (cream and milk)	1 c	242	81	315	7	28
	1 T	15	81	20	Trace	2
Light, coffee, or table	1 c	240	74	470	6	46
	1 T	15	74	30	Trace	3

NOTE: Dashes (—) denote lack of reliable data for a constituent believed to be present in measurable amount.
Footnotes for this table can be found on page 704.

NUTRIENTS IN INDICATED QUANTITY

SATURATED (TOTAL) (g)	UNSATURATED OLEIC (g)	UNSATURATED LINOLEIC (g)	CARBO-HYDRATE (g)	CALCIUM (mg)	PHOS-PHORUS (mg)	IRON (mg)	POTASSIUM (mg)	VITAMIN A VALUE (IU)	THIAMINE (mg)	RIBOFLAVIN (mg)	NIACIN (mg)	ASCORBIC ACID (mg)
5.3	1.9	0.2	1	150	110	0.1	73	200	0.01	0.11	0.3	0
5.8	2.2	0.2	Trace	147	132	0.1	71	350	0.01	0.19	0.2	0
6.1	2.1	0.2	Trace	204	145	0.2	28	300	0.01	0.11	Trace	0
3.7	1.3	0.1	Trace	124	88	0.1	17	180	Trace	0.06	Trace	0
24.2	8.5	0.7	1	815	579	0.8	111	1,200	0.03	0.42	0.1	0
6.4	2.4	0.2	6	135	297	0.3	190	370	0.05	0.37	0.3	Trace
6.0	2.2	0.2	6	126	277	0.3	177	340	0.04	0.34	0.3	Trace
2.8	1.0	0.1	8	155	340	0.4	217	160	0.05	0.42	0.3	Trace
1.5	0.5	0.1	6	138	302	0.3	193	80	0.05	0.37	0.3	Trace
0.4	0.1	Trace	3	46	151	0.3	47	40	0.04	0.21	0.2	0
6.2	2.4	0.2	1	23	30	0.3	34	400	Trace	0.06	Trace	0
4.4	1.7	0.2	1	163	117	0.1	21	260	Trace	0.08	Trace	0
3.1	1.2	0.1	1	207	149	0.1	27	180	0.01	0.10	Trace	0
19.1	7.7	0.3	4	1,376	807	1.0	107	700	0.05	0.39	0.3	0
1.0	0.4	Trace	Trace	69	40	Trace	5	40	Trace	0.02	Trace	0
5.4	2.2	0.1	1	390	229	0.3	30	200	0.01	0.11	0.1	0
4.8	1.7	0.1	1	214	141	0.1	39	230	0.01	0.09	Trace	0
20.4	7.1	0.7	7	509	389	0.9	257	1,210	0.03	0.48	0.3	0
12.1	4.7	0.5	13	669	449	1.1	308	1,060	0.05	0.46	0.2	0
—	—	—	1	302	215	—	—	160	—	0.11	Trace	0
5.0	1.7	0.2	1	272	171	Trace	31	240	0.01	0.10	Trace	0
5.6	2.1	0.2	Trace	174	211	0.1	46	340	0.01	0.10	Trace	0
4.5	1.7	0.1	1	219	216	0.2	61	230	Trace	0.08	Trace	0
4.4	1.7	0.1	2	163	130	0.2	79	260	0.01	0.13	Trace	0
3.8	1.5	0.1	1	159	202	0.1	69	220	0.0	0.12	Trace	0
30.0	12.1	1.1	10	268	195	0.1	331	1,820	0.08	0.34	0.2	2
1.6	0.6	0.1	1	14	10	Trace	17	90	Trace	0.02	Trace	Trace
17.3	7.0	0.6	10	254	230	0.2	314	260	0.08	0.36	0.2	2
1.1	0.4	Trace	1	16	14	Trace	19	20	0.01	0.02	Trace	Trace
28.8	11.7	1.0	9	231	192	0.1	292	1,730	0.08	0.36	0.1	2
1.8	0.7	0.1	1	14	12	Trace	18	110	Trace	0.02	Trace	Trace

continued on next page

FOOD	APPROXIMATE MEASURES, UNITS, OR WEIGHT	WEIGHT (g)	WATER (%)	FOOD ENERGY (kcal)	PROTEIN (g)	FAT (g)
Whipped topping (pressurized)	1 c	60	61	155	2	13
	1 T	3	61	10	Trace	1
Whipping, unwhipped (volume about double when whipped):						
Heavy	1 c	238	58	820	5	88
	1 T	15	58	80	Trace	6
Light	1 c	239	64	700	5	74
	1 T	15	64	45	Trace	5
Cream products, imitation (made with vegetable fat):						
Sour dressing (imitation sour cream) made with nonfat dry milk	1 c	235	75	415	8	39
	1 T	12	75	20	Trace	2
Sweet:						
Creamers:						
Liquid (frozen)	1 c	245	77	335	2	24
	1 T	15	77	20	Trace	1
Powdered	1 c	94	2	515	5	33
	1 t	2	2	10	Trace	1
	1 T	4	50	15	Trace	1
Powdered, made with whole milk	1 c	80	67	150	3	10
	1 T	4	67	10	Trace	Trace
Pressurized	1 c	70	60	185	1	16
	1 T	4	60	10	Trace	1
Ice cream. See Milk desserts, frozen.						
Ice milk. See Milk desserts, frozen.						
Milk:						
Fluid:						
Whole (3.3% fat)	1 c	244	88	150	8	8
Lowfat (2%):						
No milk solids added	1 c	244	89	120	8	5
Milk solids added:						
Label claim less than 10 g of protein per cup	1 c	245	89	125	9	5
Label claim 10 or more grams of protein per cup (protein fortified)	1 c	246	88	135	10	5
Lowfat (1%):						
Milk solids added:						
Label claim less than 10 g of protein per cup	1 c	245	90	105	9	2
Label claim 10 or more grams of protein per cup (protein fortified)	1 c	246	89	120	10	3
No milk solids added	1 c	244	90	100	8	3

NUTRIENTS IN INDICATED QUANTITY												
FATTY ACIDS												
SATURATED (TOTAL) (g)	UNSATURATED		CARBO-HYDRATE (g)	CALCIUM (mg)	PHOS-PHORUS (mg)	IRON (mg)	POTASSIUM (mg)	VITAMIN A VALUE (IU)	THIAMINE (mg)	RIBOFLAVIN (mg)	NIACIN (mg)	ASCORBIC ACID (mg)
	OLEIC (g)	LINOLEIC (g)										
8.3	3.4	0.3	7	61	54	Trace	88	550	0.02	0.04	Trace	0
0.4	0.2	Trace	Trace	3	3	Trace	4	30	Trace	Trace	Trace	0
54.8	22.4	2.0	7	154	149	0.1	179	3,500	0.05	0.26	0.1	1
3.5	1.4	0.1	Trace	10	9	Trace	11	200	Trace	0.02	Trace	Trace
46.2	18.3	1.5	7	166	146	0.1	231	2,690	0.06	0.30	0.1	1
2.9	1.1	0.1	Trace	10	9	Trace	15	170	Trace	0.02	Trace	Trace
31.2	4.4	1.1	11	266	205	0.1	380	20[1]	0.09	0.38	0.2	2
1.6	0.2	0.1	1	14	10	Trace	19	Trace[1]	0.01	0.02	Trace	Trace
22.8	0.3	Trace	28	23	157	0.1	467	220[1]	0	0	0	0
1.4	Trace	0	2	1	10	Trace	29	10[1]	0	0	0	0
30.6	0.9	Trace	52	21	397	0.1	763	190[1]	0	0.16[1]	0	0
0.7	Trace	0	1	Trace	8	Trace	16	Trace[1]	0	Trace	0	0
16.3	1.0	0.2	17	5	6	0.1	14	650[1]	0	0	0	0
0.9	0.1	Trace	1	Trace	Trace	Trace	1	30[1]	0	0	0	0
8.5	0.6	0.1	13	72	69	Trace	121	290[1]	0.02	0.09	Trace	1
0.4	Trace	Trace	1	4	3	Trace	6	10[1]	Trace	Trace	Trace	Trace
13.2	1.4	0.2	11	4	13	Trace	13	330[1]	0	0	0	0
0.8	0.1	Trace	1	Trace	1	Trace	1	20[1]	0	0	0	0
5.1	2.1	0.2	11	291	228	0.1	370	310[2]	0.09	0.40	0.2	2
2.9	1.2	0.1	12	297	232	0.1	377	500	0.10	0.40	0.2	2
2.9	1.2	0.1	12	313	245	0.1	397	500	0.10	0.42	0.2	2
3.0	1.2	0.1	14	352	276	0.1	447	500	0.11	0.48	0.2	2
1.5	0.6	0.1	12	313	245	0.1	397	500	0.10	0.42	0.2	2
1.8	0.7	0.1	14	349	273	0.1	444	500	0.11	0.47	0.2	3
1.6	0.7	0.1	12	300	235	0.1	381	500	0.10	0.41	0.2	2

continued on next page

Table B-1
continued

FOOD	APPROXIMATE MEASURES, UNITS, OR WEIGHT	WEIGHT (g)	WATER (%)	FOOD ENERGY (kcal)	PROTEIN (g)	FAT (g)
Nonfat (skim):						
Milk solids added:						
Label claim less than 10 g of protein per cup	1 c	245	90	90	9	1
Label claim 10 or more grams of protein per cup (protein fortified)	1 c	246	89	100	10	1
No milk solids added	1 c	245	91	85	8	Trace
Buttermilk	1 c	245	90	100	8	2
Canned:						
Evaporated, unsweetened:						
Whole milk	1 c	252	74	340	17	19
Skim milk	1 c	255	79	200	19	1
Sweetened, condensed	1 c	306	27	980	24	27
Dried:						
Buttermilk	1 c	120	3	465	41	7
Nonfat instant:						
Envelopes	3.2 oz (net weight)	91	4	325	32	1
Cup	1 c	68[7]	4	245	24	Trace
Milk beverages:						
Chocolate milk (commercial):						
Regular	1 c	250	82	210	8	8
Lowfat (2%)	1 c	250	84	180	8	5
Lowfat (1%)	1 c	250	85	160	8	3
Eggnog (commercial)	1 c	254	74	340	10	19
Malted milk, home-prepared with 1 c of whole milk and 2 to 3 heaping teaspoons of malted milk powder (about ¾ oz)						
Chocolate	1 c of milk plus ¾ oz of powder	265	81	235	9	9
Natural	1 c of milk plus ¾ oz of powder	265	81	235	11	10
Shakes, thick:[8]						
Chocolate, container	10.6 oz	300	72	355	9	8
Vanilla, container	11 oz	313	74	350	12	9
Milk desserts, frozen:						
Ice cream:						
Regular (about 11% fat):						
Hardened	½ gal	1,064	61	2,155	38	115
	1 c	133	61	270	5	14
	3-fl-oz container	50	61	100	2	5
Soft serve (frozen custard)	1 c	173	60	375	7	23
Rich (about 16% fat), hardened	½ gal	1,188	59	2,805	33	190
	1 c	148	59	350	4	24

| | FATTY ACIDS | | | | | | | | | | | |
| | UNSATURATED | | | | | | | | | | | |
SATURATED (TOTAL) (g)	OLEIC (g)	LINOLEIC (g)	CARBO-HYDRATE (g)	CALCIUM (mg)	PHOS-PHORUS (mg)	IRON (mg)	POTASSIUM (mg)	VITAMIN A VALUE (IU)	THIAMINE (mg)	RIBOFLAVIN (mg)	NIACIN (mg)	ASCORBIC ACID (mg)
						NUTRIENTS IN INDICATED QUANTITY						
0.4	0.1	Trace	12	316	255	0.1	418	500	0.10	0.43	0.2	2
0.4	0.1	Trace	14	352	275	0.1	446	500	0.11	0.48	0.2	3
0.3	0.1	Trace	12	247	247	0.1	406	500	0.09	0.34	0.2	2
1.3	0.5	Trace	12	285	219	0.1	371	80[3]	0.08	0.38	0.1	2
11.6	5.3	0.4	25	657	510	0.5	764	610[3]	0.12	0.80	0.5	5
0.3	0.1	Trace	29	738	497	0.7	845	1,000[3]	0.11	0.79	0.4	3
16.8	6.7	0.7	166	868	775	0.6	1,136	1,000[3]	0.28	1.27	0.6	8
4.3	1.7	0.2	59	1,421	1,119	0.4	1,910	260[3]	0.47	1.90	1.1	7
0.4	0.1	Trace	47	1,120	896	0.3	1,552	2,160[6]	0.38	1.59	0.8	5
0.3	0.1	Trace	35	837	670	0.2	1,160	1,610[6]	0.28	1.19	0.6	4
5.3	2.2	0.2	26	280	251	0.6	417	300[3]	0.09	0.41	0.3	2
3.1	1.3	0.1	26	284	254	0.6	422	500	0.10	0.42	0.33	2
1.5	0.7	0.1	26	287	257	0.6	426	500	0.10	0.40	0.2	2
11.3	5.0	0.6	34	330	278	0.5	420	890	0.09	0.48	0.3	4
5.5	—	—	29	304	265	0.5	500	330	0.14	0.43	0.7	2
6.0	—	—	27	347	307	0.3	529	380	0.20	0.54	1.3	2
5.0	2.0	0.2	63	396	378	0.9	672	260	0.14	0.67	0.4	0
5.9	2.4	0.2	56	457	361	0.3	572	360	0.09	0.61	0.5	0
71.3	28.8	2.6	254	1,406	1,075	1.0	2,052	4,340	0.42	2.63	1.1	6
8.9	3.6	0.3	32	176	134	0.1	257	540	0.05	0.33	0.1	1
3.4	1.4	0.1	12	66	51	Trace	96	200	0.02	0.12	0.1	Trace
13.5	5.9	0.6	38	236	199	0.4	338	790	0.08	0.45	0.2	1
118.3	47.8	4.3	256	1,213	927	0.8	1,771	7,200	0.36	2.27	0.9	5
14.7	6.0	0.5	32	151	115	0.1	221	900	0.04	0.28	0.1	1

continued on next page

Table B-1
continued

FOOD	APPROXIMATE MEASURES, UNITS, OR WEIGHT	WEIGHT (g)	WATER (%)	FOOD ENERGY (kcal)	PROTEIN (g)	FAT (g)
Ice milk:						
Hardened (about 4.3% fat)	½ gal	1,048	69	1,470	41	45
	1 c	131	69	185	5	6
Soft serve (about 2.6% fat)	1 c	175	70	225	8	5
Sherbet (about 2% fat)	½ gal	1,542	66	2,160	17	31
	1 c	193	66	270	2	4
Milk desserts, other:						
Custard, baked	1 c	265	77	305	14	15
Puddings:						
From home recipe:						
Starch base:						
Chocolate	1 c	260	66	385	8	12
Vanilla (blancmange)	1 c	255	76	285	9	10
Tapioca cream	1 c	165	72	220	8	8
From mix (chocolate) and milk:						
Regular (cooked)	1 c	260	70	320	9	8
Instant	1 c	260	69	325	8	7
Yogurt:						
With added milk solids:						
Made with lowfat milk:						
Fruit-flavored[9]	8 oz	227	75	230	10	3
Plain	8 oz	227	85	145	12	4
Made with nonfat milk	8 oz	227	85	125	13	Trace
Without added milk solids:						
Made with whole milk	8 oz	227	88	140	8	7
Eggs						
Eggs, large (24 oz per dozen):						
Raw:						
Whole, without shell	1	50	75	80	6	6
White	1	33	88	15	3	Trace
Yolk	1	17	49	65	3	6
Cooked, whole:						
Fried in butter	1	46	72	85	5	6
Hard-cooked, shell removed	1	50	75	80	6	6
Poached	1	50	74	80	6	6
Scrambled (milk added) in butter (also omelet)	1	64	76	95	6	7
Fats, Oils; Related products						
Butter:						
Regular (1 brick or 4 sticks per pound)						
Stick (½ c)	1 stick	113	16	815	1	92
Tablespoon (about ⅛ stick)	1 T	14	16	100	Trace	12
Pat (1-in. square, ⅓ in. high; 90 per pound)	1 pat	5	16	35	Trace	4

	NUTRIENTS IN INDICATED QUANTITY											
FATTY ACIDS												
SATURATED (TOTAL) (g)	UNSATURATED OLEIC (g)	LINOLEIC (g)	CARBO-HYDRATE (g)	CALCIUM (mg)	PHOS-PHORUS (mg)	IRON (mg)	POTASSIUM (mg)	VITAMIN A VALUE (IU)	THIAMINE (mg)	RIBOFLAVIN (mg)	NIACIN (mg)	ASCORBIC ACID (mg)
28.1	11.3	1.0	232	1,409	1,035	1.5	2,117	1,710	0.61	2.78	0.9	6
3.5	1.4	0.1	29	176	129	0.1	265	210	0.08	0.35	0.1	1
2.9	1.2	0.1	38	274	202	0.3	412	180	0.12	0.54	0.2	1
19.0	7.7	0.7	469	827	594	2.5	1,585	1,480	0.26	0.71	1.0	31
2.4	1.0	0.1	59	103	74	0.3	198	190	0.03	0.09	0.1	4
6.8	5.4	0.7	29	297	310	1.1	387	930	0.11	0.50	0.3	1
7.6	3.3	0.3	67	250	255	1.3	445	390	0.05	0.36	0.3	1
6.2	2.5	0.2	41	298	232	Trace	352	410	0.08	0.41	0.3	2
4.1	2.5	0.5	28	173	180	0.7	223	480	0.07	0.30	0.2	2
4.3	2.6	0.2	59	265	247	0.8	354	340	0.05	0.39	0.3	2
3.6	2.2	0.3	63	374	237	1.3	335	340	0.08	0.39	0.3	2
1.8	0.6	0.1	42	343	269	0.2	439	120[10]	0.08	0.40	0.2	1
2.3	0.8	0.1	16	415	326	0.2	531	150[10]	0.10	0.49	0.3	2
0.3	0.1	Trace	17	452	355	0.2	579	20[10]	0.11	0.53	0.3	2
4.8	1.7	0.1	11	274	215	0.1	351	280	0.07	0.32	0.2	1
1.7	2.0	0.6	1	28	90	1.0	65	260	0.04	0.15	Trace	0
0	0	0	Trace	4	4	Trace	45	0	Trace	0.09	Trace	0
1.7	2.1	0.6	Trace	26	86	0.9	15	310	0.04	0.07	Trace	0
2.4	2.2	0.6	1	26	80	0.9	58	290	0.03	0.13	Trace	0
1.7	2.0	0.6	1	28	90	1.0	65	260	0.04	0.14	Trace	0
1.7	2.0	0.6	1	28	90	1.0	65	260	0.04	0.13	Trace	0
2.8	2.3	0.6	1	47	97	0.9	85	310	0.04	0.16	Trace	0
57.3	23.1	2.1	Trace	27	26	0.2	29	3,470[11]	0.01	0.04	Trace	0
7.2	2.9	0.3	Trace	3	3	Trace	4	430[11]	Trace	Trace	Trace	0
2.5	1.0	0.1	Trace	1	1	Trace	1	150[11]	Trace	Trace	Trace	0

continued on next page

Table B-1
continued

FOOD	APPROXIMATE MEASURES, UNITS, OR WEIGHT	WEIGHT (g)	WATER (%)	FOOD ENERGY (kcal)	PROTEIN (g)	FAT (g)
Whipped (6 sticks or two 8-oz containers per pound)						
Stick (½ c)	1 stick	76	16	540	1	61
Tablespoon (about ⅛ stick)	1 T	9	16	65	Trace	8
Pat (1¼-in. square, ⅓ in. high; 120 per pound)	1 pat	4	16	25	Trace	3
Fats, cooking (vegetable shortenings)	1 c	200	0	1,770	0	200
	1 T	13	0	110	0	13
Lard	1 c	205	0	1,850	0	205
	1 T	13	0	115	0	13
Margarine:						
Regular (1 brick or 4 sticks per pound):						
Stick (½ c)	1 stick	113	16	815	1	92
Tablespoon (about ⅛ stick)	1 T	14	16	100	Trace	12
Pat (1-in. square, ⅓ in. high; 90 per pound)	1 pat	5	16	35	Trace	4
Soft, two 8-oz containers per pound	8 oz	227	16	1,635	1	184
	1 T	14	16	100	Trace	12
Whipped (6 sticks per pound):						
Stick (½ c)	1 stick	76	16	545	Trace	61
Tablespoon (about ⅛ stick)	1 T	9	16	70	Trace	8
Oils, salad or cooking:						
Corn	1 c	218	0	1,925	0	218
	1 T	14	0	120	0	14
Olive	1 c	216	0	1,910	0	216
	1 T	14	0	120	0	14
Peanut	1 c	216	0	1,910	0	216
	1 T	14	0	120	0	14
Safflower	1 c	218	0	1,925	0	218
	1 T	14	0	120	0	14
Soybean oil, hydrogenated (partially hardened)	1 c	218	0	1,925	0	218
	1 T	14	0	120	0	14
Soybean-cottonseed oil blend, hydrogenated	1 c	218	0	1,925	0	218
	1 T	14	0	120	0	14
Salad dressings:						
Commercial:						
Blue cheese:						
Regular	1 T	15	32	75	1	8
Low calorie (5 kcal per teaspoon)	1 T	16	84	10	Trace	1
French:						
Regular	1 T	16	39	65	Trace	6
Low calorie (5 kcal per teaspoon)	1 T	16	77	15	Trace	1
Italian:						
Regular	1 T	15	28	85	Trace	9
Low calorie (2 kcal per teaspoon)	1 T	15	90	10	Trace	1

	FATTY ACIDS											
		NUTRIENTS IN INDICATED QUANTITY										
SATURATED (TOTAL) (g)	UNSATURATED OLEIC (g)	UNSATURATED LINOLEIC (g)	CARBO-HYDRATE (g)	CALCIUM (mg)	PHOS-PHORUS (mg)	IRON (mg)	POTASSIUM (mg)	VITAMIN A VALUE (IU)	THIAMINE (mg)	RIBOFLAVIN (mg)	NIACIN (mg)	ASCORBIC ACID (mg)
38.2	15.4	1.4	Trace	18	17	0.1	20	2,310[11]	Trace	0.03	Trace	0
4.7	1.9	0.2	Trace	2	2	Trace	2	290[11]	Trace	Trace	Trace	0
1.9	0.8	0.1	Trace	1	1	Trace	1	120[11]	0	Trace	Trace	0
48.8	88.2	48.4	0	0	0	0	0	—	0	0	0	0
3.2	5.7	3.1	0	0	0	0	0	—	0	0	0	0
81.0	83.8	20.5	0	0	0	0	0	0	0	0	0	0
5.1	5.3	1.3	0	0	0	0	0	0	0	0	0	0
16.7	42.9	24.9	Trace	27	26	0.2	29	3,750[12]	0.01	0.04	Trace	0
2.1	5.3	3.1	Trace	3	3	Trace	4	470[12]	Trace	Trace	Trace	0
0.7	1.9	1.1	Trace	1	1	Trace	1	170[12]	Trace	Trace	Trace	0
32.5	71.5	65.4	Trace	53	52	0.4	59	7,500[12]	0.01	0.08	0.1	0
2.0	4.5	4.1	Trace	3	3	Trace	4	470[12]	Trace	Trace	Trace	0
11.2	28.7	16.7	Trace	18	17	0.1	20	2,500[12]	Trace	0.03	Trace	0
1.4	3.6	2.1	Trace	2	2	Trace	2	310[12]	Trace	Trace	Trace	0
27.7	53.6	125.1	0	0	0	0	0	—	0	0	0	0
1.7	3.3	7.8	0	0	0	0	0	—	0	0	0	0
30.7	154.4	17.7	0	0	0	0	0	—	0	0	0	0
1.9	9.7	1.1	0	0	0	0	0	—	0	0	0	0
37.4	98.5	67.0	0	0	0	0	0	—	0	0	0	0
2.3	6.2	4.2	0	0	0	0	0	—	0	0	0	0
20.5	25.9	159.8	0	0	0	0	0	—	0	0	0	0
1.3	1.6	10.0	0	0	0	0	0	—	0	0	0	0
31.8	93.1	75.6	0	0	0	0	0	—	0	0	0	0
2.0	5.8	4.7	0	0	0	0	0	—	0	0	0	0
38.2	63.0	99.6	0	0	0	0	0	—	0	0	0	0
2.4	3.9	6.2	0	0	0	0	0	—	0	0	0	0
1.6	1.7	3.8	1	12	11	Trace	6	30	Trace	0.02	Trace	Trace
0.5	0.3	Trace	1	10	8	Trace	5	30	Trace	0.01	Trace	Trace
1.1	1.3	3.2	3	2	2	0.1	13	—	—	—	—	—
0.1	0.1	0.4	2	2	2	0.1	13	—	—	—	—	—
1.6	1.9	4.7	1	2	1	Trace	2	Trace	Trace	Trace	Trace	—
0.1	0.1	0.4	Trace	Trace	1	Trace	2	Trace	Trace	Trace	Trace	—

continued on next page

Table B-1
continued

FOOD	APPROXIMATE MEASURES, UNITS, OR WEIGHT	WEIGHT (g)	WATER (%)	FOOD ENERGY (kcal)	PROTEIN (g)	FAT (g)
Mayonnaise	1 T	14	15	100	Trace	11
Mayonnaise type:						
Regular	1 T	15	41	65	Trace	6
Low calorie (8 kcal per teaspoon)	1 T	16	81	20	Trace	2
Tartar sauce, regular	1 T	14	34	75	Trace	8
Thousand Island:						
Regular	1 T	16	32	80	Trace	8
Low calorie (10 kcal per teaspoon)	1 T	15	68	25	Trace	2
Homemade:						
Cooked type[13]	1 T	16	68	25	1	2
Fish, shellfish, meat, poultry; related products						
Fish and shellfish:						
Bluefish, baked with butter or margarine	3 oz	85	68	135	22	4
Clams:						
Raw, meat only	3 oz	85	82	65	11	1
Canned, solids and liquid	3 oz	85	86	45	7	1
Crabmeat (white or king), canned, not pressed down	1 c	135	77	135	24	3
Fish stick, breaded, cooked, frozen (4 × 1½ in.)	1 fish stick or 1 oz	28	66	50	5	3
Haddock, breaded, fried[14]	3 oz	85	66	140	17	5
Ocean perch, breaded fried[14]	1 fillet	85	59	195	16	11
Oysters, raw, meat only (13–19 medium selects)	1 c	240	85	160	20	4
Salmon, pink, canned, solids and liquid	3 oz	85	71	120	17	5
Sardines, Atlantic, canned in oil, drained solids	3 oz	85	62	175	20	9
Scallops, frozen, breaded, fried, reheated	6	90	60	175	16	8
Shad, baked with butter or margarine and bacon	3 oz	85	64	170	20	10
Shrimp:						
Canned meat	3 oz	85	70	100	21	1
French fried[16]	3 oz	85	57	190	17	9
Tuna, canned in oil, drained solids	3 oz	85	61	170	24	7
Tuna salad[17]	1 c	205	70	350	30	22
Meat and meat products:						
Bacon (20 slices per pound, raw), broiled or fried, crisp	2 slices	15	8	85	4	8
Beef, canned:						
Corned beef	3 oz	85	59	185	22	10
Corned beef hash	1 c	220	67	400	19	25
Beef,[18] cooked:						
Cuts braised, simmered, or pot-roasted:						
Lean and fat (piece, 2½ × x 2½ × ¾ in.)	3 oz	85	53	245	23	16
Lean only	2.5 oz	72	62	140	22	5

					NUTRIENTS IN INDICATED QUANTITY							
	FATTY ACIDS											
	UNSATURATED											
SATURATED (TOTAL) (g)	OLEIC (g)	LINOLEIC (g)	CARBO-HYDRATE (g)	CALCIUM (mg)	PHOS-PHORUS (mg)	IRON (mg)	POTASSIUM (mg)	VITAMIN A VALUE (IU)	THIAMINE (mg)	RIBOFLAVIN (mg)	NIACIN (mg)	ASCORBIC ACID (mg)
2.0	2.4	5.6	Trace	3	4	0.1	5	40	Trace	0.01	Trace	—
1.1	1.4	3.2	2	2	4	Trace	1	30	Trace	Trace	Trace	—
0.4	0.4	1.0	2	3	4	Trace	1	40	Trace	Trace	Trace	—
1.5	1.8	4.1	1	3	4	0.1	11	30	Trace	Trace	Trace	Trace
1.4	1.7	4.0	2	2	3	0.1	18	50	Trace	Trace	Trace	Trace
0.4	0.4	1.0	2	2	3	0.1	17	50	Trace	Trace	Trace	Trace
0.5	0.6	0.3	2	14	15	0.1	19	80	0.01	0.03	Trace	Trace
—	—	—	0	25	244	0.6	—	40	0.09	0.08	1.6	—
—	—	—	2	59	138	5.2	154	90	0.08	0.15	1.1	8
0.2	Trace	Trace	2	47	116	3.5	119	—	0.01	0.09	0.9	—
0.6	0.4	0.1	1	61	246	1.1	149	—	0.11	0.11	2.6	—
—	—	—	2	3	47	0.1	—	0	0.01	0.02	0.5	—
1.4	2.2	1.2	5	34	210	1.0	296	—	0.03	0.06	2.7	2
2.7	4.4	2.3	6	28	192	1.1	242	—	0.10	0.10	1.6	—
1.3	0.2	0.1	8	226	343	13.2	290	740	0.34	0.43	6.0	—
0.9	0.8	0.1	0	167[15]	243	0.7	307	60	0.03	0.16	6.8	—
3.0	2.5	0.5	0	372	424	2.5	502	190	0.02	0.17	4.6	—
—	—	—	9	—	—	—	—	—	—	—	—	—
—	—	—	0	20	266	0.5	320	30	0.11	0.22	7.3	—
0.1	0.1	Trace	1	98	224	2.6	104	50	0.01	0.03	1.5	—
2.3	3.7	2.0	9	61	162	1.7	195	—	0.03	0.07	2.3	—
1.7	1.7	0.7	0	7	199	1.6	—	70	0.04	0.10	10.1	—
4.3	6.3	6.7	7	41	291	2.7	—	590	0.08	0.23	10.3	2
2.5	3.7	0.7	Trace	2	34	0.5	35	0	0.08	0.05	0.8	—
4.9	4.5	0.2	0	17	90	3.7	—	—	0.01	0.20	2.9	—
11.9	10.9	0.5	24	29	147	4.4	440	—	0.02	0.20	4.6	—
6.8	6.5	0.4	0	10	114	2.9	184	30	0.04	0.18	3.6	—
2.1	1.8	0.2	0	10	108	2.7	176	10	0.04	0.17	3.3	—

continued on next page

FOOD	APPROXIMATE MEASURES, UNITS, OR WEIGHT	WEIGHT (g)	WATER (%)	FOOD ENERGY (kcal)	PROTEIN (g)	FAT (g)
Ground beef, broiled:						
Lean with 10% fat patty	3 oz	85	60	185	23	10
Lean with 21% fat patty	2.9 oz	82	54	235	20	17
Roast, oven-cooked, no liquid added:						
Relatively fat, such as rib:						
Lean and fat (2 pieces, 4⅛ × 2¼ × ¼ in.)	3 oz	85	40	375	17	33
Lean only	1.8 oz	51	57	125	14	7
Relatively lean, such as heel of round:						
Lean and fat (2 pieces, 4⅛ × 2¼ × ¼ in.)	3 oz	85	62	165	25	7
Lean only from item 168	2.8 oz	78	65	125	24	3
Steak:						
Relatively fat, such as sirloin, broiled:						
Lean and fat (piece, 2½ × 2½ × ¾ in.)	3 oz	85	44	330	20	27
Lean only	2.0 oz	56	59	115	18	4
Relatively lean, such as round, braised:						
Lean and fat (piece, 4⅛ × 2¼ × ½ in.)	3 oz	85	55	220	24	13
Lean only	2.4 oz	68	61	130	21	4
Beef, dried, chipped	2½-oz	71	48	145	24	4
Beef and vegetable stew	1 c	245	82	220	16	11
Beef potpie (homemade), baked[19] (piece, ⅓ of 9-in.-diam. pie)	1 piece	210	55	515	21	30
Chili con carne with beans, canned	1 c	255	72	340	19	16
Chop suey with beef and pork (homemade)	1 c	250	75	300	26	17
Heart, beef, lean, braised	3 oz	85	61	160	27	5
Lamb, cooked:						
Chop, rib (cut 3 per pound with bone), broiled:						
Lean and fat	3.1 oz	89	43	360	18	32
Lean only	2 oz	57	60	120	16	6
Leg, roasted:						
Lean and fat (2 pieces, 4⅛ × 2¼ × ¼ in.)	3 oz	85	54	235	22	16
Lean only	2.5 oz	71	62	130	20	5
Shoulder, roasted:						
Lean and fat (3 pieces, 2½ × 2½ × ¼ in.)	3 oz	85	50	285	18	23
Lean only	2.3 oz	64	61	130	17	6
Liver, beef, fried[20] (slice, 6½ × 2⅜ × ⅜ in.)	3 oz	85	56	195	22	9
Pork, cured, cooked:						
Ham, light cure, lean and fat, roasted (2 pieces, 4⅛ × 2¼ × ¼ in.)[22]	3 oz	85	54	245	18	19

NUTRIENTS IN INDICATED QUANTITY

| FATTY ACIDS | | | | | | | | | | | | |
SATURATED (TOTAL) (g)	UNSATURATED OLEIC (g)	LINOLEIC (g)	CARBO-HYDRATE (g)	CALCIUM (mg)	PHOS-PHORUS (mg)	IRON (mg)	POTASSIUM (mg)	VITAMIN A VALUE (IU)	THIAMINE (mg)	RIBOFLAVIN (mg)	NIACIN (mg)	ASCORBIC ACID (mg)
4.0	3.9	0.3	0	10	196	3.0	261	20	0.08	0.20	5.1	—
7.0	6.7	0.4	0	9	159	2.6	221	30	0.07	0.17	4.4	—
14.0	13.6	0.8	0	8	158	2.2	189	70	0.05	0.13	3.1	—
3.0	2.5	0.3	0	6	131	1.8	161	10	0.04	0.11	2.6	—
2.8	2.7	0.2	0	11	208	3.2	279	10	0.06	0.19	4.5	—
1.2	1.0	0.1	0	10	199	3.0	268	Trace	0.06	0.18	4.3	—
11.3	11.1	0.6	0	9	162	2.5	220	50	0.05	0.15	4.0	—
1.8	1.6	0.2	0	7	146	2.2	202	10	0.05	0.14	3.6	—
5.5	5.2	0.4	0	10	213	3.0	272	20	0.07	0.19	4.8	—
1.7	1.5	0.2	0	9	182	2.5	238	10	0.05	0.16	4.1	—
2.1	2.0	0.1	0	14	287	3.6	142	—	0.05	0.23	2.7	0
4.9	4.5	0.2	15	29	184	2.9	613	2,400	0.15	0.17	4.7	17
7.9	12.8	6.7	39	29	149	3.8	334	1,720	0.30	0.30	5.5	6
7.5	6.8	0.3	31	82	321	4.3	594	150	0.08	0.18	3.3	—
8.5	6.2	0.7	13	60	248	4.8	425	600	0.28	0.38	5.0	33
1.5	1.1	0.6	1	5	154	5.0	197	20	0.21	1.04	6.5	1
14.8	12.1	1.2	0	8	139	1.0	200	—	0.11	0.19	4.1	—
2.5	2.1	0.2	0	6	121	1.1	174	—	0.09	0.15	3.4	—
7.3	6.0	0.6	0	9	177	1.4	241	—	0.13	0.23	4.7	—
2.1	1.8	0.2	0	9	169	1.4	227	—	0.12	0.21	4.4	—
10.8	8.8	0.9	0	9	146	1.0	206	—	0.11	0.20	4.0	—
3.6	2.3	0.2	0	8	140	1.0	193	—	0.10	0.18	3.7	—
2.5	3.5	0.9	5	9	405	7.5	323	45,390[21]	0.22	3.56	14.0	23
6.8	7.9	1.7	0	8	146	2.2	199	0	0.40	0.15	3.1	—

continued on next page

Table B-1
continued

FOOD	APPROXIMATE MEASURES, UNITS, OR WEIGHT	WEIGHT (g)	WATER (%)	FOOD ENERGY (kcal)	PROTEIN (g)	FAT (g)
Luncheon meat:						
Boiled ham, slice	1 oz	28	59	65	5	5
Canned, spiced or unspiced:						
Slice, 3 × 2 × ½ in.	1 slice	60	55	175	9	15
Pork, fresh, cooked:[18]						
Chop, loin (cut 3 per pound with bone), broiled:						
Lean and fat	2.7 oz	78	42	305	19	25
Lean only	2 oz	56	53	150	17	9
Roast, oven-cooked, no liquid added:						
Lean and fat (piece, 2½ × 2½ × ¾ in.)	3 oz	85	46	310	21	24
Lean only	2.4 oz	68	55	175	20	10
Shoulder cut, simmered:						
Lean and fat (3 pieces, 2½ × 2½ × ¼ in.)	3 oz	85	46	320	20	26
Lean only	2.2 oz	63	60	135	18	6
Sausages (see also Luncheon meat):						
Bologna, slice	1 oz	28	56	85	3	8
Braunschweiger, slice	1 oz	28	53	90	4	8
Brown-and-serve (10 to 11 per 8-oz package), browned	1 link	17	40	70	3	6
Deviled ham, canned	1 T	13	51	45	2	4
Frankfurter (8 per 1-lb package), cooked (reheated)	1	56	57	170	7	15
Meat, potted (beef, chicken, turkey), canned	1 T	13	61	30	2	2
Pork link (16 per 1-lb package), cooked	1 link	13	35	60	2	6
Salami:						
Dry type, slice (12 per 4-oz package)	1 slice	10	30	45	2	4
Cooked type, slice (8 per 8-oz package)	1 slice	28	51	90	5	7
Vienna sausage (7 per 4-oz can)	1	16	63	40	2	3
Veal, medium fat, cooked, bone removed:						
Cutlet (4⅛ × 2¼ × ½ in.), braised or broiled	3 oz	85	60	185	23	9
Rib (2 pieces, 4⅛ × 2¼ × ¼ in.), roasted	3 oz	85	55	230	23	14
Poultry and poultry products:						
Chicken, cooked:						
Breast, fried,[23] bones removed, ½ breast (3.3 oz with bones)	2.8 oz	79	58	160	26	5
Drumstick, fried,[23] bones removed (2 oz with bones)	1.3 oz	38	55	90	12	4
Half broiler, broiled, bones removed (10.4 oz with bones)	6.2 oz	176	71	240	42	7
Chicken, canned, boneless	3 oz	85	65	170	18	10
Chicken a la king, cooked (homemade)	1 c	245	68	470	27	34
Chicken and noodles, cooked (homemade)	1 c	240	71	365	22	18

| | FATTY ACIDS | | | | | | | | | | | |
| | UNSATURATED | | | | | | | | | | | |
SATURATED (TOTAL) (g)	OLEIC (g)	LINOLEIC (g)	CARBO-HYDRATE (g)	CALCIUM (mg)	PHOS-PHORUS (mg)	IRON (mg)	POTASSIUM (mg)	VITAMIN A VALUE (IU)	THIAMINE (mg)	RIBOFLAVIN (mg)	NIACIN (mg)	ASCORBIC ACID (mg)
1.7	2.0	0.4	0	3	47	0.8	—	0	0.12	0.04	0.7	—
5.4	6.7	1.0	1	5	65	1.3	133	0	0.19	0.13	1.8	—
8.9	10.4	2.2	0	9	209	2.7	216	0	0.75	0.22	4.5	—
3.1	3.6	0.8	0	7	181	2.2	192	0	0.63	0.18	3.8	—
8.7	10.2	2.2	0	9	218	2.7	233	0	0.78	0.22	4.8	—
3.5	4.1	0.8	0	9	211	2.6	224	0	0.73	0.21	4.4	—
9.3	10.9	2.3	0	9	118	2.6	158	0	0.46	0.21	4.1	—
2.2	2.6	0.6	0	8	111	2.3	146	0	0.42	0.19	3.7	—
3.0	3.4	0.5	Trace	2	36	0.5	65	—	0.05	0.06	0.7	—
2.6	3.4	0.8	1	3	69	1.7	—	1,850	0.05	0.41	2.3	—
2.3	2.8	0.7	Trace	—	—	—	—	—	—	—	—	—
1.5	1.8	0.4	0	1	12	0.3	—	0	0.02	0.01	0.2	—
5.6	6.5	1.2	1	3	57	0.8	—	—	0.08	0.11	1.4	—
—	—	—	0	—	—	—	—	—	Trace	0.03	0.2	—
2.1	2.4	0.5	Trace	1	21	0.3	35	0	0.10	0.04	0.5	—
1.6	1.6	0.1	Trace	1	28	0.4	—	—	0.04	0.03	0.5	—
3.1	3.0	0.2	Trace	3	57	0.7	—	—	0.07	0.07	1.2	—
1.2	1.4	0.2	Trace	1	24	0.3	—	—	0.01	0.02	0.4	—
4.0	3.4	0.4	0	9	196	2.7	258	—	0.06	0.21	4.6	—
6.1	5.1	0.6	0	10	211	2.9	259	—	0.11	0.26	6.6	—
1.4	1.8	1.1	1	9	218	1.3	—	70	0.04	0.17	11.6	—
1.1	1.3	0.9	Trace	6	89	0.9	—	50	0.03	0.15	2.7	—
2.2	2.5	1.3	0	16	355	3.0	483	160	0.09	0.34	15.5	—
3.2	3.8	2.0	0	18	210	1.3	117	200	0.03	0.11	3.7	3
12.7	14.3	3.3	12	127	358	2.5	404	1,130	0.10	0.42	5.4	12
5.9	7.1	3.5	26	26	247	2.2	149	430	0.05	0.17	4.3	Trace

NUTRIENTS IN INDICATED QUANTITY

continued on next page

Table B-1
continued

FOOD	APPROXIMATE MEASURES, UNITS, OR WEIGHT	WEIGHT (g)	WATER (%)	FOOD ENERGY (kcal)	PROTEIN (g)	FAT (g)
Chicken chow mein:						
Canned	1 c	250	89	95	7	Trace
Homemade	1 c	250	78	255	31	10
Chicken potpie (homemade), baked,[19] piece (⅓ of 9-in.-diam. pie)	1 piece	232	57	545	23	31
Turkey, roasted, flesh without skin:						
Dark meat, piece, 2½ × 1⅝ × ¼ in.	4 pieces	85	61	175	26	7
Light and dark meat:						
Chopped or diced	1 c	140	61	265	44	9
Pieces (1 slice white meat, 4 × 2 × ¼ in., and 2 slices dark meat, 2½ × 1⅝ × ¼ in.)	3 pieces	85	61	160	27	5
Light meat, piece, 4 × 2 × ¼ in.	2 pieces	85	62	150	28	3
Fruits and fruit products						
Apples, raw, unpeeled, without cores:						
2¾-in. diam. (about 3 per pound with cores)	1	138	84	80	Trace	1
3¼-in. diam. (about 2 per pound with cores)	1	212	84	125	Trace	1
Applejuice, bottled or canned[24]	1 c	248	88	120	Trace	Trace
Applesauce, canned:						
Sweetened	1 c	255	76	230	1	Trace
Unsweetened	1 c	244	89	100	Trace	Trace
Apricots:						
Raw, without pits (about 12 per pound with pits)	3	107	85	55	1	Trace
Canned in heavy syrup (halves and syrup)	1 c	258	77	220	2	Trace
Dried:						
Uncooked (28 large or 37 medium halves per cup)	1 c	130	25	340	7	1
Cooked, unsweetened, fruit and liquid	1 c	250	76	215	4	1
Apricot nectar, canned	1 c	251	85	145	1	Trace
Avocados, raw, whole, without skins and seeds:						
California, mid- and late-winter (with skin and seed, 3⅛-in. diam.; 10 oz)	1	216	74	370	5	37
Florida, late summer and fall (with skin and seed, 3⅝-in. diam.; 1 lb)	1	304	78	390	4	33
Banana, without peel (about 2.6 per pound with peel)	1	119	76	100	1	Trace
Banana flakes	1 T	6	3	20	Trace	Trace
Blackberries, raw	1 c	144	85	85	2	1
Blueberries, raw	1 c	145	83	90	1	1
Cantaloupe. See Muskmelons.						
Cherries:						
Sour (tart), red, pitted, canned, water pack	1 c	244	88	105	2	Trace
Sweet, raw, without pits and stems	10	68	80	45	1	Trace
Cranberry juice cocktail, bottled, sweetened	1 c	253	83	165	Trace	Trace
Cranberry sauce, sweetened, canned, strained	1 c	277	62	405	Trace	1

						NUTRIENTS IN INDICATED QUANTITY						
	FATTY ACIDS											
SATURATED (TOTAL) (g)	**UNSATURATED**		**CARBO-HYDRATE (g)**	**CALCIUM (mg)**	**PHOS-PHORUS (mg)**	**IRON (mg)**	**POTASSIUM (mg)**	**VITAMIN A VALUE (IU)**	**THIAMINE (mg)**	**RIBOFLAVIN (mg)**	**NIACIN (mg)**	**ASCORBIC ACID (mg)**
	OLEIC (g)	**LINOLEIC (g)**										
—	—	—	18	45	35	1.3	418	150	0.05	0.10	1.0	13
2.4	3.4	3.1	10	58	293	2.5	473	280	0.08	0.23	4.3	10
11.3	10.9	5.6	42	70	232	3.0	343	3,090	0.34	0.31	5.5	5
2.1	1.5	1.5	0	—	—	2.0	338	—	0.03	0.20	3.6	—
2.5	1.7	1.8	0	11	351	2.5	514	—	0.07	0.25	10.8	—
1.5	1.0	1.1	0	7	213	1.5	312	—	0.04	0.15	6.5	—
0.9	0.6	0.7	0	—	—	1.0	349	—	0.04	0.12	9.4	—
—	—	—	20	10	14	0.4	152	120	0.04	0.03	0.1	6
—	—	—	31	15	21	0.6	233	190	0.06	0.04	0.2	8
—	—	—	30	15	22	1.5	250	—	0.02	0.05	0.2	2[25]
—	—	—	61	10	13	1.3	166	100	0.05	0.03	0.1	3[25]
—	—	—	26	10	12	1.2	190	100	0.05	0.02	0.1	2[25]
—	—	—	14	18	25	0.5	301	2,890	0.03	0.04	0.6	11
—	—	—	57	28	39	0.8	604	4,490	0.05	0.05	1.0	10
—	—	—	86	87	140	7.2	1,273	14,170	0.01	0.21	4.3	16
—	—	—	54	55	88	4.5	795	7,500	0.01	0.13	2.5	8
—	—	—	37	23	30	0.5	379	2,380	0.03	0.03	0.5	36[26]
5.5	22.0	3.7	13	22	91	1.3	1,303	630	0.24	0.43	3.5	30
6.7	15.7	5.3	27	30	128	1.8	1,836	880	0.33	0.61	4.9	43
—	—	—	26	10	31	0.8	440	230	0.06	0.07	0.8	12
—	—	—	5	2	6	0.2	92	50	0.01	0.01	0.2	Trace
—	—	—	19	46	27	1.3	245	290	0.04	0.06	0.6	30
—	—	—	22	22	19	1.5	117	150	0.04	0.09	0.7	20
—	—	—	26	37	32	0.7	317	1,660	0.07	0.05	0.5	12
—	—	—	12	15	13	0.3	129	70	0.03	0.04	0.3	7
—	—	—	42	13	8	0.8	25	Trace	0.03	0.03	0.1	81[27]
—	—	—	104	17	11	0.6	83	60	0.03	0.03	0.1	6

continued on next page

Table B-1
continued

FOOD	APPROXIMATE MEASURES, UNITS, OR WEIGHT	WEIGHT (g)	WATER (%)	FOOD ENERGY (kcal)	PROTEIN (g)	FAT (g)
Dates:						
Whole, without pits	10	80	23	220	2	Trace
Chopped	1 c	178	23	490	4	1
Fruit cocktail, canned, in heavy syrup	1 c	255	80	195	1	Trace
Grapefruit:						
Raw, medium, 3¾-in. diam. (about 1 lb 1 oz):						
Pink or red, with peel	½	241[28]	89	50	1	Trace
White, with peel	½	241[28]	89	45	1	Trace
Canned, sections with syrup	1 c	254	81	180	2	Trace
Grapefruit juice:						
Raw, pink, red, or white	1 c	246	90	95	1	Trace
Canned, white:						
Unsweetened	1 c	247	89	100	1	Trace
Sweetened	1 c	250	86	135	1	Trace
Frozen, concentrate, unsweetened:						
Undiluted	6 fl oz	207	62	300	4	1
Diluted with 3 parts water by volume	1 c	247	89	100	1	Trace
Dehydrated crystals, prepared with water (1 lb yields about 1 gal)	1 c	247	90	100	1	Trace
Grapes, European type (adherent skin), raw:						
Thompson seedless	10	50	81	35	Trace	Trace
Tokay and Emperor (seeded)	10	60[30]	81	40	Trace	Trace
Grape juice:						
Canned or bottled	1 c	253	83	165	1	Trace
Frozen concentrate, sweetened:						
Undiluted	6 fl oz	216	53	395	1	Trace
Diluted with 3 parts water by volume	1 c	250	86	135	1	Trace
Grape drink, canned	1 c	250	86	135	Trace	Trace
Lemon, raw, size 165, without peel and seeds (about 4 per pound with peels and seeds)	1	74	90	20	1	Trace
Lemonade concentrate, frozen:						
Undiluted	6 fl oz	219	49	425	Trace	Trace
Diluted with 4⅓ parts water by volume	1 c	248	89	105	Trace	Trace
Lemon juice:						
Raw	1 c	244	91	60	1	Trace
Canned or bottled, unsweetened	1 c	244	92	55	1	Trace
Frozen, single strength, unsweetened	6 oz	183	92	40	1	Trace
Limeade concentrate, frozen:						
Undiluted	6 fl oz	218	50	410	Trace	Trace
Diluted with 4⅓ parts water by volume	1 c	247	89	100	Trace	Trace
Lime juice:						
Raw	1 c	246	90	65	1	Trace
Canned, unsweetened	1 c	246	90	65	1	Trace
Muskmelons, raw, with rind, without seed cavity:						
Cantaloupe, orange-fleshed (with rind and seed cavity, 5-in. diam., 2⅓ lb), with rind	½	477[33]	91	80	2	Trace

	FATTY ACIDS											
		UNSATURATED										
SATURATED (TOTAL) (g)	OLEIC (g)	LINOLEIC (g)	CARBO-HYDRATE (g)	CALCIUM (mg)	PHOS-PHORUS (mg)	IRON (mg)	POTASSIUM (mg)	VITAMIN A VALUE (IU)	THIAMINE (mg)	RIBOFLAVIN (mg)	NIACIN (mg)	ASCORBIC ACID (mg)

NUTRIENTS IN INDICATED QUANTITY

SAT	OLEIC	LINOLEIC	CARBO	CALCIUM	PHOS	IRON	POTASSIUM	VIT A	THIAMINE	RIBOFLAVIN	NIACIN	ASCORBIC
—	—	—	58	47	50	2.4	518	40	0.07	0.08	1.8	0
—	—	—	130	105	112	5.3	1,153	90	0.16	0.18	3.9	0
—	—	—	50	23	31	1.0	411	360	0.05	0.03	1.0	5
—	—	—	13	20	20	0.5	166	540	0.05	0.02	0.2	44
—	—	—	12	19	19	0.5	159	10	0.05	0.02	0.2	44
—	—	—	45	33	36	0.8	343	30	0.08	0.05	0.5	76
—	—	—	23	22	37	0.5	399	29	0.10	0.05	0.5	93
—	—	—	24	20	35	1.0	400	20	0.07	0.05	0.5	84
—	—	—	32	20	35	1.0	405	30	0.08	0.05	0.	78
—	—	—	72	70	124	0.8	1,250	60	0.29	0.12	1.4	286
—	—	—	24	25	42	0.2	420	20	0.10	0.04	0.5	96
—	—	—	24	22	40	0.2	412	20	0.10	0.05	0.5	91
—	—	—	9	6	10	0.2	87	50	0.03	0.02	0.2	2
—	—	—	10	7	11	0.2	99	60	0.03	0.02	0.2	2
—	—	—	42	28	30	0.8	293	—	0.10	0.05	0.5	Trace[25]
—	—	—	100	22	32	0.9	255	40	0.13	0.22	1.5	32[31]
—	—	—	33	8	10	0.3	85	10	0.05	0.08	0.5	10[31]
—	—	—	35	8	10	0.3	88	—	0.03[32]	0.03[32]	0.3	[32]
—	—	—	6	19	12	0.4	102	10	0.03	0.01	0.1	39
—	—	—	112	9	13	0.4	153	40	0.05	0.06	0.7	66
—	—	—	28	2	3	0.1	40	10	0.01	0.02	0.2	17
—	—	—	20	17	24	0.5	344	50	0.07	0.02	0.2	112
—	—	—	19	17	24	0.5	344	50	0.07	0.02	0.2	102
—	—	—	13	13	16	0.5	258	40	0.05	0.02	0.2	81
—	—	—	108	11	13	0.2	129	Trace	0.02	0.02	0.2	26
—	—	—	27	3	3	Trace	32	Trace	Trace	Trace	Trace	6
—	—	—	22	22	27	0.5	256	20	0.05	0.02	0.2	79
—	—	—	22	22	27	0.5	256	20	0.05	0.02	0.2	52
—	—	—	20	38	44	1.1	682	9,240	0.11	0.08	1.6	90

Table B-1
continued

FOOD	APPROXIMATE MEASURES, UNITS, OR WEIGHT	WEIGHT (g)	WATER (%)	FOOD ENERGY (kcal)	PROTEIN (g)	FAT (g)
Honeydew (with rind and seed cavity, 6½-in. diam., 5¼ lb), with rind	1/10	226[33]	91	50	1	Trace
Oranges, all commercial varieties, raw:						
Whole, 2⅝-in. diam., without peel and seeds (about 2½ per pounds with peel and seeds)	1	131	86	65	1	Trace
Sections without membranes	1 c	180	86	90	2	Trace
Orange juice:						
Raw, all varieties	1 c	248	88	110	2	Trace
Canned, unsweetened	1 c	249	87	120	2	Trace
Frozen concentrate:						
Undiluted	6 fl oz	213	55	360	5	Trace
Diluted with 3 parts water by volume	1 c	249	87	120	2	Trace
Dehydrated crystals, prepared with water (1 lb yields about 1 gal)	1 c	248	88	115	1	Trace
Orange and grapefruit juice:						
Frozen concentrate:						
Undiluted	6 fl oz	210	59	330	4	1
Diluted with 3 parts water by volume	1 c	248	88	110	1	Trace
Papayas, raw, ½-in. cubes	1 c	140	89	55	1	Trace
Peaches:						
Raw:						
Whole, 2½-in. diam., peeled, pitted (about 4 per pound with peels and pits)	1	100	89	40	1	Trace
Sliced	1 c	170	89	65	1	Trace
Canned, yellow-fleshed, solids and liquids (halves or slices):						
Syrup pack	1 c	256	79	200	1	Trace
Water pack	1 c	244	91	75	1	Trace
Dried:						
Uncooked	1 c	160	25	420	5	1
Cooked, unsweetened, halves and juice	1 c	250	77	205	3	1
Frozen, sliced, sweetened:						
10-oz container	1 container	284	77	250	1	Trace
Cup	1 c	250	77	220	1	Trace
Pears:						
Raw, with skin, cored:						
Anjou, 3-in. diam. (about 2 per pound with cores and stems)	1	200	83	120	1	1
Bartlett, 2½-in. diam. (about 2½ per pound with cores and stems)	1	164	83	100	1	1
Bosc, 2½-in. diam. (about 3 per pound with cores and stems)	1	141	83	85	1	1
Canned, solids and liquids, syrup pack, heavy (halves or slices)	1 c	255	80	195	1	1

NUTRIENTS IN INDICATED QUANTITY

| FATTY ACIDS | | | | | | | | | | | | |
SATURATED (TOTAL) (g)	UNSATURATED OLEIC (g)	LINOLEIC (g)	CARBO-HYDRATE (g)	CALCIUM (mg)	PHOS-PHORUS (mg)	IRON (mg)	POTASSIUM (mg)	VITAMIN A VALUE (IU)	THIAMINE (mg)	RIBOFLAVIN (mg)	NIACIN (mg)	ASCORBIC ACID (mg)
—	—	—	11	21	24	0.6	374	60	0.06	0.04	0.9	34
—	—	—	16	54	26	0.5	263	260	0.13	0.05	0.5	66
—	—	—	22	74	36	0.7	360	360	0.18	0.07	0.7	90
—	—	—	26	27	42	0.5	496	500	0.22	0.07	1.0	124
—	—	—	28	25	45	1.0	496	500	0.17	0.05	0.7	100
—	—	—	87	75	126	0.9	1,500	1,620	0.68	0.11	2.8	360
—	—	—	29	25	42	0.2	503	540	0.23	0.03	0.9	120
—	—	—	27	25	40	0.5	518	500	0.20	0.07	1.0	109
—	—	—	78	61	99	0.8	1,308	800	0.48	0.06	2.3	302
—	—	—	26	20	32	0.2	439	270	0.15	0.02	0.7	102
—	—	—	14	28	22	0.4	328	2,450	0.06	0.06	0.4	78
—	—	—	10	9	19	0.5	202	1,330[34]	0.02	0.05	1.0	7
—	—	—	16	15	32	0.9	343	2,260[34]	0.03	0.09	1.7	12
—	—	—	51	10	31	0.8	333	1,100	0.03	0.05	1.5	8
—	—	—	20	10	32	0.7	334	1,100	0.02	0.07	1.5	7
—	—	—	109	77	187	9.6	1,520	6,240	0.02	0.30	8.5	29
—	—	—	54	38	93	4.8	743	3,050	0.01	0.15	3.8	5
—	—	—	64	11	37	1.4	352	1,850	0.03	0.11	2.0	116[35]
—	—	—	57	10	33	1.3	310	1,630	0.03	0.10	1.8	103[35]
—	—	—	31	16	22	0.6	260	40	0.04	0.08	0.2	8
—	—	—	25	13	18	0.5	213	30	0.03	0.07	0.2	7
—	—	—	22	11	16	0.4	83	30	0.03	0.06	0.1	6
—	—	—	50	13	18	0.5	214	10	0.03	0.05	0.3	3

continued on next page

Table B-1
continued

FOOD	APPROXIMATE MEASURES, UNITS, OR WEIGHT	WEIGHT (g)	WATER (%)	FOOD ENERGY (kcal)	PROTEIN (g)	FAT (g)
Pineapple:						
Raw, diced	1 c	155	85	80	1	Trace
Canned, heavy syrup pack, solids and liquid:						
Crushed, chunks, tidbits	1 c	255	80	190	1	Trace
Slices and liquid:						
Large	1 slice; 2¼ T liquid	105	80	80	Trace	Trace
Medium	1 slice; 1¼ T liquid	58	80	45	Trace	Trace
Pineapple juice, unsweetened, canned	1 c	250	86	140	1	Trace
Plums:						
Raw, without pits:						
Japanese and hybrid (2⅛-in. diam., about 6½ per pound with pits)	1	66	87	30	Trace	Trace
Prune-type (1½-in. diam., about 15 per pound with pits)	1	28	79	20	Trace	Trace
Canned, heavy syrup pack (Italian prunes), with pits and liquid:						
Cup	1 c[36]	272	77	215	1	Trace
Portion	3; 2¾ T liquid[36]	140	77	110	1	Trace
Prunes, dried, "softenized," with pits:						
Uncooked	4 extra large or 5 large	49[36]	28	110	1	Trace
Cooked, unsweetened, all sizes, fruit and liquid	1 c	250[36]	66	255	2	1
Prune juice, canned or bottles	1 c	256	80	195	1	Trace
Raisins, seedless:						
Cup, not pressed down	1 c	145	18	420	4	Trace
Packet, ½ oz (1½ T)	1 packet	14	18	40	Trace	Trace
Raspberries, red:						
Raw, capped, whole	1 c	123	84	70	1	1
Frozen, sweetened	10 oz	284	74	280	2	1
Rhubarb, cooked, added sugar:						
From raw	1 c	270	63	380	1	Trace
From frozen, sweetened	1 c	270	63	385	1	1
Strawberries:						
Raw, whole berries, capped	1 c	149	90	55	1	1
Frozen, sweetened:						
Sliced	10 oz	284	71	310	1	1
Whole	1 lb (about 1¾ c)	454	76	415	2	1
Tangerine, raw, 2⅜-in. diam., size 176, without peel (about 4 per pound with peels and seeds)	1	86	87	40	1	Trace
Tangerine juice, canned, sweetened	1c	249	87	125	1	Trace
Watermelon, raw, 4 × 8 in. wedge with rind and seeds (¹⁄₁₆ of 32⅔-lb melon, 10 × 16 in.)	1	926[37]	93	110	2	1

| | FATTY ACIDS | | | | | | | | | | | |
| SATURATED (TOTAL) (g) | UNSATURATED | | CARBO-HYDRATE (g) | CALCIUM (mg) | PHOS-PHORUS (mg) | IRON (mg) | POTASSIUM (mg) | VITAMIN A VALUE (IU) | THIAMINE (mg) | RIBOFLAVIN (mg) | NIACIN (mg) | ASCORBIC ACID (mg) |
	OLEIC (g)	LINOLEIC (g)										
—	—	—	21	26	12	0.8	226	110	0.14	0.05	0.3	26
—	—	—	49	28	13	0.8	245	130	0.20	0.05	0.5	18
—	—	—	20	12	5	0.3	101	50	0.08	0.02	0.2	7
—	—	—	11	6	3	0.2	56	30	0.05	0.01	0.1	4
—	—	—	34	38	23	0.8	373	130	0.13	0.05	0.5	80[27]
—	—	—	8	8	12	0.3	112	160	0.02	0.02	0.3	4
—	—	—	6	3	5	0.1	48	80	0.01	0.01	0.1	1
—	—	—	56	23	26	2.3	367	3,130	0.05	0.05	1.0	5
—	—	—	29	12	13	1.2	189	1,610	0.03	0.03	0.5	3
—	—	—	29	22	34	1.7	298	690	0.04	0.07	0.7	1
—	—	—	67	51	79	3.8	695	1,590	0.07	0.15	1.5	2
—	—	—	49	36	51	1.8	602	—	0.03	0.03	1.0	5
—	—	—	112	90	146	5.1	1,106	30	0.16	0.12	0.7	1
—	—	—	11	9	14	0.5	107	Trace	0.02	0.01	0.1	Trace
—	—	—	17	27	27	1.1	207	160	0.04	0.11	1.1	31
—	—	—	70	37	48	1.7	284	200	0.06	0.17	1.7	60
—	—	—	97	211	41	1.6	548	220	0.05	0.14	0.8	16
—	—	—	98	211	32	1.9	475	190	0.03	0.11	0.5	16
—	—	—	13	31	31	1.5	244	90	0.04	0.10	0.9	88
—	—	—	79	40	48	2.0	318	90	0.06	0.17	1.4	151
—	—	—	107	59	73	2.7	472	140	0.09	0.27	2.3	249
—	—	—	10	34	15	0.3	108	360	0.05	0.02	0.1	27
—	—	—	30	44	35	0.5	440	1,040	0.15	0.05	0.2	54
—	—	—	27	30	43	2.1	426	2,510	0.13	0.13	0.9	30

continued on next page

FOOD	APPROXIMATE MEASURES, UNITS, OR WEIGHT	WEIGHT (g)	WATER (%)	FOOD ENERGY (kcal)	PROTEIN (g)	FAT (g)
Grain products						
Bagel, 3-in. diam.:						
Egg	1	55	32	165	6	2
Water	1	55	29	165	6	1
Barley, pearled, light, uncooked	1 c	200	11	700	16	2
Biscuits, baking powder, 2-in. diam. (enriched flour, vegetable shortening):						
Homemade	1	28	27	105	2	5
From mix	1	28	29	90	2	3
Bread crumbs (enriched):[38]						
Dry, grated	1 c	100	7	390	13	5
Soft. See Bread, White.						
Bread:						
Boston brown bread, canned, slice, 3¼ × ½ in.[38]	1 sl	45	45	95	2	1
Cracked wheat (¾ enriched wheat flour, ¼ cracked wheat):[38]						
Loaf	1 lb	454	35	1,195	39	10
Slice (18 per loaf)	1 sl	25	35	65	2	1
French or Vienna, enriched:[38]						
Loaf	1 lb	454	31	1,315	41	14
Slice:						
French (5 × 2½ × 1 in.)	1 sl	35	31	100	3	1
Vienna (4¾ × 4 × ½ in.)	1 sl	25	31	75	2	1
Italian, enriched:						
Loaf	1 lb	454	32	1,250	41	4
Slice, 4½ × 3¼ × ¾ in.	1 sl	30	32	85	3	Trace
Raisin, enriched:[38]						
Loaf	1 lb	454	35	1,190	30	13
Slice (18 per loaf)	1 sl	25	35	65	2	1
Rye:						
American, light (⅔ enriched wheat flour, ⅓ rye flour):						
Loaf	1 lb	454	36	1,100	41	5
Slice (4¾ × 3¾ × 7/16 in.)	1 sl	25	36	60	2	Trace
Pumpernickel (⅔ rye flour, ⅓ enriched wheat flour):						
Loaf	1 lb	454	34	1,115	41	5
Slice (5 × 4 × ⅜ in.)	1 sl	32	34	80	3	Trace
White, enriched:[38]						
Soft-crumb type:						
Loaf	1 lb	454	36	1,225	39	15
Slice (18 per loaf)	1 sl	25	36	70	2	1
Toast	1 sl	22	25	70	2	1
Slice (22 per loaf)	1 sl	20	36	55	2	1
Toast	1 sl	17	25	55	2	1

NUTRIENTS IN INDICATED QUANTITY

| FATTY ACIDS | | | | | | | | | | | | |
SATURATED (TOTAL) (g)	UNSATURATED OLEIC (g)	UNSATURATED LINOLEIC (g)	CARBO-HYDRATE (g)	CALCIUM (mg)	PHOS-PHORUS (mg)	IRON (mg)	POTASSIUM (mg)	VITAMIN A VALUE (IU)	THIAMINE (mg)	RIBOFLAVIN (mg)	NIACIN (mg)	ASCORBIC ACID (mg)
0.5	0.9	0.8	28	9	43	1.2	41	30	0.14	0.10	1.2	0
0.2	0.4	0.6	30	8	41	1.2	42	0	0.15	0.11	1.4	0
0.3	0.2	0.8	158	32	378	4.0	320	0	0.24	0.10	6.2	0
1.2	2.0	1.2	13	34	49	0.4	33	Trace	0.08	0.08	0.7	Trace
0.6	1.1	0.7	15	19	65	0.6	32	Trace	0.09	0.08	0.8	Trace
1.0	1.6	1.4	73	122	141	3.6	152	Trace	0.35	0.35	4.8	Trace
0.1	0.2	0.2	21	41	72	0.9	131	0[39]	0.06	0.04	0.7	0
2.2	3.0	3.9	236	399	581	9.5	608	Trace	1.52	1.13	14.4	Trace
0.1	0.2	0.2	13	22	32	0.5	34	Trace	0.08	0.06	0.8	Trace
3.2	4.7	4.6	251	195	386	10.0	408	Trace	1.80	1.10	15.0	Trace
0.2	0.4	0.4	19	15	30	0.8	32	Trace	0.14	0.08	1.2	Trace
0.2	0.3	0.3	14	11	21	0.6	23	Trace	0.10	0.06	0.8	Trace
0.6	0.3	1.5	256	77	349	10.0	336	0	1.80	1.10	15.0	0
Trace	Trace	0.1	17	5	23	0.7	22	0	0.12	0.07	1.0	0
3.0	4.7	3.9	243	322	395	10.0	1,057	Trace	1.70	1.07	10.7	Trace
0.2	0.3	0.2	13	18	22	0.6	58	Trace	0.09	0.06	0.6	Trace
0.7	0.5	2.2	236	340	667	9.1	658	0	1.35	0.98	12.9	0
Trace	Trace	0.1	13	19	37	0.5	36	0	0.07	0.05	0.7	0
0.7	0.5	2.4	241	381	1,039	11.8	2,059	0	1.30	0.93	8.5	0
0.1	Trace	0.2	17	27	73	0.8	145	0	0.09	0.07	0.6	0
3.4	5.3	4.6	229	381	440	11.3	476	Trace	1.80	1.10	15.0	Trace
0.2	0.3	0.3	13	21	24	0.6	26	Trace	0.10	0.06	0.8	Trace
0.2	0.3	0.3	13	21	24	0.6	26	Trace	0.08	0.06	0.8	Trace
0.2	0.2	0.2	10	17	19	0.5	21	Trace	0.08	0.05	0.7	Trace
0.2	0.2	0.2	10	17	19	0.5	21	Trace	0.06	0.05	0.7	Trace

continued on next page

Table B-1
continued

FOOD	APPROXIMATE MEASURES, UNITS, OR WEIGHT	WEIGHT (g)	WATER (%)	FOOD ENERGY (kcal)	PROTEIN (g)	FAT (g)
Loaf	1½ lb	680	36	1,835	59	22
Slice (24 per loaf)	1 sl	28	36	75	2	1
Toast	1 sl	24	25	75	2	1
Slice (28 per loaf)	1 sl	24	36	65	2	1
Toast	1 sl	21	25	65	2	1
Crumbs	1 c	45	36	120	4	1
Cubes	1 c	30	36	80	3	1
Firm-crumb type:						
Loaf	1 lb	454	35	1,245	41	17
Slice (20 per loaf)	1 sl	23	35	65	2	1
Toast	1 sl	20	24	65	2	1
Loaf	2 lb	907	35	2,495	82	34
Slice (34 per loaf)	1 sl	27	35	75	2	1
Toast	1 sl	23	24	75	2	1
Whole wheat:						
Soft-crumb type:[38]						
Loaf	1 lb	454	36	1,095	41	12
Slice (16 per loaf)	1 sl	28	36	65	3	1
Toast	1 sl	24	24	65	3	1
Firm-crumb type:[38]						
Loaf	1 lb	454	36	1,100	48	14
Slice (18 per loaf)	1 sl	25	36	60	3	1
Toast	1 sl	21	24	60	3	1
Breakfast cereals:						
Hot type, cooked:						
Corn (hominy) grits, degermed:						
Enriched	1 c	245	87	125	3	Trace
Unenriched	1 c	245	87	125	3	Trace
Farina, quick-cooking, enriched	1 c	245	89	105	3	Trace
Oatmeal or rolled oats	1 c	240	87	130	5	2
Wheat, rolled	1 c	240	80	180	5	1
Wheat, whole meal	1 c	245	88	110	4	1
Ready-to-eat:						
Bran flakes (40% bran), added sugar, salt, iron, vitamins	1 c	35	3	105	4	1
Bran flakes with raisins, added sugar, salt, iron, vitamins	1 c	50	7	145	4	1
Corn flakes:						
Plain, added sugar, salt, iron, vitamins	1 c	25	4	95	2	Trace
Sugar-coated, added salt, iron, vitamins	1 c	40	2	155	2	Trace
Corn, oat flour, puffed, added sugar, salt, iron, vitamins	1 c	20	4	80	2	1
Corn, shredded, added sugar, salt, iron, thiamine, niacin	1 c	25	3	95	2	Trace

				NUTRIENTS IN INDICATED QUANTITY								
FATTY ACIDS												
SATURATED (TOTAL) (g)	UNSATURATED		CARBO-HYDRATE (g)	CALCIUM (mg)	PHOS-PHORUS (mg)	IRON (mg)	POTASSIUM (mg)	VITAMIN A VALUE (IU)	THIAMINE (mg)	RIBOFLAVIN (mg)	NIACIN (mg)	ASCORBIC ACID (mg)
	OLEIC (g)	LINOLEIC (g)										
5.2	7.9	6.9	343	571	660	17.0	714	Trace	2.70	1.65	22.5	Trace
0.2	0.3	0.3	14	24	27	0.7	29	Trace	0.11	0.07	0.9	Trace
0.2	0.3	0.3	14	24	27	0.7	29	Trace	0.09	0.07	0.9	Trace
0.2	0.3	0.2	12	20	23	0.6	25	Trace	0.10	0.06	0.8	Trace
0.2	0.3	0.2	12	20	23	0.6	25	Trace	0.08	0.06	0.8	Trace
0.3	0.5	0.5	23	38	44	1.1	47	Trace	0.18	0.11	1.5	Trace
0.2	0.3	0.3	15	25	29	0.8	32	Trace	0.12	0.07	1.0	Trace
3.9	5.9	5.2	228	435	463	11.3	549	Trace	1.80	1.10	15.0	Trace
0.2	0.3	0.3	12	22	23	0.6	28	Trace	0.09	0.06	0.8	Trace
0.2	0.3	0.3	12	22	23	0.6	28	Trace	0.07	0.06	0.8	Trace
7.7	11.8	10.4	455	871	925	22.7	1,097	Trace	3.60	2.20	30.0	Trace
0.2	0.3	0.3	14	26	28	0.7	33	Trace	0.11	0.06	0.9	Trace
0.2	0.3	0.3	14	26	28	0.7	33	Trace	0.09	0.06	0.9	Trace
2.2	2.9	4.2	224	381	1,152	13.6	1,161	Trace	1.37	0.45	12.7	Trace
0.1	0.2	0.2	14	24	71	0.8	72	Trace	0.09	0.03	0.8	Trace
0.1	0.2	0.2	14	24	71	0.8	72	Trace	0.07	0.03	0.8	Trace
2.5	3.3	4.9	216	449	1,034	13.6	1,238	Trace	1.17	0.54	12.7	Trace
0.1	0.2	0.3	12	25	57	0.8	68	Trace	0.06	0.03	0.7	Trace
0.1	0.2	0.3	12	25	57	0.8	68	Trace	0.05	0.03	0.7	Trace
Trace	Trace	0.1	27	2	25	0.7	27	Trace[40]	0.10	0.07	1.0	0
Trace	Trace	0.1	27	2	25	0.2	27	Trace[40]	0.05	0.02	0.5	0
Trace	Trace	0.1	22	147	113[41]	[42]	25	0	0.12	0.07	1.0	0
0.4	0.8	0.9	23	22	137	1.4	146	0	0.19	0.05	0.2	0
—	—	—	41	19	182	1.7	202	0	0.17	0.07	2.2	0
—	—	—	23	17	127	1.2	118	0	0.15	0.05	1.5	0
—	—	—	28	19	125	5.6	137	1,540	0.46	0.52	6.2	0
—	—	—	40	28	146	7.9	154	2,200[43]	[44]	[44]	[44]	0
—	—	—	21	[44]	9	[44]	30	[44]	[44]	[44]	[44]	13[45]
—	—	—	37	1	10	[44]	27	1,760	0.53	0.60	7.1	21[45]
—	—	—	16	4	18	5.7	—	880	0.26	0.30	3.5	11
—	—	—	22	1	10	0.6	—	0	0.33	0.05	4.4	13

continued on next page

Table B-1
continued

FOOD	APPROXIMATE MEASURES, UNITS, OR WEIGHT	WEIGHT (g)	WATER (%)	FOOD ENERGY (kcal)	PROTEIN (g)	FAT (g)
Oats, puffed, added sugar, salt, minerals, vitamins	1 c	25	3	100	3	1
Rice, puffed:						
Plain, added iron, thiamine, niacin	1 c	15	4	60	1	Trace
Presweetened, added salt, iron, vitamins	1 c	28	3	115	1	0
Wheat flakes, added sugar, salt, iron, vitamins	1 c	30	4	105	3	Trace
Wheat, puffed:						
Plain, added iron, thiamine, niacin	1 c	15	3	55	2	Trace
Presweetened, added salt, iron, vitamins	1 c	38	3	140	3	Trace
Wheat, shredded, plain	1 oblong biscuit or ½ spoon-size biscuits	25	7	90	2	1
Wheat germ, without salt and sugar, toasted	1 T	6	4	25	2	1
Buckwheat flour, light, sifted	1 c	98	12	340	6	1
Bulgur, canned, seasoned	1 c	135	56	245	8	4
Cake icings. See Sugars and Sweets.						
Cakes made from cake mixes with enriched flour:[46]						
Angel food:						
Whole cake (9¾-in. diam. tube cake)	1	635	34	1,645	36	1
Piece, ¹⁄₁₂ of cake	1	53	34	135	3	Trace
Coffee cake:						
Whole cake (7¾ × 5⅝ × 1¼ in.)	1	430	30	1,385	27	41
Piece, ⅙ of cake	1	72	30	230	5	7
Cupcake, made with egg, milk, 2½-in. diam.:						
Without icing	1	25	26	90	1	3
With chocolate icing	1	36	22	130	2	5
Devil's food with chocolate icing:						
Whole, 2-layer cake (8- or 9-in. diam.)	1	1,107	24	3,755	49	136
Piece, ¹⁄₁₆ of cake	1	69	24	235	3	8
Cupcake, 2½-in. diam.	1	35	24	120	2	4
Gingerbread:						
Whole cake (8-in. square)	1	570	37	1,575	18	39
Piece, ⅑ of cake	1	63	37	175	2	4
White, 2-layer with chocolate icing:						
Whole cake (8- or 9-in. diam.)	1	1,140	21	4,000	44	122
Piece, ¹⁄₁₆ of cake	1	71	21	250	3	8
Yellow, 2-layer with chocolate icing:						
Whole cake (8- or 9-in. diam.)	1	1,108	26	3,735	45	125
Piece, ¹⁄₁₆ of cake	1	69	26	235	3	8
Cakes made from home recipes using enriched flour:[47]						
Boston cream pie with custard filling:						
Whole cake (8-in. diam.)	1	825	35	2,490	41	78
Piece, ¹⁄₁₂ of cake	1	69	35	210	3	6

								NUTRIENTS IN INDICATED QUANTITY				
SATURATED (TOTAL) (g)	UNSATURATED OLEIC (g)	LINOLEIC (g)	CARBO-HYDRATE (g)	CALCIUM (mg)	PHOS-PHORUS (mg)	IRON (mg)	POTASSIUM (mg)	VITAMIN A VALUE (IU)	THIAMINE (mg)	RIBOFLAVIN (mg)	NIACIN (mg)	ASCORBIC ACID (mg)
—	—	—	19	44	102	4.0	—	1,100	0.33	0.38	4.4	13
—	—	—	13	3	14	0.3	15	0	0.07	0.01	0.7	0
—	—	—	26	3	14	[44]	43	1,240[45]	[44]	[44]	[44]	15[45]
—	—	—	24	12	83	4.8	81	1,320	0.40	0.45	5.3	16
—	—	—	12	4	48	0.6	51	0	0.08	0.03	1.2	0
—	—	—	33	7	52	[44]	63	1,680	0.50	0.57	6.7	20[45]
—	—	—	20	11	97	0.9	87	0	0.06	0.03	1.1	0
—	—	—	3	3	70	0.5	57	10	0.11	0.05	0.3	1
0.2	0.4	0.4	78	11	86	1.0	314	0	0.08	0.04	0.4	0
—	—	—	44	27	263	1.9	151	0	0.08	0.05	4.1	0
—	—	—	377	603	756	2.5	381	0	0.37	0.95	3.6	0
—	—	—	32	50	63	0.2	32	0	0.03	0.08	0.3	0
11.7	16.3	8.8	225	262	748	6.9	469	690	0.82	0.91	7.7	1
2.0	2.7	1.5	38	44	125	1.2	78	120	0.14	0.15	1.3	Trace
0.8	1.2	0.7	14	40	59	0.3	21	40	0.05	0.05	0.4	Trace
2.0	1.6	0.6	21	47	71	0.4	42	60	0.05	0.06	0.4	Trace
50.0	44.9	17.0	645	653	1,162	16.6	1,439	1,660	1.06	1.65	10.1	1
3.1	2.8	1.1	40	41	72	1.0	90	100	0.07	0.10	0.6	Trace
1.6	1.4	0.5	20	21	37	0.5	46	50	0.03	0.05	0.3	Trace
9.7	16.6	10.0	291	513	570	8.6	1,562	Trace	0.84	1.00	7.4	Trace
1.1	1.8	1.1	32	57	63	0.9	173	Trace	0.09	0.11	0.8	Trace
48.2	46.4	20.0	716	1,129	2,041	11.4	1,322	680	1.50	1.77	12.5	2
3.0	2.9	1.2	45	70	127	0.7	82	40	0.09	0.11	0.8	Trace
47.8	47.8	20.3	638	1,008	2,017	12.2	1,208	1,550	1.24	1.67	10.6	2
3.0	3.0	1.3	40	63	126	0.8	75	100	0.08	0.10	0.7	Trace
23.0	30.1	15.2	412	553	833	8.2	734[48]	1,730	1.04	1.27	9.6	2
1.9	2.5	1.3	34	46	70	0.7	61[48]	140	0.09	0.11	0.8	Trace

continued on next page

Table B-1
continued

FOOD	APPROXIMATE MEASURES, UNITS, OR WEIGHT	WEIGHT (g)	WATER (%)	FOOD ENERGY (kcal)	PROTEIN (g)	FAT (g)
Fruitcake, dark:						
Loaf, 1 lb (7½ × 2 × 1½ in.)	1 lb	454	18	1,720	22	69
Slice, 1/30 of loaf	1 slice	15	18	55	1	2
Plain, sheet cake:						
Without icing:						
Whole cake (9-in. square)	1	777	25	2,830	35	108
Piece, 1/9 of cake	1	86	25	315	4	12
With uncooked white icing:						
Whole cake (9-in. square)	1	1,096	21	4,020	37	129
Piece, 1/9 of cake	1	121	21	445	4	14
Pound:[49]						
Loaf, 8½ × 3½ × 3¼ in.	1	565	16	2,725	31	170
Slice, 1/17 of loaf	1	33	16	160	2	10
Sponge cake:						
Whole cake (9¾-in. diam. tube cake)	1	790	32	2,345	60	45
Piece, 1/12 of cake	1	66	32	195	5	4
Cookies made with enriched flour:[50 51]						
Brownie with nuts:						
Homemade, 1¾ × 1¾ × 7/8 in.:						
From home recipe	1	20	10	95	1	6
From commercial recipe	1	20	11	85	1	4
Frozen, with chocolate icing,[52] 1½ × 1¾ × 7/8 in.	1	25	13	105	1	5
Chocolate chip:						
Commercial, 2¼-in. diam., 3/8 in. thick	4	42	3	200	2	9
Homemade, 2⅓-in. diam.	4	40	3	205	2	12
Fig bars, square (1⅝ × 1⅝ × 3/8 in.) or rectangular (1½ × 1¾ × ½ in.)	4	56	14	200	2	3
Gingersnaps, 2-in. diam., ¼ in. thick	4	28	3	90	2	2
Macaroons, 2¾-in. diam., ¼ in. thick	2	38	4	180	2	9
Oatmeal with raisins, 2⅝-in. diam., ¼ in. thick	4	52	3	235	3	8
Plain, prepared from commercial chilled dough, 2½-in. diam., ¼ in. thick	4	48	5	240	2	12
Sandwich type (chocolate or vanilla), 1¾-in. diam., 3/8 in. thick	4	40	2	200	2	9
Vanilla wafers, 1¾-in. diam., ¼ in. thick	10	40	3	185	2	6
Cornmeal:						
Whole-grain, unbolted, dry form	1 c	122	12	435	11	5
Bolted (nearly whole grain), dry form	1 c	122	12	440	11	4
Degermed, enriched:						
Dry form	1 c	138	12	500	11	2
Cooked	1 c	240	88	120	3	Trace
Degermed, unenriched:						
Dry form	1 c	138	12	500	11	2
Cooked	1 c	240	88	120	3	Trace

| | FATTY ACIDS | | | | | | | | | | | |
| | UNSATURATED | | | | | | | | | | | |
SATURATED (TOTAL) (g)	OLEIC (g)	LINOLEIC (g)	CARBO-HYDRATE (g)	CALCIUM (mg)	PHOS-PHORUS (mg)	IRON (mg)	POTASSIUM (mg)	VITAMIN A VALUE (IU)	THIAMINE (mg)	RIBOFLAVIN (mg)	NIACIN (mg)	ASCORBIC ACID (mg)
14.4	33.5	14.8	271	327	513	11.8	2,250	540	0.72	0.73	4.9	2
0.5	1.1	0.5	9	11	17	0.4	74	20	0.02	0.02	0.2	Trace
29.5	44.4	23.9	434	497	793	8.5	614[48]	1,320	1.21	1.40	10.2	2
3.3	4.9	2.6	48	55	88	0.9	68[48]	150	0.13	0.15	1.1	Trace
42.2	49.5	24.4	694	548	822	8.2	669[48]	2,190	1.22	1.47	10.2	2
4.7	5.5	2.7	77	61	91	0.8	74[48]	240	0.14	0.16	1.1	Trace
42.9	73.1	39.6	273	107	418	7.9	345	1,410	0.90	0.99	7.3	0
2.5	4.3	2.3	16	6	24	0.5	20	80	0.05	0.06	0.4	0
13.1	15.8	5.7	427	237	885	13.4	687	3,560	1.10	1.64	7.4	Trace
1.1	1.3	0.5	36	20	74	1.1	57	300	0.09	0.14	0.6	Trace
1.5	3.0	1.2	10	8	30	0.4	38	40	0.04	0.03	0.2	Trace
0.9	1.4	1.3	13	9	27	0.4	34	20	0.03	0.02	0.2	Trace
2.0	2.2	0.7	15	10	31	0.4	44	50	0.03	0.03	0.2	Trace
2.8	2.9	2.2	29	16	48	1.0	56	50	0.10	0.17	0.9	Trace
3.5	4.5	2.9	24	14	40	0.8	47	40	0.06	0.06	0.5	Trace
0.8	1.2	0.7	42	44	34	1.0	111	60	0.04	0.14	0.9	Trace
0.7	1.0	0.6	22	20	13	0.7	129	20	0.08	0.06	0.7	0
—	—	—	25	10	32	0.3	176	0	0.02	0.06	0.2	0
2.0	3.3	2.0	38	11	53	1.4	192	30	0.15	0.10	1.0	Trace
3.0	5.2	2.9	31	17	35	0.6	23	30	0.10	0.08	0.9	0
2.2	3.9	2.2	28	10	96	0.7	15	0	0.06	0.10	0.7	0
—	—	—	30	16	25	0.6	29	50	0.10	0.09	0.8	0
0.5	1.0	2.5	90	24	312	2.9	346	620[53]	0.46	0.13	2.4	0
0.5	0.9	2.1	91	21	272	2.2	303	590[53]	0.37	0.10	2.3	0
0.2	0.4	0.9	108	8	137	4.0	166	610[53]	0.61	0.36	4.8	0
Trace	0.1	0.2	26	2	34	1.0	38	140[53]	0.14	0.10	1.2	0
0.2	0.4	0.9	108	8	137	1.5	166	610[53]	0.19	0.07	1.4	0
Trace	0.1	0.2	26	2	34	0.5	38	140[53]	0.05	0.02	0.2	0

continued on next page

Table B-1
continued

FOOD	APPROXIMATE MEASURES, UNITS, OR WEIGHT	WEIGHT (g)	WATER (%)	FOOD ENERGY (kcal)	PROTEIN (g)	FAT (g)
Crackers:[38]						
Graham, plain, 2½-in. square	2	14	6	55	1	1
Rye wafers, whole grain, 1⅞ × 3½ in.	2	13	6	45	2	Trace
Saltines, made with enriched flour	4 crackers	11	4	50	1	1
Danish pastry (enriched flour), plain without fruit or nuts:[54]						
Ounce	1 oz	28	22	120	2	7
Packaged ring, 12 oz	1	340	22	1,435	25	80
Round piece, about 4¼-in. diam. × 1 in.	1 pastry	65	22	275	5	15
Doughnut, made with enriched flour:[38]						
Cake type, plain, 2½-in. diam., 1 in. high	1	25	24	100	1	5
Yeast-leavened, glazed, 3¾-in. diam., 1¼ in. high	1	50	26	205	3	11
Macaroni, enriched, cooked (cut lengths, elbows, shells):						
Firm stage (hot)	1 c	130	64	190	7	1
Tender stage:						
Cold	1 c	105	73	115	4	Trace
Hot	1 c	140	73	155	5	1
Macaroni (enriched) and cheese:						
Canned[55]	1 c	240	80	230	9	10
Homemade (served hot)[56]	1 c	200	58	430	17	22
Muffin made with enriched flour:[38]						
Homemade:						
Blueberry, 2⅜-in. diam., 1½ in. high	1	40	39	110	3	4
Bran	1	40	35	105	3	4
Corn (enriched, degermed cornmeal and flour), 2⅜-in. diam., 1½ in. high	1	40	33	125	3	4
Plain, 3-in. diam., 1½ in. high	1	40	38	120	3	4
From mix, egg, milk:						
Corn, 2⅜-in. diam., 1½ in. high[58]	1	40	30	130	3	4
Noodles, chow mein, canned	1 c	45	1	220	6	11
Noodles (egg noodles), enriched, cooked	1 c	160	71	200	7	2
Pancakes, (4-in. diam.):[38]						
Buckwheat, made from mix (with buckwheat and enriched flours), egg and milk added	1 cake	27	58	55	2	2
Plain:						
Homemade with enriched flour	1 cake	27	50	60	2	2
Made from mix with enriched flour; egg and milk added	1 cake	27	51	60	2	2
Pies, piecrust made with enriched flour and vegetable shortening (9-in. diam.):						
Apple:						
Whole	1 pie	945	48	2,420	21	105
Sector, ⅐ of pie	1 sector	135	48	345	3	15

					NUTRIENTS IN INDICATED QUANTITY							

FATTY ACIDS												
SATURATED (TOTAL) (g)	UNSATURATED		CARBO-HYDRATE (g)	CALCIUM (mg)	PHOS-PHORUS (mg)	IRON (mg)	POTASSIUM (mg)	VITAMIN A VALUE (IU)	THIAMINE (mg)	RIBOFLAVIN (mg)	NIACIN (mg)	ASCORBIC ACID (mg)
	OLEIC (g)	LINOLEIC (g)										
0.3	0.5	0.3	10	6	21	0.5	55	0	0.02	0.08	0.5	0
—	—	—	10	7	50	0.5	78	0	0.04	0.03	0.2	0
0.3	0.5	0.4	8	2	10	0.5	13	0	0.05	0.05	0.4	0
2.0	2.7	1.4	13	14	31	0.5	32	90	0.08	0.08	0.7	Trace
24.3	31.7	16.5	155	170	371	6.1	381	1,050	0.97	1.01	8.6	Trace
4.7	6.1	3.2	30	33	71	1.2	73	200	0.18	0.19	1.7	Trace
1.2	2.0	1.1	13	10	48	0.4	23	20	0.05	0.05	0.4	Trace
3.3	5.8	3.3	22	16	33	0.6	34	25	0.10	0.10	0.8	0
—	—	—	39	14	85	1.4	103	0	0.23	0.13	1.8	0
—	—	—	24	8	53	0.9	64	0	0.15	0.08	1.2	0
—	—	—	32	11	70	1.3	85	0	0.20	0.11	1.5	0
4.2	3.1	1.4	26	199	182	1.0	139	260	0.12	0.24	1.0	Trace
8.9	8.8	2.9	40	362	322	1.8	240	860	0.20	0.40	1.8	Trace
1.1	1.4	0.7	17	34	53	0.6	46	90	0.09	0.10	0.7	Trace
1.2	1.4	0.8	17	57	162	1.5	172	90	0.07	0.10	1.7	Trace
1.2	1.6	0.9	19	42	68	0.7	54	120[57]	0.10	0.10	0.7	Trace
1.0	1.7	1.0	17	42	60	0.6	50	40	0.09	0.12	0.9	Trace
1.2	1.7	0.9	20	96	152	0.6	44	100[57]	0.08	0.09	0.7	Trace
—	—	—	26	—	—	—	—	—	—	—	—	—
—	—	—	37	16	94	1.4	70	110	0.22	0.13	1.9	0
0.8	0.9	0.4	6	59	91	0.4	66	60	0.04	0.05	0.2	Trace
0.5	0.8	0.5	9	27	38	0.4	33	30	0.06	0.07	0.5	Trace
0.7	0.7	0.3	9	58	70	0.3	42	70	0.04	0.06	0.2	Trace
27.0	44.5	25.2	360	76	208	6.6	756	280	1.06	0.79	9.3	9
3.9	6.4	3.6	51	11	30	0.9	108	40	0.15	0.11	1.3	2

continued on next page

Table B-1
continued

FOOD	APPROXIMATE MEASURES, UNITS, OR WEIGHT	WEIGHT (g)	WATER (%)	FOOD ENERGY (kcal)	PROTEIN (g)	FAT (g)
Banana cream:						
Whole	1 pie	910	54	2,010	41	85
Sector, 1/7 of pie	1 sector	130	54	285	6	12
Blueberry:						
Whole	1 pie	945	51	2,285	23	102
Sector, 1/7 of pie	1 sector	135	51	325	3	15
Cherry:						
Whole	1 pie	945	47	2,465	25	107
Sector, 1/7 of pie	1 sector	135	47	350	4	15
Custard:						
Whole	1 pie	910	58	1,985	56	101
Sector, 1/7 of pie	1 sector	130	58	285	8	14
Lemon meringue:						
Whole	1 pie	840	47	2,140	31	86
Sector, 1/7 of pie	1 sector	120	47	305	4	12
Mince:						
Whole	1 pie	945	43	2,560	24	109
Sector, 1/7 of pie	1 sector	135	43	365	3	16
Peach:						
Whole	1 pie	945	48	2,410	24	101
Sector, 1/7 of pie	1 sector	135	48	345	3	14
Pecan:						
Whole	1 pie	825	20	3,450	42	189
Sector, 1/7 of pie	1 sector	118	20	495	6	27
Pumpkin:						
Whole	1 pie	910	59	1,920	36	102
Sector, 1/7 of pie	1 sector	130	59	275	5	15
Piecrust (homemade) made with enriched flour and vegetable shortening, baked, 9-in. diam.	1 shell	180	15	900	11	60
Piecrust mix with enriched flour and vegetable shortening, 10-oz. package prepared and baked, 9-in. diam.	1 shell (2-crust pie)	320	19	1,485	20	93
Pizza (cheese) baked, 4¾-in. sector; ⅛ of 12-in.-diam. pie[19]	1 sector	60	45	145	6	4
Popcorn, popped:						
Plain, large kernel	1 c	6	4	25	1	Trace
With oil (coconut) and salt added, large kernel	1 c	9	3	40	1	2
Sugar coated	1 c	35	4	135	2	1
Pretzels, made with enriched flour:						
Dutch, twisted, 2¾ × 2⅝ in.	1	16	5	60	2	1
Thin, twisted, 3¼ × 2¼ × ¼ in.	10	60	5	235	6	3
Stick, 2¼ in. long	10	3	5	10	Trace	Trace

								NUTRIENTS IN INDICATED QUANTITY				
	FATTY ACIDS											
SATURATED (TOTAL) (g)	UNSATURATED		CARBO-HYDRATE (g)	CALCIUM (mg)	PHOS-PHORUS (mg)	IRON (mg)	POTASSIUM (mg)	VITAMIN A VALUE (IU)	THIAMINE (mg)	RIBOFLAVIN (mg)	NIACIN (mg)	ASCORBIC ACID (mg)
	OLEIC (g)	LINOLEIC (g)										
26.7	33.2	16.2	279	601	746	7.3	1,847	2,280	0.77	1.51	7.0	9
3.8	4.7	2.3	40	86	107	1.0	264	330	0.11	0.22	1.0	1
24.8	43.7	25.1	330	104	217	9.5	614	280	1.03	0.80	10.0	28
3.5	6.2	3.6	47	15	31	1.4	88	40	0.15	0.11	1.4	4
28.2	45.0	25.3	363	132	236	6.6	992	4,160	1.09	0.84	9.8	Trace
4.0	6.4	3.6	52	19	34	0.9	142	590	0.16	0.12	1.4	Trace
33.9	38.5	17.5	213	874	1,028	8.2	1,247	2,090	0.79	1.92	5.6	0
4.8	5.5	2.5	30	125	147	1.2	178	300	0.11	0.27	0.8	0
26.1	33.8	16.4	317	118	412	6.7	420	1,430	0.61	0.84	5.2	25
3.7	4.8	2.3	45	17	59	1.0	60	200	0.09	0.12	0.7	4
28.0	45.9	25.2	389	265	359	13.3	1,682	20	0.96	0.86	9.8	9
4.0	6.6	3.6	56	38	51	1.9	240	Trace	0.14	0.12	1.4	1
24.8	43.7	25.1	361	95	274	8.5	1,408	6,900	1.04	0.97	14.0	28
3.5	6.2	3.6	52	14	39	1.2	201	990	0.15	0.14	2.0	4
27.8	101.0	44.2	423	388	850	25.6	1,015	1,320	1.80	0.95	6.9	Trace
4.0	14.4	6.3	61	55	122	3.7	145	190	0.26	0.14	1.0	Trace
37.4	37.5	16.6	223	464	628	7.3	1,456	22,480	0.78	1.27	7.0	Trace
5.4	5.4	2.4	32	66	90	1.0	208	3,210	0.11	0.18	1.0	Trace
14.8	26.1	14.9	79	25	90	3.1	89	0	0.47	0.40	5.0	0
22.7	39.7	23.4	141	131	272	6.1	179	0	1.07	0.79	9.9	0
1.7	1.5	0.6	22	86	89	1.1	67	230	0.16	0.18	1.6	4
Trace	0.1	0.2	5	1	17	0.2	—	—	—	0.01	0.1	0
1.5	0.2	0.2	5	1	19	0.2	—	—	—	0.01	0.2	0
0.5	0.2	0.4	30	2	47	0.5	—	—	—	0.02	0.4	0
—	—	—	12	4	21	0.2	21	0	0.05	0.04	0.7	0
—	—	—	46	13	79	0.9	78	0	0.20	0.15	2.5	0
—	—	—	2	1	4	Trace	4	0	0.01	0.01	0.1	0

continued on next page

Table B-1
continued

FOOD	APPROXIMATE MEASURES, UNITS, OR WEIGHT	WEIGHT (g)	WATER (%)	FOOD ENERGY (kcal)	PROTEIN (g)	FAT (g)
Rice, white, enriched:						
Instant, ready-to-serve, hot	1 c	165	73	180	4	Trace
Long grain:						
Raw	1 c	185	12	670	12	1
Cooked, served hot	1 c	205	73	225	4	Trace
Parboiled:						
Raw	1 c	185	10	685	14	1
Cooked, served hot	1 c	175	73	185	4	Trace
Roll, enriched:[38]						
Commercial:						
Brown-and-serve (1 oz), browned	1	26	27	85	2	2
Cloverleaf or pan, 2½-in. diam., 2 in. high	1	28	31	85	2	2
Frankfurter and hamburger (8 per 11½-oz package)	1	40	31	120	3	2
Hard, 3¾-in. diam., 2 in. high	1	50	25	155	5	2
Hoagie or submarine, 11½ × 3 × 2½ in.	1	135	31	390	12	4
Homemade:						
Cloverleaf, 2½-in. diam., 2 in. high	1	35	26	120	3	3
Spaghetti, enriched, cooked:						
Firm stage, *al dente*, served hot	1 c	130	64	190	7	1
Tender stage, served hot	1 c	140	73	155	5	1
Spaghetti (enriched) in tomato sauce with cheese:						
Canned	1 c	250	80	190	6	2
Homemade	1 c	250	77	260	9	9
Spaghetti (enriched) with meat balls and tomato sauce:						
Canned	1 c	250	78	260	12	10
Homemade	1 c	248	70	330	19	12
Toaster pastry	1	50	12	200	3	6
Waffles, made with enriched flour, 7-in. diam.:[38]						
Homemade	1	75	41	210	7	7
From mix, egg and milk added	1	75	42	205	7	8
Wheat flour:						
All-purpose or family flour, enriched:						
Sifted, spooned	1 c	115	12	420	12	1
Unsifted, spooned	1 c	125	12	455	13	1
Cake or pastry flour, enriched, sifted, spooned	1 c	96	12	350	7	1
Self-rising, enriched, unsifted, spooned	1 c	125	12	440	12	1
Whole wheat, from hard wheats, stirred	1 c	120	12	400	16	2
Legumes (dry), nuts, seeds; related products						
Almonds, shelled:						
Chopped (about 130 almonds)	1 c	130	5	775	24	70
Slivered, not pressed down (about 115 almonds)	1 c	115	5	690	21	62

NUTRIENTS IN INDICATED QUANTITY

SATURATED (TOTAL) (g)	UNSATURATED OLEIC (g)	UNSATURATED LINOLEIC (g)	CARBO-HYDRATE (g)	CALCIUM (mg)	PHOS-PHORUS (mg)	IRON (mg)	POTASSIUM (mg)	VITAMIN A VALUE (IU)	THIAMINE (mg)	RIBOFLAVIN (mg)	NIACIN (mg)	ASCORBIC ACID (mg)
Trace	Trace	Trace	40	5	31	1.3	—	0	0.21	[59]	1.7	0
0.2	0.2	0.2	149	44	174	5.4	170	0	0.81	0.06	6.5	0
0.1	0.1	0.1	50	21	57	1.8	57	0	0.23	0.02	2.1	0
0.2	0.1	0.2	150	111	370	5.4	278	0	0.81	0.07	6.5	0
0.1	0.1	0.1	41	33	100	1.4	75	0	0.19	0.02	2.1	0
0.4	0.7	0.5	14	20	23	0.5	25	Trace	0.10	0.06	0.9	Trace
0.4	0.6	0.4	15	21	24	0.5	27	Trace	0.11	0.07	0.9	Trace
0.5	0.8	0.6	21	30	34	0.8	38	Trace	0.16	0.10	1.3	Trace
0.4	0.6	0.5	30	24	46	1.2	49	Trace	0.20	0.12	1.7	Trace
0.9	1.4	1.4	75	58	115	3.0	122	Trace	0.54	0.32	4.5	Trace
0.8	1.1	0.7	20	16	36	0.7	41	30	0.12	0.12	1.2	Trace
—	—	—	39	14	85	1.4	103	0	0.23	0.13	1.8	0
—	—	—	32	11	70	1.3	85	0	0.20	0.11	1.5	0
0.5	0.3	0.4	39	40	88	2.8	303	930	0.35	0.28	4.5	10
2.0	5.4	0.7	37	80	135	2.3	408	1,080	0.25	0.18	2.3	13
2.2	3.3	3.9	29	53	113	3.3	245	1,000	0.15	0.18	2.3	5
3.3	6.3	0.9	39	124	236	3.7	665	1,590	0.25	0.30	4.0	22
—	—	—	36	54[60]	67[60]	1.9	74[60]	500	0.16	0.17	2.1	[60]
2.3	2.8	1.4	28	85	130	1.3	109	250	0.17	0.23	1.4	Trace
2.8	2.9	1.2	27	179	257	1.0	146	170	0.14	0.22	0.9	Trace
0.2	0.1	0.5	88	18	100	3.3	109	0	0.74	0.46	6.1	0
0.2	0.1	0.5	95	20	109	3.6	119	0	0.80	0.50	6.6	0
0.1	0.1	0.3	76	16	70	2.8	91	0	0.61	0.38	5.1	0
0.2	0.1	0.5	93	331	583	3.6	—	0	0.80	0.50	6.6	0
0.4	0.2	1.0	85	49	446	4.0	444	0	0.66	0.14	5.2	0
5.6	47.7	12.8	25	304	655	6.1	1,005	0	0.31	1.20	4.6	Trace
5.0	42.2	11.3	22	269	580	5.4	889	0	0.28	1.06	4.0	Trace

continued on next page

Table B-1
continued

FOOD	APPROXIMATE MEASURES, UNITS, OR WEIGHT	WEIGHT (g)	WATER (%)	FOOD ENERGY (kcal)	PROTEIN (g)	FAT (g)
Beans, dry:						
Common varieties as Great Northern, navy, and others:						
Canned, solids and liquid:						
White with—						
Frankfurters (sliced)	1 c	255	71	365	19	18
Pork and sweet sauce	1 c	255	66	385	16	12
Pork and tomato sauce	1 c	255	71	310	16	7
Red kidney	1 c	255	76	230	15	1
Cooked, drained:						
Great Northern	1 c	180	69	210	14	1
Pea (navy)	1 c	190	69	225	15	1
Lima, cooked, drained	1 c	190	64	260	16	1
Black-eyed peas, dry, cooked (with residual cooking liquid)	1 c	250	80	190	13	1
Brazil nuts, shelled (6–8 large kernels)	1 oz	28	5	185	4	19
Cashew nuts, roasted in oil	1 c	140	5	785	24	64
Coconut meat, fresh:						
Piece, about 2 × 2 × ½ in.	1	45	51	155	2	16
Shredded or grated, not pressed down	1 c	80	51	275	3	28
Filberts (hazelnuts), chopped (about 80 kernels)	1 c	115	6	730	14	72
Lentils, whole, cooked	1 c	200	72	210	16	Trace
Peanuts, roasted in oil, salted (whole, halves, chopped)	1 c	144	2	840	37	72
Peanut butter	1 T	16	2	95	4	8
Peas, split, dry, cooked	1 c	200	70	230	16	1
Pecans, chopped or pieces (about 120 large halves)	1 c	118	3	810	11	84
Pumpkin and squash kernels, dry, hulled	1 c	140	4	775	41	65
Sunflower seeds, dry, hulled	1 c	145	5	810	35	69
Walnuts:						
Black:						
Chopped or broken kernels	1 c	125	3	785	26	74
Ground (finely)	1 c	80	3	500	16	47
Persian or English, chopped (about 60 halves)	1 c	120	4	780	18	77
Sugars and sweets						
Cake icings:						
Boiled, white:						
Plain	1 c	94	18	295	1	0
With coconut	1 c	166	15	605	3	13
Uncooked:						
Chocolate made with milk and butter	1 c	275	14	1,035	9	38
Creamy fudge from mix and water	1 c	245	15	830	7	16
White	1 c	319	11	1,200	2	21

NUTRIENTS IN INDICATED QUANTITY

FATTY ACIDS												
	UNSATURATED											
SATURATED (TOTAL) (g)	OLEIC (g)	LINOLEIC (g)	CARBO-HYDRATE (g)	CALCIUM (mg)	PHOS-PHORUS (mg)	IRON (mg)	POTASSIUM (mg)	VITAMIN A VALUE (IU)	THIAMINE (mg)	RIBOFLAVIN (mg)	NIACIN (mg)	ASCORBIC ACID (mg)
—	—	—	32	94	303	4.8	668	330	0.18	0.15	3.3	Trace
4.3	5.0	1.1	54	161	291	5.9	—	—	0.15	0.10	1.3	—
2.4	2.8	0.6	48	138	235	4.6	536	330	0.20	0.08	1.5	5
—	—	—	42	74	278	4.6	673	10	0.13	0.10	1.5	—
—	—	—	38	90	266	4.9	749	0	0.25	0.13	1.3	0
—	—	—	40	95	281	5.1	790	0	0.27	0.13	1.3	0
—	—	—	49	55	293	5.9	1,163	—	0.25	0.11	1.3	—
—	—	—	35	43	238	3.3	573	30	0.40	0.10	1.0	—
4.8	6.2	7.1	3	53	196	1.0	203	Trace	0.27	0.03	0.5	—
12.9	36.8	10.2	41	53	522	5.3	650	140	0.60	0.35	2.5	—
14.0	0.9	0.3	4	6	43	0.8	115	0	0.02	0.01	0.2	1
24.8	1.6	0.5	8	10	76	1.4	205	0	0.04	0.02	0.4	2
5.1	55.2	7.3	19	240	388	3.9	810	—	0.53	—	1.0	Trace
—	—	—	39	50	238	4.2	498	40	0.14	0.12	1.2	0
13.7	33.0	20.7	27	107	577	3.0	971	—	0.46	0.19	24.8	0
1.5	3.7	2.3	3	9	61	0.3	100	—	0.02	0.02	2.4	0
—	—	—	42	22	178	3.4	592	80	0.30	0.18	1.8	—
7.2	50.5	20.0	17	86	341	2.8	712	150	1.01	0.15	1.1	2
11.8	23.5	27.5	21	71	1,602	15.7	1,386	100	0.34	0.27	3.4	—
8.2	13.7	43.2	29	174	1,214	10.3	1,334	70	2.84	0.33	7.8	—
6.3	13.3	45.7	19	Trace	713	7.5	575	380	0.28	0.14	0.9	—
4.0	8.5	29.2	12	Trace	456	4.8	368	240	0.18	0.09	0.6	—
8.4	11.8	42.2	19	119	456	3.7	540	40	0.40	0.16	1.1	2
0	0	0	75	2	2	Trace	17	0	Trace	0.03	Trace	0
11.0	0.9	Trace	124	10	50	0.8	277	0	0.02	0.07	0.3	0
23.4	11.7	1.0	185	165	305	3.3	536	580	0.06	0.28	0.6	1
5.1	6.7	3.1	183	96	218	2.7	238	Trace	0.05	0.20	0.7	Trace
12.7	5.1	0.5	260	48	38	Trace	57	860	Trace	0.06	Trace	Trace

continued on next page

Table B-1
continued

FOOD	APPROXIMATE MEASURES, UNITS, OR WEIGHT	WEIGHT (g)	WATER (%)	FOOD ENERGY (kcal)	PROTEIN (g)	FAT (g)
Candy:						
Caramels, plain or chocolate	1 oz	28	8	115	1	3
Chocolate:						
Milk, plain	1 oz	28	1	145	2	9
Semisweet, small pieces (60 per ounce)	1 c or 6 oz	170	1	860	7	61
Chocolate-covered peanuts	1 oz	28	1	160	5	12
Fondant, uncoated (mints, candy corn, other)	1 oz	28	8	105	Trace	1
Fudge, chocolate, plain	1 oz	28	8	115	1	3
Gumdrops	1 oz	28	12	100	Trace	Trace
Hard	1 oz	28	1	110	0	Trace
Marshmallows	1 oz	28	17	90	1	Trace
Chocolate-flavored beverage powders (about 4 heaping teaspoons per ounce):						
With nonfat milk	1 oz	28	2	100	5	1
Without milk	1 oz	28	1	100	1	1
Honey, strained or extracted	1 T	21	17	65	Trace	0
Jams and preserves	1 T	20	29	55	Trace	Trace
	1 packet	14	29	40	Trace	Trace
Jellies	1 T	18	29	50	Trace	Trace
	1 packet	14	29	40	Trace	Trace
Syrups:						
Chocolate-flavored syrup or topping:						
Fudge type	1 fl oz or 2 T	38	25	125	2	5
Thin type	1 fl oz or 2 T	38	32	90	1	1
Molasses, cane:						
Light (first extraction)	1 T	20	24	50	—	—
Blackstrap (third extraction)	1 T	20	24	45	—	—
Sorghum	1 T	21	23	55	—	—
Table blends, chiefly corn, light and dark	1 T	21	24	60	0	0
Sugar:						
Brown, pressed down	1 c	220	2	820	0	0
White:						
Granulated	1 c	200	1	770	0	0
	1 T	12	1	45	0	0
	1 packet	6	1	23	0	0
Powdered, sifted, spooned into cup	1 c	100	1	385	0	0
Vegetables and vegetable products						
Asparagus, green:						
Cooked, drained:						
Cuts and tips, 1½- to 2-in. lengths:						
From raw	1 c	145	94	30	3	Trace
From frozen	1 c	180	93	40	6	Trace
Spears, ½-in. diam. at base:						
From raw	4	60	94	10	1	Trace
From frozen	4	60	92	15	2	Trace
Canned, spears, ½-in. diam. at base	4	80	93	15	2	Trace

NUTRIENTS IN INDICATED QUANTITY

SATURATED (TOTAL) (g)	UNSATURATED OLEIC (g)	UNSATURATED LINOLEIC (g)	CARBO-HYDRATE (g)	CALCIUM (mg)	PHOS-PHORUS (mg)	IRON (mg)	POTASSIUM (mg)	VITAMIN A VALUE (IU)	THIAMINE (mg)	RIBOFLAVIN (mg)	NIACIN (mg)	ASCORBIC ACID (mg)
1.6	1.1	0.1	22	42	35	0.4	54	Trace	0.01	0.05	0.1	Trace
5.5	3.0	0.3	16	65	65	0.3	109	80	0.02	0.10	0.1	Trace
36.2	19.8	1.7	97	51	255	4.4	553	30	0.02	0.14	0.9	0
4.0	4.7	2.1	11	33	84	0.4	143	Trace	0.10	0.05	2.1	Trace
0.1	0.3	0.1	25	4	2	0.3	1	0	Trace	Trace	Trace	0
1.3	1.4	0.6	21	22	24	0.3	42	Trace	0.01	0.03	0.1	Trace
—	—	—	25	2	Trace	0.1	1	0	0	Trace	Trace	0
—	—	—	28	6	2	0.5	1	0	0	0	0	0
—	—	—	23	5	2	0.5	2	0	0	Trace	Trace	0
0.5	0.3	Trace	20	167	155	0.5	227	10	0.04	0.21	0.2	1
0.4	0.2	Trace	25	9	48	0.6	142	—	0.01	0.03	0.1	0
0	0	0	17	1	1	0.1	11	0	Trace	0.01	0.1	Trace
—	—	—	14	4	2	0.2	18	Trace	Trace	0.01	Trace	Trace
—	—	—	10	3	1	0.1	12	Trace	Trace	Trace	Trace	Trace
—	—	—	13	4	1	0.3	14	Trace	Trace	0.01	Trace	1
—	—	—	10	3	1	0.2	11	Trace	Trace	Trace	Trace	1
3.1	1.6	0.1	20	48	60	0.5	107	60	0.02	0.08	0.2	Trace
0.5	0.3	Trace	24	6	35	0.6	106	Trace	0.01	0.03	0.2	0
—	—	—	13	33	9	0.9	183	—	0.01	0.01	Trace	—
—	—	—	11	137	17	3.2	585	—	0.02	0.04	0.4	—
0	—	—	14	35	5	2.6	—	—	—	0.02	Trace	—
0	0	0	15	9	3	0.8	1	0	0	0	0	0
0	0	0	212	187	42	7.5	757	0	0.02	0.07	0.4	0
0	0	0	199	0	0	0.2	6	0	0	0	0	0
0	0	0	12	0	0	Trace	Trace	0	0	0	0	0
0	0	0	6	0	0	Trace	Trace	0	0	0	0	0
0	0	0	100	0	0	0.1	3	0	0	0	0	0
—	—	—	5	30	73	0.9	265	1,310	0.23	0.26	2.0	38
—	—	—	6	40	115	2.2	396	1,530	0.25	0.23	1.8	41
—	—	—	2	13	30	0.4	110	540	0.10	0.11	0.8	16
—	—	—	2	13	40	0.7	143	470	0.10	0.08	0.7	16
—	—	—	3	15	42	1.5	133	640	0.05	0.08	0.6	12

Table B-1
continued

FOOD	APPROXIMATE MEASURES, UNITS, OR WEIGHT	WEIGHT (g)	WATER (%)	FOOD ENERGY (kcal)	PROTEIN (g)	FAT (g)
Beans:						
Lima, immature seeds, frozen, cooked, drained:						
Thick-seeded types (Fordhooks)	1 c	170	74	170	10	Trace
Thin-seeded types (baby limas)	1 c	180	69	210	13	Trace
Snap:						
Green:						
Canned, drained solids (cuts)	1 c	135	92	30	2	Trace
Cooked, drained:						
From raw (cuts and French style)	1 c	125	92	30	2	Trace
From frozen:						
Cuts	1 c	135	92	35	2	Trace
French style	1 c	130	92	35	2	Trace
Yellow or wax:						
Cooked, drained:						
From raw (cuts and French style)	1 c	125	93	30	2	Trace
From frozen (cuts)	1 c	135	92	35	2	Trace
Canned, drained solids (cuts)	1 c	135	92	30	2	Trace
Beans, mature. See Beans, dry, and Black-eyed peas, dry.						
Bean sprouts (mung):						
Raw	1 c	105	89	35	4	Trace
Cooked, drained	1 c	125	91	35	4	Trace
Beets:						
Canned, drained, solids:						
Whole, small	1 c	160	89	60	2	Trace
Diced or sliced	1 c	170	89	65	2	Trace
Cooked, drained, peeled:						
Whole, 2-in. diam.	2	100	91	30	1	Trace
Diced or sliced	1 c	170	91	55	1	Trace
Beet greens, leaves and stems, cooked, drained	1 c	145	94	25	2	Trace
Black-eyed peas, immature seeds, cooked and drained:						
From raw	1 c	165	72	180	13	1
From frozen	1 c	170	66	220	15	1
Broccoli, cooked, drained:						
From raw:						
Stalk, medium size	1	180	91	45	6	1
Stalks cut into ½-in. pieces	1 c	155	91	40	5	Trace
From frozen:						
Chopped	1 c	185	92	50	5	1
Stalk, 4½ to 5 in. long	1	30	91	10	1	Trace
Brussels sprouts, cooked, drained:						
From raw, 7–8 sprouts (1¼- to 1½-in. diam.)	1 c	155	88	55	7	1
From frozen	1 c	155	89	50	5	Trace

NUTRIENTS IN INDICATED QUANTITY

| FATTY ACIDS | | | | | | | | | | | |
| SATURATED (TOTAL) (g) | UNSATURATED | | CARBO-HYDRATE (g) | CALCIUM (mg) | PHOS-PHORUS (mg) | IRON (mg) | POTASSIUM (mg) | VITAMIN A VALUE (IU) | THIAMINE (mg) | RIBOFLAVIN (mg) | NIACIN (mg) | ASCORBIC ACID (mg) |
	OLEIC (g)	LINOLEIC (g)										
—	—	—	32	34	153	2.9	724	390	0.12	0.09	1.7	29
—	—	—	40	63	227	4.7	709	400	0.16	0.09	2.2	22
—	—	—	7	61	34	2.0	128	630	0.04	0.07	0.4	5
—	—	—	7	63	46	0.8	189	680	0.09	0.11	0.4	15
—	—	—	8	54	43	0.9	205	780	0.09	0.12	0.5	7
—	—	—	8	49	39	1.2	177	690	0.08	0.10	0.4	9
—	—	—	6	63	46	0.8	189	290	0.09	0.11	0.6	16
—	—	—	8	47	42	0.9	221	140	0.09	0.11	0.5	8
—	—	—	7	61	34	2.0	128	140	0.04	0.07	0.4	7
—	—	—	7	20	67	1.4	234	20	0.14	0.14	0.8	20
—	—	—	7	21	60	1.1	195	30	0.11	0.13	0.9	8
—	—	—	14	30	29	1.1	267	30	0.02	0.05	0.2	5
—	—	—	15	32	31	1.2	284	30	0.02	0.05	0.2	5
—	—	—	7	14	23	0.5	208	20	0.03	0.04	0.3	6
—	—	—	12	24	39	0.9	354	30	0.05	0.07	0.5	10
—	—	—	5	144	36	2.8	481	7,400	0.10	0.22	0.4	22
—	—	—	30	40	241	3.5	625	580	0.50	0.18	2.3	28
—	—	—	40	43	286	4.8	573	290	0.68	0.19	2.4	15
—	—	—	8	158	112	1.4	481	4,500	0.16	0.36	1.4	162
—	—	—	7	136	96	1.2	414	3,880	0.14	0.31	1.2	140
—	—	—	9	100	104	1.3	392	4,810	0.11	0.22	0.9	105
—	—	—	1	12	17	0.2	66	570	0.02	0.03	0.2	22
—	—	—	10	50	112	1.7	423	810	0.12	0.22	1.2	135
—	—	—	10	33	95	1.2	457	880	0.12	0.16	0.9	126

continued on next page

FOOD	APPROXIMATE MEASURES, UNITS, OR WEIGHT	WEIGHT (g)	WATER (%)	FOOD ENERGY (kcal)	PROTEIN (g)	FAT (g)
Cabbage:						
Common varieties:						
Raw:						
Coarsely shredded or sliced	1 c	70	92	15	1	Trace
Finely shredded or chopped	1 c	90	92	20	1	Trace
Cooked, drained	1 c	145	94	30	2	Trace
Red, raw, coarsely shredded or sliced	1 c	70	90	20	1	Trace
Savoy, raw, coarsely shredded or sliced	1 c	70	92	15	2	Trace
Cabbage, celery (also called pe-tsai or wongbok), raw, 1-in. pieces	1 c	75	95	10	1	Trace
Cabbage, white mustard (also called bokchoy or pakchoy), cooked, drained	1 c	170	95	25	2	Trace
Carrots:						
Raw, without crowns and tips, scraped:						
Grated	1 c	110	88	45	1	Trace
Whole, 7½ by 1⅛ in. or strips, 2½ to 3 in. long	1 carrot or 18 strips	72	88	30	1	Trace
Canned:						
Sliced, drained solids	1 c	155	91	45	1	Trace
Strained or junior (baby food)	1 oz (1¾ to 2 T)	28	92	10	Trace	Trace
Cooked (crosswise cuts), drained	1 c	155	91	50	1	Trace
Cauliflower:						
Raw, chopped	1 c	115	91	31	3	Trace
Cooked, drained:						
From raw (flower buds)	1 c	125	93	30	3	Trace
From frozen (flowerets)	1 c	180	94	30	3	Trace
Celery, Pascal type, raw:						
Pieces, diced	1 c	120	94	20	1	Trace
Stalk, large outer, 8 by 1½ in. at root end	1	40	94	5	Trace	Trace
Collards, cooked, drained:						
From raw (leaves without stems)	1 c	190	90	65	7	1
From frozen (chopped)	1 c	170	90	50	5	1
Corn, sweet:						
Cooked, drained:						
From raw, ear, 5 by 1¾ in.	1	140[61]	74	70	2	1
From frozen:						
Ear, 5 in. long	1	229[61]	73	120	4	1
Kernels	1 c	165	77	130	5	1
Canned:						
Cream style	1 c	256	76	210	5	2
Whole kernel:						
Vacuum pack	1 c	210	76	175	5	1
Wet pack, drained solids	1 c	165	76	140	4	1
Cowpeas. See Black-eyed peas.						

NUTRIENTS IN INDICATED QUANTITY

SATURATED (TOTAL) (g)	UNSATURATED OLEIC (g)	LINOLEIC (g)	CARBO-HYDRATE (g)	CALCIUM (mg)	PHOS-PHORUS (mg)	IRON (mg)	POTASSIUM (mg)	VITAMIN A VALUE (IU)	THIAMINE (mg)	RIBOFLAVIN (mg)	NIACIN (mg)	ASCORBIC ACID (mg)
—	—	—	4	34	20	0.3	163	90	0.04	0.04	0.2	33
—	—	—	5	44	26	0.4	210	120	0.05	0.05	0.3	42
—	—	—	6	64	29	0.4	236	190	0.06	0.06	0.4	48
—	—	—	5	29	25	0.6	188	30	0.06	0.04	0.3	43
—	—	—	3	47	38	0.6	188	140	0.04	0.06	0.2	39
—	—	—	2	32	30	0.5	190	110	0.04	0.03	0.5	19
—	—	—	4	252	56	1.0	364	5,270	0.07	0.14	1.2	26
—	—	—	11	41	40	0.8	375	12,100	0.07	0.06	0.7	9
—	—	—	7	27	26	0.5	246	7,930	0.04	0.04	0.4	6
—	—	—	10	47	34	1.1	186	23,250	0.03	0.05	0.6	3
—	—	—	2	7	6	0.1	51	3,690	0.01	0.01	0.1	1
—	—	—	11	51	48	0.9	344	16,280	0.08	0.08	0.8	9
—	—	—	6	29	64	1.3	339	70	0.13	0.12	0.8	90
—	—	—	5	26	53	0.9	258	80	0.11	0.10	0.8	69
—	—	—	6	31	68	0.9	373	50	0.07	0.09	0.7	74
—	—	—	5	47	34	0.4	409	320	0.04	0.04	0.4	11
—	—	—	2	16	11	0.1	136	110	0.01	0.01	0.1	4
—	—	—	10	357	99	1.5	498	14,820	0.21	0.38	2.3	144
—	—	—	10	299	87	1.7	401	11,560	0.10	0.24	1.0	56
—	—	—	16	2	69	0.5	151	310[62]	0.09	0.08	1.1	7
—	—	—	27	4	121	1.0	291	440[62]	0.18	0.10	2.1	9
—	—	—	31	5	120	1.3	304	580[62]	0.15	0.10	2.5	8
—	—	—	51	8	143	1.5	248	840[62]	0.08	0.13	2.6	13
—	—	—	43	6	153	1.1	204	740[62]	0.06	0.13	2.3	11
—	—	—	33	8	81	0.8	160	580[62]	0.05	0.08	1.5	7

continued on next page

FOOD	APPROXIMATE MEASURES, UNITS, OR WEIGHT	WEIGHT (g)	WATER (%)	FOOD ENERGY (kcal)	PROTEIN (g)	FAT (g)
Cucumber slices, ⅛ in. thick (large, 2⅛-in. diam.; small, 1¾-in. diam.):						
With peel	6 large or 8 small	28	95	5	Trace	Trace
Without peel	6½ large or 9 small pieces	28	96	5	Trace	Trace
Dandelion greens, cooked, drained	1 c	105	90	35	2	1
Endive, curly (including escarole), raw, small pieces	1 c	50	93	10	1	Trace
Kale, cooked, drained:						
From raw (leaves without stems and midribs)	1 c	110	88	45	5	1
From frozen (leaf style)	1 c	130	91	40	4	1
Lettuce, raw:						
Butter head, as Boston types:						
Head, 5-in. diam.	1	220[63]	95	25	2	Trace
Leaves	1 outer, 2 inner, or 3 heart leaves	15	95	Trace	Trace	Trace
Crisp head, as iceberg:						
Head, 6-in. diam.	1	567[64]	96	70	5	1
Wedge, ¼ of head	1	135	96	20	1	Trace
Pieces, chopped or shredded	1 c	55	96	5	Trace	Trace
Loose leaf (bunching varieties including romaine), chopped or shredded pieces	1 c	55	94	10	1	Trace
Mushrooms, raw, sliced, or chopped	1 c	70	90	20	2	Trace
Mustard greens, without stems and midribs, cooked, drained	1 c	140	93	30	3	1
Okra pods, 3 by ⅝ in., cooked	10	106	91	30	2	Trace
Onions:						
Mature:						
Raw:						
Chopped	1 c	170	89	65	3	Trace
Sliced	1 c	115	89	45	2	Trace
Cooked (whole or sliced) drained	1 c	210	92	60	3	Trace
Young green, bulb (⅜-in. diam.) and white portion of top	6 onions	30	88	15	Trace	Trace
Parsley, raw, chopped	1 T	4	85	Trace	Trace	Trace
Parsnips, cooked (diced or 2-in. lengths)	1 c	155	82	100	2	1
Peas, green:						
Canned:						
Whole, drained solids	1 c	170	77	150	8	1
Strained (baby food)	1 oz (1¾–2 T)	28	86	15	1	Trace
Frozen, cooked, drained	1 c	160	82	110	8	Trace
Peppers, hot, red, without seeds, dried (ground chili powder, added seasonings)	1 t	2	9	5	Trace	Trace
Peppers, sweet (about 5 per pound, whole), stem and seeds removed:						
Raw	1 pod	74	93	15	1	Trace
Cooked, boiled, drained	1 pod	73	95	15	1	Trace

NUTRIENTS IN INDICATED QUANTITY

| FATTY ACIDS | | | | | | | | | | | | |
SATURATED (TOTAL) (g)	UNSATURATED OLEIC (g)	LINOLEIC (g)	CARBO-HYDRATE (g)	CALCIUM (mg)	PHOS-PHORUS (mg)	IRON (mg)	POTASSIUM (mg)	VITAMIN A VALUE (IU)	THIAMINE (mg)	RIBOFLAVIN (mg)	NIACIN (mg)	ASCORBIC ACID (mg)
—	—	—	1	7	8	0.3	45	70	0.01	0.01	0.1	3
—	—	—	1	5	5	0.1	45	Trace	0.01	0.01	0.1	3
—	—	—	7	147	44	1.9	244	12,290	0.14	0.17	—	19
—	—	—	2	41	27	0.9	147	1,650	0.04	0.07	0.3	5
—	—	—	7	206	64	1.8	243	9,130	0.11	0.20	1.8	102
—	—	—	7	157	62	1.3	251	10.660	0.08	0.20	0.9	49
—	—	—	4	57	42	3.3	430	1,580	0.10	0.10	0.5	13
—	—	—	Trace	5	4	0.3	40	150	0.01	0.01	Trace	1
—	—	—	16	108	118	2.7	943	1,780	0.32	0.32	1.6	32
—	—	—	4	27	30	0.7	236	450	0.08	0.08	0.4	8
—	—	—	2	11	12	0.3	96	180	0.03	0.03	0.2	3
—	—	—	2	37	14	0.8	145	1,050	0.03	0.04	0.2	10
—	—	—	3	4	81	0.6	290	Trace	0.07	0.32	2.9	2
—	—	—	6	193	45	2.5	308	8,120	0.11	0.20	0.8	67
—	—	—	6	98	43	0.5	184	520	0.14	0.19	1.0	21
—	—	—	15	46	61	0.9	267	Trace[65]	0.05	0.07	0.3	17
—	—	—	10	31	41	0.6	181	Trace[65]	0.03	0.05	0.2	12
—	—	—	14	50	61	0.8	231	Trace[65]	0.06	0.06	0.4	15
—	—	—	3	12	12	0.2	69	Trace	0.02	0.01	0.1	8
—	—	—	Trace	7	2	0.2	25	300	Trace	0.01	Trace	6
—	—	—	23	70	96	0.9	587	50	0.11	0.12	0.2	16
—	—	—	29	44	129	3.2	163	1,170	0.15	0.10	1.4	14
—	—	—	3	3	18	0.3	28	140	0.02	0.03	0.3	3
—	—	—	19	30	138	3.0	216	960	0.43	0.14	2.7	21
—	—	—	1	5	4	0.3	20	1,300	Trace	0.02	0.2	Trace
—	—	—	4	7	16	0.5	157	310	0.06	0.06	0.4	94
—	—	—	3	7	12	0.4	109	310	0.05	0.05	0.4	70

continued on next page

FOOD	APPROXIMATE MEASURES, UNITS, OR WEIGHT	WEIGHT (g)	WATER (%)	FOOD ENERGY (kcal)	PROTEIN (g)	FAT (g)
Potatoes, cooked:						
Baked, peeled after baking (about 2 per pound, raw)	1	156	75	145	4	Trace
Boiled (about 3 per pound, raw):						
Peeled after boiling	1	137	80	105	3	Trace
Peeled before boiling	1	135	83	90	3	Trace
French-fries, 2 to 3½ in. long:						
Prepared from raw	10	50	45	135	2	7
Frozen, oven heated	10	50	53	110	2	4
Hashed brown, prepared from frozen	1 c	155	56	345	3	18
Mashed, prepared from—						
Raw:						
Milk added	1 c	210	83	135	4	2
Milk and butter added	1 c	210	80	195	4	9
Dehydrated flakes (without milk), water, milk, butter, and salt added	1 c	210	79	195	4	7
Potato chips, 1¾ by 2½ in. oval cross section	10	20	2	115	1	8
Potato salad, made with cooked salad dressing	1 c	250	76	250	7	7
Pumpkin, canned	1 c	245	90	80	2	1
Radishes, raw (prepackaged) stem ends, rootlets cut off	4	18	95	5	Trace	Trace
Sauerkraut, canned, solids, and liquid	1 c	235	93	40	2	Trace
Southern peas. See Black-eyed peas.						
Spinach:						
Raw, chopped	1 c	55	91	15	2	Trace
Canned, drained solids	1 c	205	91	50	6	1
Cooked, drained:						
From raw	1 c	180	92	40	5	1
From frozen:						
Chopped	1 c	205	92	45	6	1
Leaf	1 c	190	92	45	6	1
Squash, cooked:						
Summer (all varieties), diced, drained	1 c	210	96	30	2	Trace
Winter (all varieties), baked, mashed	1 c	205	81	130	4	1
Sweet potatoes:						
Candied, 2½ × 2 in. piece	1 piece	105	60	175	1	3
Canned						
Solid pack (mashed)	1 c	255	72	275	5	1
Vacuum pack, 2¾ × 1 in. piece	1 piece	40	72	45	1	Trace
Cooked (raw, 5 × 2 in.; about 2½ per pound):						
Baked in skin, peeled	1	114	64	160	2	1
Boiled in skin, peeled	1	151	71	170	3	1
Tomatoes:						
Raw, 2⅗-in. diam. (3 per 12-oz package)	1	135[66]	94	25	1	Trace
Canned, solids and liquid	1 c	241	94	50	2	Trace

					NUTRIENTS IN INDICATED QUANTITY							

FATTY ACIDS												
SATURATED (TOTAL) (g)	UNSATURATED		CARBO-HYDRATE (g)	CALCIUM (mg)	PHOS-PHORUS (mg)	IRON (mg)	POTASSIUM (mg)	VITAMIN A VALUE (IU)	THIAMINE (mg)	RIBOFLAVIN (mg)	NIACIN (mg)	ASCORBIC ACID (mg)
	OLEIC (g)	LINOLEIC (g)										
—	—	—	33	14	101	1.1	782	Trace	0.15	0.07	2.7	31
—	—	—	23	10	72	0.8	556	Trace	0.12	0.05	2.0	22
—	—	—	20	8	57	0.7	385	Trace	0.12	0.05	1.6	22
1.7	1.2	3.3	18	8	56	0.7	427	Trace	0.07	0.04	1.6	11
1.1	.8	2.1	17	5	43	0.9	326	Trace	0.07	0.01	1.3	11
4.6	3.2	9.0	45	28	78	1.9	439	Trace	0.11	0.03	1.6	12
0.7	0.4	Trace	27	50	103	0.8	548	40	0.17	0.11	2.1	21
5.6	2.3	0.2	26	50	101	0.8	525	360	0.17	0.11	2.1	19
3.6	2.1	0.2	30	65	99	0.6	601	270	0.08	0.08	1.9	11
2.1	1.4	4.0	10	8	28	0.4	226	Trace	0.04	0.01	1.0	3
2.0	2.7	1.3	41	80	160	1.5	798	350	0.20	0.18	2.8	28
—	—	—	19	61	64	1.0	588	15,680	0.07	0.12	1.5	12
—	—	—	1	5	6	0.2	58	Trace	0.01	0.01	0.1	5
—	—	—	9	85	42	1.2	329	120	0.07	0.09	0.5	33
—	—	—	2	51	28	1.7	259	4,460	0.06	0.11	0.3	28
—	—	—	7	242	53	5.3	513	16,400	0.04	0.25	0.6	29
—	—	—	6	167	68	4.0	583	14,580	0.13	0.25	0.9	50
—	—	—	8	232	90	4.3	683	16,200	0.14	0.31	0.8	39
—	—	—	7	200	84	4.8	688	15,390	0.15	0.27	1.0	53
—	—	—	7	53	53	0.8	296	820	0.11	0.17	1.7	21
—	—	—	32	57	98	1.6	945	8,610	0.10	0.27	1.4	27
2.0	0.8	0.1	36	39	45	0.9	200	6,620	0.06	0.04	0.4	11
—	—	—	63	64	105	2.0	510	19,890	0.13	0.10	1.5	36
—	—	—	10	10	16	0.3	80	3,120	0.02	0.02	0.2	6
—	—	—	37	46	66	1.0	342	9,230	0.10	0.08	0.8	25
—	—	—	40	48	71	1.1	367	11,940	0.14	0.09	0.9	26
—	—	—	6	16	33	0.6	300	1,110	0.07	0.05	0.9	28[67]
—	—	—	10	14[68]	46	1.2	523	2,170	0.12	0.07	1.7	41

continued on next page

Table B-1
continued

FOOD	APPROXIMATE MEASURES, UNITS, OR WEIGHT	WEIGHT (g)	WATER (%)	FOOD ENERGY (kcal)	PROTEIN (g)	FAT (g)
Tomato catsup	1 c	273	69	290	5	1
	1 T	15	69	15	Trace	Trace
Tomato juice, canned:						
Cup	1 c	243	94	45	2	Trace
Glass	6 fl oz	182	94	35	2	Trace
Turnips, cooked, diced	1 c	155	94	35	1	Trace
Turnip greens, cooked, drained:						
From raw (leaves and stems)	1 c	145	94	30	3	Trace
From frozen (chopped)	1 c	165	93	40	4	Trace
Vegetables, mixed, frozen, cooked	1 c	182	83	115	6	1
Miscellaneous items						
Baking powders for home use:						
Sodium aluminum sulfate:						
With monocalcium phosphate monohydrate	1 t	3.0	2	5	Trace	Trace
With monocalcium phosphate monohydrate, calcium sulfate	1 t	2.9	1	5	Trace	Trace
Straight phosphate	1 t	3.8	2	5	Trace	Trace
Low sodium	1 t	4.3	2	5	Trace	Trace
Barbecue sauce	1 c	250	81	230	4	17
Beverages, alcoholic:						
Beer	12 fl oz	360	92	150	1	0
Gin, rum, vodka, whisky:						
80 proof	1½-fl oz (jigger)	42	67	95	—	—
86 proof	1½-fl oz (jigger)	42	64	105	—	—
90 proof	1½-fl oz (jigger)	42	62	110	—	—
Wines:						
Dessert	3½ fl oz	103	77	140	Trace	0
Table	3½ fl oz	102	86	85	Trace	0
Beverages, carbonated, sweetened, nonalcoholic:						
Carbonated water	12 fl oz	366	92	115	0	0
Cola type	12 fl oz	369	90	145	0	0
Fruit-flavored sodas and Tom Collins mixer	12 fl oz	372	88	170	0	0
Ginger ale	12 fl oz	366	92	115	0	0
Root beer	12 fl oz	370	90	150	0	0
Chili powder. See Peppers, hot, red.						
Chocolate:						
Bitter or baking	1 oz	28	2	145	3	15
Semisweet, see Candy: Chocolate.						
Gelatin, dry	7 g	7	13	25	6	Trace
Gelatin dessert prepared with gelatin dessert powder and water	1 c	240	84	140	4	0
Mustard, prepared, yellow	1 t or individual serving pouch or cup	5	80	5	Trace	Trace

NUTRIENTS IN INDICATED QUANTITY

SATURATED (TOTAL) (g)	UNSATURATED OLEIC (g)	LINOLEIC (g)	CARBO-HYDRATE (g)	CALCIUM (mg)	PHOS-PHORUS (mg)	IRON (mg)	POTASSIUM (mg)	VITAMIN A VALUE (IU)	THIAMINE (mg)	RIBOFLAVIN (mg)	NIACIN (mg)	ASCORBIC ACID (mg)
—	—	—	69	60	137	2.2	991	3,820	0.25	0.19	4.4	41
—	—	—	4	3	8	0.1	54	210	0.01	0.01	0.2	2
—	—	—	10	17	44	2.2	552	1,940	0.12	0.07	1.9	39
—	—	—	8	13	33	1.6	413	1,460	0.09	0.05	1.5	29
—	—	—	8	54	37	0.6	291	Trace	0.06	0.08	0.5	34
—	—	—	5	252	49	1.5	—	8,270	0.15	0.33	0.7	68
—	—	—	6	195	64	2.6	246	11,390	0.08	0.15	0.7	31
—	—	—	24	46	115	2.4	348	9,010	0.22	0.13	2.0	15
0	0	0	1	58	87	—	5	0	0	0	0	0
0	0	0	1	183	45	—	—	0	0	0	0	0
0	0	0	1	239	359	—	6	0	0	0	0	0
0	0	0	2	207	314	—	471	0	0	0	0	0
2.2	4.3	10.0	20	53	50	2.0	435	900	0.03	0.03	0.8	13
0	0	0	14	18	108	Trace	90	—	0.01	0.11	2.2	—
0	0	0	Trace	—	—	—	1	—	—	—	—	—
0	0	0	Trace	—	—	—	1	—	—	—	—	—
0	0	0	Trace	—	—	—	1	—	—	—	—	—
0	0	0	8	8	—	—	77	—	0.01	0.02	0.2	—
0	0	0	4	9	10	0.4	94	—	Trace	0.01	0.1	—
0	0	0	29	—	—	—	—	0	0	0	0	0
0	0	0	37	—	—	—	—	0	0	0	0	0
0	0	0	45	—	—	—	—	0	0	0	0	0
0	0	0	29	—	—	—	0	0	0	0	0	0
0	0	0	39	—	—	—	0	0	0	0	0	0
8.9	4.9	0.4	8	22	109	1.9	235	20	0.01	0.07	0.4	0
0	0	0	0	—	—	—	—	—	—	—	—	—
0	0	0	34	—	—	—	—	—	—	—	—	—
—	—	—	Trace	4	4	0.1	7	—	—	—	—	—

continued on next page

Table B-1
continued

FOOD	APPROXIMATE MEASURES, UNITS, OR WEIGHT	WEIGHT (g)	WATER (%)	FOOD ENERGY (kcal)	PROTEIN (g)	FAT (g)
Olives, pickled, canned:						
Green:	4 medium, 3 extra large, or 2 giant	16[69]	78	15	Trace	2
Ripe, Mission	3 small or 2 large	10[69]	73	15	Trace	2
Pickles, cucumber:						
Dill, medium, whole, 3¾ in. long, 1¼-in. diam.	1 pickel	65	93	5	Trace	Trace
Fresh pack, slices 1½-in. diam., ¼ in. thick	2 slices	15	79	10	Trace	Trace
Sweet, gherkin, small, whole, about 2½ in. long, ¾-in. diam.	1 pickle	15	61	20	Trace	Trace
Relish, finely chopped, sweet	1 T	15	63	20	Trace	Trace
Popcorn. See items 476-478.						
Popsicle	3 fl oz	95	80	70	0	0
Soups:						
Canned, condensed:						
Prepared with equal volume of milk:						
Cream of chicken	1 c	245	85	180	7	10
Cream of mushroom	1 c	245	83	215	7	14
Tomato	1 c	250	84	175	7	7
Prepared with equal volume of water:						
Bean with pork	1 c	250	84	170	8	6
Beef broth, bouillon, consommé	1 c	240	96	30	5	0
Beef noodle	1 c	240	93	65	4	3
Clam chowder, Manhattan type (with tomatoes, without milk)	1 c	245	92	80	2	3
Cream of chicken	1 c	240	92	95	3	6
Cream of mushroom	1 c	240	90	135	2	10
Minestrone	1 c	245	90	105	5	3
Split pea	1 c	245	85	145	9	3
Tomato	1 c	245	91	90	2	3
Vegetable beef	1 c	245	92	80	5	2
Vegetarian	1 c	245	92	80	2	2
Dehydrated:						
Bouillon cube, ½ in.	1 cube	4	4	5	1	Trace
Mixes:						
Unprepared:						
Onion	1½ oz	43	3	150	6	5
Prepared with water:						
Chicken noodle	1 c	240	95	55	2	1
Onion	1 c	240	96	35	1	1
Tomato vegetable with noodles	1 c	240	93	65	1	1
Vinegar, cider	1 T	15	94	Trace	Trace	0
White sauce, medium, with enriched flour	1 c	250	73	405	10	31
Yeast:						
Baker's, dry, active	1 package	7	5	20	3	Trace
Brewer's, dry	1 T	8	5	25	3	Trace

NUTRIENTS IN INDICATED QUANTITY

| FATTY ACIDS | | | | | | | | | | | | |
SATURATED (TOTAL) (g)	UNSATURATED OLEIC (g)	LINOLEIC (g)	CARBO-HYDRATE (g)	CALCIUM (mg)	PHOS-PHORUS (mg)	IRON (mg)	POTASSIUM (mg)	VITAMIN A VALUE (IU)	THIAMINE (mg)	RIBOFLAVIN (mg)	NIACIN (mg)	ASCORBIC ACID (mg)
0.2	1.2	0.1	Trace	8	2	0.2	7	40	—	—	—	—
0.2	1.2	0.1	Trace	9	1	0.1	2	10	Trace	Trace	—	—
—	—	—	1	17	14	0.7	130	70	Trace	0.01	Trace	4
—	—	—	3	5	4	0.3	—	20	Trace	Trace	Trace	1
—	—	—	5	2	2	0.2	—	10	Trace	Trace	Trace	1
—	—	—	5	3	2	0.1	—	—	—	—	—	—
0	0	0	18	0	—	Trace	—	0	0	0	0	0
4.2	3.6	1.3	15	172	152	0.5	260	610	0.05	0.27	0.7	2
5.4	2.9	4.6	16	191	169	0.5	279	250	0.05	0.34	0.7	1
3.4	1.7	1.0	23	168	155	0.8	418	1,200	0.10	0.25	1.3	15
1.2	1.8	2.4	22	63	128	2.3	395	650	0.13	0.08	1.0	3
0	0	0	3	Trace	31	0.5	130	Trace	Trace	0.02	1.2	—
0.6	0.7	0.8	7	7	48	1.0	77	50	0.05	0.07	1.0	Trace
0.5	0.4	1.3	12	34	47	1.0	184	880	0.02	0.02	1.0	—
1.6	2.3	1.1	8	24	34	0.5	79	410	0.02	0.05	0.5	Trace
2.6	1.7	4.5	10	41	50	0.5	98	70	0.02	0.12	0.7	Trace
0.7	0.9	1.3	14	37	59	1.0	314	2,350	0.07	0.05	1.0	—
1.1	1.2	0.4	21	29	149	1.5	270	440	0.25	0.15	1.5	1
0.5	0.5	1.0	16	15	34	0.7	230	1,000	0.05	0.05	1.2	12
—	—	—	10	12	49	0.7	162	2,700	0.05	0.05	1.0	—
—	—	—	13	20	39	1.0	172	2,940	0.05	0.05	1.0	—
—	—	—	Trace	—	—	—	4	—	—	—	—	—
1.1	2.3	1.0	23	42	49	0.6	238	30	0.05	0.03	0.3	6
—	—	—	8	7	19	0.2	19	50	0.07	0.05	0.5	Trace
—	—	—	6	10	12	0.2	58	Trace	Trace	Trace	Trace	2
—	—	—	12	7	19	0.2	29	480	0.05	0.02	0.5	5
0	0	0	1	1	1	0.1	15	—	—	—	—	—
19.3	7.8	0.8	22	288	233	0.5	348	1,150	0.12	0.43	0.7	2
—	—	—	3	3	90	1.1	140	Trace	0.16	0.38	2.6	Trace
—	—	—	3	17[70]	140	1.4	152	Trace	1.25	0.34	3.0	Trace

continued on next page

Appendix B

Footnotes for Table B-1

[1]Vitamin A value is largely from β-carotene used for coloring. Riboflavin value for powdered creamers apply to products with added riboflavin.

[2]Applies to product without added vitamin A. With added vitamin A, value is 500 IU.

[3]Applies to product without vitamin A added.

[4]Applies to product with added vitamin A. Without added vitamin A, value is 20 IU.

[5]Yields 1 qt of fluid milk when reconstituted according to package directions.

[6]Applies to product with added vitamin A.

[7]Weight applies to product with label claim of 1⅓ cups equal 3.2 oz.

[8]Applies to products made from thick shake mixes with no added ice cream. Products made from milk shake mixes are higher in fat and usually contain added ice cream.

[9]Content of fat, vitamin A, and carbohydrate varies. Consult the label when precise values are needed for special diets.

[10]Applies to product made with milk containing no added vitamin A.

[11]Based on year-round average.

[12]Based on average vitamin A content of fortified margarine. Federal specifications for fortified margarine require a minimum of 15,000 IU of vitamin A per pound.

[13]Fatty acid values apply to product made with regular margarine.

[14]Dipped in egg, milk or water, and bread crumbs; fried in vegetable shortening.

[15]If bones are discarded, value for calcium will be greatly reduced.

[16]Dipped in egg, bread crumbs, and flour or batter.

[17]Prepared with tuna, celery, salad dressing (mayonnaise type), pickle, onion, and egg.

[18]Outer layer of fat on the cut removed to within approximately ½ in. of the lean. Deposits of fat within the cut not removed.

[19]Crust made with vegetable shortening and enriched flour.

[20]Regular margarine used.

[21]Value varies widely.

[22]About one-fourth of the outer layer of fat on the cut removed. Deposits of fat within the cut not removed.

[23]Vegetable shortening used.

[24]Also applies to pasteurized apple cider.

[25]Applies to product without added ascorbic acid. For value of product with added ascorbic acid, refer to label.

[26]Based on product with label claim of 45% of U.S. RDA in 6 fl oz.

[27]Based on product with label claim of 100% of U.S. RDA in 6 fl oz.

[28]Weight includes peel and membranes between sections. Without these parts, the weight of the edible portion is 123 g for pink or red grapefruit and 118 g for white.

[29]For white-fleshed varieties, value is about 20 IU per cup; for red-fleshed varieties, 1,080 IU.

[30]Weight includes seeds. Without seeds, weight of the edible portion is 57 g.

[31]Applies to product without added ascorbic acid. With added ascorbic acid, based on claim that 6 fl oz of reconstituted juice contain 45% or 50% of the U.S. RDA, value is 108 or 120 mg for a 6-fl-oz can and 36 or 40 mg for 1 c of diluted juice.

[32]For products with added thiamine and riboflavin but without added ascorbic acid, values in milligrams would be 0.60 for thiamine, 0.80 for riboflavin, and a trace for ascorbic acid. For products with only ascorbic acid added, value varies with the brand. Consult the label.

[33]Weight includes rind. Without rind, the weight of the edible portion is 272 g for cantaloupe and 149 g for honeydew.

[34]Represents yellow-fleshed varieties. For white-fleshed varieties, value is 50 IU for 1 peach and 90 IU for 1 c of slices.

[35]Value represents products with added ascorbic acid. For products without added ascorbic acid, the values are highly variable; e.g., 10–25 mg for a 10-oz container, and 15–35 mg for 1 c.

[36]Weight includes pits. After removal of the pits, the weight of the edible portion is 258 g for a cup and 133 g for a portion, 43 g for uncooked prunes, and 213 g for cooked prunes.

[37]Weight includes rind and seeds. Without rind and seeds, weight of the edible portion is 426 g.

[38]Made with vegetable shortening.

[39]Applies to product made with white cornmeal. With yellow cornmeal, value is 30 IU.

[40]Applies to white varieties. For yellow varieties, value is 150 IU.

[41]Applies to products that do not contain disodium phosphate. If disodium phosphate is an ingredient, value is 162 mg.

[42]Value may range from less than 1 mg to about 8 mg, depending on the brand. Consult the label.

[43]Applies to product with added nutrient. Without added nutrient, value is trace.

[44]Value varies with the brand. Consult the label.

[45]Applies to product with added nutrient. Without added nutrient, value is trace.

[46]Except for angel food cake, cakes were made from mixes containing vegetable shortening; icings made from butter.

[47]Except for sponge cake, vegetable shortening used for cake portion; butter, for icing. If butter or margarine used for cake portion, vitamin A values are higher.

[48]Applies to product made with a sodium-aluminum-sulfate-type baking powder. With a low-sodium baking powder containing potassium, value would be about twice the amount shown.

[49]Equal weights of flour, sugar, eggs, and vegetable shortening.

[50]Products are commercial unless otherwise specified.

[51]Made with enriched flour and vegetable shortening except for macaroons, which do not contain flour or shortening.

[52]Icing made with butter.

[53]Applies to yellow varieties; white varieties contain only a trace.

[54] Contains vegetable shortening and butter.

[55] Made with corn oil.

[56] Made with regular margarine.

[57] Applies to product made with yellow cornmeal.

[58] Made with enriched degermed cornmeal and enriched flour.

[59] Product may or may not be enriched with riboflavin. Consult the label.

[60] Value varies with the brand. Consult the label.

[61] Weight includes cob. Without cob, weight is 77 g for a raw ear and 126 g for a frozen ear.

[62] Based on yellow varieties. For white varieties, value is trace.

[63] Weight includes refuse of outer leaves and core. Without these parts, weight is 163 g.

[64] Weight includes core. Without core, weight is 539 g.

[65] Value based on white-fleshed varieties. For yellow-fleshed varieties, value is 70 IU for chopped raw onions, 50 IU for sliced raw onions, and 80 IU for cooked onions.

[66] Weight includes cores and stem ends. Without these parts, weight is 123 g.

[67] Based on year-round average. For tomatoes marketed from November through May, value is about 12 mg; from June through October, 32 mg.

[68] Applies to product without calcium salts added. Value for products with calcium salts added may be as much as 63 mg for whole tomatoes, 241 mg for cut forms.

[69] Weight includes pits. Without pits, weight is 13 g for green olives and 9 g for Mission ripe olives.

[70] Value may vary from 6 to 60 mg.

Table B-2
Cholesterol Content of Foods

FOOD AND DESCRIPTION	HOUSEHOLD MEASURE WEIGHT AND/OR UNIT	CHOLESTEROL (mg)
Beef, composite of retail cuts		
Total edible, cooked, bone removed	85 g (3 oz)	(80)
Lean, trimmed of separable fat		
Raw		
Cooked	85 g (3 oz)	(77)
Beef and vegetable stew		
Cooked (homemade, with lean beef chuck)	245 (1 c)	63
Canned	245 g (1 c)	36
Beef, dried, chipped, creamed	245 g (1 c)	65
Beef potpie		
Homemade, baked	210 g	44
Commercial, frozen, unheated	216 g	38
Bread pudding with raisins	265 g (1 c)	170
Butter		
Regular (4 sticks/lb)	14 g (1 T or ⅛ stick)	35
	113 g (½ c or 1 stick)	282
Whipped (6 sticks/lb or in containers)	9 g (1 T or ⅛ stick)	22
	76 g (½ c or 1 stick)	190

SOURCE: R. M. Feeley, "Cholesterol Contents of Foods," *Journal of The American Dietetic Association* 61 (1972):136–146.

NOTE: Numbers in parentheses denote imputed values.

[1] Cholesterol accounts for about 40% of the total sterol content of clams.

[2] Prepared with bread cubes, margarine, parsley, eggs, lemon juice, and catsup.

[3] Prepared with margarine, flour, milk, onion, green pepper, eggs, and lemon juice.

[4] Prepared with butter, egg yolks, sherry, and cream.

[5] Amount needed for reconstitution to 1 qt.

[6] Cholesterol accounts for about 40% of total sterol of oysters.

[7] Cholesterol accounts for about 30% of total sterol of scallops.

continued on next page

Table B-2
continued

FOOD AND DESCRIPTION	HOUSEHOLD MEASURE WEIGHT AND/OR UNIT	CHOLESTEROL (mg)
Buttermilk, fluid, cultured, made from nonfat fluid milk	245 g (1 c)	5
Cakes		
Baked, from home recipes		
Chocolate (devil's food), 2-layer, with chocolate frosting	75 g (1 sl)	32
Fruitcake, dark	15 g (1 sl)	7
Sponge	66 g (1 sl)	162
Yellow, 2-layer, with chocolate frosting	75 g (1 sl)	33
Baked, from mixes		
Angel food, made with water and flavorings	53 g (1 sl)	0
Chocolate (devil's food), 2-layer, made with eggs, water, chocolate frosting	Piece (69 g) (1 sl)	33
	Cupcake (36 g)	17
Gingerbread, made with water	63 g (1 sl)	Trace
White, 2-layer, made with eggs, water, chocolate frosting	71 g (1 sl)	1
Yellow, 2-layer, made with eggs, water, chocolate frosting	75 g (1 sl)	36
Caviar, sturgeon, granular	16 g (1 T)	>48
Cheeses, natural and processed; cheese foods; cheese spreads		
Natural cheeses		
Blue	28 g (1 oz)	(24)
	135 g (1 c)	(117)
Brick	28 g (1 oz)	(25)
Camembert	28 g (1 oz)	(26)
	38 g (1⅓ oz)	(35)
Cheddar, mild or sharp	28 g (1 oz)	28
	113 g (1 c shredded)	112
Colby	28 g (1 oz)	(27)
Cottage (large or small curd)		
Creamed		
1% fat	267 g (1 c packed)	23
4% fat	245 g (1 c packed)	48
Uncreamed	200 g (1 c packed)	13
Cream cheese	14 g (1 T)	16
	85 g (3 oz)	94
Edam	28 g (1 oz)	(29)
Limburger	28 g (1 oz)	(28)
Mozzarella, low moisture, part skim	28 g (1 oz)	18
Muenster	28 g (1 oz)	(25)
Neufchâtel	85 g (3 oz)	(64)
Parmesan	28 g (1 oz)	(27)
Grated	100 g (1 c not packed)	(113)
Provolone	28 g (1 oz)	(28)
Ricotta	28 g (1 oz)	(14)
Part skim	28 g (1 oz)	(9)
Swiss	35 g (1¼ oz)	35
Pasteurized process cheese		
American	28 g (1 oz)	(25)

FOOD AND DESCRIPTION	HOUSEHOLD MEASURE WEIGHT AND/OR UNIT	CHOLESTEROL (mg)
Swiss	28 g (1 oz)	(26)
Pasteurized process cheese food, American	14 g (1 T)	(10)
	28 g (1 oz)	(20)
Pasteurized process cheese spread, American	14 g (1 T)	(9)
	28 g (1 oz)	(18)
	113 g (1 c shredded, packed)	(73)
Cheese sauce	250 g (1 c)	44
Cheese soufflé, homemade	110 g	184
Cheese straws	60 g	19
Chicken, all classes		
Whole, cooked, flesh and skin only	624 g	542
Cut-up parts		
Breast		
Cooked		
Total edible	92 g	74
Meat only	80 g	63
Drumstick		
Cooked		
Total edible	52 g	47
Meat only	43 g	39
Chicken à la king, cooked, homemade	245 g (1 c)	185
Chicken fricassee, cooked, homemade	240 g (1 c)	96
Chicken potpie		
Homemade, baked	232 g	71
Commercial, frozen, unheated	227 g	29
Chicken and noodles, cooked, homemade	240 g (1 c)	96
Chop suey, with meat		
Cooked, homemade	250 g (1 c)	64
Canned	85 g (3 oz)	10
Chow mein, chicken (without noodles)		
Cooked, homemade	250 g (1 c)	77
Canned	250 g (1 c)	7
Clams[1]		
Raw		
In shell		
Soft (refuse: shell and liquid, 65%)	143 g (5 oz)	72
Hard or round (refuse: shell and liquid, 83%)	389 g (13.7 oz)	194
Meat only	227 g (1 c)	114
Canned, drained solids	80 g (½ c)	(50)
Fritters[1]	1 (40 g)	51
Cod, dried, salted	80 g	(66)
Cookies		
Brownies with nuts, baked, homemade	1 (20 g)	17
Ladyfingers	4 (44 g)	157
Corn pudding	245 g (1 c)	102
Cornbread		
Baked, homemade, made with degermed cornmeal	83 g	58

continued on next page

FOOD AND DESCRIPTION	HOUSEHOLD MEASURE WEIGHT AND/OR UNIT	CHOLESTEROL (mg)
Baked, from mix, made with egg and milk	Muffin (40 g)	28
	Piece (55 g)	38
Crab, all kinds		
Steamed, meat only	125 g (1 c)	125
Canned, meat only	160 g (1 c packed)	(161)
Crab, deviled[2]	240 g (1 c)	244
Crab imperial[3]	220 g (1 c)	308
Cream		
Half and half (cream and milk)	15 g (1 T)	6
	242 g (1 c)	105
Light, coffee, or table	15 g (1 T)	10
	240 g (1 c)	158
Sour	12 g (1 T)	8
	230 g (1 c)	152
Whipped topping (pressurized)	60 g (1 c)	51
Whipping, heavy	15 g (1 T)	20
	238 g (2 c)	316
Cream puffs with custard filling	130 g (1 cream puff)	188
Custard, baked	265 g (1 c)	278
Eggs, chicken		
Whole		
Raw or cooked with nothing added (refuse: shell, 11%)	1 large (50 g)	252
Scrambled or omelet with milk and fat	1 large (64 g)	263
Yolks, raw or cooked with nothing added	From large egg (17 g)	252
Gizzard		
Chicken, all classes, cooked	354 g (12½ oz)	(690)
Turkey, all classes, cooked	361 g (12¾ oz)	827
Halibut, cooked, flesh only, broiled with vegetable shortening	125 g	(75)
Heart		
Beef, cooked	145 g (1 c chopped or diced pieces)	(398)
Chicken, all classes, cooked	145 g (1 c chopped or diced pieces)	(335)
Turkey, all classes, cooked	145 g (1 c chopped or diced pieces)	345
Herring, canned, plain, solids and liquid	425 g (15 oz)	(412)
Ice cream		
Regular, approx. 10% fat	133 g (1 c)	53
	1,064 g (½ gal)	426
Rich, approx. 16% fat	148 g (1 c)	85
	1,188 g (½ gal)	682
Frozen custard or French ice cream	133 g (1 c)	97
	1,064 g (½ gal)	777
Ice milk		
Hardened	131 g (1 c)	26
	1,048 g (½ gal)	213
Soft-serve	175 g (1 c)	36
Kidneys, all kinds (beef, calf, hog, lamb), cooked	140 g (1 sl)	(1,125)

FOOD AND DESCRIPTION	HOUSEHOLD MEASURE WEIGHT AND/OR UNIT	CHOLESTEROL (mg)
Lamb		
Composite of retail cuts		
Total edible, cooked, bone removed	85 g (3 oz)	(83)
Lean, trimmed of separable fat, cooked	85 g (3 oz)	(85)
Lard	205 g (1 c)	195
Liver		
Beef, calf, hog, or lamb; cooked	85 g (3 oz)	(372)
Chicken, all classes, cooked	25 g (1 oz)	(187)
Turkey, all classes, cooked	140 g (1 c chopped)	839
Lobster, cooked, meat only	145 g	123
Lobster Newburg[4]	250 g (1 c)	456
Macaroni and cheese, baked, homemade	200 g (1 c)	42
Mackerel		
Canned, solids and liquid	425 g (15 oz)	(399)
Cooked, flesh only, broiled with vegetable shortening	105 g (3.8 oz)	(106)
Margarine		
All vegetable fat		
⅔ animal fat, ⅓ vegetable fat	14 g (1 T or ⅛ stick)	7
	113 g (½ c or 1 stick)	56
Milk		
Fluid		
Whole	244 g (1 c)	34
Low-fat		
1% fat with 1% to 2% nonfat milk solids added	246 g (1 c)	14
2% fat with 1% to 2% nonfat milk solids added	246 g (1 c)	22
Nonfat (skim)	245 g (1 c)	5
Canned, concentrated, undiluted		
Evaporated, unsweetened	252 g (1 c)	79
Condensed, sweetened	306 g (1 c)	105
Dry		
Whole, instant	120 g (1¾ c)[5]	131
Nonfat, instant	91 g (1⅓ c low-density or ⅞ c high-density)[5]	20
Chocolate beverages		
Commercial		
Chocolate-flavored milk drink with 2% added butterfat	250 g (1 c)	20
Chocolate-flavored milk	250 g (1 c)	32
Homemade		
Hot chocolate	250 g (1 c)	31
Hot cocoa	250 g (1 c)	35
Muffins, plain, homemade	1 (40 g)	21
Noodles		
Whole egg		
Dry form	227 g (8 oz)	213
Cooked	160 g (1 c)	50
Chow mein, canned	45 g (1 c)	5

continued on next page

FOOD AND DESCRIPTION	HOUSEHOLD MEASURE WEIGHT AND/OR UNIT	CHOLESTEROL (mg)
Oysters[6]		
Raw		
In shell, Eastern, select (medium) size (refuse: shell and liquid, 90%)	180 g (6⅓ oz)	90
Meat only, Eastern and Pacific	240 g (1 c)	120
Canned, solids and liquid	85 g (3 oz)	(38)
Oyster stew, home prepared[6]		
1 part oysters to 2 parts milk by volume	240 g (1 c)	63
1 part oysters to 3 parts milk by volume	240 g (1 c)	57
Pancakes, baked from mix, made with egg and milk	73 g	54
Pepper, sweet, stuffed with beef and crumbs	1 with 1⅛ stuffing (185 g)	56
Pies, baked		
Custard	114 g (4 oz)	120
Lemon chiffon	81 g (3 oz)	137
Lemon meringue	105 g (3.8 oz)	98
Pumpkin	114 g (4 oz)	70
Popovers, baked from home recipe	1 (40 g)	59
Pork, composite of lean retail cuts, total edible		
Cooked, bone removed	85 g (3 oz)	(76)
Lean, trimmed of separable fat, cooked	85 g (3 oz)	(75)
Potatoes		
Au gratin, made with milk and cheese	245 g (1 c)	36
Scalloped, made with milk	245 g (1 c)	14
Potato salad, homemade, with mayonnaise and hard-cooked eggs	250 g (1 c)	162
Puddings, cooked		
Chocolate, made from mix	260 g (1 c)	30
Vanilla (blanc mange), homemade	255 g (1 c)	35
Rabbit, domesticated, flesh only, cooked	140 g (1 c chopped or diced)	(127)
Rice pudding with raisins	265 g (1 c)	29
Roe, salmon, raw	28 g (1 oz)	101
Salad dressings		
Mayonnaise, commercial	14 g (1 T)	10
	220 g (1 c)	154
Salad dressing		
Cooked, homemade	16 g (1 T)	12
	255 g (1 c)	190
Mayonnaise-type, commercial	15 g (1 T)	8
	235 g (1 c)	118
Salmon, sockeye or red		
Cooked, broiled with vegetable shortening, steak (refuse: bone, 12%)	145 g (5 oz)	(59)
Canned, solids and liquid	454 g (16 oz)	159
Sardines, canned in oil		
Solids and liquid	106 g (3¾ oz)	(127)
Drained solids	92 g (3¼ oz)	129
Sausage, frankfurter, all meat, cooked	1 (56 g)	(34)

FOOD AND DESCRIPTION	HOUSEHOLD MEASURE WEIGHT AND/OR UNIT	CHOLESTEROL (mg)
Scallops, muscle only, steamed[7]	85 g (3 oz)	(45)
Shrimp, canned, drained solids	128 g (1 c)	192
Spaghetti with meat balls in tomato sauce		
Homemade	248 g (1 c)	75
Canned	250 g (1 c)	39
Sweetbreads (thymus), cooked	85 g (3 oz)	(396)
Tapioca cream pudding	165 g (1 c)	159
Tartar sauce, regular	14 g (1 T)	7
	230 g (1 c)	118
Tuna		
Canned in oil		
Solids and liquid	184 g (6½ oz)	(100)
Drained solids	157 g (5½ oz)	102
Canned in water, solids and liquid	184 g (6½ oz)	(116)
Turkey, all classes		
Whole, cooked		
Flesh, skin, and giblets	3,680 (8.1 lb)	3,864
Flesh and skin only	3,530 g (7.8 lb)	3,283
Light meat without skin, cooked	85 g (3 oz)	65
Dark meat without skin, cooked	85 g (3 oz)	86
Turkey potpie		
Homemade, baked	232 g	71
Commercial, frozen, unheated	227 g (8 oz)	20
Veal		
Composite of retail cuts		
Total edible, cooked, bone removed	85 g (3 oz)	(86)
Lean, trimmed of separable fat, cooked	85 g (3 oz)	(84)
Waffles, baked from mix, made with egg and milk	1 (200 g)	119
Welsh rarebit	232 g (1 c)	71
White sauce		
Thin	250 g (1 c)	36
Medium	250 g (1 c)	33
Thick	250 g (1 c)	30
Yogurt, made from fluid and dry milk		
Plain or vanilla	227 g (8 oz)	17
Fruit flavored (all kinds)	227 g (8 oz)	15

Table B-3
Sodium and Potassium Content of Foods

	UNIT	WEIGHT (g)	SODIUM (mg)	POTASSIUM (mg)
Dairy and egg products				
Butter, regular	1 T	14.2	140	3
Buttermilk	1 c	245	319	343
Cheese, blue or roquefort	1 c	135	380	70
Cheese, cheddar or American	1 oz	28	197	23
Cheese, cottage, uncreamed	1 c	226	918	194
Cheese, parmesan, grated	1 T	5	93	5
Cream, coffee	1 c	240	103	293
Cream, half-and-half	1 c	242	111	312
Cream, heavy	1 c	238	76	212
Eggs	1	50	54	57
Ice cream	1 c	133	84	241
Margarine	1 T	9.4	93	2
Milk, dry, nonfat, instant	1 envelope	91	479	1,570
Milk, dry, nonfat, regular	1 c	120	638	2,094
Milk, dry, whole, regular, instant	1 lb	454	11,837	6,033
Milk, low-fat	1 c	246	150	431
Milk, skim	1 c	245	127	355
Milk, whole	1 c	244	122	351
Yogurt, skim milk	8 oz	226	115	323
Meat and meat products				
Bacon, Canadian	1 slice	21	537	91
Beef, chuck, braised	3½ oz	100	60	370
Beef, corned, cooked	1 lb	454	4,277	272
Beef, hamburger, lean	1 patty	86	41	480
Beef, rib roast	2 slices	41	17	169
Beef, round, stew	¼ lb	133	68	563
Beef, sirloin tip	1 slice	44	19	199
Chicken, canned	1 c	205	—	283
Chicken, dark meat	1 c	140	120	449
Chicken, light meat	1 c	140	90	575
Gizzard, chicken	1 c	145	83	306
Heart, beef	1 c	145	151	336
Kidney, beef	1 c	140	354	454
Lamb, chop	3.4 oz	95	51	234
Lamb, leg	1 c	140	87	396
Liver, beef	1 slice	85	156	323
Pork, chops	8.6 oz	244	147	670
Pork, spareribs	6.3	180	65	299
Pork, ham	10.9 oz	308	173	793
Rabbit, meat	1 c	140	57	515
Sausages, frankfurter	1	50	550	110
Sausages, Italian	1 slice	28	161	81
Sausages, knockwurst	3½ oz	100	—	—

SOURCE: Adapted from *Composition of Foods—Raw, Processed, Prepared,* Agriculture Handbook no. 8, U.S. Department of Agriculture (Washington, D.C., 1963).

NOTE: A dash means the level varies with the product.

	UNIT	WEIGHT (g)	SODIUM (mg)	POTASSIUM (mg)
Sausages, Polish	1 slice	30	—	—
Sausages, pork link	3½ oz	100	740	140
Sausages, salami	1 slice	30	—	—
Sausages, Vienna	1	18	590	150
Tongue, beef	1 slice	20	12	33
Turkey, meat	1 c	140	115	575
Veal	9.5 oz	269	174	795
Seafood				
Bluefish	1 lb	454	662	722
Caviar, sturgeon	1 T	16	352	29
Clams	1 pt (1 lb)	454	163	1,066
Cod, cooked with margarine	1 fillet	65	72	265
Crab, canned	1 c	135	1,350	149
Flounder, baked with margarine	1 oz	28	67	166
Haddock, fried	1 fillet	110	195	383
Halibut, broiled with butter	1 fillet	125	168	656
Lobster, northern	1 c	145	305	261
Lobster, Newburg	1 c	250	573	428
Ocean perch, Atlantic	1 oz	28	43	81
Oysters	1 c	240	175	210
Rockfish	1 fillet	115	78	513
Salmon, broiled with butter	1 steak	145	148	565
Sardines, Atlantic, canned, oil	1 lb	454	3,733	2,676
Scallops	1 lb	454	1,202	2,159
Shad, baked	12.8 oz	365	288	1,376
Shrimp	1 lb	454	844	1,039
Sturgeon	1 lb	454	490	1,066
Tuna, canned in oil	1 can	198	1,584	596
Tuna, canned in water	1 can	99	41	276
Whitefish, lake	1 oz	28	55	82
Grain and grain products				
Barley, pearl	1 c	200	—	592
Biscuits, from mix	1	28	272	32
Biscuits, with baking powder	1	28	175	33
Boston brown bread	1 piece	45	113	131
Bran	1 c	60	493	466
Bread, French	1 slice	35	203	32
Bread, raisin	1 slice	25	91	58
Bread, white, enriched	1 slice	28	142	29
Bread, whole wheat	1 slice	25	132	68
Cereals, hot				
Ralston	⅔ c	28	4	107
Cream of wheat, instant	1 c	38	96	—
Cream of rice	1 c	245	0	65
Oats and wheat	1 c	245	412	—
Malt-O-Meal	¾ c	28	1	16

continued on next page

Table B-3
continued

	UNIT	WEIGHT (g)	SODIUM (mg)	POTASSIUM (mg)
Farina, instant	1 c	245	461	32
Oatmeal with raisins and spices, dry, instant	½ c	40	214	133
Oatmeal, rolled oats	1 c	236	1	130
Cereals, ready-to-eat				
Natural, 100% Quaker	1 oz	28	18	146
Wheaties, General Mills	1 c	28	315	—
Shredded wheat	1 biscuit	25	1	87
Puffed Rice, Quaker	1 c	14	1	15
Corn Flakes, Kellogg	1 c	22	216	26
Cheerios, General Mills	1 c	25	260	83
Bran flakes, 40%	1 c	35	207	137
All Bran, Kellogg	1 c	56	567	517
Cookies, assorted	1 lb	454	1,656	304
Cookies, butter	10	50	209	30
Cookies, chocolate chip	10	105	421	141
Cookies, molasses	1	32.5	125	45
Cookies, oatmeal with raisins	4	52	84	192
Cookies, peanut	4	49	85	86
Cookies, sugar	10	80	254	61
Cornbread	1 piece	83	491	130
Corn grits	1 c	245	502	27
Crackers, animal	10	26	79	25
Crackers, cheese	10	31	325	34
Crackers, graham	1 piece	14	95	55
Crackers, soda	10	28	312	34
Doughnut	1	42	99	34
Muffin	1	40	176	50
Noodles, egg	1 c	160	3	70
Pancake	1	73	412	112
Popcorn, buttered, salted	1 c	9	175	—
Rice, brown	1 c	195	550	137
Rice, white, enriched	1 c	205	767	57
Rolls, brown-and-serve	1	28	157	28
Rolls, dinner	1	17	83	—
Rolls, hamburger	1	30	152	28
Rolls, hard	1	35	219	34
Spaghetti	1 c	130	1	103
Waffles, baked	1	75	356	109
Wheat flour	1 c	137	3	130
Wheat flour, self-rising	1 c	115	1,241	—
Wild rice	1 c	160	11	352
Zwieback	1 package	170	425	255
Nuts and nut products				
Almonds, shelled	1 c	142	1	241
Brazil nuts, shelled	1 c	140	1	1,001
Cashew nuts	1 c	140	21	650

	UNIT	WEIGHT (g)	SODIUM (mg)	POTASSIUM (mg)
Filberts, hazelnuts	1 c	115	2	810
Peanut butter	1 T	16	97	100
Peanuts, roasted, salted	1 c	144	602	971
Pecans, halves	1 c	108	Trace	651
Walnuts, black, shelled	1 c	125	4	575
Vegetables and juices				
Artichokes	1 bud	300	36	361
Asparagus	4 spears	60	1	110
Beans, lima	1 c	170	5	1,914
Beans, mung	1 c	125	5	195
Beans, navy	1 c	190	13	790
Beans, red kidney	1 c	185	6	629
Beans, snap, green	1 c	125	5	189
Beans, snap, yellow or wax	1 c	110	4	189
Beets, red	1 c	170	73	354
Beet greens	1 c	145	110	481
Broccoli, stalks	1	180	18	481
Brussels sprouts	1 c	155	16	423
Cabbage, Chinese	1 c	75	17	190
Cabbage, common	1 c	90	18	210
Carrots	1	81	34	246
Cauliflower	1 c	100	13	295
Celery, stalks	1	40	50	136
Chard, Swiss	1 c	145	125	465
Corn, sweet	1 c	165	Trace	272
Coleslaw, with mayonnaise	1 c	120	144	239
Cowpeas	1 c	165	2	625
Cress	1 lb	454	64	2,749
Cucumbers	1 c	105	6	168
Dandelion greens	1 c	105	46	244
Eggplant	1 c	200	2	300
Kale, leaves	1 c	110	195	1,002
Kohlrabi	1 c	165	10	429
Lentils	1 c	200	—	498
Lettuce	1 wedge	135	12	236
Mushrooms	1 c	70	11	290
Okra	1 c	160	3	278
Onions	1 c	170	17	267
Onions, young green	1 c	100	5	231
Parsley	1 c	60	27	436
Parsnips	1 c	155	12	587
Peas, green, frozen	1 c	145	187	218
Peas, split	1 c	200	26	592
Peas and carrots	1 c	160	134	251
Peppers, sweet	1 c	100	13	213
Potato, baked	1	202	5	782

continued on next page

Table B-3
continued

	UNIT	WEIGHT (g)	SODIUM (mg)	POTASSIUM (mg)
Potato, french fries	10	78	5	665
Potato chips	10	20	—	226
Pumpkin, canned	1 c	245	5	588
Rhubarb	1 c	270	5	548
Rutabaga	1	170	7	284
Sauerkraut, canned	1 c	235	1,755	329
Squash, summer	1 c	180	2	254
Spinach	1 c	55	39	259
Squash, crookneck and straight neck	1 c	180	2	254
Squash, zucchini and cocozelle	1 c	180	2	254
Soybeans	1 c	180	4	972
Soybean curd (tofu)	1 piece	120	8	50
Succotash, frozen	1 c	170	65	418
Sweet potato, baked	1	146	14	342
Tomato, ripe	1	135	4	300
Tomato juice, canned	1 c	243	486	552
Tomato juice cocktail, canned	1 c	243	486	537
Tomato paste, canned	1 c	262	100	2,237
Tomato puree, canned	1 can	822	3,280	3,502
Vegetables, mixed	1 c	182	96	348
Vegetable juice, cocktail, canned	1 can	182	364	402
Yam, tuber	1 lb	454	—	2,341
Watercress	1 c	35	18	99
Water chestnuts, Chinese	1 lb	454	70	1,747
Fruits and juices				
Apple	1	230	2	218
Apple, dehydrated	1 c	255	3	270
Apple butter	1 c	282	6	711
Apple juice, canned	1 c	248	2	250
Applesauce, canned	1 c	255	5	166
Apricots	3	114	1	301
Apricots, canned	1 c	254	3	604
Apricots, dehydrated	1 c	300	24	897
Apricot nectar	1 c	251	Trace	379
Avocado	½	125	5	680
Banana	1	175	1	440
Blackberries, canned	1 c	244	2	281
Blueberries	1 c	145	1	117
Cherries	1 c	130	2	223
Cherries, canned	1 c	244	5	317
Coconut cream	1 c	240	203	185
Coconut meat	1 piece	45	10	115
Cranberries	1 c	110	2	90
Dates	10	92	1	518
Fig	1	50	1	97
Fruit salad, canned	1 lb	454	5	631

	UNIT	WEIGHT (g)	SODIUM (mg)	POTASSIUM (mg)
Grape juice, canned	1 c	253	5	293
Grapes, American	1 c	153	3	160
Grapefruit	½	184	1	132
Grapefruit juice, frozen concentrate	1 c	247	2	420
Grapefruit juice and orange juice, blended	1 c	248	Trace	439
Lemonade concentrate, frozen	1 c	248	1	40
Lemon juice	1 T	15.2	Trace	21
Lime juice	1 c	246	2	256
Mangos	1 c	165	12	312
Marmalade, citrus	1 T	20	37	—
Muskmelon	½	477	33	682
Nectarine	1	150	8	406
Oranges	1	180	1	263
Orange juice	1 c	247	2	509
Orange juice concentrate, frozen	1 can	213	4	1,500
Papaya	1	454	9	711
Peach nectar	1 c	249	2	194
Peach	1	175	2	308
Pear	1	180	3	213
Persimmon	1	200	10	292
Pineapple	1 c	155	2	226
Pineapple juice, canned	1 c	250	3	373
Pineapple juice and grapefruit juice drink	1 c	250	Trace	155
Plums	10	110	2	299
Prunes, dehydrated	1 c	100	11	940
Prune juice, canned	1 c	256	5	602
Raisins	1 c	145	39	1,106
Raspberries	1 c	123	1	207
Strawberries	1 c	149	1	244
Tangerine	1	136	2	127
Tangerine juice, canned	1 can	185	2	329
Watermelon	1 piece	926	4	426
Soups				
Bean with pork, canned	1 c	265	2,136	837
Beef broth, bouillon, consommé	1 c	245	1,872	157
Beef noodle, condensed	1 c	245	1,872	157
Clam chowder, canned	1 c	250	1,915	375
Cream of asparagus, canned	1 c	245	2,009	245
Cream of celery, canned	1 c	245	1,950	221
Cream of chicken	1 c	245	1,982	162
Cream of mushroom, canned	1 c	245	1,948	201
Minestrone, canned	1 c	250	2,033	638
Tomato, canned	1 c	250	1,980	470
Vegetable beef, canned	1 c	250	2,135	328
Beverages				
Beer	12 fl oz	360	25	90

continued on next page

Table B-3
continued

	UNIT	WEIGHT (g)	SODIUM (mg)	POTASSIUM (mg)
Beverages, alcoholic (gin, rum, vodka, whiskey)	1 jigger	42	Trace	1
Cocoa and chocolate-flavored powder	1 oz or 4 t	28	149	227
Coffee, instant	1 T	3.5	3	114
Soft drinks (cola, cream soda, ginger ale, root beer)	12 fl oz	369	—	—
Wine	1 gallon	103	4	77
Candy				
Caramel	1 oz	28	65	54
Chocolate, milk	1 oz	28	27	109
Fondant, mints	1 piece	8.8	19	Trace
Fudge, chocolate	1 oz	28	54	42
Gumdrops	1 oz	28	10	1
Jelly beans	1 oz	28	26	2
Marshmallow	1	7.2	3	Trace
Peanut brittle	1 oz	28	9	43
Desserts				
Cake, angel food	1 piece	60	170	53
Cake, coffee	1 piece	108	465	118
Cake, fruitcake	1 sl	15	24	74
Cake, plain	1 cupcake	33	99	26
Cake, sponge	1 piece	66	110	57
Custard	1 c	265	209	387
Gelatin dessert, from powder	1 c	240	122	—
Jellies	1 T	18	3	14
Pie, apple	1 sl	158	476	126
Pie, custard	1 sl	152	436	208
Pie, lemon	1 sl	140	395	70
Pie, mince	1 sl	158	708	281
Pie, pumpkin	1 sl	152	325	243
Pudding	1 c	260	335	354
Sherbet, orange	1 c	193	19	42
Tapioca cream pudding	1 c	165	257	223
Condiments				
Horseradish	1 T	15	14	44
Mustard	1 t	5	65	7
Pickle, cucumber, dill	1	135	1,928	270
Radishes	10	90	15	261
Relish, pickle, sweet	1 c	245	1,744	—
Salt, table	1 t	5.5	2,132	Trace
Soy sauce	1 T	18	1,319	66
Tartar sauce, regular	1 c	230	1,626	179
Tomato catsup, canned	1 can (12 oz)	340	3,543	1,234
Tomato chili sauce	1 c	273	3,653	1,010

	UNIT	WEIGHT (g)	SODIUM (mg)	POTASSIUM (mg)
Miscellaneous				
Baking chocolate	1 oz	28	1	235
Baking powder, phosphate	1 t	3.8	312	6
Barbecue sauce	1 c	250	2,038	435
Bouillon cube	1	4	960	4
Cornstarch	1 T	8	Trace	Trace
Fats	1 c	200	0	0
Molasses, blackstrap	1 c	328	315	9,601
French salad dressing	1 T	16	219	13
Honey, strained or extracted	1 c	339	17	173
Jams and preserves	1 T	20	2	18
Mayonnaise	1 T	14	84	5
Pretzels, twisted	1	16	269	21
Sugar, brown	1 c	145	44	499
Sugar, granulated	1 c	200	2	6
Syrup, corn	1 bottle (1½ lb)	657	447	26
Vinegar, cider	1 c	240	2	240
Yeast, brewer's, debittered	1 T	8	10	152

Table B-4
Carbohydrate, Alcohol, and Calorie Content of Alcoholic Beverages

ALCOHOLIC BEVERAGE	WEIGHT (g)	SERVING SIZE	CARBOHYDRATE (g)	ALCOHOL (g)	KILOCALORIES
Cocktails					
Daiquiri	100	1 cocktail glass	5.2	15.2	126
Highball	240	8 oz	Unknown	20–30	139–208
Manhattan	100	1 cocktail glass	8.0	19.1	164
Martini	100	1 cocktail glass	0.3	18.5	140
Mint julep	300	10 oz	2.8	29.0	212
Old-fashioned	100	4 oz	3.4	23.9	179
Rum sour	100	4 oz	4.0	22.0	168
Tom Collins	300	10 oz	9.1	21.0	182
Whiskey sour	75	1 cocktail glass	7.6	15.0	134
Wines					
Champagne	120	1 wine glass	3.0	11.0	85
Madeira	100	1 wine glass	1.0	15.0	105
Sauterne, California	100	1 wine glass	4.0	10.5	85
Sherry, dry	60	1 wine glass	4.8	9.0	85
Vermouth, dry	100	1 wine glass	1.0	15.0	105
Wine, red, California	100	1 wine glass	3.9	10.0	85
Wine, table	100	1 wine glass	4.2	10.5	90
American malt liquors					
Ale, mild	345	12 oz	12.2	13.0	139
Beer	360	12 oz	15.0	14.0	157
Beer, Budweiser	360	12 oz	14.0	17.6	150
Beer, Lite	360	12 oz	2.8	12.1	96
Beer, Michelob	360	12 oz	16.0	18.0	160
Beer, Natural Light	360	12 oz	6.0	14.4	100
Distilled spirits					
Liqueurs					
Benedictine	20	1 cordial glass	6.6	6.6	70
Cognac brandy	30	1 brandy glass	0.0	10.5	73
Creme de menthe	20	1 cordial glass	6.0	7.0	67
Curaçao	20	1 cordial glass	6.0	6.0	55
Others (vodka, rum, gin)					
80 proof	45	1 jigger	0.0	15.0	104
86 proof	45	1 jigger	0.0	16.2	112
100 proof	45	1 jigger	0.0	19.1	133

NOTE: Data obtained by direct calculation from beverage label and other literature. In the body, 1 g of carbohydrate supplies 4 kcal, and 1 g of alcohol supplies 6.93 kcal. Volume contents of glassware for alcoholic beverages: 1 cordial glass = 20 mL; 1 brandy glass = 30 mL; 1 sherry glass = 60 mL; 1 cocktail glass = 90 mL; 1 burgundy glass = 120 mL; 1 champagne glass = 150 mL; 1 tumbler = 240–360 mL; 1 mixing glass = 360 mL; 1 jigger = 45 mL.

Table B-5
Approximate Caffeine Content of Beverages and Some Nonprescription Drugs

ITEM	CAFFEINE CONTENT (mg)	ITEM	CAFFEINE CONTENT (mg)
Beverage		*Nonprescription drugs*	
Coffee		Aspirin-containing preparations	30–35/tablet
Decaffeinated	2–70/cup	Excedrin	60/tablet
Ground	85–200/cup	Stimulants, nonprescription	80–150/tablet
Instant	30–80/cup		
Cola	40–60/glass		
Tea	20–150/cup		

Appendix C Weights and Measures

Table C-1
Common Weights and Measures

MEASURE	EQUIVALENT	MEASURE	EQUIVALENT
3 t	1 T	1 fl oz	30 g
2 T	1 oz	½ c	120 g
4 T	¼ c	1 c	240 g
8 T	½ c	1 lb	454 g
16 T	1 c		
		1 g	1 mL
2 c	1 pt	1 t	5 mL
4 c	1 qt	1 T	15 mL
4 qt	1 gal	1 fl oz	30 mL
		1 c	240 mL
1 t	5 g	1 pt	480 mL
1 T	15 g	1 qt	960 mL
1 oz	28.35 g	1 L	1,000 mL

Table C-2
Weights and Measures Conversions

U.S. SYSTEM TO METRIC		METRIC TO U.S. SYSTEM	
U.S. MEASURE	METRIC MEASURE	METRIC MEASURE	U.S. MEASURE
Length		*Length*	
1 in.	25.0 mm	1 mm	0.04 in.
1 ft	0.3 m	1 m	3.3 ft
Mass		*Mass*	
1 gr	64.8 mg	1 mg	0.015 gr
1 oz	28.0 g	1 g	0.035 oz
1 lb	0.45 kg	1 kg	2.2 lb
1 short ton	907.1 kg	1 metric ton	1.102 short tons
Volume		*Volume*	
1 cu. in.	16.0 cm^3	1 cm^3	0.06 in.^{3}
1 t	5.0 mL	1 mL	0.2 t
1 T	15.0 mL	1 mL	0.07 T
1 fl oz	30.0 mL	1 mL	0.03 oz
1 c	0.24 L	1 L	4.2 c
1 pt	0.47 L	1 L	2.1 pt
1 qt (liq)	0.95 L	1 L	1.1 qt
1 gal	0.004 m^3	1 m^3	264.0 gal
1 pk	0.009 m^3	1 m^3	113.0 pk
1 bu	0.04 m^3	1 m^3	28.0 bu
Energy		*Energy*	
1 cal	4.18 J	1 J	0.24 cal

To convert Celsius degrees into Fahrenheit, multiply by ⁹∕₅ and add 32. To convert Fahrenheit degrees into Celcius, subtract 32 and multiply by ⁵∕₉. For example:

$$30\,°C = \left(30 \times \frac{9}{5} + 32\right)°F = (54 + 32)\,°F = 86\,°F$$

$$90\,°F = (90 - 32) \times \frac{5}{9}\,°C = 58 \times \frac{5}{9}\,°C = 32.2\,°C$$

Table C-3
Milligrams and Milliequivalents Conversions

SODIUM (EQUIVALENT WEIGHT 23)		POTASSIUM (EQUIVALENT WEIGHT 39)		
MILLIGRAMS	GRAMS	MILLIGRAMS	GRAMS	MILLIEQUIVALENTS
230	0.23	390	0.39	10
460	0.46	780	0.78	20
—	—	1,000	1.00	25.6
690	0.69	1,170	1.17	30
920	0.92	1,560	1.56	40
1,000	1.00	—	—	43.5
1,150	1.15	1,950	1.95	50
1,380	1.38	2,340	2.34	60
1,610	1.61	2,730	2.73	70
1,840	1.84	3,170	3.17	80
2,170	2.17	3,510	3.51	90
2,300	2.30	3,900	3.9	100
—	—	5,000	5.0	128
5,000	5.00	—	—	217.5
—	—	10,000	10.0	256
10,000	10.00	—	—	435

NOTE: To convert milligrams to milliequivalents: milliequivalents of sodium or potassium = milligrams of sodium or potassium ÷ equivalent weight in milligrams
To convert milliequivalents to milligrams: milligrams of sodium or potassium = milliequivalents of sodium or potassium × equivalent weight in milligrams

Table D-1
Desirable Weight in Relation to Height, Frame, and Age*

MEN					WOMEN				
HEIGHT		SMALL	MEDIUM	LARGE	HEIGHT		SMALL	MEDIUM	LARGE
FEET	INCHES	FRAME	FRAME	FRAME	FEET	INCHES	FRAME	FRAME	FRAME
5	2	128–134	131–141	138–150	4	10	102–111	109–121	118–131
5	3	130–136	133–143	140–153	4	11	103–113	111–123	120–134
5	4	132–138	135–145	142–156	5	0	104–115	113–126	122–137
5	5	134–140	137–148	144–160	5	1	106–118	115–129	125–140
5	6	136–142	139–151	146–164	5	2	108–121	118–132	128–143
5	7	138–145	142–154	149–168	5	3	111–124	121–135	131–147
5	8	140–148	145–157	152–172	5	4	114–127	124–138	134–151
5	9	142–151	148–160	155–176	5	5	117–130	127–141	137–155
5	10	144–154	151–163	158–180	5	6	120–133	130–144	140–159
5	11	146–157	154–166	161–184	5	7	123–136	133–147	143–163
6	0	149–160	157–170	164–188	5	8	126–139	136–150	146–167
6	1	152–164	160–174	168–192	5	9	129–142	139–153	149–170
6	2	155–168	164–178	172–197	5	10	132–145	142–156	152–173
6	3	158–172	167–182	176–202	5	11	135–148	145–159	155–176
6	4	162–176	171–187	181–207	6	0	138–151	148–162	158–179

SOURCE: Reproduced with permission of Metropolitan Life Insurance Company, 1983. Source of basic data: 1979 Build Study, Society of Actuaries and Association of Life Insurance Medical Directors of America, 1980.

*Weights at ages 25–29 in indoor clothing; includes shoes with 1-inch heels.

Table D-2
Average Weights by Height and Age (Graduated Weights in Indoor Clothings in Pounds)

	HEIGHT (IN SHOES)	AGE GROUPS							
		15–16	17–19	20–24	25–29	30–39	40–49	50–59	60–69
MEN	4'10"	93	106	112	116	120	121	122	121
	11"	98	110	117	121	124	126	127	126
	5'0"	102	115	121	125	129	131	132	130
	1"	107	119	126	130	133	135	136	135
	2"	112	124	130	134	138	140	141	140
	3"	116	129	136	140	143	144	145	144
	4"	121	132	139	143	147	149	150	149
	5"	127	137	143	147	151	154	155	153
	6"	133	141	148	152	156	158	159	158
	7"	137	145	153	156	160	163	164	163
	8"	143	150	157	161	165	167	168	167
	9"	148	155	163	166	170	172	173	172
	10"	153	159	167	171	174	176	177	176
	11"	159	164	171	175	179	181	182	181
	6'0"	162	168	176	181	184	186	187	186
	1"	168	174	182	186	190	192	193	191
	2"	173	179	187	191	195	197	198	196
	3"	178	185	193	197	201	203	204	200
	4"	184	190	198	202	206	208	209	207
	5"	189	195	203	207	211	213	214	212
	6"	195	201	209	213	217	219	220	218
	7"	201	207	215	219	223	225	226	224
WOMEN	4'6"	85	87	89	95	101	105	109	111
	7"	89	91	93	98	104	108	112	114
	8"	93	95	99	103	107	111	115	117
	9"	97	99	101	106	110	114	118	120
	10"	101	103	105	110	113	118	121	123
	11"	105	108	110	112	115	121	125	127
	5'0"	109	111	112	114	118	123	127	130
	1"	112	115	116	119	121	127	131	133
	2"	117	119	120	121	124	129	133	136
	3"	121	123	124	125	128	133	137	140
	4"	123	126	127	128	131	136	141	143
	5"	128	129	130	132	134	139	144	147
	6"	131	132	133	134	137	143	147	150
	7"	135	136	137	138	141	147	152	155
	8"	138	140	141	142	145	150	156	158
	9"	142	145	146	148	150	155	159	161
	10"	146	148	149	150	153	158	162	163
	11"	149	150	155	156	159	162	166	167
	6'0"	152	154	157	159	164	168	171	172
	1"	155	157	159	163	168	172	175	176
	2"	158	160	162	166	172	176	179	180
	3"	161	163	165	170	176	180	183	184

SOURCE: 1979 Build and Blood Pressure Study by the Society of Actuaries and the Association of Life Insurance Medical Directors of America. Reproduced by permission.

Appendix D

Table D-3
Guidelines for Body Weight According to the National Institutes of Health

METRIC

HEIGHT* (m)	MEN WEIGHT (kg)* AVER-AGE	ACCEPTABLE WEIGHT		WOMEN WEIGHT (kg)* AVER-AGE	ACCEPTABLE WEIGHT	
1.45				46.0	42	53
1.48				46.5	42	54
1.50				47.0	43	55
1.52				48.5	44	57
1.54				49.5	44	58
1.56				50.4	45	58
1.58	55.8	51	64	51.3	46	59
1.60	57.6	52	65	52.6	48	61
1.62	58.6	53	66	54.0	49	62
1.64	59.6	54	67	55.4	50	64
1.66	60.6	55	69	56.8	51	65
1.68	61.7	56	71	58.1	52	66
1.70	63.5	58	73	60.0	53	67
1.72	65.0	59	74	61.3	55	69
1.74	66.5	60	75	62.6	56	70
1.76	68.0	62	77	64.0	58	72
1.78	69.4	64	79	65.3	59	74
1.80	71.0	65	80			
1.82	72.6	66	82			
1.84	74.2	67	84			
1.86	75.8	69	86			
1.88	77.6	71	88			
1.90	79.3	73	90			
1.92	81.0	75	93			

NONMETRIC

HEIGHT* (ft in)	MEN WEIGHT (lb)* AVER-AGE	ACCEPTABLE WEIGHT		WOMEN WEIGHT (lb)* AVER-AGE	ACCEPTABLE WEIGHT	
4 10				102	92	119
4 11				104	94	122
5 0				107	96	125
5 1				110	99	128
5 2	123	112	141	113	102	131
5 3	127	115	144	116	105	134
5 4	130	118	148	120	108	138
5 5	133	121	152	123	111	142
5 6	136	124	156	128	114	146
5 7	140	128	161	132	118	150
5 8	145	132	166	136	122	154
5 9	149	136	170	140	126	158
5 10	153	140	174	144	130	163
5 11	158	144	179	148	134	168
6 0	162	148	184	152	138	173
6 1	166	152	189			
6 2	171	156	194			
6 3	176	160	199			
6 4	181	164	204			

SOURCE: "Obesity in America," edited by G. A. Bray, U.S. Department of Health, Education, and Welfare, Public Health Service, National Institutes of Health, NIH Publication No. 80-359, 1980, page 7.

*Height without shoes, weight without clothes.

Table D-4
Growth Charts with Reference Percentiles for Girls
Birth to 36 Months of Age

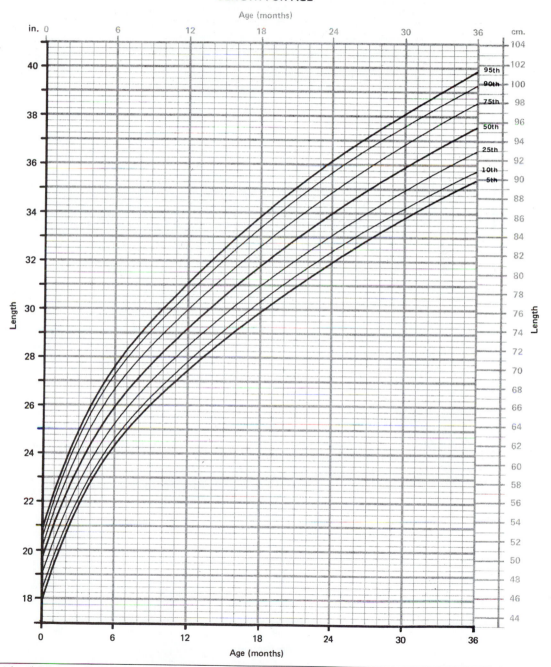

GIRLS FROM BIRTH TO 36 MONTHS
LENGTH FOR AGE

Tables D-4 through D-7 courtesy Centers for Disease Control, Atlanta, Georgia.

Table D-4
continued

GIRLS FROM BIRTH TO 36 MONTHS

WEIGHT FOR AGE

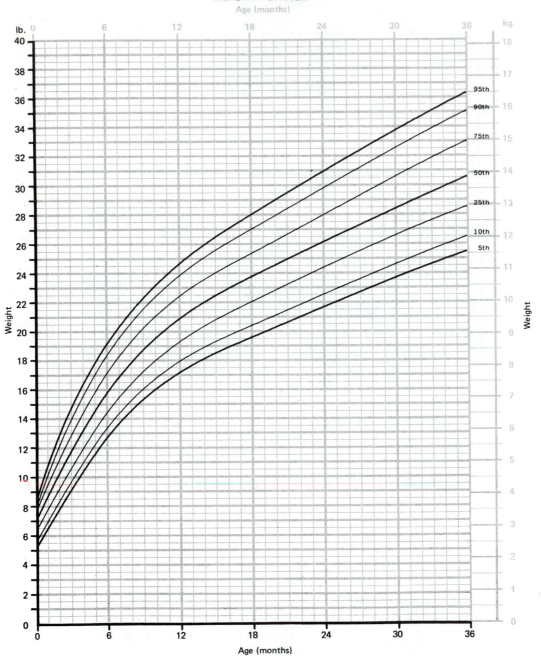

Table D-4
continued

GIRLS FROM BIRTH TO 36 MONTHS

HEAD CIRCUMFERENCE FOR AGE

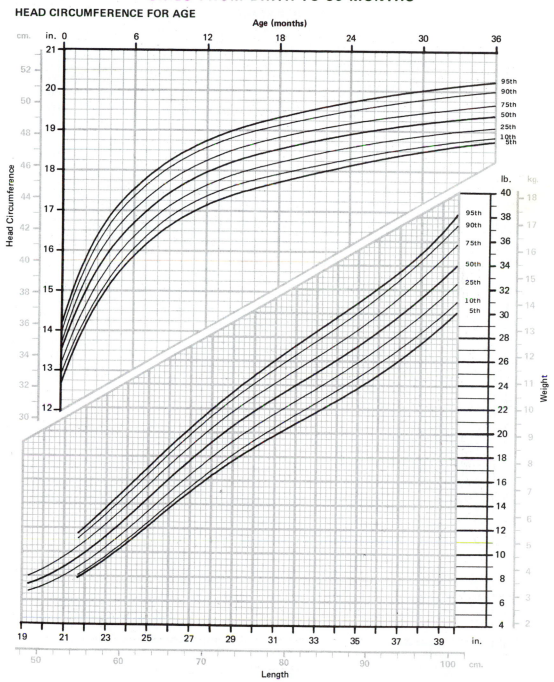

Table D-5
Growth Charts with Reference Percentiles for Boys
Birth to 36 Months of Age

BOYS FROM BIRTH TO 36 MONTHS
LENGTH FOR AGE

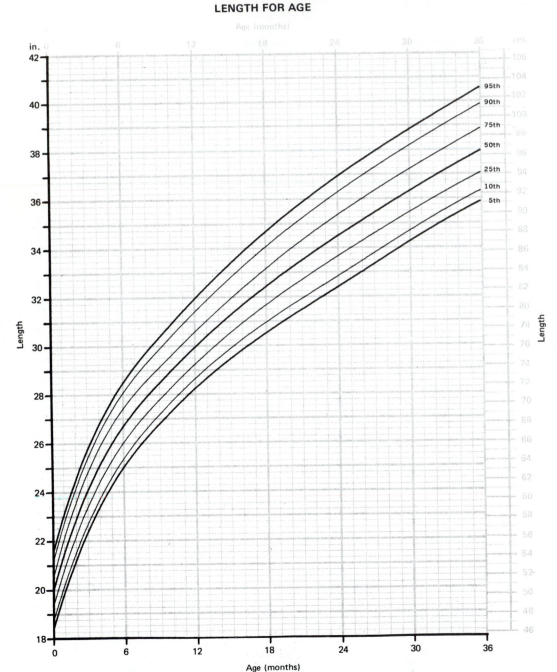

Table D-5
continued

BOYS FROM BIRTH TO 36 MONTHS
WEIGHT FOR AGE

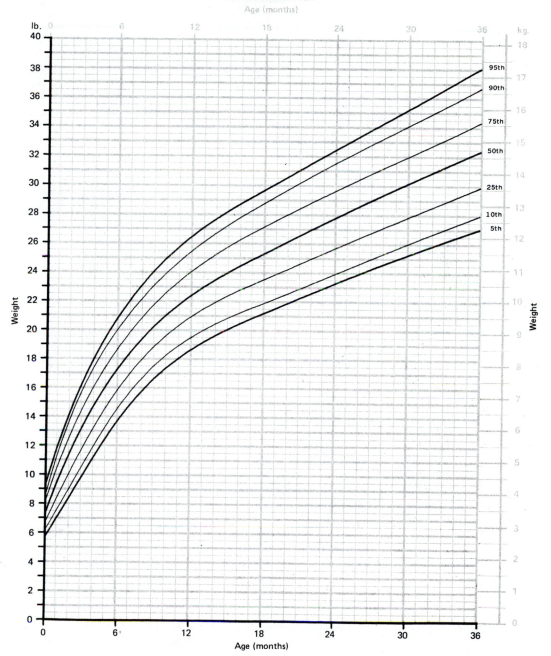

Table D-5
continued

BOYS FROM BIRTH TO 36 MONTHS

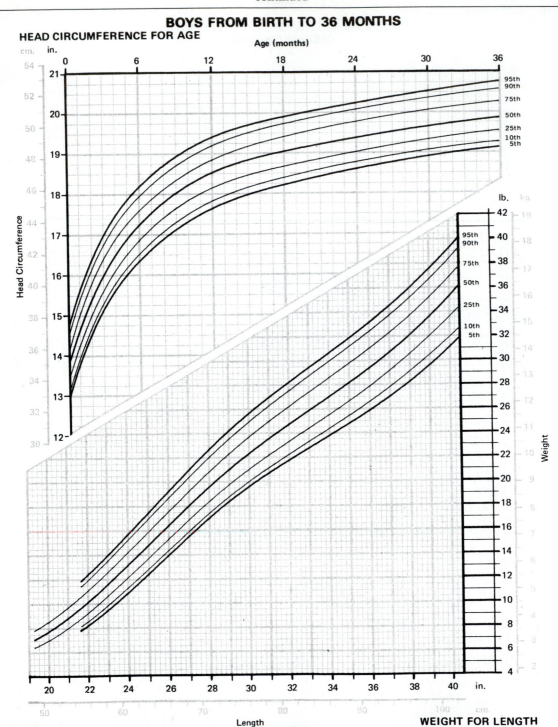

HEAD CIRCUMFERENCE FOR AGE

WEIGHT FOR LENGTH

Table D-6
**Growth Charts with Reference Percentiles for Girls
2 to 18 Years of Age**

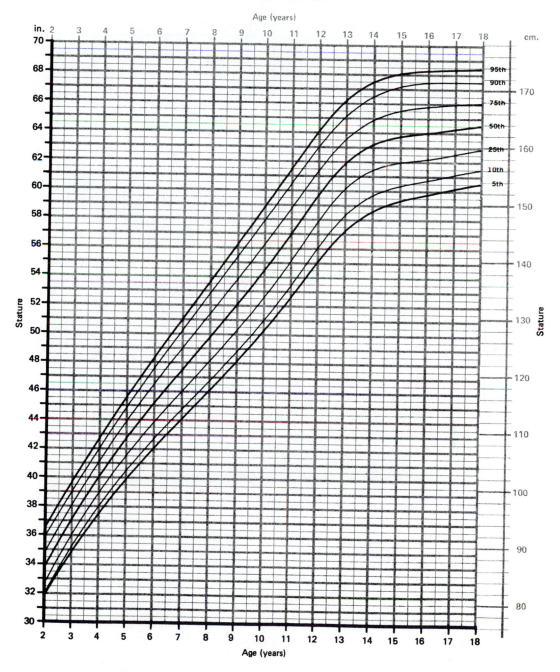

GIRLS FROM 2 TO 18 YEARS
STATURE FOR AGE

GIRLS FROM 2 TO 18 YEARS
WEIGHT FOR AGE

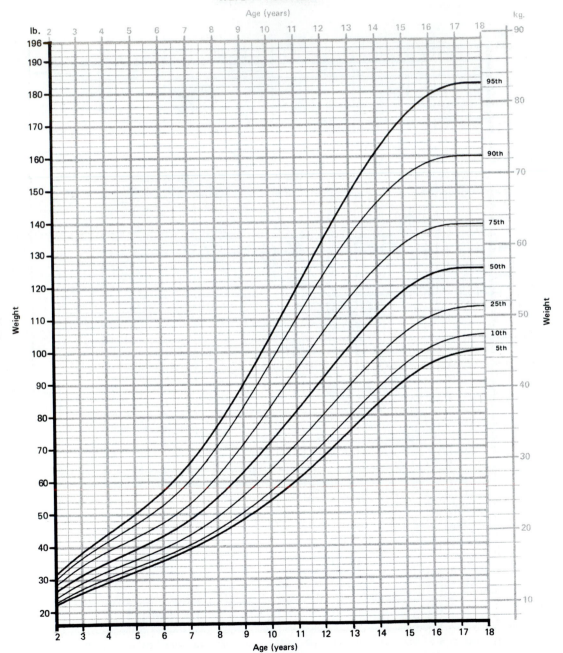

Table D-6
continued

PRE-PUBERTAL GIRLS FROM 2 TO 10 YEARS

WEIGHT FOR STATURE

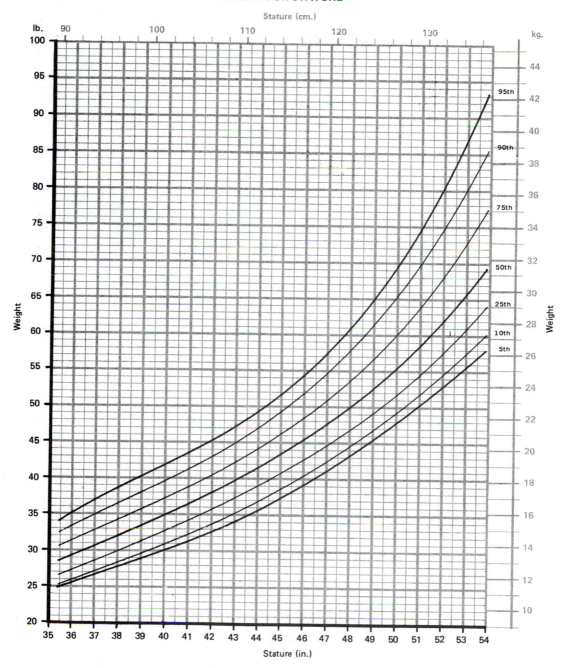

Table D-7
Growth Charts with Reference Percentiles for Boys
2 to 18 Years of Age

BOYS FROM 2 TO 18 YEARS
STATURE FOR AGE

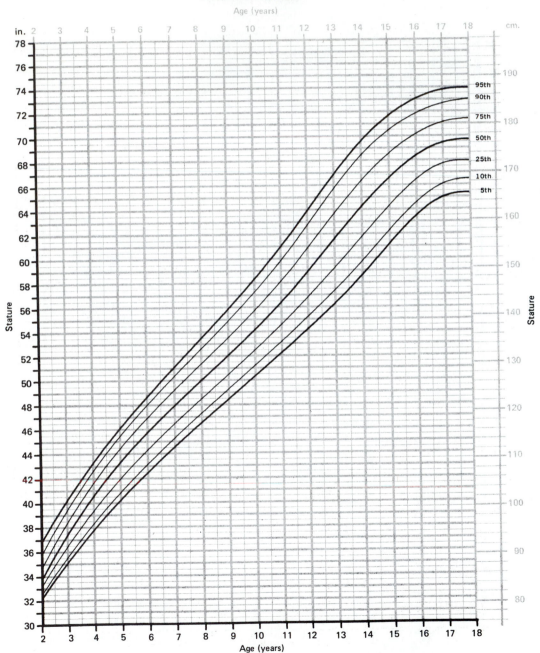

Table D-7
continued

BOYS FROM 2 TO 18 YEARS
WEIGHT FOR AGE

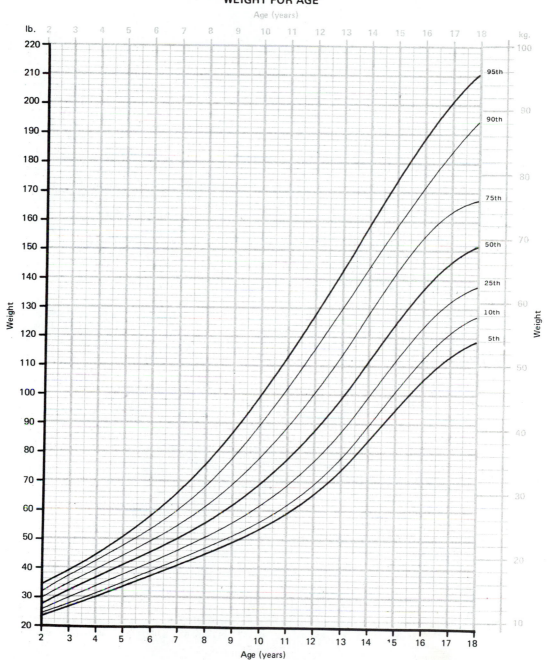

PRE-PUBERTAL BOYS FROM 2 TO 11½ YEARS
WEIGHT FOR STATURE

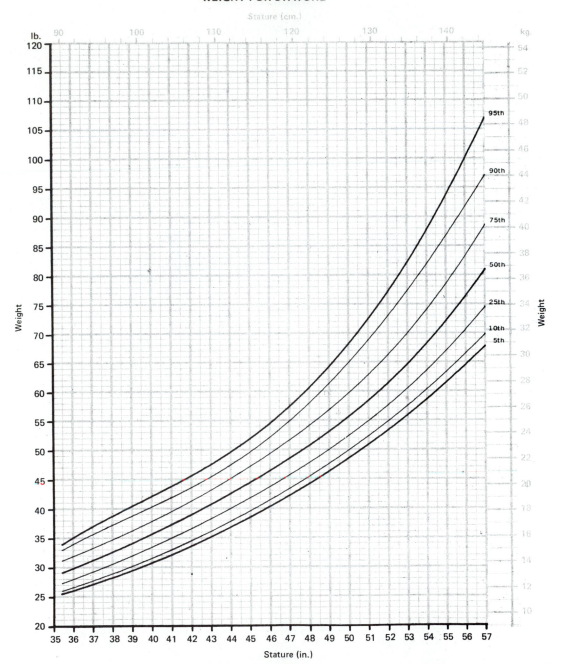

Amino Acids

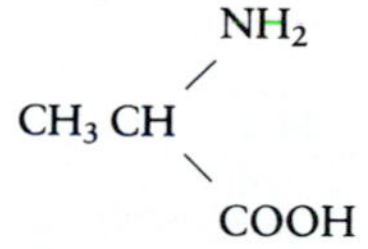

$$CH_3\ \underset{|}{\overset{NH_2}{CH}}$$
$$COOH$$

Alanine

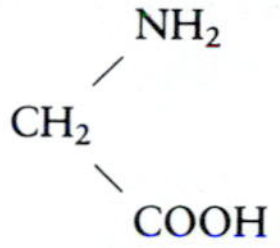

$$\underset{|}{\overset{NH_2}{CH_2}}$$
$$COOH$$

Glycine

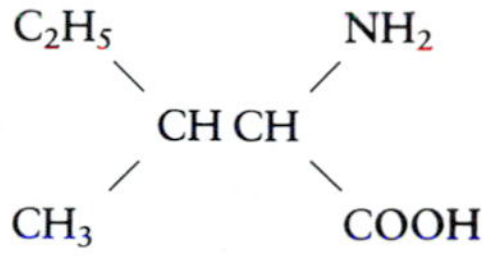

$$C_2H_5 \qquad NH_2$$
$$\underset{|}{CH}\ CH$$
$$CH_3 \qquad COOH$$

Isoleucine

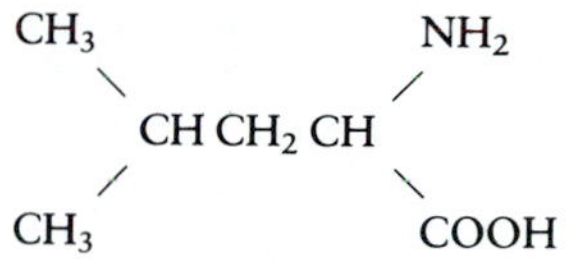

$$CH_3 \qquad\qquad NH_2$$
$$CH\ CH_2\ CH$$
$$CH_3 \qquad\qquad COOH$$

Leucine

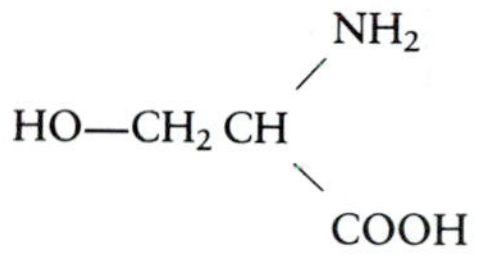

$$NH_2$$
$$HO\!-\!CH_2\ CH$$
$$COOH$$

Serine

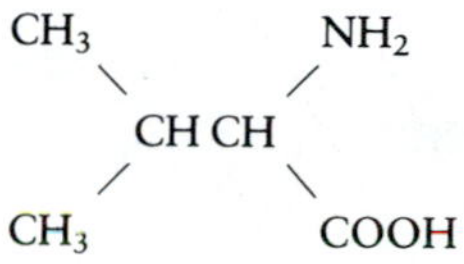

$$CH_3 \qquad NH_2$$
$$CH\ CH$$
$$CH_3 \qquad COOH$$

Valine

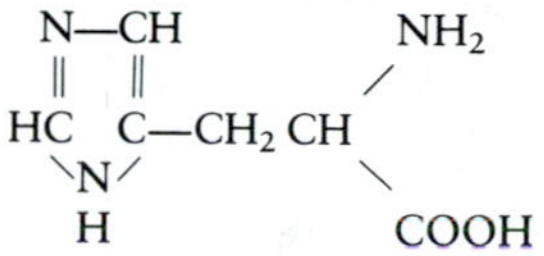

$$N\!-\!CH \qquad\quad NH_2$$
$$HC \quad C\!-\!CH_2\ CH$$
$$N$$
$$H \qquad\qquad COOH$$

Histidine

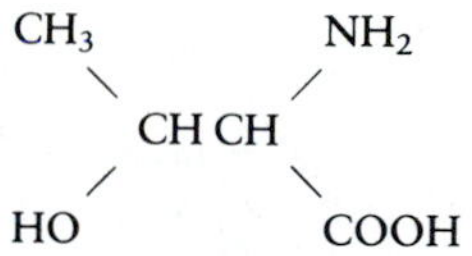

$$CH_3 \qquad NH_2$$
$$CH\ CH$$
$$HO \qquad COOH$$

Threonine

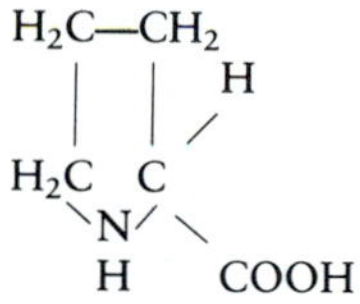

$$H_2C\!-\!CH_2$$
$$\qquad\qquad H$$
$$H_2C \quad C$$
$$N$$
$$H \quad COOH$$

Proline

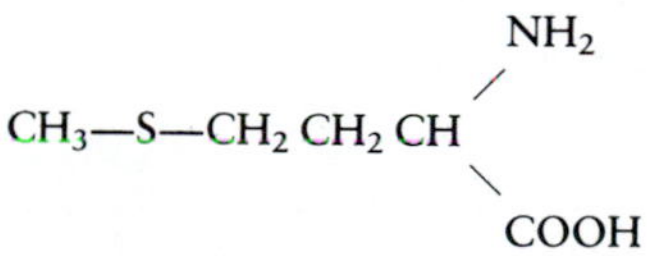

$$CH_3\!-\!S\!-\!CH_2\ CH_2\ CH$$
$$NH_2$$
$$COOH$$

Methionine

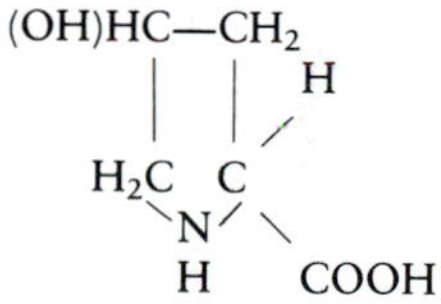

$$(OH)HC\!-\!CH_2$$
$$\qquad\qquad H$$
$$H_2C \quad C$$
$$N$$
$$H \quad COOH$$

Hydroxyproline

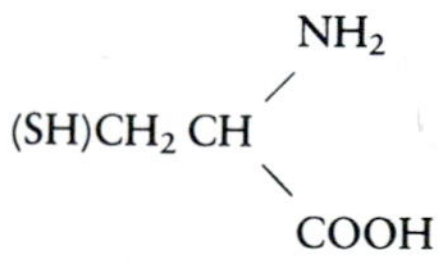

$$(SH)CH_2\ CH$$
$$NH_2$$
$$COOH$$

Cysteine

$$(NH_2)CH_2\ (CH_2)_3\ CH$$
$$NH_2$$
$$COOH$$

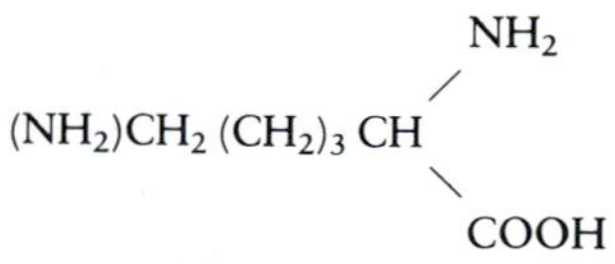

Lysine

Amino Acids
continued

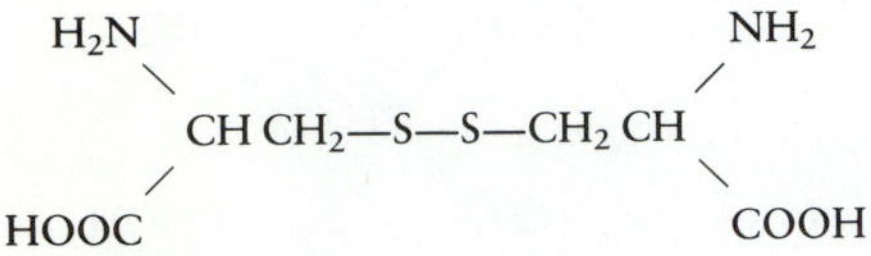

H_2N $CH\ CH_2$—S—S—$CH_2\ CH$ NH_2
HOOC $\qquad$ COOH

Cystine

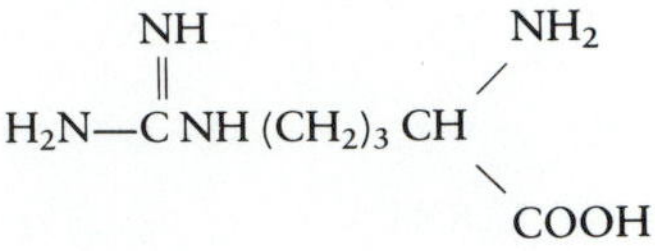

NH
H_2N—$C\ NH\ (CH_2)_3\ CH$ NH_2
$\qquad$ COOH

Arginine

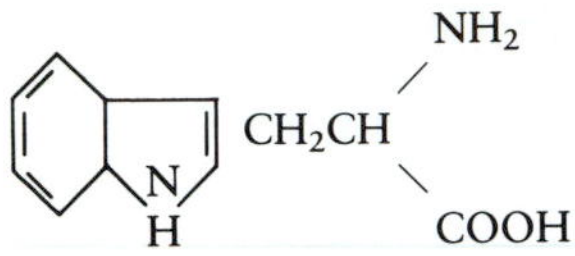

CH_2CH NH_2
$\qquad$ COOH

Tryptophan

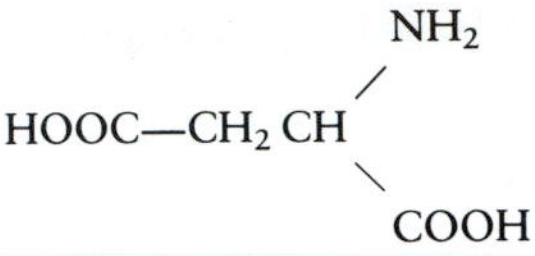

$HOOC$—$CH_2\ CH$ NH_2
$\qquad$ COOH

Aspartic acid

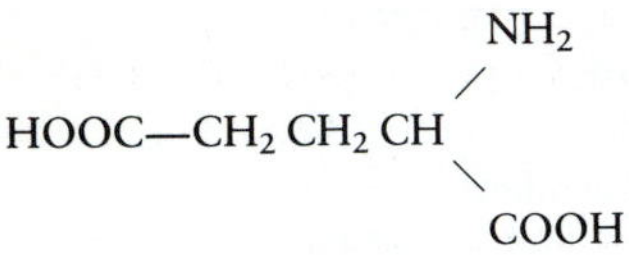

$HOOC$—$CH_2\ CH_2\ CH$ NH_2
$\qquad$ COOH

Glutamic acid

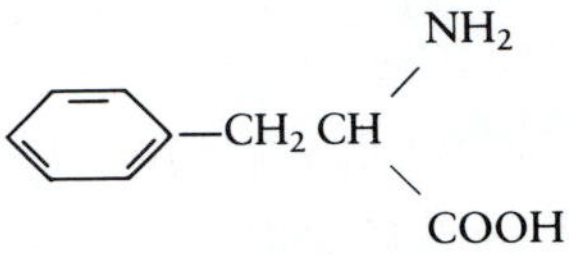

—$CH_2\ CH$ NH_2
$\qquad$ COOH

Phenylalanine

OH —$CH_2\ CH$ NH_2
$\qquad$ COOH

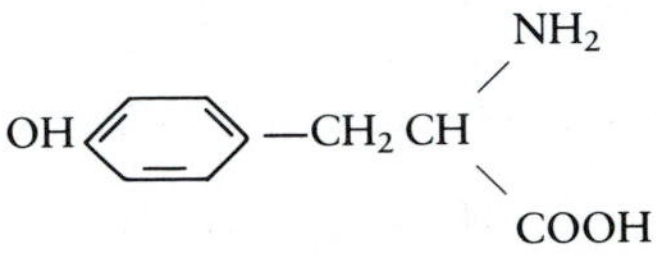

Tyrosine

Fats (Lipids)
Glycerides

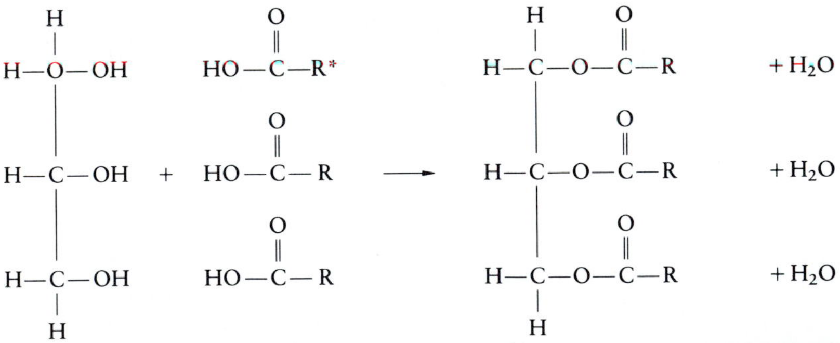

$$H-O-OH \quad + \quad HO-\overset{\overset{\displaystyle O}{\|}}{C}-R^* \quad \longrightarrow \quad H-\overset{\displaystyle H}{\underset{}{C}}-O-\overset{\overset{\displaystyle O}{\|}}{C}-R \quad + H_2O$$

$$H-\overset{}{C}-OH \quad + \quad HO-\overset{\overset{\displaystyle O}{\|}}{C}-R \quad \longrightarrow \quad H-\overset{}{C}-O-\overset{\overset{\displaystyle O}{\|}}{C}-R \quad + H_2O$$

$$H-\overset{}{\underset{\overset{}{H}}{C}}-OH \quad HO-\overset{\overset{\displaystyle O}{\|}}{C}-R \quad H-\overset{}{\underset{\overset{}{H}}{C}}-O-\overset{\overset{\displaystyle O}{\|}}{C}-R \quad + H_2O$$

Glycerol $\qquad$ 3 fatty acids $\qquad$ Fat (triglyceride) $\qquad$ 3 H_2O (water)

*R = radical (rest of molecule)

Fats (Lipids)
continued

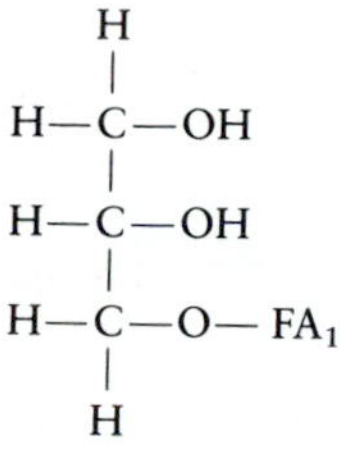

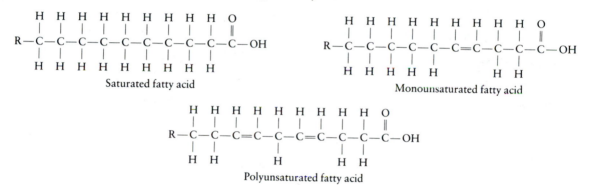

H
|
H—C—OH
|
H—C—OH
|
H—C—O— FA$_1$
|
H
Monoglyceride

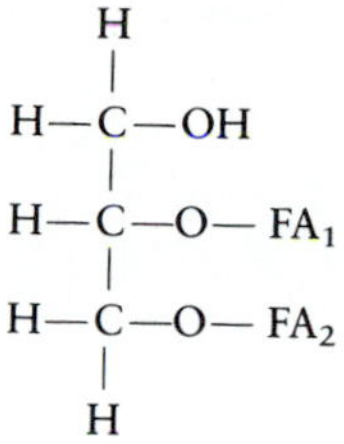

H
|
H—C—OH
|
H—C—O— FA$_1$
|
H—C—O— FA$_2$
|
H
Diglyceride

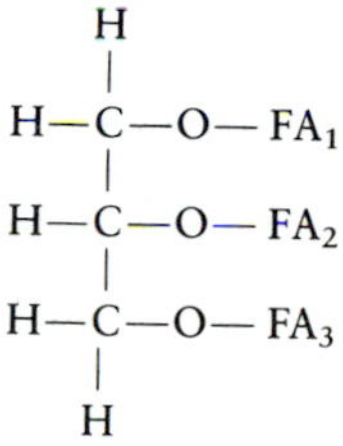

H
|
H—C—O— FA$_1$
|
H—C—O— FA$_2$
|
H—C—O— FA$_3$
|
H
Mixed triglyceride

Types of Fatty Acids

Saturated fatty acid

Monounsaturated fatty acid

Polyunsaturated fatty acid

Vitamins

Water-Soluble Vitamins

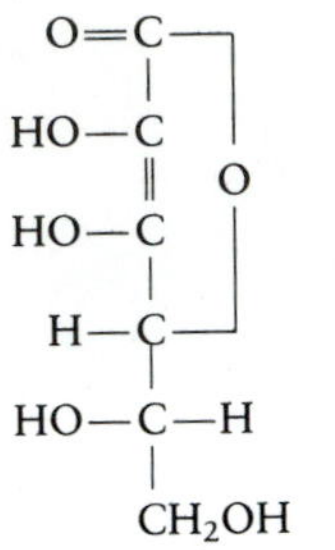

Ascorbic acid (vitamin C)

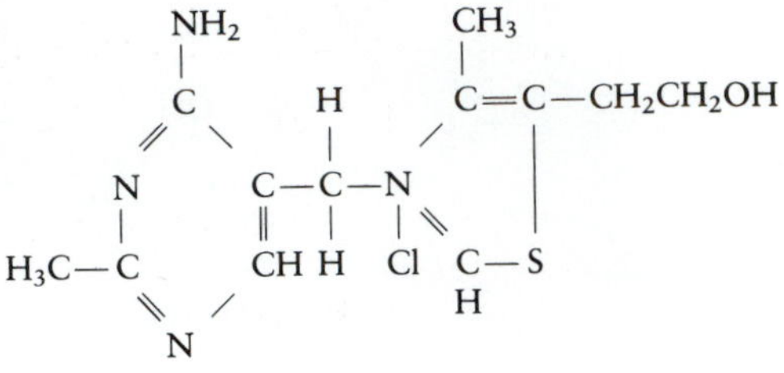

Thiamine (vitamin B$_1$)

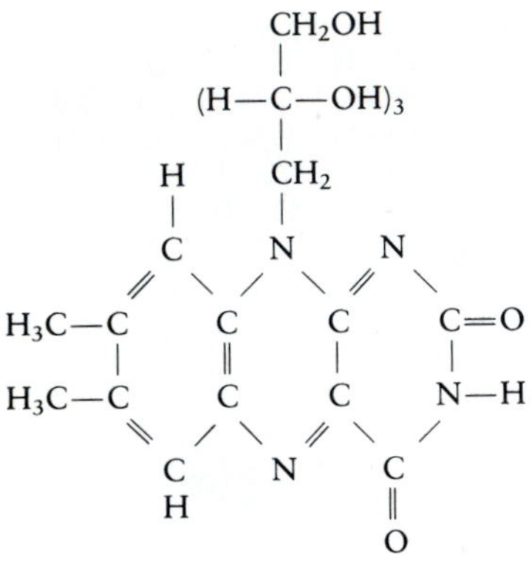

Riboflavin (vitamin B$_2$)

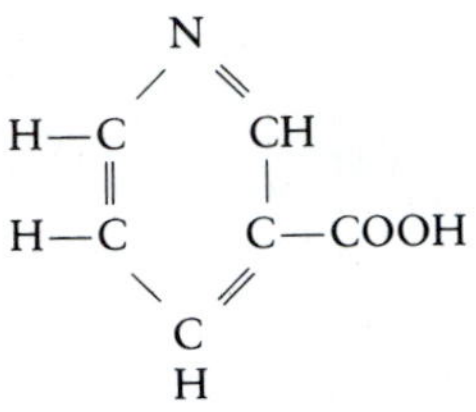

Nicotinic acid

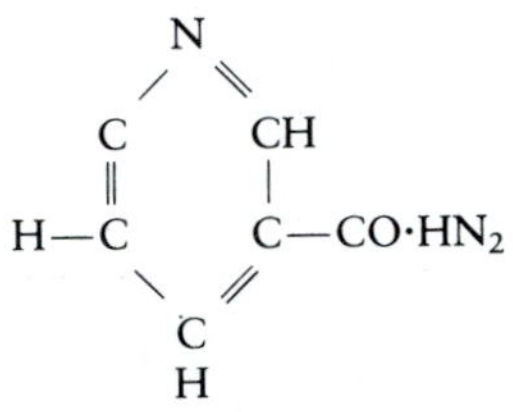

Nicotinamide

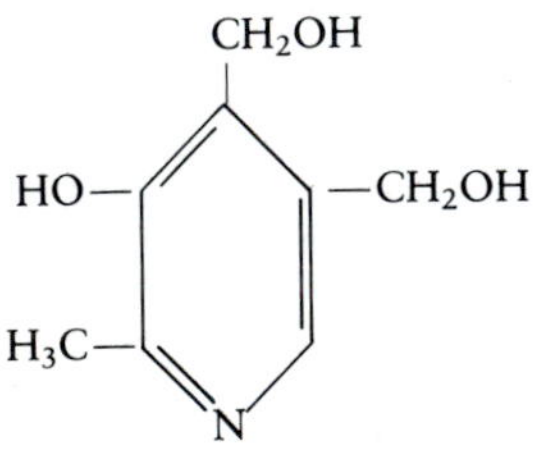

Pyridoxine

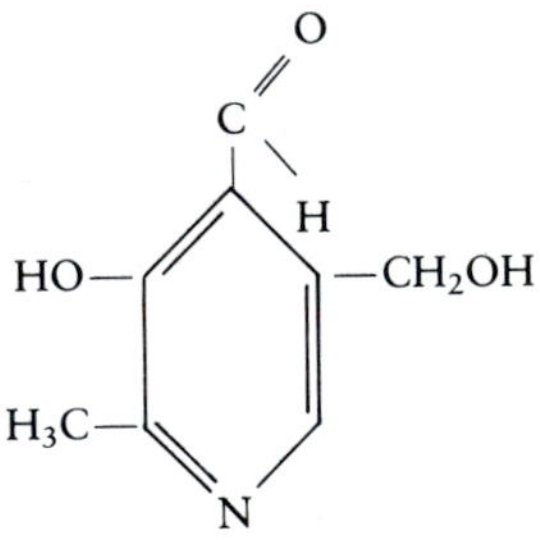

Pyridoxal

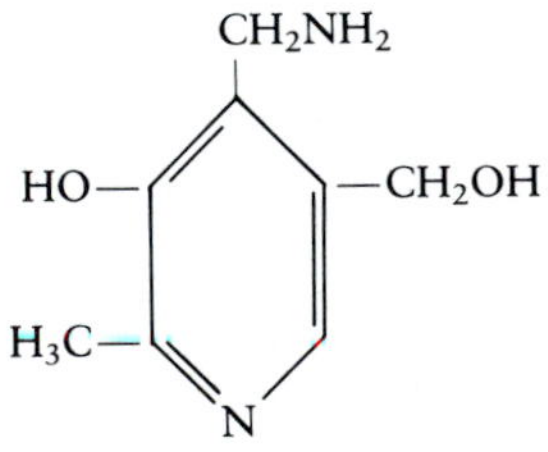

Pyridoxamine

Vitamins
continued

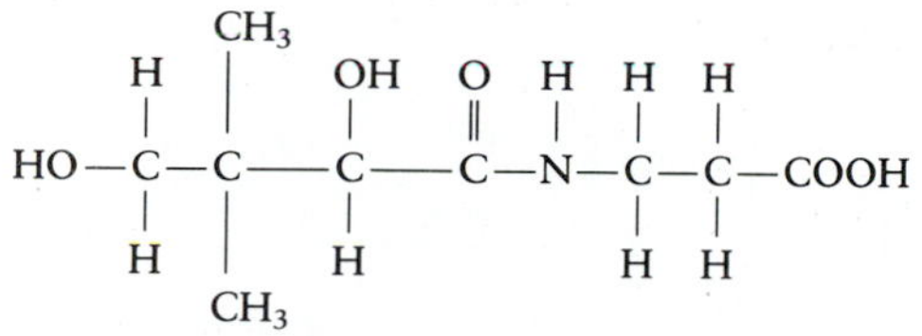

$$HO-\underset{\underset{H}{|}}{\overset{\overset{H}{|}}{C}}-\underset{\underset{CH_3}{|}}{\overset{\overset{CH_3}{|}}{C}}-\underset{\underset{H}{|}}{\overset{\overset{OH}{|}}{C}}-\overset{\overset{O}{\|}}{C}-\underset{H}{N}-\underset{\underset{H}{|}}{\overset{\overset{H}{|}}{C}}-\underset{\underset{H}{|}}{\overset{\overset{H}{|}}{C}}-COOH$$

Pantothenic acid

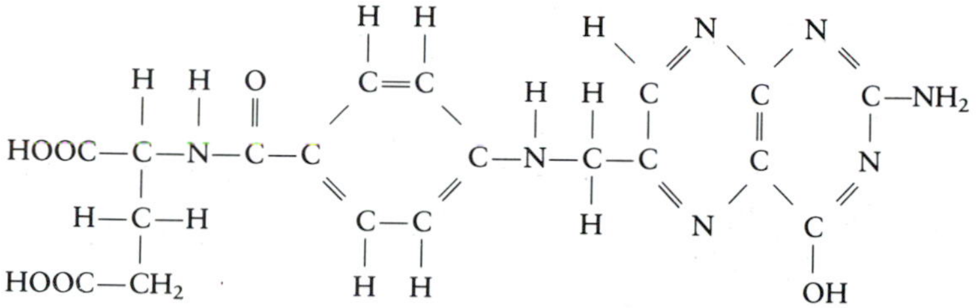

Folacin (monopteroylglutamic acid)

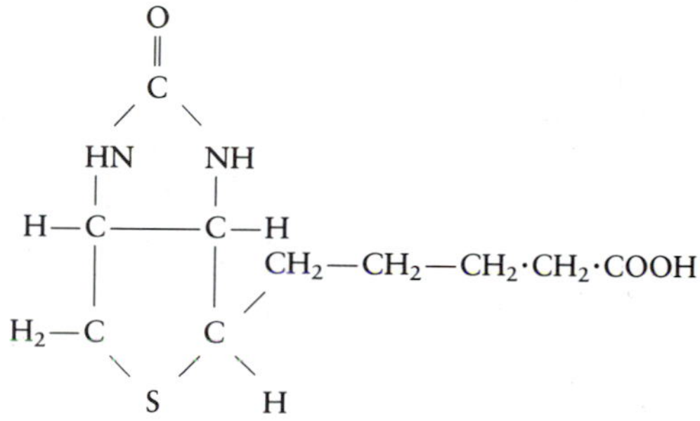

Biotin

Vitamins
continued

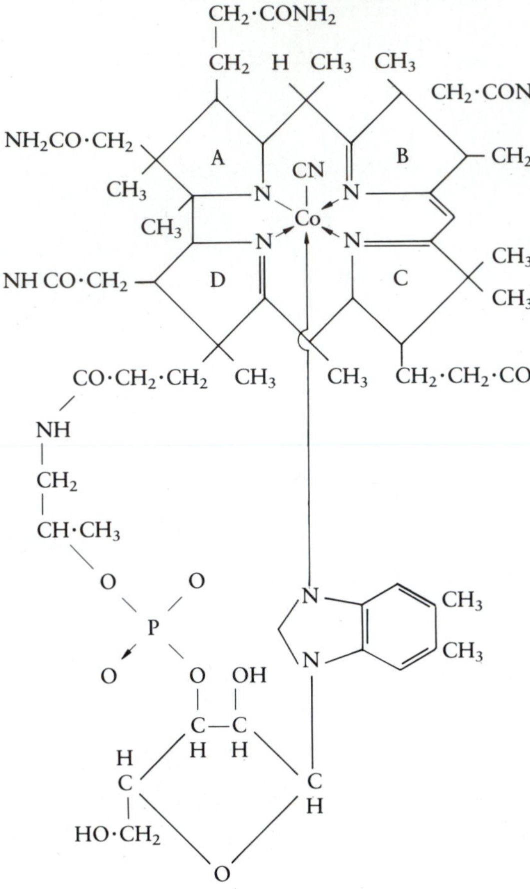
CH₂·CONH₂
CH₂
H
CH₃
CH₃
CH₂·CONH₂
NH₂CO·CH₂
A
B
CN
CH₂·CH₂·CONH₂
CH₃
N
N
Co
CH₃
N
N
CH₃
NH CO·CH₂
D
C
CH₃
CO·CH₂·CH₂
CH₃
CH₃
CH₂·CH₂·CONH₂
NH
CH₂
CH·CH₃
O
O
P
O
O
OH
N
CH₃
CH₃
N
C—C
H H
H
C
C
H
HO·CH₂
O

Cyanocobalamin (vitamin B_{12})

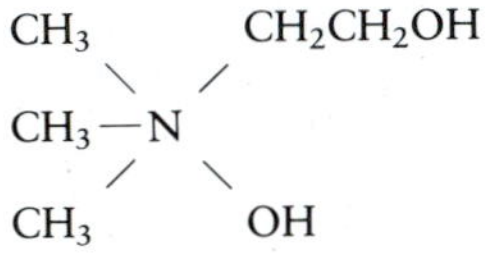
CH₃
CH₂CH₂OH
CH₃—N
CH₃
OH

Choline

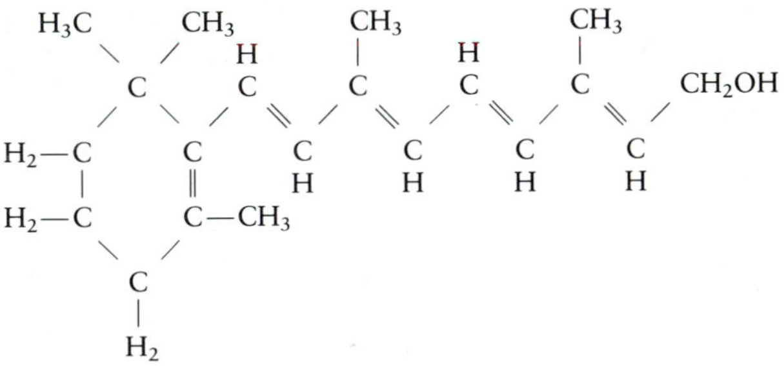
H₃C
CH₃
H
C
CH₃
C
H
CH₃
C
CH₂OH
H₂—C
H₂—C
C—CH₃
H₂

Vitamin A (retinol)

Vitamin D (cholecalciferol, vitamin D$_3$)

Vitamin E (α-tocopherol)

Vitamin K (phytylmenaquinone, vitamin K$_1$)

Glossary

A

acetyl CoA A chemical substance serving as the meeting ground of carbohydrate, fat, and protein metabolism

acid/base balance The relationship of acidity to alkalinity in the body fluids, normally slightly alkaline

acidosis High acidity in body fluids

acrodermatitis enteropathica A rare genetic disorder involving a severe zinc deficiency (from malabsorption?)

adenosine triphosphate The high-energy phosphate molecule which is the major form of stored energy in the human body. Abbreviated "ATP"

alanine A nonessential amino acid

albumin An important blood protein, also found in egg white, milk, etc.

alimentary canal The mucous-membrane lined tube of the digestive system, from mouth to the anus

alkalosis Excess alkalinity of body fluids

allergen The substance that triggers an allergic reaction. Also called "antigen"

allergy An altered immunological state in which pathological reactions are induced by an antigen

Amanita The major family of toxic mushrooms in the United States

amino acids The structural units of protein molecules

amylopectin A constituent of starch, composed of many glucose units joined in branching patterns

amylose A constituent of starch, consisting of many glucose units joined linearly without branching

anabolism The metabolic process within the cells whereby metabolites (e.g., nutrients) are used to synthesize new materials for cellular growth, maintenance, or repair

anemia Pathological deficiency of oxygen-carrying material in the blood

anion A negatively charged electrolyte

anorexia The loss of appetite

anorexia nervosa A disorder in which a person refuses food and loses a lot of weight

anthropometric The physical measurements of parts of the body, e.g., height, weight, head circumference, chest circumference, etc.

antioxidant A chemical that can prevent oxidation

arachidic acid A saturated fatty acid

arachidonic acid An essential polyunsaturated fatty acid

arginine An amino acid known to be essential for infants and children

ash The non-combustible mineral residue left after a substance has been oxidized

asparagine A nonessential amino acid

aspartic acid A nonessential amino acid

atherosclerosis Thickening of the lining of blood vessels as lipid materials are deposited and covered by fibrous connective tissues

atrophy The wasting of tissues

avidin A heat-sensitive glycoprotein found in raw egg white, which can complex with biotin, rendering it unavailable for absorption.

B

basal metabolic rate The least amount of energy required by an individual's body at rest to keep the essential life processes functioning; abbreviated "BMR"

behenic acid A saturated fatty acid

beriberi A syndrome describing vitamin B_1 deficiency

BHA Butylated hydroxyanisole, a controversial antioxidant used commercially to prevent rancidity in fats

BHT Butylated hydroxytoluene, a controversial antioxidant used commercially to prevent rancidity in fats

bile The substance stored in the gallbladder and is especially important in fat digestion

bioflavonoids Substances in fruits and vegetables for which certain therapeutic effects have been claimed but not substantiated

biological value The degree to which a protein contains all essential amino acids in the proportions needed by the body

biotin A water-soluble vitamin and part of the B vitamin complex

bomb calorimeter A device in which food samples are oxidized to determine their energy content

botulism Food poisoning caused by ingestion of *Clostridium botulinum*, a bacterium found mainly in improperly home-canned foods. Can be fatal

butyric acid A saturated fatty acid

C

cachexia General wasting of the body, especially during chronic disease

calorie The amount of heat energy that will raise the temperature of 1 gm of water from 15°C to 16°C

capric acid A saturated fatty acid

caproic acid A saturated fatty acid

caprylic acid A saturated fatty acid

carbohydrate An organic compound containing carbon, hydrogen, and oxygen, with a ratio of carbon to hydrogen to oxygen atoms of 1:2:1

carcinogenic Cancer-causing

cardiovascular Involving the heart and blood vessels

carotene The precursor of vitamin A, found in plant products

casein Major protein in milk, cheese, and eggs

catabolism Conversion of larger (organized) substances in body into smaller (simpler) ones. The destructive part of metabolism (= catabolism + anabolism)

cation A positively charged electrolyte

cellulose A polysaccharide made of many glucose molecules and not digestible by man

cheilosis Cracks at the corners of the mouth with yellow crusts, a symptom of deficiency of vitamin B_2, folic acid, vitamin B_{12}, or niacin

cholecalciferol One chemical form of vitamin D

cholesterol One chemical form of fat, found only in animal products and suspected to play a role in heart disease

choline A substance normally synthesized in the body, important in the biochemistry of metabolism and closely associated with the physiology of vitamins

chylomicron A large, low-density molecule consisting mostly of triglycerides. Its main function is to transport fat in the body, primarily in the form of triglycerides

citric acid cycle The series of chemical reactions whereby carbohydrate, fat, and/or protein are completely oxidized to carbon dioxide, water, and energy. Also called the "Krebs cycle"

Clostridium perfringens A bacterium which, when present in great numbers in food, may cause nausea, diarrhea, and acute inflammation of the stomach and intestines

cobalamin Vitamin B_{12}, important in all cell metabolism, tissue growth, and maintenance of the central nervous system

cobamide coenzyme The biologically active form of vitamin B_{12}

coenzyme An accessory substance that facilitates the working of an enzyme, largely by acting as a carrier for products of the chemical reaction

coenzyme A A critical substance in the metabolism of fat, protein, and carbohydrate (it participates in the citric acid cycle and permits the release of energy) which also has other essential functions in the body. Abbreviated CoA. Also see CoQ or Coenzyme Q

coenzyme Q A fat-soluble vitamin-like substance found in most living cells. A perfect biological catalyst, it is an important component of the respiratory chain. Abbreviated CoQ

collagen An insoluble protein that holds together the cells and tissues of skin, cartilage, tendons, ligaments, bones, teeth, and blood vessels

colostrum The thick yellowish fluid that precedes white breast milk, suspected to provide infant with passive immunity

complementary proteins Protein foods which are individually incomplete but which when combined correct each other's deficiencies in essential amino acids

core eating plan On a weight loss diet, specification of the approximate number of servings of each category of food to be consumed daily

creatine A nitrogenous chemical derived from three amino acids. In its phosphorylated form, it supplies energy for muscle contraction

creatinine A nitrogenous substance in the urine derived from the catabolism of creatine

cretinism Retardation of infants and children in physical and mental development, associated with a lack of iodine

cysteine A nonessential amino acid

cystine Though classified as a nonessential amino acid, a substance derived from the essential amino acid methionine

D

daily food guide A translation of Recommended Daily Allowances into simple-to-follow recommendations of the kinds and amounts of food needed for good nutrition

dehydration Excessive loss of water from the body; also called "underhydration"

dextran A polysaccharide made of many glucose molecules, with potential clinical usages. Does not occur naturally in food

dextrin A small polysaccharide of five to six glucose units, found in the leaves of starch-forming plants and in the human alimentary canal as a product of starch digestion

diabetes mellitus A disease characterized by excess blood sugar and urine sugar. Caused mostly by a malfunctioning pancreas

diffusion Movement of a substance from a location of higher concentration to one of lower concentration

digestion The breaking down of ingested foods into particles of a size and chemical composition that the body can readily absorb

digestive system The long tube including the mouth, esophagus, stomach, small intestine, colon, rectum, and associated organs such as pancreas. These structural units and their secretions break food down into units absorbable by the body

diglyceride A glyceride with two molecules of fatty acids

dipeptide Two amino acids chemically joined

disaccharide A carbohydrate composed of two monosaccharides

disaccharidase An enzyme responsible for hydrolysis of disaccharides to monosaccharides in the duodenum, jejunum, and ileum

diuretic A substance that increases urine excretion

diverticulum A blind pouch in the colon, usually developed from some clinical disorders

E

edema The presence of an abnormally high amount of fluid in the intercellular spaces; also called "overhydration"

electrolyte A substance that is a charged particle or is separated into charged particles when dissolved in fluid

-emia A suffix indicating the blood

emulsifier A substance that helps foods to mix

energy The capacity to do work

enrichment The addition of nutrients to foods; for example, to restore what has been lost through processing

enzyme A protein that catalyzes a specific chemical reaction or a few specific reactions in the body

epidemiology The study of the incidence, distribution, and control of a certain disease or pathogen in a population

ergosterol The form of vitamin D found in plant products

erucic acid A monounsaturated fatty acid

Escherichia coli A pathogenic bacterium which can cause intestinal infection

essential Referring to a nutrient that the body needs but is unable to synthesize from ordinary foods

essential amino acid One of the 8 to 10 amino acids that the human body cannot manufacture and that must therefore be consumed in foods

essential fatty acids The polyunsaturated fatty acids lineoleic acid and linolenic acid, which cannot be synthesized by the body and must therefore be consumed in the diet

extracellular Located outside a cell or cells

F

fat An organic compound whose molecules contain glycerol and fatty acids. Also used in referring to adipose tissue

fatty acid A constituent of fat, a simple lipid containing only carbon, hydrogen, and oxygen

fiber Indigestible carbohydrate found in plant foods and connective tissues of meats. Also known as "roughage" or "bulk"

flavor enhancer A substance that can modify or magnify the flavor of foods without contributing any flavor of its own, such as MSG

folic acid Part of the B vitamin complex, a substance which participates in many essential biological reactions in its coenzyme form; also called "folacin"

Food Exchange Lists Groups of food in which each group or list contains selected foods, each of which contributes approximately equal amounts of certain nutrients and calories. The American Diabetes Association and the American Dietetic Association originated the Food Exchange Lists for diabetic patients

foodborne infection The consumption of food containing enough live bacteria to produce sufficient toxin in the intestine to poison the person who has eaten it

foodborne intoxication The consumption of a food in which pathogenic bacteria have released toxins capable of poisoning the person who eats the food

fortification The addition of nutrients to foods to improve their nutritional value

foundation diet A diet consisting only of the recommended numbers of servings from the Four Food Groups

the Four Food Groups Milk and milk products, meats or meat equivalents, fruits and vegetables, and breads and cereals—the main groups of food now recommended for daily consumption

free amino acid An amino acid existing singly or in free form

fructose A simple carbohydrate found in many fruits, honey, and plant saps. One of the two monosaccharides forming sucrose (table sugar); also called "fruit sugar" or "levulose"

G

galactose A six-carbon monosaccharide usually occurring as one of the two components of lactose, or milk sugar

gastrointestinal bypass Surgical stapling of a portion of the stomach or removal of part of the intestine to reduce the amount of food eaten and/or absorbed and thus reduce caloric intake

gastrointestinal system See digestive system

glossitis A smooth red tongue with flat, swollen or pebbled papillae, associated with deficiencies of vitamin B_2, folic acid, vitamin B_{12}, or niacin

glucagon A hormone that can stimulate insulin secretion

glucose A six-carbon monosaccharide found mostly in the blood in the human body, where it provides fuel for immediate energy when oxidized; also called "D-glucose," "fruit sugar," "corn sugar," and "dextrose"

glucose tolerance test A test used to ascertain how well a person tolerates an influx of glucose into the bloodstream, used to determine the presence of hyperglycemia or hypoglycemia. Abbreviated "GTT"

glutamic acid A nonessential amino acid

glutamine A nonessential amino acid

glyceride A simple lipid, an ester of fatty acids and glycerol

glycine A nonessential amino acid

glycogen The polysaccharide form in which energy is stored in an animal; sometimes called "animal starch"

glycolysis The degradation of glucose to pyruvate and/or lactate

goiter A lack of iodine, resulting in enlargement of the thyroid gland

goitrogen A substance capable of inducing goiter

H

hematuria Blood in the urine

hemocellulose A form of indigestible carbohydrate found in plant foods

hemoglobin The iron-containing protein in red blood cells which carries oxygen to the tissues

hemolysis The hemolytic process

hemolytic Causing blood elements (e.g., red blood cells) to disintegrate

hexoses Six-carbon sugars, such as glucose, fructose, galactose, and mannose

high density lipoprotein One type of cholesterol carrier in the blood: that which removes deposited cholesterol and carries it away for excretion

high nutrient diet A diet made of nutritionally potent liquids and semi-solid foods of a consistency that can be taken as a beverage or through a straw. Also called "modified full liquid diet"

histidine An amino acid known to be essential for infants and children, and perhaps essential for adults as well

humectant A substance that helps food products maintain moistness

hydrogenation The commercial process by which oils with a high level of unsaturated fatty acids are turned into fats with soft to hard texture

hydrolyze To break down a chemical compound by adding water

hyper- A prefix indicating an abnormal excess

hyperglycemia A high blood "sugar" (glucose) level

hyperkalemia An elevated serum level of potassium

hyperlipidemia An elevated level of lipids in the blood serum

hyperlipoproteinemia An elevated level of certain lipoproteins in the blood

hypertension Sustained elevation of systolic and/or diastolic arterial blood pressure

hypo- A prefix indicating an abnormal insufficiency

hypocalcemia A low level of calcium in the blood

hypoglycemia A low blood "sugar" (glucose) level

hypokalemia A decreased serum potassium level

hypoproteinemia An abnormal decrease of protein in the blood

I

incomplete protein A protein in which one or more of the essential amino acids is missing or occurs in limited quantity

inorganic Composed of material other than plant or animal in origin

inositol An alcohol form of glucose sometimes called "muscle sugar" because of its high concentration in hair and muscle tissues. Its exact function in the human body is unknown

insensible loss The constant but invisible evaporation of moisture from the skin surface

insulin A pancreatic hormone which controls the body's use of glucose

intra- A prefix meaning within or inside of

intracellular Located inside a cell or cells

intravenous Within a blood vein or veins

intrinsic factor A mucoprotein in the gastric juice which combines with vitamin B_{12} and makes its absorption possible; lack of this substance results in pernicious anemia

isoleucine An essential amino acid

J

Joule One thousand joules: the amount of mechanical energy required when a force of 1 Newton moves 1 kilogram by a distance of 1 meter; preferred by some professionals over the heat energy measurements of the calorie system for calculating food energy. Sometimes referred to as "kilojoule," "Kilojoule," "kJ," or "KJ"

K

keratinization Degeneration of the epithelial cells (which cover most internal surfaces and organs and the outer surface of the body), a condition associated with vitamin A deficiency

ketone body Describes the three chemicals, acetone, acetoacetic acid, and β-hydroxybutyric acid

ketonuria The presence of ketone bodies in the urine

ketosis A condition in which fatty acids are incompletely oxidized, with resulting accumulation of ketone bodies

kilocalorie The preferred unit of measurement for food energy, equivalent to one thousand calories. Referred to as "Kilocalorie," "Calorie," "Kcal," or "Cal."

Kilojoule See *Joule*

koilonchia A condition in which fingernails and perhaps toenails become thin, flattened, lusterless, and spoon-shaped; associated with long-term iron deficiency

kwashiorkor The syndrome resulting from a severe deficiency in dietary protein, mild to moderate lack of other essential nutrients, but an adequate or even excessive intake of calories

L

lact-, lacto- A prefix indicating milk

lactase The enzyme that digests lactose in the intestine

lactation Milk secretion; child suckling; period of milk secretion

lacteal system Tiny lymph-carrying vessels that convey finely emulsified fat from the intestine to the thoracic duct

lacto-ovo-vegetarian An individual whose diet contains no meat, poultry, or fish, but does include milk and eggs

lactose The disaccharide made of glucose and galactose; often called "milk sugar"

L-ascorbic acid The chemically active form of vitamin C, a monosaccharide-like six-carbon substance

lathyrism Food poisoning from eating certain peas of the lathyrus family

lauric acid A saturated fatty acid

lean body mass In determining body composition, what is left after body fat is subtracted from the total body weight. Also referred to as the "fat-free body" or "body cell mass"

leavening agent A substance that helps dough to rise when baked

leucine An essential amino acid

lignins Certain forms of indigestible carbohydrate found in plant foods

limiting amino acids The amino acids that are deficient or missing in vegetable proteins, determining the extent to which the other amino acids present can be used by the body

linoleic acid An essential polyunsaturated fatty acid

linolenic acid An essential polyunsaturated fatty acid

lipectomy Surgical excision of a mass of subcutaneous fat tissue

lipids A term for fats

lipoic acid A substance not now classified as an essential vitamin for humans. Although it is a participant in many biochemical reactions, it can be synthesized in apparently adequate amounts by the body

lipoprotein A fat combined with a protein, forming a compound which transports both in the blood circulation

liver cirrhosis A serious disease characterized by reduction and death of liver cells, derangement of blood circulation in the liver, and scarring of remaining tissues in the liver

low density lipoprotein One type of cholesterol carrier in the blood: that which carries cholesterol and deposits it in the blood vessels

lumen The open inner space of a tubular organ, such as an intestine or blood vessel

lymphatic system The system of vessels and spaces between organs and tissues through which lymph is circulated in the body

lysine An essential amino acid

M

macrocytic anemia A form of anemia involving immature red blood cells, resulting from lack of folic acid and/or vitamin B_{12}

macroelements Minerals needed by the body in relatively large quantity: sodium, potassium, calcium, phosphorus, magnesium, chlorine, and sulfur

malabsorption syndrome Failure of the small intestine to absorb nutrients properly

malnutrition Refers to bad (= mal) nutrition. For example: lack of food or eating too much

maltose The disaccharide whose units are each composed of two molecules of glucose; also called "malt sugar"

mannose A six-carbon monosaccharide which sometimes occurs as a free sugar

marasmus The syndrome resulting from a deficiency of calories and nearly all other essential nutrients

megaloblastosis Failure of red blood cells to mature, resulting in a form of anemia which may be associated with deficiency of folic acid and/or vitamin B_{12}

metabolism The complex of processes which food nutrients undergo after absorption, including both their breaking down for energy or excretion or their use in synthesizing new materials for cellular growth, maintenance, or repair

methionine An essential amino acid

microcytic anemia Anemia resulting from a lack of iron and/or other nutrients

microelements Minerals needed by the body in very small amounts; iron, iodine, zinc, fluorine, copper, and other trace elements

mono- A prefix meaning "one"

monoglyceride A glyceride with only one molecule of fatty acid

monosaccharide One of the simplest carbohydrate molecules, for it cannot be split into simpler forms

monosodium glutamate An amino acid used as a flavor enhancer. Abbreviated "MSG"

monounsaturated fatty acid An unsaturated fatty acid with one double bond

mucin A component of saliva that lubricates food

mucosa The mucous membrane that lines the tubes and body cavities which open to the outside of the body

mutagen A substance that alters genetic materials so that the change is passed on to the offspring, usually with adverse effects

myristic acid A saturated fatty acid

N

negative nitrogen balance The condition in which nitrogen losses from the body exceed nitrogen intake

niacin (nicotinic acid) A watersoluble B vitamin that can be synthesized in limited amounts in the body if the amino acid tryptophan is present in an adequate amount

niacinamide The amide of nicotinic acid (niacin)

nitrogen equilibrium The normal condition in which nitrogen intake is equal to nitrogen loss from the body

nonessential amino acid One of the amino acids that can be manufactured in the human body if the proper building blocks are available. These compounds are nonetheless necessary in the diet, in a certain relationship to the "essential" amino acids

normoglycemia A normal level of blood "sugar" (glucose)

nutrient A nourishing organic or inorganic substance in food that can be digested, absorbed, and metabolized by the body

nutrition (1) The sum of the processes by which an animal or plant takes in and utilizes food substances: ingestion, digestion, absorption, and assimilation (2) The scientific study of these processes

O

obesity The condition of weighing 15% to 25% more than one's ideal body weight, with the excess consisting of fat rather than water, muscle, or bones

oleic acid A monounsaturated fatty acid

oligosaccharide A carbohydrate containing many units, each made of two to ten chemically joined monosaccharides

oliguria Abnormally low excretion of urine

organic Derived from living organisms

osmolality The concentration of a solute in a solution per unit of solvent

osmolarity The concentration of a solute in a solution per unit volume of the solution

osmosis Passage of dissolved molecules through a semipermeable membrane from an area of higher concentration to an area of lower concentration until the concentration is equal on both sides of the membrane

osteomalacia Bone softening because of impaired mineralization

osteoporosis A clinical disorder characterized by a reduction in the total quantity of bone in the body

overweight The body weighs more than an accepted norm. The excess can be fat, bone, muscle, water, etc.

ovo-vegetarian An individual whose diet contains no meat, poultry, fish, milk, or milk products, but does include eggs

oxalic acid A substance occurring naturally in vegetables such as chard, rhubarb, and spinach which can chelate calcium in the intestinal tract, rendering it unavailable for absorption

oxidation The process in which a substrate takes up oxygen or loses hydrogen

P

palmitic acid A saturated fatty acid, usually solid at room temperature

palmitoleic acid A monounsaturated fatty acid

pantothenic acid A B vitamin

parietal cell A cell of a gastric gland which secretes hydrochloric acid and intrinsic factor

pellagra The niacin (a vitamin) deficiency syndrome, characterized by dermatitis, diarrhea, and dementia

pentoses Five-carbon sugars that play an important role in energy release and formation but are not themselves sources of energy

pepsin A protein-digesting enzyme in the gastric juice of the stomach

peptic ulcer An inflammatory lesion found in the lower end of the esophagus, or in any part of the stomach or duodenum

peptide A compound composed of two or more amino acids joined to each other

peritoneum The membrane that lines the walls of the abdominal cavity and encloses the internal organs

pernicious anemia One form of anemia caused by vitamin B_{12} deficiency, due to a lack of intrinsic factor to facilitate its absorption

phenylalanine An essential amino acid

phospholipid A fat containing glycerol, two fatty acids, phosphate, and a variable chemical, which serves as a structural component of cell membranes

photolytic conversion A chemical reaction made possible by light

phytic acid A substance found in the outer husks of cereals that can complex with certain minerals including calcium and zinc, making them unavailable for absorption

plaque (1) A deposit of fat and/or fibrous matter in the wall of a blood vessel
(2) a mucus film providing a home for bacteria on a tooth

poly- A prefix meaning "many"

polypeptide 50 to 100 amino acids chemically joined

polysaccharide A carbohydrate containing many units, each made of hundreds to thousands of chemically joined monosaccharides

polyunsaturated fatty acid An unsaturated fatty acid in which two or more carbon atoms have formed double bonds, with each holding only one hydrogen atom; abbreviated "PUFA"

polyuria Excessive urination

positive nitrogen balance The condition in which nitrogen intake exceeds nitrogen losses from the body

precursor A substance from which another substance is derived. Niacin (a vitamin), for instance, can be made from the precursor tryptophan (an amino acid)

preformed vitamins One form of a group of vitamins that the body can synthesize partially. This term applies to niacin and vitamins A and D. Preformed refers to the presence of these vitamins in readily utilizable forms, e.g., in food

proline A nonessential amino acid

protein Any of the large nitrogen-containing organic compounds built of amino acids and found in the cells of all living organisms

protein efficiency ratio In determining protein quality, the gram of body weight gained by experimental animals per gram of a particular protein food eaten; abbreviated "PER"

proteinuria The abnormal presence of protein in the urine

prothrombin A protein important to blood clotting; synthesized in the liver, requiring the presence of vitamin K

provitamins One form of a group of vitamins that the body can synthesize partially. The vitamins include niacin and vitamins A and D. For example, the body can make vitamin A from carotene (found in carrot). Carotene is the provitamin A

ptyalin A digestive enzyme in saliva

pulses The edible seeds of certain pod-bearing plants, such as beans and peas

purine A nitrogen-containing structural component of all cells

pyridoxine A term used for vitamin B_6, most important for serving as a coenzyme in many metabolic processes

R

RDA Recommended Dietary Allowances—the amounts of specific nutrients established by the National Research Council of the National Academy of Sciences as appropriate for daily consumption by people of specific age and sex groups

reduction The process by which a substrate loses oxygen or accepts hydrogen

relactation Stimulation of milk production in women who have not been breastfeeding

rhodopsin The red light sensitive pigment in the retinal rods of the eyes, whose formation requires vitamin A. Also called "visual purple," it is responsible for the ability to see at night

riboflavin Vitamin B_2, important in facilitating many biological reactions

rickets The syndrome caused by vitamin D and/or calcium deficiency, characterized by bone deformities

S

saccharin A controversial artificial sweetener

Salmonella A bacterium capable of causing food poisoning, with symptoms ranging from severe headache, vomiting, diarrhea, abdominal cramps, and fever, to death

satiety The satisfying feeling of being full

saturated fatty acid A fatty acid in which each carbon is joined with four other atoms, thus tying up all potential carbon/hydrogen linkages except the carbons at the "carboxyl" end of the chain

scurvy The vitamin C deficiency syndrome characterized by bleeding gums, pain in joints, bone malformation in childhood, and other problems

serine A nonessential amino acid

serum The clear, yellowish fluid within blood, obtained when whole blood is separated into its solid and liquid constituents

sorbitol A six-carbon sugar alcohol, often used to sweeten "diabetic" products because it has little immediate effect on blood glucose level

Staphylococcus aureus A bacterium capable of causing foodborne intoxication

starch A polysaccharide of many units, each containing hundreds or thousands of glucose molecules; the major form in which energy is stored in plants

stearic acid A saturated fatty acid, usually solid at room temperature

steatorrhea The condition in which the fecal waste is bulky, clay-colored, and fatty because fat has not been properly digested and absorbed

sterol Solid alcohol of the steroid group, found in animals and plants

stomatitis Inflammation of the oral mucous tissue

subcutaneous Beneath the skin

sucrose The disaccharide composed of glucose and fructose, often called "table sugar"

systemic blood circulation The vessels carrying blood between the heart and the body tissues with the exception of the lungs

T

teratogen A substance with the potential of causing birth defects

tetany A syndrome resulting from a decreased serum ionizable calcium level, characterized by symptoms such as uncontrolled muscular contractions, seizures, confusion, and increased nervous excitability

thiamine The original chemical name for vitamin B_1, especially important in carbohydrate metabolism

thiaminase An enzyme antagonist of the vitamin thiamin, occurring in some vegetables

threonine An essential amino acid

tocopherol One chemical form of vitamin E. The term implies "antisterile"

toxemia A pathological condition that develops in some pregnant women, characterized by raised blood pressure, edema, nausea, vomiting, liver enlargement and tenderness, headache, the presence of protein in the urine, reduced urine excretion, dizziness, irritability, and sometimes convulsions and coma

triglyceride A fat made of glycerol and three fatty acids; sometimes called a "neutral fat"

trypsin A pancreatic enzyme that breaks down protein molecules

tryptophan An essential amino acid and a precursor of niacin

tyrosine Although classified as a nonessential amino acid, it must be derived from the essential amino acid phenylalanine

U

undernutrition The lack of essential nutrients in the human body as a result of insufficient food

unsaturated fatty acid A fatty acid in which two or more carbon atoms are not joined with all the hydrogen atoms they can hold. If so, the bond between any two such carbons is called a double bond

urea A nonprotein nitrogen-containing substance produced when protein is metabolized in the liver; the main nitrogenous component of urine

-uria A suffix indicating the abnormal presence of a specified substance in the urine

uric acid A nitrogenous substance formed when purines are metabolized, excreted in urine

USRDA The highest level of recommended intakes for population groups excluding pregnant and nursing mothers, described in the 1968 Recommended Dietary Allowances. Used by the Food & Drug Administration in food labeling

V

valine An essential amino acid

vegan An individual whose diet contains no meat, poultry, fish, milk, milk products, or eggs: a "strict vegetarian"

vitamin An organic compound the body requires in very small amounts to perform its essential functions

vitamin antagonist A substance which can destroy or replace a specific vitamin in the body; also called "antivitamin," "antimetabolite," or "pseudovitamin"

vitamin B complex All known water-soluble vitamins except vitamin C: B_1, B_2, B_6, niacin, folic acid, B_{12}, pantothenic acid, and biotin

W

Wernicke-Korsakoff syndrome The neurological problems from vitamin B_1 deficiency that develop in alcoholics, pregnant women experiencing excessive vomiting, and patients deficient in thiamin who are given glucose intravenously

X

xylitol A five-carbon sugar with potential clinical applications such as use as a sweetener for diabetic patients

Index